Women's Health Nursing
Toward Evidence-Based Practice

Women's Health Nursing
Toward Evidence-Based Practice

Eileen T. Breslin, PhD, RN
Dean and Professor, School of Nursing
University of Massachusetts—Amherst
Amherst, Massachusetts

Vicki A. Lucas, PhD, RN
Vice President, Women's Services
MedStar Health
Baltimore, Maryland and Washington, D.C.

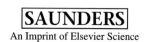
SAUNDERS
An Imprint of Elsevier Science

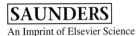

SAUNDERS

An Imprint of Elsevier Science

11830 Westline Industrial Drive
St. Louis, Missouri 63146

NOTICE

Nursing is an ever-changing field. Standard safety precautions must be followed, but as new research and clinical experience broaden our knowledge, changes in treatment and drug therapy may become necessary or appropriate. Readers are advised to check the most current product information provided by the manufacturer of each drug to be administered to verify the recommended dose, the method and duration of administration, and contraindications. It is the responsibility of the licensed prescriber, relying on experience and knowledge of the patient, to determine dosages and the best treatment for each individual patient. Neither the publisher nor the author assumes any liability for any injury and/or damage to persons or property arising from this publication.

The Publisher

International Standard Book Number 0-7216-7423-2

Executive Editor: Michael S. Ledbetter
Senior Developmental Editor: Laurie K. Muench
Publishing Services Manager: John Rogers
Project Manager: Helen Hudlin
Senior Designer: Kathi Gosche
Designer: Dana Peick
Cover Designer: Dana Peick

Printed in the United States of America

Last digit is the print number: 9 8 7 6 5 4 3 2 1

This work is dedicated to my parents, Charles and Theresa Breslin, with love,
respect, and gratitude.
Eileen T. Breslin

I dedicate my work to the most influential women in my life:
my mother, Mary Louise Brown Lucas, and my grandmother, Samantha Areford Lucas.
I also dedicate my work to the generations of women to follow
as revealed to me through the eyes of my daughters,
Chelsea Lucas Kaj
and
Bridget Lucas Kaj,
the true loves of my life.
Vicki A. Lucas

Contributors

Maria Alvarez Amaya, PhD, RNC, WHNP
Professor, School of Nursing
Wakefield Professor of Health Sciences
University of Texas at El Paso
El Paso, Texas

Linda A. Bernhard, PhD, RN
Associate Dean, Undergraduate Studies
Associate Professor
Ohio State University
Columbus, Ohio

Virginia Blankenship, PhD
Professor of Psychology
College of Social and Behavioral Sciences
Department of Nursing
Northern Arizona University
Flagstaff, Arizona

Margaret Burns, PhD, RN
Director of Inpatient Services
Northeast Health Systems
Beverly, Massachusetts

Catherine Ingram Fogel, PhD, RNC, WHCNP, FAAN
Professor, School of Nursing
University of North Carolina at Chapel Hill
Chapel Hill, North Carolina

Roxana Huebscher, PhD, FNPC, HNC
Associate Professor
College of Nursing
University of Wisconsin—Oshkosh
Oshkosh, Wisconsin

Carole Kanusky, MSN, RN, CNS
Clinical Educator, Education Resource Specialist III
Memorial Hermann Southwest Hospital
Houston, Texas

Susan Bragg Leight, EdD, RNCS, CRNP
Assistant Professor
Department of Nursing
Fairmont State College
Fairmont, West Virginia

Erin Miller, BS, ACE
Group Exercise Instructor/Personal Trainer
Lifestyle and Weight Management Consultant
Baltimore, Maryland

Susan Miller, MPA, RD
Registered Dietitian
Flagstaff, Arizona

Thelma Patrick, PhD, RN
Assistant Professor, Department of Health Promotion and Development
Assistant Investigator, Magee-Women's Research Institute
University of Pittsburgh School of Nursing
Pittsburgh, Pennsylvania

Judith Bunnell Sellers, DNSc, APRN, BC, FNP
Chair and Associate Professor, Department of Nursing
Northern Arizona University
Flagstaff, Arizona

Leslie Skillman-Hull, PhD, RNC
New Jersey Center for Visual Arts
Summit, New Jersey

Karen C. Smith, MD
Section Lead, General Internal Medicine
Virginia Mason Medical Center
Seattle, Washington

Michelle Teschendorf, MSN, RNC, PNCNS
Assistant Professor of Nursing
St. Louis Community College
St. Louis, Missouri

Michele J. Upvall, PhD, BScN, FNP
Professor and Director
The Aga Khan University School of Nursing
Karachi, Pakistan

Preface

The genesis for this book occurred during the Women, Health and Healing Summer Institute 1986, directed by Virginia Olesen, Sheryl Ruzek, and Adele Clarke and supported by the U.S. Fund for the Improvement of Post-Secondary Education. At that event the editors met with other colleagues and engaged in dialogue about the complexities associated with women's health. We struggled with diversity issues, how social forces affect health, and how caring facilitates health and healing. From that experience, the notion that women's health is intrinsically embedded within the context of a woman's life took hold. Nurses need to move beyond the traditional biomedical paradigm and embrace a more holistic approach to examining women's health issues. We subsequently presented a series of women's health continuing education programs for the Association of Women's Health, Obstetric and Neonatal Nurses. Our conversations extended to nurses nationwide within this forum and enhanced our understanding of the complexities of delivering care to women within an ever-changing delivery system.

Since the U.S. General Accounting Office issued its landmark report in 1990, citing the historical inequities in research and health care services for women, increased attention has focused on women's health. The literature in this new discipline is emerging and examines the complexities involved in women's health experience. Many disciplines such as psychology, anthropology, women's studies, social work, and medicine are making contributions to the scholarship of women's health.

The nursing profession, with its holistic lens, has taken a lead role in articulating issues facing women and in valuing lessons learned from women's health experiences. Nurses have proposed both a re-visioning and a reexamination of the definition of women's health (Dan, 1994; Chinn, 1994; Writing Group of the 1996 American Academy of Nursing, Expert Panel on Women's Health, 1997; Association of Women's Health, Obstetric and Neonatal Nurses, 1999). Nurses have challenged us to avoid over-simplification and generalization of the woman's experience and to transform the delivery of health services to women (Munhill, 1994, 1995; Taylor & Woods, 1999). Health promotion, health maintenance, and health restoration across the lifespan have been key elements.

Association of Women's Health, Obstetric and Neonatal Nurses. (1999). Association of Women's Health, Obstetric and Neonatal Nurses' Health for Women and Newborns' program, *Nursing Outlook, 47*(1), 37–38.

Chinn, P. (1994). *Developing nursing's perspectives in women's health.* Gaithersburg, MD: Aspen.

Dan, A. (Ed.). (1994). *Reframing women's health: Multidisciplinary research and practice.* Thousand Oaks, CA: Sage.

Munhill, P. L. (1994). *In women's experience.* Vol. I. New York: National League for Nursing.

Munhill, P.L. (1995). *In women's experience.* Vol. II. New York: National League for Nursing.

Taylor, D., & Woods, N.F. (1999) Changing women's health, changing nursing practice. *Advancing Evidence-Based Practice: Women's Health, Supplement to JOGNN, 28*(6), 1–12.

Writing Group of the 1996 American Academy of Nursing, Expert Panel on Women's Health. (1997). Women's health and women's health care: Recommendations of the 1996 AAN Expert Panel on Women's Health. *Nursing Outlook, 45*(1), 7–15.

This book attempts the daunting task of painting the broad landscape of women's health and, at the same time, providing guidance to the practicing nurse. The purpose of the book is to propose a core curriculum, based on evidence-based information, for the care of women across the lifespan. The nature of women's health demands nurses care for the woman in the context of her daily life experience and challenges the traditional biomedical approach to the health care of women.

Each chapter within the book elaborates on core knowledge essential to delivering safe, competent, and sensitive care to women. The book purposefully departs from the outline format of other core curriculum texts by closing the multidisciplinary conceptual gap evident in most women's health textbooks. Further, we emphasize the broader contextual foundations influencing woman's health. We place this core curriculum within a health promotion/disease prevention, health maintenance/restoration framework, taking a developmental approach

The first seven chapters comprise Unit I. These chapters provide the reader with a wide and broad perspective, taking into account the environmental influences affecting a woman's health. They also move from the general to specific. The next three chapters comprise Unit II and cover the essentials of the health database, health history, physical examination, and diagnostic screening. Unit III is comprised of the four chapters basic to health promotion: nutrition, exercise, immunization, and sexuality. Unit IV, the next four chapters, focuses on the major life stages: adolescence, reproductive years, middle years, and elder years from a health promotion, disease prevention, and health maintenance perspective. Unit V is the chapter on the business of women's health. It provides resources for the planning and development of women's health services.

Breslin in Chapter 1 provides an organizing framework for the women's health core curriculum. Essential to understanding where we must go in the future is an examination of where we have been in the past. The first section of this chapter sets the stage by focusing on women's health scholarship and activism. The second section of the chapter speaks to the development of evidence-based practice, what it is, how it can contribute to current women's health nursing practice. Current status indicators that may influence woman's health are reviewed in the third chapter section. The final section of the chapter provides the reader with a health promotion/disease prevention model that comes from an empowerment perspective.

Bernhard in Chapter 2 discusses, through a feminist lens, patriarchy and its effects on women and women's health. She proposes feminism as a strategy for transforming the world. Understanding the invisible nature of patriarchy, what it is, its structure, and how it permeates our western culture and influences the provision of women's health is essential. She assists us in understanding the complexities of human sex and gender while at the same time fostering an appreciation of the distinctiveness of individuals.

Upvall in Chapter 3 provides a comprehensive framework for examining the concept of culture. The impact of poverty on ethnicity, race, and health is acknowledged. She defines culture as a "process of determining our reality," guiding our conscious and unconscious decisions. She cautions us not to use a cookbook approach, clarifies common misunderstandings, and presents key questions for cultural assessments. She outlines specific information regarding social organization and environmental control for African-American, Hispanic, Middle Eastern, American Indian/Alaskan Native, and Asian American/Pacific Islander women. Additionally she also presents the unique concerns of such special populations as homeless women, immigrant and refugee women in America, and rural women.

Amaya in Chapter 4 discusses environmental effects on women's health as an environmental justice issue. She highlights the interaction between culture and geography as mediators of toxic risk. Amaya captures the unique environmental issues involved with women and the work setting, citing the nursing profession as an exemplar. She provides an overview of hazardous agents and advocates for a community approach to comprehensive risk assessment and identification of sentinel events and clusters. She proposes a primary prevention approach for risk management and lists relevant web resources.

Huebscher in Chapter 5 describes the natural/alternative/complementary health care (NAC) modalities, specifically focusing on NAC practices for women's common symptoms and concerns across the lifespan. As more and more women are seeking care, comfort, and healing with these practices, it is incumbent for the women's health care nurse to be knowledgeable about NAC modalities. Huebscher presents definitions and the rationale for NAC use and provides a rich resource listing for NAC practices. She is inclusive of both self-care and provider-based practices and is sensitive to a multiplicity of practices. She addresses the specific women's issues of premenstrual syndrome, dysmenorrhea, pregnancy, breast concerns, and menopause.

Blankenship in Chapter 6 provides a rich description of women's psychosocial development from girlhood to the elderly. She explores three main aspects of women's personalities and motivation: achievement, intimacy, and power. Women's health nurses will benefit from understanding how intimacy, power, and achievement correspond to women's lives and relationships. This new perspective departs from the traditional biomedical model. Blankenship questions whether current common models of psychosocial development are adequate to address and reflect the complexity of women's psychological health.

Patrick in Chapter 7 also departs from the traditional approach of examining the physical development from solely a reproductive perspective. She moves from a hierarchy of simple to complex, starting with the cell. She covers the cell, gene expression, communication within and between cells, hormones as chemical messengers, and the cellular processes involved in growth and development, particularly physical development of the female. The intentional emphasis on the cell and molecular events provides us with core knowledge from which to understand the future nature of clinical treatments as well as areas of illness prevention, health promotion, and health restoration.

Leight in Chapter 8 talks to us of the importance of establishing a caring therapeutic relationship with the woman, reviewing pertinent literature. She highlights use of narratives as a means to connect via the woman's voice. The sharing of power during the health history interview is a way to communicate respect. Leight provides us with a very comprehensive approach to establishing a relationship with the patient, specific communication tips, and conducting and documenting the comprehensive health history of a well woman.

Burns in Chapters 9 and 10 provides essential information for screening and diagnostic testing and conducting a well woman physical examination. She begins in Chapter 9 by providing a comprehensive overview of preventive care and evaluation of preventive services. She encourages dialogue and discussion with the woman about each screening and diagnostic test. She succinctly covers the recommended screening and diagnostic tests for women across the lifespan. In Chapter 10 she provides a systematic approach to the conduct of the physical examination of the well woman. She highlights for the reader the normal range of findings specific for particular age groups. She guides the reader through a comprehensive head to toe examination, paying particular attention to the pelvic examination.

Susan Miller in Chapter 11 maintains that nutrition is central to a woman's health and is essential to a health agenda. The specific nutrient needs for the woman across the lifespan are given. Emphasis is placed on special needs for the adolescent, reproductive, middle, and elder years. Nutrition designed for disease prevention is the key message of this chapter.

Erin Miller in Chapter 12 provides us with a plan of action to guard against sedentary living. She outlines how American culture has contributed to the growing problem of overweight and obese individuals within American society. The multiple benefits of exercise, both cardiovascular and strength training, are given. Specific suggestions for assisting a woman who is planning to start and maintain an exercise regimen are presented in a clear format. Additionally, a summary table of specific exercise recommendations for women across the lifespan simplifies recommended activities as well as the appropriate amount of time to engage in such physical activity.

Smith in Chapter 13 reminds us that comprehensive women's health care includes use of immunizations within health promotion programs. Currently, immunization rates are being used as quality assurance indicators and as a means to increase compliance with current recommendations. Smith reviews the immunization recommendations for the well woman across the lifespan, giving appropriate screening and counseling information.

Fogel in Chapter 14 explores the many dimensions of female sexuality. Viewing sexual health promotion as an essential nursing function, she focuses on both the physiological and psychological processes involved in sexual development across the lifespan. She captures the complexities involved with sexual desire, the women's view of self, and subsequent presentations to society. She provides a discussion of the multiple aspects of sexual response and a framework for the management of specific sexual concerns.

Skillman-Hull in Chapter 15 provides a comprehensive approach to the care of the adolescent. She emphasizes the need to take into consideration the contextual impact of adolescence—the environment, the physical self, and the emotional, intellectual self. She elaborates on the special assessment needs of the adolescent, with special emphasis on the first pelvic examination. Health promotion content includes nutrition, exercise, and contraceptive options. The health restoration focus provides information about specific conditions affecting the physical and emotional well-being of the female adolescent.

Teschendorf in Chapter 16 discusses the unique health needs of women during the reproductive years. She begins the chapter by presenting the myriad of choices women have today and the various family structures that evolve from those choices. A comprehensive assessment of reproductive age women is followed by health promotion in the form of preconception planning. An in-depth clinical guideline is presented for the management of normal and complicated pregnancies across the entire maternity experience. The clinical management of infertility is followed by a discussion of clinical guidelines for the common gynecologic problems of reproductive age women. The entire chapter is based on health promotion in reproductive age women within the context of social roles and decisions.

Kanusky in Chapter 17 presents the reader with the viewpoint that midlife can present the woman with many positive opportunities. The midlife transition provides the woman with time for personal introspection. It may be a time to assess health risks and engage in more health promotion/disease prevention activities. Kanusky broadens the health issues typically discussed, including not only menopause, but choosing such areas as osteoporosis, breast cancer, and other gynecological cancers where risk identification and lifestyle modification can have an impact on outcomes. She provides us with key information regarding the midlife woman's sexuality and mental health, giving essential guidance for the clinician.

Sellers in Chapter 18 provides us with pertinent demographic information emphasizing the changing nature of the aging woman population. Implications for changing family structures as a result of this trend are also summarized. Specific normal physiologic changes related to aging and a review of comprehensive geriatric assessments are detailed. Health promotion activities are related to screening activities, nutrition, and exercise. Sellers concludes the chapter by addressing the quality of life issues necessary for the clinician providing care to this particular population.

Lucas in Chapter 19 makes the case that the reason women's health care has been the focus of increased attention is simple economics. Because women use more health services and are the key decision makers in families, the development of a variety of health services for women and their families is no surprise. She outlines a model of women's health leadership in which the woman—the consumer of care—is the leader of the team. Business trends influencing the provision of care are clearly articulated from both a legislative and managed care perspective. Lucas articulates the need for integration of women's health services and concludes the chapter with ethical and legal issues unique to the provision of services.

Clearly, this book is a departure from previous AWHONN core curriculum formats. Purposefully, we have chosen a narrative format as opposed to an outline format. Each author writes from her expertise, experience, and heart. Each individual voice is now heard.

Lyon (1996) states nurses cannot expect women in the health care system to achieve a voice "unless the voice of women healthcare workers is clear and loud, emphasizing the value of caring for all. That caring must begin on a horizontal plane; however, nurses cannot care for others from a voiceless and powerless position. Finding a voice will be a process of growth for nurses, as well as other women in the health care system, a chance to obtain a sense of autonomy and a voice unmuffled by fear and powerlessness" (pp. 257-258). This book is dedicated to all nurses who care for women, their families, and their communities.

Lyon, D. (1996). Women as individuals. In J. Lewis & J. Bernstein (Eds.), *Women's health: A relational perspective across the life cycle* (pp. 241–259). Boston, MA: Jones and Bartlett.

Eileen T. Breslin
Vicki A. Lucas

Acknowledgments

We acknowledge that no book such as this could be undertaken without the inspiration of our patients, teachers, and colleagues. It is difficult to single out the many talented faculty and colleagues who have influenced our thinking. However, we would like to acknowledge Denise Webster and Reva Rubin, who, by their own scholarship, gave us new understanding about women's health experiences. Typing and organizational assistance were given by Amy Kapadia and Ann York. We appreciated their phenomenal skills, patience, and good humor. Michael Ledbetter, Laurie K. Muench, and Helen Hudlin at Elsevier Science were a pleasure to work with and guided us well. We are most grateful to all.

Eileen T. Breslin
Vicki A. Lucas

Contents

Chapter 1

Women's Health: Challenges and Opportunities

Eileen Breslin

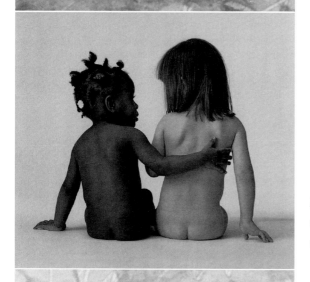

If you come here to help me, you are wasting your time. But if you come here because your liberation is bound up in mine, let us begin.

Lila Watson

INTRODUCTION

Nurses, the largest group of health care providers and predominately female, have contributed much to women's health. Building on the pioneering work of Margaret Sanger and the midwives of the rural Frontier Nursing Service, nurses have established a rich tradition of caring for women's issues. Through partnership and collaboration, women's health nurses are changing today's health care delivery system. In meeting the challenges ahead, we will transform our profession and ourselves.

The notion of women's health is barely a generation old. Traditionally, the focus within the medical community was on women's reproductive function. McBride and McBride (1982) advocated taking women's lived experience as a starting point for all women's health efforts and looking at the woman's entire life. Women's health today does not focus specifically on the reproductive role or the unique health concerns of women, but rather takes into account the quality of women's life experiences in relation to health.

To set the stage for examining women's health, it is necessary to acknowledge the complexity and diversity of women's lives. Within the past 20 years, a commitment to understanding women's health has evolved from multidisciplinary perspectives. This interest has generated a plethora of comment (Allen & Phillips, 1997; Clarke & Olesen,

1999; Dan, 1994; Olshansky, 2000; Ruzek, 1993: Ruzek, Olesen, & Clarke, 1997; Star, Lommel, & Shannon, 1995; Taylor & Woods, 1996; Writing Group of the 1996 AAN Expert Panel on Women's Health, 1997).

What emerges from the literature is the idea that women's health is a complex phenomenon. Just as every woman's life experience is unique, so also is her health experience. There are many lived health experiences of women. Diversity and disparity are key elements. Women's health is no longer synonymous with reproductive health but incorporates health promotion, health maintenance, and health restoration across the lifespan. Functional aspects of health, including the ability to perform multiple roles, are important dimensions highly valued by women themselves (Writing Group of the 1996 AAN Expert Panel on Women's Health, 1997).

Fundamental to our understanding of women's health is acknowledging the influence of race and class. Disparities in earned wages and income levels, educational opportunities, housing, and other areas influence a woman's perception of health (Ruzek, 1997) and contribute to her experience of health as well.

Voices of women from special populations are no longer silenced. Society hears from women with disabilities, homeless women, lesbian women, women struggling with addictions and abuse, incarcerated women, and women survivors of violence (Campbell, 1986; Fennelly & Lacy, 1997; Gill, 1997; Gill & Brown, 2000; Hughes, 1990; Krotoski, Nosek, & Turk, 1996; Lucas, 1993; Smith & Dailard, 1997; Stevens, 1993; Stoller, 1997; Trippet & Bain, 1993). Women from diverse cultural backgrounds have also felt devalued and discriminated against by the health care system. These women have expressed their sense of invisibility along with other women (Bair & Cayleff, 1993). Their voices are now heard.

Seeking to understand such diverse and disparate health and illness experiences embedded within individual, familial, and community perceptions will inevitably create conflict. Yet, it is our charge as nurses within this specialty to listen carefully and hear all voices, advocating for the provision of women's health for all.

Although diverse in many ways, women have many shared experiences. Caring for themselves and caring for others have been common themes for most women. Women have long been acknowledged as the primary caregivers for families and friends, and they have made a priority of promoting and maintaining health for themselves and others.

Women's health nurses have traditionally challenged prevailing medical paradigms by advocating and examining health issues within the context of a woman's life (Dan, 1994; MacPherson, 1981, 1985; Olshansky, 2000). Raising questions in the professional nursing literature, such as whether motherhood is good for women, indicates that nurses within the specialty are ready to lead and challenge the current culture of oppression within the hierarchical and patriarchal health care delivery system (Kirkley, 2000).

This chapter begins by examining the history of women's health scholarship and activism. The next section speaks to the need for evidence-based practice and provides resources for the practicing nurse. A general discussion of the health status of women and the factors influencing health follows, and the chapter concludes by presenting a health promotion/disease prevention framework from an empowerment perspective.

HISTORY OF WOMEN'S HEALTH SCHOLARSHIP AND ACTIVISM

An examination of the scholarship on women and health reveals that the revolution has just begun; the scholarship is just a generation old. Friedman (1994) states that increased attention to women's health issues was concurrent with the arrival of the second wave of the feminist movement during the 1960s. Grassroots efforts such as self-help groups called attention to dissatisfaction with women's health care in general. This phase of the women's movement brought a closer examination of women's health issues. Because the biomedical model did not serve women and their families well, women consumers demanded more sensitive care.

During the 1960s and the 1970s, the Women's Health Movement took form and shape (Marieskind, 1975). Not surprisingly, the issues galvanizing this generation of grassroots activists centered on reproductive rights, including abortion and childbirth practices. With the publication of *Our Bodies, Ourselves* by the Boston Women's Health Book Collective (1970, 1976), women gave voice to their health experiences as they related to reproductive care. They validated that the process of telling their story was as important as the facts. This movement, however, has been criticized as being led primarily by white middle-class college-educated women (Ruzek, 1997).

In 1975 the National Women's Health Network came into existence. The national membership of this advocacy organization had two primary goals: to provide a resource for balanced information on women's health and to give a strong voice for women in the political arena (National Women's Health Network, 1986). The norm during this period was to make global statements regarding the health of women as a group with little attention given to differences related to age, race, and socioeconomic status. Subsequently, during the 1970s and 1980s, organizations such as the National Black Women's Health Project, the Gray Panthers, and the Project on Health and Women and Disability were founded to raise awareness and advocate for the unique needs of these populations.

The 1980s also proved to be a more politically conservative period. During this time the federal government became involved in women's health issues (Nichols, 2000). In 1985, the United States Public Health Service issued the first report on women's health. This landmark report, the first attempt to set a national agenda for women's health issues, outlined specific health concerns to be addressed at the federal level. It called attention to the need for safe and healthful physical and social environments; for disease prevention and treatment; for more research and evaluation of women's health issues; for education, recruitment, and training of health personnel; and for informed guidance on legislation and regulatory measures related to women (Women's Health, 1985). Typical of that era, the report did not address the issue of diversity within special populations of women.

According to Haseltine and Greenburg-Jacobson (1997), menopause became a "safe issue" for public discussion during this period, as politically powerful groups so concerned about controlling the sexual behavior of younger women "basically neutered" menopausal women. A move was made to examine health issues apart from reproductive issues. Other health issues such as breast cancer, which primarily affects older women, came to the forefront.

In the early 1990s, health professionals focused their attention on the disparities in health care provided to men and women. Gender differences in health status became more apparent. Gender gaps were beginning to be identified, solutions proposed, and research agendas identified. Research findings supported the notion that compared to men, women experience more severe first acute myocardial infarction, undergo fewer diagnostic and therapeutic procedures for coronary heart disease, and have higher morbidity and lower mortality rates (Ayanian & Epstein, 1991; Clancy & Massion, 1992; Council on Ethical and Judicial Affairs, 1991; Rodin & Ickovics, 1990; Steingart et al., 1991).

Prior to the 1990s, much of what was known about women's health was extrapolated from studies done primarily on men, by men, and for men. New scholarship was necessary to understand all conditions influencing women's health status. Research traditionally focused on the specific conditions that affect only women, such as menstruation, pregnancy, menopause, and reproductive cancers, whereas health conditions experienced more frequently by women, such as depression, osteoporosis, and autoimmune diseases, needed special attention. Additionally, certain conditions such as heart disease and substance abuse were found to manifest themselves differently in women, requiring further study (Haseltine & Greenburg-Jacobson, 1997).

Pressure from advocacy groups and recognition of the systematic exclusion of women from clinical trials contributed to the formation in 1991 of the Office of Research on Women's Health at the National Institutes of Health (NIH). Although the establishment of such an office was a milestone, marginalization and tokenism remained possibilities, given the history of the women's health movement. Integrating a women's research agenda throughout NIH became essential.

The goals of the NIH Office of Research on Women's Health are threefold: to strengthen and develop research related to women, to ensure representation of women in federally sponsored research, and to increase the number of women in biomedical careers. The Public Health Service affirmed women's health as a priority within the government by publishing the Action Plan for Women's Health in 1991, which outlined an agenda to improve the quality of life of women.

Challenges remain, however, despite the increased federal commitment to systematically investigate women's health across the lifespan and to increase funding. Narrigan, Sprague-Jones, Worchester, and Grad (1997) succinctly identified and addressed five factors contributing to the inequities in women's research: (1) health research has been conducted primarily by white middle-class men; (2) the quantitative scientific method used in clinical trials has frequently excluded women from studies by citing a need for homogeneity in samples (implying that the menstrual cycle is a methodological problem); (3) research to specifically benefit diverse populations has not been considered a priority; (4) funds for health care research have been scarce in comparison to other governmental priorities; and (5) there has been a lack of women, notably of color, in positions of authority and policy making in academic and governmental institutions.

Johnson and Fee (1997) cited several additional reasons for excluding women from research studies. First, the research community has not kept pace with changing social, legal, and demographic changes that reflect the multiplicity of women's roles within employment settings. A greater variety of opportunities for longer employment exists for women today than ever before. Second, a perception exists that women are harder to recruit into studies because of childcare concerns. Third, there is a fear of harming pregnant women and their fetuses. Lastly, the authors claim that the medical establishment subconsciously believes that women's health issues are of secondary importance.

With federal funding of the multimillion dollar Women's Health Initiative (WHI), a long-term national health study begun in 1991, a major commitment was made to understand older women's health issues. The WHI, a 15-year project sponsored by the National Institutes of Health (NIH) and the National Heart, Lung, and Blood Institute, involves approximately 168,000 women aged 50 to 79 at 40 clinical centers. The study focuses on the prevention of four major disorders (cardiovascular disease, breast and colorectal cancers, and osteoporosis) that affect a woman's life during the postmenopausal years and are the major causes of death, disability, and frailty in older women.

The WHI has three major components: a randomized controlled clinical trial of promising disease prevention studies (approximately 68,000 women), an observational study to identify predictors of disease (approximately 100,000 women), and a study of community approaches to develop health-enhancing behaviors in women aged 40 or older. The latter component is a multidisciplinary, cooperative venture of eight university-based prevention centers, the Centers for Disease Control and Prevention, and the National Institutes of Health.

The clinical trial examines the benefits and risks of long-term hormone replacement therapy and the role of fat reduction and other dietary modifications, behavioral change, and calcium and vitamin D supplements in preventing disease among postmenopausal women. Women, if eligible, chose to enroll in one, two, or all three study components. The observational study examines the relationship among lifestyle, risk factors, and specific disease outcomes. Recruitment for this study was completed in 1998, and these women will be followed for 8 to 12 years. The community prevention study conducts and evaluates health programs designed to encourage women of all races and socioeconomic backgrounds to adopt healthy lifestyles in order to develop model programs for community-wide distribution (*www.nhlbi.nih.gov/whi/factsht*, 2000).

Preliminary data are available on the demographic characteristics of women enrolled in the Women's Health Study (WHS) clinical trial. This randomized, double-blind placebo-controlled trial was designed to evaluate the benefits and risks of low-dose aspirin and vitamins in the primary prevention of cardiovascular disease and cancer in women. Baseline characteristics of the study sample indicate that the 39,876 women participants are healthier in some respects than the general population and comparable with respect to obesity, hypertension, and elevated cholesterol (Rexrode et al., 2000).

More recently, the estrogen and progesterone therapy component of the WHI study was stopped for postmenopausal women who had not had a hysterectomy before joining the WHI study. In its review of study data, the WHI Data and Safety Monitoring Board found increased risk of breast cancer, and the risk for heart attack, strokes, and pulmonary embolism remained high (*www.nhlbi.nih.gov/whi/hrtupd*).

Nichols (2000) cites four major achievements of the women's health movement: women have more control over their reproductive rights, gender-based research has become an integral part of biomedicine, research on cardiovascular disease in women has progressed, and violence and discrimination are recognized worldwide as significant health issues. Much more work remains to be done, however, as new questions and opportunities present themselves to all women. Promoting scholarship that examines the diversity, complexity, and disparities of women's health will continue to be a priority in women's health research and advocacy. Nurses within this specialty must continue their advocacy for research that reflects the complexity of the woman's health/illness experience and supports meaningful nursing interventions.

EVIDENCE-BASED PRACTICE

An international movement is occurring within the health care field to develop guidelines for practice and clinical decision making that are grounded in scientific evidence. This evidence-based approach to examining clinical decision making can indeed inform women's health. Such an evidence-based approach relies on examining the scientific literature and identifying and reviewing key articles to determine the value of a particular diagnosis, treatment, or test, rather than relying solely on expert opinion. Both quantitative and qualitative data will need to be considered in a systematic manner to determine the quality of the evidence used to support decisions. An explosion of new knowledge and increased access to multiple data sources present unique challenges for the practicing nurse, as does the relative lack of research on women's health.

The Association of Women's Health, Obstetric, and Neonatal Nursing (AWHONN) has developed several evidence-based practice guidelines (Box 1-1). The American Nursing Association's *Manual to Develop Guidelines* (Marek, 1995) provides a framework to guide the process. Quantitative studies are evaluated by categories such as the problem or question under study, sampling and measurement techniques, internal validity, external validity, construct validity, statistical conclusion validity, and justification for the conclusions. Qualitative studies are evaluated on the basis of descriptive vividness, methodological congruence, analytical precision, theoretical connectedness, and heuristic relevance. Parameters for assessing the quality of the evidence rating are given in the United States Preventive Services Task Force's *Guide to Clinical Preventive*

Box 1-1 AWHONN'S EVIDENCE-BASED GUIDELINES

- Continence for women (2000)
- Nursing management of second-stage labor (2000)
- Breast-feeding support: parental care through the first years (2001)
- Nursing care of women receiving regional analgesia/anesthesia (2001)
- Emotional well-being of midlife women (2001)
- Cardiovascular health for women: primary prevention (2001)

From AWHONN (*www.Awhonn.org*).

Services (1996) presented in Box 1-2. Resources for women's health care providers can be found following the reference section.

DeGeorges (1999) has provided a useful guide for finding one's way through the World Wide Web in search of evidence-based information. Web-based resources provide quick access to evidence-based information. Consulting with the literature through web access or library services is mandatory, given the rapid pace at which information is currently transmitted. Considering the length of time needed to produce textbooks, their information may not always be up to date.

DeGeorges 1999 lists two web sites, *Health Web: Evidence-Based Health Care* (*www.healthweb.org*), and the *National Guideline Clearinghouse* (*www.guidelines.gov*), as practice resource sites. *Health Web* is a collaborative project of over 20 health sciences libraries, supported by the National Library of Medicine. Libraries of the Greater Midwest Region of the National Network of Libraries of Medicine and the Committee for Institutional Cooperation are involved in this project, which provides organized access to evaluated noncommercial, health-related, Internet-accessible resources. The *National Guideline Clearinghouse,* a public resource for evidence-based clinical practice guidelines, is sponsored by the Agency for Healthcare Research and Quality in partnership with the American Medical Association and the American Association of Health Plans. Clinicians can search for information based on disease/condition, treatment/intervention, or both.

Clinical Evidence (*www.clinicalevidence.org.*), an international resource that provides evidence for clinicians and patients to use in jointly deciding on health care interventions, is updated every 6 months and is available for a fee. It is considered complementary to the Cochrane Collaboration, an international multidisciplinary organization dedicated to systematically reviewing randomized clinical trials for evidence-based practice. Seven review groups specialize in women's health issues, such as breast cancer, gynecological care, incontinence, pregnancy, childbirth, fertility, and menstrual disorders (Callister & Hobbins-Garbett, 2000).

Critically evaluating the rationale for interventions in clinical practice can create quality care for women and actually challenge existing paradigms. As an example, a metaanalysis by Thacker, Stroup, and Peterson (1995) examined the safety and efficacy

Box 1-2 QUALITY OF EVIDENCE RATING

I. Evidence obtained from at least one properly designed randomized controlled trial.

II-1. Evidence obtained from well-designed controlled trials without randomization.

II-2. Evidence obtained from well-designed cohort or case control analytic studies, preferably from more than one center or research group.

II-3. Evidence from multiple time series with or without the intervention. Dramatic results in uncontrolled experiments (such as the results of the introduction of penicillin treatment in the 1940s) could also be regarded as this type of evidence.

III. Opinions of respected authorities, based on clinical experiences, descriptive studies, or reports of expert committees.

From United States Preventive Services Task Force. (1996). *Guide to clinical preventive services* (2nd ed). Baltimore, MD: Williams & Wilkins.

of intrapartum electronic fetal monitoring. By aggregating data from a randomized clinical controlled trial with 58,855 women and 59,324 infants, the authors found an increase in the number of cesarean and operative deliveries. They also found a significant reduction in neonatal seizures, which did not affect long-term neurological outcomes. Consequently, the United States Preventive Services Task Force now states that fair evidence does not support routine fetal monitoring for low-risk pregnant women.

Another example can be found in the use of oral contraceptives. In most countries, oral contraceptives are routinely prescribed without a Pap smear. The World Health Organization and outside experts reviewed over 2000 articles on adverse effects and contraindications to oral contraceptives and developed four criteria for their use. They also created a classification system for medical tests and procedures to be given prior to dispensing oral contraceptives and concluded that only family and personal medical history and blood pressure measurement are necessary (Hannaford & Webb, 1996).

As more evidence-based data accumulate, it is essential that nurses remain in the vanguard in translating the best available evidence into practice. As patients gain greater access to health care information through such sources as the Internet, nurses will increasingly be called upon to translate and interpret the information.

STATUS INDICATORS OF WOMEN'S HEALTH

When one considers women's health status, it is important to understand how women themselves perceive their health. In 1993, 60% of white women believed they were in excellent health as compared to 48% of Hispanic women and 44% of African-American women. Thirty-three percent of African-American women and 29% of Hispanic women indicated that they were in good health. Twenty-three percent of both African-American and Hispanic women reported themselves to be in poor health, while only 12% of white women did (Hartmann, Kuriansky, & Owens, 1996).

As of 1995, there were 134 million women living in the United States. According to census data, in which women checked multiple categories, a majority of women categorized themselves as white (83%). Next in frequency were African-Americans (13%) and Hispanics (10%), followed by Asian and Pacific Islanders (4%) and American Indians, Eskimos, and Aleuts (1%) (U.S. Bureau of the Census, 1995). Women of color have been typically defined as Asian, African-American, Hispanic, or Native American. Within the United States, cultural experiences and personal circumstances greatly affect the life expectancies and health status of women in these four groups. Federal government policies currently support a goal of zero disparity in health care access and quality among all ethnic and racial groups.

The health of women varies substantially by age and race/ethnicity. The Office of Minority and Women's Health was established in 1994 to develop and promote specific activities to reduce disparities in health care for women from minority populations. Life expectancy, the average number of years of life remaining to an individual at a given age if death rates remain constant, is often used as a summary indicator of the overall health in a particular population. In 1997, the life expectancy at birth was 79 years for all American women, as opposed to 75 for men (*www.agingstas.gov/chartbook2000/healthstatus.html*, 2000). Although these statistics do not take into account the diversity of women, it remains true that most women can expect to outlive their male counterparts. Asian subpopulations have the longest life expectancies, while American Indian/Alaska Native and African-American women have the shortest.

In examining the major causes of death for women, diseases of the heart rank first for all females except for Asian and Pacific Islanders, for whom they are the second most frequent cause of death. Cancer is the second major cause of death for women, with the exception of Asian and Pacific Islanders for whom it is first. African-American women have the highest death rates from both heart disease and cancer. Noteworthy is that some conditions cause death more frequently only among women of color. Conditions such as HIV infection, suicide, homicide, and chronic liver disease are among the top ten causes of death among women of color (National Center for Health Statistics, 1995). (A more detailed discussion of the health status of women of color occurs in Chapter 5).

Women are also known to be more likely than men to use health services throughout their life cycle. Interestingly, Bartman, Clancy, Moy, and Langenberg (1996) found that if a woman has an internist as a primary care provider rather than an obstetrician-gynecologist or a family physician, she is likely to make more visits and incur higher total outpatient care costs. Common chronic diseases for all women under the age of 65 include asthma, hypertension, diabetes, and thyroid disorders (National Center for Health Statistics, 1997). Women are more likely than men to experience chronic health problems related to arthritis, hypertension, and osteoporosis (Kramerow, Lentzner, Rookes, Weeks, & Sayday, 1999; Watts, 1999; *www.agingstas.gov/chartbook2000/healthstatus.htm*).

Access to health care involves not only health insurance but also the availability of competent care providers and facilities that are conveniently located, provide child care, and are readily accessible by public transportation. Two thirds of women do receive their health insurance benefits from their own or their spouse's employer (U.S. Bureau of Census, 2000). Women who are uninsured are less likely to get the necessary care than those with insurance coverage. Additionally, these women are less likely to receive care from specialists and to fill prescriptions (Collins et al., 1999).

Access to quality care can further be diminished by the woman's own life experience. Specific subpopulations within the health care system, such as lesbians and women with disabilities, have had negative encounters with the health care system, resulting in delayed help-seeking and fear of discrimination.

Research has indicated that caregivers hold preconceived stereotypical notions about lesbians, are ignorant of their needs, and create nontherapeutic environments for delivery of care (Hall, 1993; Kenney & Tash, 1993; Stoller, 1997). Common barriers to seeking health care services include a lack of financial resources or insurance, no access to a partner's coverage, and lack of services sensitive to the unique needs of lesbians.

Finding good health information can be particularly difficult for the more than 28 million women with disabilities. Disabled women may be limited by transportation problems, architectural barriers, and financial constraints. Lacking the support necessary to run errands or go to appointments that millions of other women take for granted, some women with disabilities find it difficult to leave their homes. Even those who do have the ability and resources to search for information often cannot find helpful information that addresses their special unique needs. Two themes predominate: invisibility and genderlessness. The lack of access to health care services because of gender inequity and service barriers remains.

Sexuality may also be invalidated and reproductive health needs are at times ignored for these women. Abuse has been documented and is only just beginning to be publicly addressed by scholars. Mental health issues such as stress and an increased risk for depression and suicide indicate a need for screening and preventive services. Privacy concerns and negligence of medical providers persist (Nosek, Howland, Rintala, Young, & Chanpong, 1997).

To overlook the effect of social factors on health would be a mistake. The social milieu in which a woman functions is complex. Both social factors (education, employment, earnings, and marital status) and reproductive factors (fertility rates, birth rates, and out-of-wedlock births) have roles in determining health status and opportunities. The ways that women chose to live their lives are also changing. The number of women delaying marriage and/or choosing a single life has increased. There has been a noticeable rise in the longevity of women and there has been a tripling of the proportion of women aged 30 to 34 from 1970 to 1994 (Slauter, 1987; U.S. Bureau of the Census, 1995). With aging comes more health concerns. Women health care providers will have increasingly greater numbers of older women to care for than in the past.

Although the participation of women in the labor force has increased since 1950, almost doubling from 30% to 59%, women still earn less than men, making only 76% of men's medium income in 1998 (U.S. Department of Labor 1999). Research has indicated that some aspects of the work environment have contributed to health problems in some women (Pugliesi, 1995; Ross & Mirowsky, 1995; Verbrugge, 1985). Other research has indicated that chronic disease may be exacerbated by employment stresses (Brett, Strogatz, & Savitz, 1997).

The intersection of women, work, and health has just begun to be examined (Frankenhaeuser, Lundberg, & Chesney, 1991). Cultural biases associated with work need to be re-examined. For instance, Guendelman and Sliber (1993) refute previous studies that view maquiladora work as hazardous. They found that this work may actually afford these women more economic alternatives to early marriage and childbearing. They reported that the maquiladora perceptions of working conditions were more predictive of health status than the actual conditions. In general, as the population has aged, more women have entered the workforce for the first time at midlife, changing careers and anticipating working longer than previous generations (AWHONN, 2000).

Another societal change that has influenced health status is the increasing number of women living in poverty. Ruzek (1993) has suggest that health care providers should routinely include low income and lack of education as risk factors for poor health. For example, the health status of American Indian women is affected by the fact that poverty (27%) and unemployment rates are higher for them than for any other U.S. ethnic population. Ruzek has also challenged the health care system to consider economic development, education, and housing as public health investments.

As previously stated, financial barriers also play a significant role in the health status of women, who have lower incomes than men. Despite their larger numbers in the workforce, women are overrepresented in lower paying positions. Women of color are more likely to be economically disadvantaged and to have lower education levels, contributing to poorer health status and barriers to care (Salganicoff et al., 2002).

The women's health nurse must consider women's perceptions regarding risk and exposure to disease. In addition, social and cultural issues, such as access to care, choice of care provider, types of care, poverty, violence, hunger, and environmental toxins, have yet to be fully explored in light of their relationship to women's health status. Poverty remains one of the major factors that affects women's health. Further scholarship is necessary to understand the complex relationship among these social and cultural variables influencing women's health.

HEALTH PROMOTION AND DISEASE PREVENTION

Nurses have historically focused on health promotion and disease prevention as essential components of nursing care (Pender , Barkauskas, Hayman, Rice, & Anderson, 1992). Prevention has become an increasingly important part of health care, particularly with respect to chronic disease. In the United States, preventable disease and injuries are thought to cost $450 billion dollars a year (Centers for Disease Control and Prevention, 1998). Estimates indicate that approximately 60% of chronic diseases are preventable and that consumers are interested in pursuing healthier lifestyles (McGuinnes & Foege, 1993).

Throughout their life cycle women may experience a chronic disease that limits activity. Well women visits are a prime time to assess risk and screen for chronic disease. Risk factors for chronic disease include poor nutrition, smoking, physical inactivity, and stress (Misra, Inglis-Baldy, & Ruderman, 1998).

Health promotion, health maintenance, and disease prevention are viewed by American society as a personal responsibility. The expectation is that the individual will make responsible lifestyle choices, care for his or her body, and limit potential harm to others. There has also been increased recognition of the need to manage environmental risks (Peterson & Lupton, 1996). Economics drives the perception that each American is responsible for maintaining his or her own health.

Lifestyle choices such as a nutritious diet, regular exercise, and avoidance of smoking may prevent chronic diseases later in life. How and why individuals actively engage in healthy lifestyles is only beginning to be understood. Research findings to date have been compromised by limited internal and external validity measurement, design problems, and a lack of attention to gender- and age-related concerns. The cultural context of health promotion and disease prevention activities has not been systematically addressed. Working and living conditions, as well as environmental risks, need to be taken into account. Nonetheless, there is a growing interest in understanding what activities are meaningful for women's health.

Nurses in ambulatory health care can contribute greatly to a better understanding of health promotion and disease prevention. The nursing profession has taken proactive stances on disease prevention and health promotion and is clear about the nurse's role in those activities (Knollmueller, 1993). Nurses in advanced practice roles may be in key positions to form alliances with minority women to develop gender-related and culturally sensitive health promotional activities. Health promotion, which has been defined as "the process of enabling people to increase control over, and to improve, their health" (WHO, 1986), has as its goal the enhancement of health and the prevention of ill health (Downie, Tannahill, & Tannahill, 1996). Nurses have generally preferred a broad definition of health, taking into consideration physical, emotional, social, political, and environmental concerns.

The United States adopted a national prevention strategy to significantly improve the health of the American people by focusing on goals that increase the lifespan, reduce health disparities, and achieve preventive services for everyone. Now into its third decade, the U.S. Department of Health and Human Services (USDHHS) launched its report, *Healthy People 2010* (U.S. Department of Health and Human Services, 2000), which built upon the work of two previous major initiatives, *Healthy People: The Surgeon General's Report on Health Promotion and Disease Prevention* (U.S. Department of Health, Education, and Welfare, 1979) and *Healthy People 2000* (U.S. Department of Health and Human Services, 1991).

Healthy People 2010 has two main goals: to increase the quality and years of healthy life and to eliminate health disparities. Its 467 objectives (an increase from 226 objectives in *Healthy People 2000*) are designed to assist the American public in improving health. These objectives will be monitored though 28 focus areas. A limited set of objectives, known as leading indicators, focuses on physical activity, overweight and obesity, tobacco use, substance abuse, responsible sexual behavior, mental health, injury and violence, environmental quality, immunization, and access to health care. Inherent in these goals is the need to place special attention on health education for women. Women are more likely than men to pursue health as a personal goal and also are the primary caregivers for families and others in need. Assisting women to create healthier lifestyles will likely have the overall result of improving the health of the population (Murray & Zentner, 1993).

MacDonald and Bunton (1992) state that health promotion is comprised fundamentally of strategies aimed at individual (lifestyle) and structural (fiscal/ecological) elements to promote the health of populations. The role of health promotion is to empower individuals. Raeburn and Rootman (1996) propose that empowerment may occur at multiple social levels, not only through developing personal skills, self care, small group development but also by creating supportive environments, community building, and public health policy. Resources for addressing leading health indicators for *Healthy People 2010* are found in Box 1-3.

Box 1-3 LEADING HEALTH INDICATOR RESOURCES

Physical Activity
- President's Council on Physical Fitness and Sports 202-690-9000: *www.fitness.gov*
- Centers for Disease Control and Prevention (CDC) 888-232-3228: *www.cdc.gov/nccdphp/dnpa*

Overweight and Obesity
- Obesity Education Initiative, National Heart, Lung, and Blood Institute Information Center 301-592-8573: *www.nhlbi.nih.gov/about/oei/index.htm*
- The Weight-Control Information Network, National Institutes of Health (NIH) 877-946-4627: *www.niddk.nih.gov/health/nutrit/win.htm*

Tobacco Use
- Office of Smoking Health, National Center for Chronic Disease Prevention and Health Promotion, CDC 800-CDC-1311: *www.cdc.gov/tobacco*
- Cancer Information Service, NIH 800-4-CANCER: *cis.nci.nih.gov*

Substance Abuse
- National Clearinghouse for Alcohol and Drug Information, Substance Abuse and Mental Health Services Administration (SAMHSA) 800-729-6686; 800-487-4889 (TDD): *www.health.org*
- National Institute on Drug Abuse, NIH: *www.nida.nih.gov*
- National Institute on Alcohol Abuse and Alcoholism, NIH 201-443-3860: *www.niaaa.nih.gov*

Responsible Sexual Behavior
- CDC National AIDS Hotline 800-342-AIDS (800-342-2437): *www.cdc.gov/hiv/hivinfo/nah.htm*
- CDC National Sexually Transmitted Disease (STD) Hotline 800-227-8922: *www.cdc.gov/nchstp/dstd/dstdp.html*
- CDC National Prevention Information Network 800-458-5231: *www.cdcnpin.org*
- Office of Population Affairs 301-654-6190: *opa.osophs.dhhs.gov*

Mental Health
- Center for Mental Health Service, SAMHSA: *www.mentalhealth.org/cmhs/index.htm*
- Knowledge Exchange Network, SAMHSA: *www.mentalhealth.org*
- National Institute of Mental Health Information Line, NIH 800-421-4211: *www.nimh.nih.gov/publicat/depressionmenu.cfm*

Injury and Violence
- National Center for Injury Prevention and Control, CDC 770-488-1506: *www.cdc.gov/ncipc/ncipchm.htm*
- Office of Justice Programs, U.S. Department of Justice 202-307-0703: *www.ojp.usdoj.gov/home.htm*
- National Highway Traffic Safety Administration, U.S. Department of Transportation Auto Safety Hotline 888-DASH-2-DOT (888-327-4236): *www.nhtsa.dot.gov/hotline*

Environmental Quality
- Indoor Air Quality Information Clearinghouse, U.S. Environmental Protection Agency 800-438-4318 (IAQ hotline) 800-SALUD-12 (725-8312) Spanish: *www.epa.gov/iaq/iaqinfo.html*
- Information Resources Center (IRC), U.S. Environmental Protection Agency 202-260-5922: *www.epa.gov/natlibra/hqirc/about.htm*
- Agency for Toxic Substances and Disease Registry, CDC 888-442-8737: *www.atsdr.cdc.gov*

Immunization
- National Immunization Program, CDC 888-232-2522 (English); 888-232-0233 (Spanish); 888-CDC FAXX (Fax-back): *www.cdc/gov/nip*

Continued

Box 1-3 LEADING HEALTH INDICATOR RESOURCES—CONT'D

Health Care Access
- Agency for Healthcare Research and Quality, Office of Healthcare Information 301-594-1264 *www.ahrq.gov/consumer/index.html#plans*
- "Insure Kids Now" Initiative, Health Care Financing Administration (HCFA) 877-KIDS NOW (800-543-7669): *www.insurekidsnow.gov*: *www.hcfa.gov/init/outreach/outhome.htm*
- Healthy Start National Resource Center, Health Resources and Services Administration 800-311-BABY; 800-514-7081: *www.healthystart.net*
- Office of Beneficiary Relations HCFA 800-444-4606 (Customer Service Center) 800-MED-ICARE (Info Line): *www.medicare.gov*

Labonte (1989) clearly outlines the levels at which empowerment occurs. At the intrapersonal level, one experiences a potent sense of self—the power within an experience of choice. At the interpersonal level, one feels power with an experience of interdependency. At the intergroup level, individuals cultivate resources and strategies for personal and sociopolitical gains, enhancing advocacy and participatory democracy, creating greater social equity; the power between becomes an experience of generosity. For nurses engaging with women of diverse backgrounds, it is helpful to recognize the importance of empowerment and its role in health promotion.

Preventive services have long been essential components of nursing care. Primary prevention refers to those interventions designed to reduce disease or the negative consequences thereof by delaying age of onset. Such measures may be exercise, better nutrition, improved sleep habits, and specific protection for populations, such as immunization. Simply, primary prevention prevents disease, disability, or ill health. Secondary prevention is aimed at detecting problems early and intervening quickly. Intervention strategies at this level are designed to reduce the prevalence of a disease by shortening its course and duration. Taking a complete health history and physical examination are simple tools to diagnose disease and promote health. Tertiary prevention focuses on limitations of disability and rehabilitation with the goal of limiting distress. An example would be speech therapy for stroke victims. The *Clinician's Handbook of Preventive Services* (U.S. Department of Health and Human Services, 1998) is the cornerstone of the federal government's campaign Putting Prevention in Practice. This resource offers practical tools for putting prevention into practice. Recommendations by major authorities, basic content for educational counseling, as well as provider and patient resources are all listed.

Knowledge about prevention activities related specifically to women has just begun to be gathered and published. In the area of primary prevention, Rosenberg and Gollub (1992) have recommended that prevention messages designed for sexually transmitted diseases place more emphasis on female-controlled contraceptive methods, such as the diaphragm and spermicides. With respect to secondary prevention activities, such as health histories and physicals, it is recognized that women are traditionally underexamined. It is not uncommon to find in a woman's medical record, "breast exam, pelvic exam, and rectal exam deferred." The standard for a comprehensive examination of the breasts is 3 minutes per breast (Meisler, 2000). Only within the past few years has there been a systematic analysis of research addressing the interactions among biological, psychological, and social forces that affect women's health status (Stanton & Gallant, 1995).

Eleven known behavioral health risk factors were studied in U.S. women aged 18 years and older (Hahn et al., 1998). Behavior Risk Surveillance System data from 1992 to 1994 were analyzed to determine the prevalence of smoking, obesity, diabetes, heavy alcohol consumption, sedentary lifestyle and the inadequate use of seatbelts, Pap smears, consumption of fruits or vegetables, mammography, and colorectal screening and immunizations. The results indicated that African-Americans and Native Americans have relatively high prevalences of every major risk factor and that Pacific Islanders have relatively low prevalence of most risk factors. Interestingly, when socioeconomic factors were accounted for, the prevalence of risk factors among racial/ethnic groups was diminished but not eliminated (Hahn et al., 1998).

Women's health concerns necessitate health promotion and disease prevention activities directed toward specific conditions and population needs. For instance, cervical and breast cancer screening programs might target African-American women, given their increased mortality rate when compared to white women. Prenatal education and parenting assistance might be tailored to be targeted to adolescent needs. Given the increased number of new AIDS cases among Hispanic and African-American women, increased prevention efforts may be warranted (Centers for Disease Control and Prevention, 1999).

It is difficult to talk about health promotion and disease prevention activities without acknowledging the roles played by unemployment, underemployment, and illiteracy. Women typically move in and out of the work force on a full or part-time basis more than men and are more often employed in low paying jobs. In the United States, it has been estimated that 23 to 40 million adults are functionally illiterate; consequently, much health information is inaccessible to a large portion of the population. The gap between reading level of the general population and access to health information needs to be considered.

Ruzek (1997) raises six interesting questions for nurses to ponder when considering health promotion activities as they relate to women. How will women access behavioral assistance programs through third party reimbursement? Whose health gets promoted during care for pregnancy? How adequate is the research for health promotional activities? Do health promotion norms hurt women? What does health promotion mean for stigmatized women? Finally, do health promotion activities go too far? Ruzek calls for us to not only honor a woman's responsibility for her own health but also to consider the structural forces within our society that need to be altered before health promotion activities can occur. One important issue she raises is sharing work to increase opportunities for employment; more women working generates more income and thus more health.

Additionally, health promotion and disease prevention programs need to take into account other issues. When planning these programs, financial and cultural barriers to accessing the health care delivery system need to be considered. Trends in establishing guidelines for care have been shifting away from relatively simple classifications according to age, gender, and race to a more critical appraisal of the individual's circumstances. Poverty and lack of opportunity influence health status. The importance of being sensitive to the reality of a woman's life when discussing health-promotion activities cannot be overstated. Knowledge of risk factors associated with certain populations assists nurses in identifying those who need more intensive surveillance.

It is recognized that lifelong physical activity promotes health and well-being among women. Specific benefits include prevention of osteoporosis, heart disease, and high blood pressure; help with weight control; and functional independence as a woman ages. Mental health benefits also accrue (Brehm & Iannotta, 1998). As primary care providers, nurses can make a difference in the lives of women by prescribing the recommended daily level of moderate exercise (Burns, Camaione, & Chetterton, 2000).

Environment can be defined as all the external factors surrounding, affecting, and influencing the health of girls and women. Only within the last decade has attention been given to the relationship between women's health and the environment. Prior to the early 1990s, much of the research on the environment's effects on health focused on the occupational health of men. Scientific investigations have recently begun to examine the role of environmental disruptors of endocrine and hormonal function and female genetic predisposition to environmental exposures. In addition, occupational studies have linked work-related exposures to illness and disability (Haynes et al., 2000). The Institute of Medicine has stated the need to integrate information related to exposures across all aspects of women's lives—in the workplace, at home, and as caretakers who bring food into the home (Setlow, Lawson, & Woods, 1998).

SUMMARY

The health care delivery system is challenged to be inclusive of all, provide access to care, and offer treatment options in a wide variety of delivery settings. Women's health care nurses, in particular, continue to be at the forefront of their profession in advocating and meeting these challenges. Challenges remain as we plan for a health care sensitive to women of all ages and from all populations. La Rosa (1994) indicates that such planning will necessitate collaboration and cooperation on the part of providers, researchers, and women clients. We would posit that sensitive health care for all women demands more communication and listening by both woman clients and ourselves. We will learn how to meet every woman's health needs as we listen and seek understanding together.

REFERENCES

Allen, K., & Phillips, J. (1997). *Women's health across the lifespan.* Philadelphia: Lippincott.

Association of Women's Health, Obstetric and Neonatal Nursing (AWHONN). (1999). *Advancing evidence-based practice: Women's health.* Philadelphia: Lippincott Williams & Wilkins.

Ayanian, J., & Epstein, A. (1991). Differences in the use of procedures between women and men hospitalized for coronary disease. *New England Journal of Medicine, 325*(4), 221–225.

Bair, B., & Cayleff, S. (1993). *Wings of gauze: Women of color and the experience of health and illness.* Detroit: Wayne State Press.

Bartman, B., Clancy, C., Moy, E., & Langenberg, P. (1996). Cost differences among women's primary care physicians. *Health Affairs, 15*(4), 177–182.

Boston Women's Health Book Collective. (1970). (1976). *Our bodies, ourselves.* New York: Simon & Schuster.

Brehm, B. A., & Iannotta, J. G. (1998). Women and physical activity: Active lifestyles enhance health and well-being. *Journal of Health Education, 29*(2), 89–92.

Brett, K. M., Strogatz, D. S., & Savitz, D. A. (1997). Employment, job strain, and pre-term delivery among women in North Carolina. *American Journal of Public Health, 87*(2), 199–204.

Burns, K., Camaione, D., & Chetterton, C. (2000). Prescription of physical activity by adult nurse practitioners: A national survey. *Nursing Outlook, 48*, 28–33.

Callister, L. C., & Hobbins-Garbett, D. (2000). Cochrane Pregnancy and Childbirth Database: Resource for evidence-based practice. *Journal of Obstetric, Gynecologic, and Neonatal Nursing, 29*(2), 123–128.

Campbell, J. C. (1986). Nursing assessment for risk of homicide with battered women. *Advances in Nursing Science, 8*(4), 36–51.

Centers for Disease Control and Prevention. (1998). *Unrealized prevention opportunities: Reducing the health and economic burden of chronic disease. A Report of the National Center for Chronic Disease Prevention and Health Promotion.* Washington, DC: U.S. Department of Health and Human Services.

Centers for Disease Control and Prevention. Division of HIV/AIDS Prevention (1999). *HIV/AIDS surveillance report.* Atlanta: CDC.

Clancy, C., & Massion, C. (1992). American women's health care: A patchwork quilt with gaps. *Journal of the American Medical Association, 268*(14), 1918–1920.

Clarke, A. E., & Olesen, V. L. (1999). Revisioning women, health, and healing. In A. E. Clarke & V. L. Olesen (Eds.), *Feminist, cultural, and technoscience perspectives.* New York and London: Routledge.

Collins, K., Schoen, C., Joseph, S., Duchon, L., Simontov, E., & Yellowitz, M., (1999). *Health concerns across a woman's lifespan: The Commonwealth Fund 1998 Survey of Women's Health.* New York: The Commonwealth Fund.

Dan, A. (1994). *Reframing women's health: Multidisciplinary research and practice.* Thousand Oaks, CA: Sage Publications.

DeGeorges, K. (1999). Evidence! Show me the evidence. *Lifelines, 3*(3), 47–48.

Downie, R. S., Tannahill, C., & Tannahill, A. (1996). *Health promotion: Models and values.* Oxford: Oxford University Press.

Fennelly, C., & Lacy, B. (1997). Homelessness. In K. M. Allen & J. M. Phillips (Eds.), *Women's health across the lifespan: A comprehensive perspective.* Philadelphia: Lippincott-Raven Publishers.

Frankenhaeuser, M., Lundberg, U., & Chesney, M. (Eds.). (1991). *Women, work, and health: Stress and opportunities.* New York: Plenum Press.

Friedman, E. (Ed.). (1994). *An unfinished revolution: Women and health care in America.* New York: United Hospital Fund.

Gill, C. (1997). The last sisters: Health issues of women with disabilities. In S. Ruzek, V. Olesen, & A. Clarke (Eds.), *Women's health: complexities and differences,* Columbus, OH: Ohio State University Press.

Gill, C. J., & Brown, A. A. (2000). Overview of health issues of older women with intellectual disabilities. *Physical & Occupational Therapy in Geriatrics, 18*(1), 26–36.

Guendelman, S., & Sliber, M. J. (1993). The health consequences of maquiladora work: Women on the U.S. Mexican border. *American Journal of Public Health, 83*, 37–44.

Hall, J. (1993). An exploration of lesbian's images of recovery from alcohol problems. *Lesbian Health* pp. 91–108.

Hannaford, P. C., & Webb, A. M. C., (1996). *Evidence-guided prescribing of the pill,* London: CRC Press–Parthenon Publishers.

Hahn, R. A., Teutsch, S. M., Franks, A. L., Chang, M. H., & Lloyd, E. E. (1998). The prevalence of risk factors among women in the United States by race and age, 1992–1994: Opportunities for primary and secondary prevention. *Journal of the American Women's Association, 53*(2), 96–104, 107.

Hartmann, H. I., Kuriansky, J. A., & Owens, C. L. (1996). In M. M. Falik, & K. S. Collins (Eds.), *Women's health: The Commonwealth Fund Survey* (pp. 296–323). Baltimore: Johns Hopkins University Press.

Haseltine, F., & Greenburg-Jacobson, B. (Eds.). (1997). *Women's health research: A medical and policy primer.* Washington, DC: Health Press.

Haynes, S. G., Lynch, B. S., Biegel, R., Malliou, E., Rudick, J., & Sassaman, A. P. (2000). Women's health and the environment: Innovations in science and policy. *Journal of Women's Health & Gender-Based Medicine, 9*(3), 245–273.

Hughes, T. L. (1990). Evaluating research on chemical dependency among women: A women's health perspective. *Family & Community Health, 13*(3), 35–46.

Johnson, T., & Fee, E. (1997). Women's health research: A historical perspective. In F. Haseltine & B. Greenburg-Jacobson (Eds.), *Women's health research* (pp. 27–43). Washington, DC: Health Press.

Kenney, J., & Tash, D. (1993). Lesbian childbearing couples' dilemmas and decisions. *Lesbian Health*, pp. 119–129.

Kennie, D. (1993). *Preventive care for elderly people.* Cambridge: University Press.

Kirkley, D. L. (2000). Is motherhood good for women? A feminist exploration. *Journal of Obstetric, Gynecologic, and Neonatal Nursing, 29*(5), 459–464.

Knollmueller, R. (Ed.). (1993). *Prevention across the lifespan: Healthy people for the twenty-first century* (pp. 53–61). Washington, DC: American Nurses Publishing.

Kramerow, E., Lentzner, H., Rooks, R., Weeks, J., & Sayday, S., (1999). *Health United States. Health and aging chartbook*, Hyattsville, MD: National Center for Health Statistics.

Krotoski, D., Nosek, M. A., & Turk, M. A. (Eds.). (1996). *Women with physical disabilities: Achieving and maintaining health and well-being.* Baltimore: Paul H. Brookes, Publishers.

Labonte, R. (1989). Community and professional empowerment. *Canadian Nurse, 85*(3), 23–26.

La Rosa, J. H. (1994). Office of Research on Women's Health. National Institutes of Health and the women's health agenda. *Annals of the New York Academy of Sciences, 30*, 196–204.

Lucas, V. (1993). An investigation of the health care preferences of the lesbian population. *Lesbian Health*, pp. 131–138.

MacDonald, G., & Bunton, R. (1992). Health promotion: Discipline or disciplines? In R. Bunton & G. MacDonald (Eds.), *Health promotion: Disciplines and diversity.* New York: Routledge.

MacPherson, K. (1981). Menopause as disease: The social construction of a metaphor. *Advances in Nursing Science, 3*(2), 95–113.

MacPherson, K. (1985). Osteoporosis and menopause: A feminist analysis of the social construction of a syndrome. *Advances in Nursing Science, 7*(4), 11–22.

Marek, K. (1995). *Manual to develop guidelines. ANA Committee on Nursing Practice Standard and Guidelines.* Washington, DC: American Nurses Publishing, American Nurses Foundation/American Nurses Association.

Marieskind, H. (1975). The women's health movement. *International Journal of Health Services, 5*(2), 217–223.

McBride, A., & McBride, W. (1982). Theoretical underpinnings for women's health. *Women & Health, 6*(1/2), 37–55.

McGuinnes, J. M., & Foege, W. H. (1993). Actual causes of death in the United States. *Journal of the American Medical Association, 270*, 2207–2211.

Meisler, J. D. (2000). Toward optimal health: The experts respond to the art of diagnosis. *Journal of Women's Health & Gender-Based Medicine, 9*(3), 215–221.

Misra, D., Inglis-Baldy, S., & Ruderman (1998) *Women's experience of chronic disease.* Washington, DC: U.S. Department of Health & Human Services, Public Health Service Human Resource and Service Administration.

Murray, R. B., & Zentner, J. P. (1993). *Nursing assessment and health promotion: Strategies through the life span.* Norwalk, CT: Appleton & Lange.

Narrigan, D., Sprague-Jones, J., Worchester, N., & Grad, M. (1997). Research to improve women health: An agenda for equity. In S. Ruzek, V. Olesen, & A. Clarke (Eds.), *Women's health: Complexities and differences* (pp. 551–579). Columbus, OH: Ohio State University Press.

National Center for Health Statistics. (1995). *Vital Statistics System.* Source: Office of Statistics and Programming, National Center for Injury Prevention and Control, CDC, *webapp.cdc.gov/cgi-bin/broker.exe.*

National Institutes of Health. (1991). *Report of the National Institutes of Health: Opportunities for research on women's health.* Bethesda, MD: NIH.

National Women's Health Network. (1986). *Ten years of leadership, 1976–1986.* Washington, DC: National Women's Health Network.

Nichols, F. (2000). History of the women's health movement in the 20th century. *Journal of Obstetric, Gynecologic, and Neonatal Nursing, 29*(1), 56–64.

Nosek, M. A., Howland, C. A., Rintala, D. H., Young, M. E., & Chanpong, O. F. (1997). *National Study of Women with Physical Disabilities: Final Report.* Houston: Center for Research on Women with Disabilities.

Olshansky, E. (2000). *Integrated women's health: Holistic approaches for comprehensive care.* Rockville, MD: Aspen.

Pender, N. J., Barkarkauskas, V. H., Hayman, L., Rice, V. H., & Anderson, E. T. (1992). Health promotion and disease prevention: Toward excellence in nursing practice and education. *Nursing Outlook, 40,* 106–112.

Peterson, A., & Lupton, D. (1996). *The new public health: Health and self in the age of risk.* London: Sage Publications.

Pugliesi, K. (1995). Work and well-being: Gender differences in the psychological consequences of employment. *Journal of Health and Social Behavior, 36*(1), 57–71.

Raeburn, J., & Rootman, I. (1996). Quality of life and health promotion. In R. Renwick, I. Brown, & M. Nagler (Eds.), *Quality of life in health promotion and rehabilitation.* Thousand Oaks, CA: Sage Publications.

Rexrode, K., I-Min, L., Cook, N., Hennekens, C., & Buring, J. (2000). Baseline characteristics of participants in the Women's Health Study. *Journal of Women's Health & Gender-Based Medicine, 9*(1), 19–27.

Rodin, J., & Ickovics, J. (1990). Women's health: Review and research agenda as we approach the 21st century. *American Psychologist, 45*(9), 1018–1034.

Rosenberg, M., & Gollub, E. (1992). Commentary: Methods women can use that may prevent sexually transmitted disease, including HIV. *American Journal of Public Health, 82,* 1473–1478.

Ross, C. E., Mirowsky, J. (1995). Does employment affect health? *Journal of Health and Social Behavior, 36*(3), 230–243.

Ruzek S. (1993). Towards a more inclusive model of women's health. *American Journal of Public Health, 83*(1), 6–7.

Ruzek, S. (1997). Women, personal health behavior, and health promotion. In S. Ruzek, V. Olesen, & A. Clarke, (Eds.), *Women's health: Complexities and differences* (pp. 118–153). Columbus OH: Ohio State University Press.

Salganicoff, A., Beckerman, J. Z., The Henry Kaiser Family Foundation, Wyn, R., Ojeda, V., & University of California Los Angeles Center for Health Policy. (2002). *Women's Health in the United States: Health Coverage and Access to Care: Kaiser Women's Health Survey May 2002.* Los Angeles: The Henry J. Kaiser Family Foundation.

Setlow, V., Lawson, C., & Woods, N. (1998). *Gender differences in susceptibility to environmental factors: A priority assessment: Workshop report.* Washington, DC: National Academy Press.

Slauter, A. F. (1997). *Marital status and living arrangements. Current population reports (series P20–484).* Washington, DC: U.S. Government Printing Office.

Smith, B., & Dailard, C. (1997). Incarceration. In K. Allen & J. Phillips (Eds.), *Women's health across the lifespan* (pp. 464–477). Philadelphia: Lippincott.

Stanton, A. L., & Gallant, S. J. (1995). *The psychology of women's health: progress and challenges in research and application.* Washington, DC: American Psychological Association.

Star, W., Lommel, L., & Shannon, M. (1995). *Women's primary health care: Protocols for practice.* Washington, DC: American Nurses Publishing.

Steingart, R. M., Packer, M., Hamm, P., Coglianese, M. E., Gersh, B., Geltman, E. M., et al. (1991). Sex differences in the management of coronary artery disease. *New England Journal of Medicine, 325*(4), 226–230.

Stevens, P. (1993). Lesbian health care research: A review of the literature from 1970–1990. *Lesbian Health,* pp. 1–30.

Stoller, N. (1997). Responses to stigma and marginality: The health of lesbians, imprisoned women, and women with HIV. In S. Ruzek, V. Olesen, & A. Clarke (Eds.). *Women's health: Complexities and differences.* (pp. 451–472). Columbus, OH: Ohio State University Press.

Taylor, D., & Woods-Fugals, N. (1996). Changing women's health, changing nursing practices. *Journal of Obstetric and Neonatal Nursing, 25,* 791–802.

Thacker, S. B., Stroup, D. F., & Peterson, H. B. (1995). Efficacy and safety of intrapartum electronic fetal monitoring: An update, *Obstetrics & Gynecology, 86*(4pt1), 613–620.

Trippet, S., & Bain, J. (1993). Reasons American lesbians fail to seek traditional health care. *Lesbian Health,* pp.55–63.

U.S. Bureau of the Census. (1995). *Women in the United States: A profile. Statistical brief.* Washington, DC: Bureau of the Census, Economics and Statistics Administration, U.S. Department of Commerce.

U.S. Bureau of the Census. (2000). *UCLA Center for Health Policy Research: Analysis of the March 2000 Current Population Survey.* Washington, DC: Bureau of the Census, Economics and Statistics Administration, U.S. Department of Commerce.

U.S. Department of Health and Human Services. (1991). *Healthy people 2000.* Atlanta: Division of STD Prevention, Sexually Transmitted Disease Surveillance.

U.S. Department of Health and Human Services. (1991). *Healthy people 2000: National health promotion and disease prevention objectives.* Washington, DC: U.S. Government Printing Office.

U.S. Department of Health and Human Services. (1998). *Clinician's handbook of preventive services.* Washington, DC: U.S. Government Printing Office.

U.S. Department of Health and Human Services. (2000). *Healthy people 2010: Understanding and improving health,* Washington, DC: U.S. Government Printing Office.

U.S. Department of Health, Education, and Welfare. (1979) *Healthy people: The surgeon general's report on health promotion and disease prevention.* Washington, DC: U.S. Government Printing Office.

U.S. Department of Labor. Bureau of Labor Statistics (1999). *Highlights of women's earnings in 1998.* Washington, DC: U.S. Government Printing Office.

U.S. Preventive Services Task Force. (1996). *Guide to clinical preventive services.* Washington DC: U.S. Department of Health and Human Services.

Verbrugge, C. M. (1985). Gender and health: An update on hypothesis and evidence. *Journal of Health and Social Behavior, 26*: 156–182.

Watts, N. (1999). Postmenopausal osteoporosis. *Obstetric Gynecology Survey. 54,* 532–537.

Women's Health. (1985). Report of the Public Health Service Task Force on Women's Health Issues. *Public Health Reports, 100*(1), 73–106.

World Health Organization. (1986). *Ottawa charter for health promotion.* Ottawa, Ontario: Canadian Public Health Association.

Writing Group of the 1996 AAN Expert Panel on Women's Health. (1997). Women's health and women's health care: Recommendations of the 1996 AAN Expert Panel on Women's Health. *Nursing Outlook, 95* (1), 7–15.

RESOURCES

Office of Women's Health: *www.fda.gov/womens/default.htm*

Staying Healthy: *www.acog.org.*

Women's Health Issues: *www.4woman.gov/*

Women's Health and the Environment: *www.niehs.nih.gov/oc/factsheets/womens.htm*

Women's Health Initiative: *www.nhlbi.nih.gov/whi/index.html*

Women's Health in the United States: National Institute of Allergy and Infectious Diseases (NIAID) Research on Health Issues Affecting Women: *www.niaid.nih.gov/publications/women.htm*

CDC: Women's Health: *www.cdc.gov/health/womensmenu.htm*

FDA Office of Women's Health: *www.fda.gov/womens/default.htm*

National Women's Health Information Center: *www.4woman.org/*

FASTATS: Women's Health: *www.cdc.gov/nchs/fastats/women.htm*

Get Real: Straight Talk About Women's Health: *www.4woman.gov/owh/pub/factsheets/getreal.htm*

The National Women's Health Information Center: *www.4woman.gov./*

National Center for Chronic Disease Prevention and Health Promotion: *www.cdc.gov/nccdphp/*

National Center for Health Statistics: *www.cdc.gov/nchs/*

Hardin Meta Directory of Internet Health Sources: *www.lib.uiowa.edu/hardin/md/index.html*

Public Information and Communications Branch (National Institute of Child Health and Human Development): *www.nichd.nih.gov/*

Agency for Healthcare Research and Quality: *www.ahrq.gov*

Quality Interagency Coordinating Task Force: *www.quic.gov*

Institute of Medicine: *www.iom.edu/*

National Coordinating Council for Medication Error Reporting and Prevention: *www.nccmerp.org*

Medical Matrix: *www.medmatrix.org/index.asp*

Healthfinder: *www.healthfinder.org*

Health Web: *www.healthweb.org*

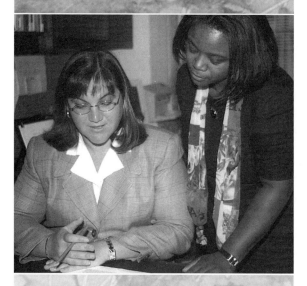

Chapter *2*

Patriarchy, Feminism, and Women's Health

Linda A. Bernhard

The feminist movement to end sexist oppression

can be successful only if we are committed to . . .

the establishment of a new social order.

bell hooks

INTRODUCTION

A world where women can achieve their full potential, where all persons live together in peace, and where all persons value each other for who they are—that is the goal of feminism, according to this writer. She is a feminist, a middle-aged nurse, and an academic who specializes in women's health. She believes that women are oppressed and that nurses are oppressed in this patriarchal society. The purpose of this chapter is to describe, within this context, patriarchy and its effects on women and women's health and to suggest feminism as a strategy for transforming the world.

PATRIARCHY

The term *patriarchy* is used in a variety of ways, but it generally refers to the structure of society with its dynamic system of social interactions. Patriarchy exists to preserve itself and the norms of a society organized for the benefit of men.

Patriarchy is an ideological explanation for male power, hierarchy, and domination. Patriarchy is sometimes called *male supremacy* or *androcentrism*. Although the term literally means "power of the father" (Rowbotham, 1981), it does not mean simply "men." Patriarchy refers to a male-dominated system that places men in control. It refers to the patterns of authority and submission that men and women exhibit, but it goes beyond what one person does to another; it is a constant pattern within society. Males control culture, thinking, and reality. All knowledge is patriarchal.

Patriarchy preceded modern society. Just as it affects people today, it affected the history, actions, experiences, and cultures of people who lived at other times. Patriarchy is thus embedded in culture; it precedes individual thought.

Patriarchy permeates life so completely that it is invisible. It is so much a part of everyday life that many people do not recognize its existence. Patriarchy is a pervasive part of the "social, political, economic, educational, and personal fabric of our lives" (Ellis & Murphy, 1994).

Patriarchy affects family relations of sex and gender and the beliefs and ideas individuals hold about themselves and others (Rowbotham, 1981). It also affects class and race relations and influences work, religion, art, and all culture.

Patriarchy and Capitalism

In the United States, patriarchy is entwined with capitalism, an economic system in which goods, industry, production, and commerce are controlled by private owners (i.e., men). Capitalists are driven by the pursuit of profit; their concept of existence is that it is always worthwhile to have more money. Marx believed that exploitation of workers is inherent in capitalism because owners (the bourgeoisie) use workers' labor to create surplus value or profit for themselves.

Eisenstein (1979) described what she called *capitalist patriarchy*, which is the relationship and operation of sexual ordering in a society with a class structure that focuses on profit. Capitalism and patriarchy exist together as a matrix of power that operates within the sexual division of labor and society.

In capitalist patriarchy, exploitation occurs through the sexual division of labor between men and women. Oppression of women and minorities is defined within patriarchal, racist, and capitalistic relationships involving both paid and unpaid labor. Women work in lower paid jobs than men (e.g., nurses compared to physicians). Men control money and keep women oppressed because self-esteem is often associated with income from employment. Capitalism uses patriarchy, and patriarchy is defined by the needs of capital, although patriarchy cannot be reduced to an economic structure (Eisenstein, 1979).

Values of Patriarchy

Johnson (1997) explains patriarchy using the metaphor of a tree (Figure 2-1). The root system of the tree contains the core values of patriarchy: male domination, male identification, and male centeredness. These roots sustain the tree, and, although the roots cannot be seen, everyone knows that they exist. The roots are deeper than anyone knows.

The trunk of the tree holds the institutions and major patterns of society, such as the economy, religion, education, and the arts (Johnson, 1997). The branches represent the communities, groups, and families in which people actually live, and, finally, the leaves are the people. Leaves both give life to the tree and draw their life from it, and they are constantly replaced.

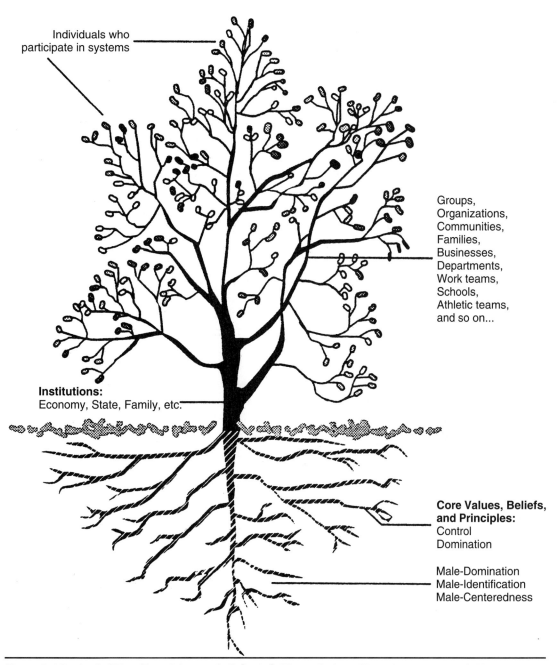

Figure 2-1 Patriarchal Tree (From Johnson, A. G. [1997]. *The gender knot: Unraveling our patriarchal legacy.* Philadelphia: Temple University Press.)

Male Domination

The components of patriarchy are too pervasive to identify completely, but patriarchy is defined by its core values, the first of which is *male domination* or *hegemony* (Johnson, 1997). Male domination refers to the power, control, and authority held by men. Power typically means the authority to make others do what you want them to do. Power differences between men and women are created as men lay claim over income and wealth, shape culture to reflect male interests, and promote male superiority.

In patriarchy, authority belongs to men through control of the political, legal, economic, labor, military, religious, educational, and other systems of society. Male dominance is seen when positions of authority are held by men (Johnson, 1997). Whatever women achieve is in spite of their inferior position in patriarchy, not because they achieve. The glass ceiling exists to keep women from gaining too much authority.

Male dominance is also observed when men feel entitled to rights and a superior place in society, which they do not think that they need to justify through virtue or merit. Men believe they are superior, and it is from that place that they justify their contempt of others (i.e., women). This sense of entitlement and superiority is also referred to as a *possessive consciousness* (Friere, 1970) and *phallism* (Frye, 1983)

Men's sense of superiority often results in *misogyny*, the hatred of women. The cultural expression of misogyny is the hatred of femaleness. Misogyny allows men to justify violence against women, by keeping women "in their place" (which is wherever men want them), where they can be ignored.

Exploitation. Exploitation is a part of male dominance, usually in the areas of work and production. Workers are exploited by the dominant class to create profit. Exploitation requires that those exploited be mobile and self-maintaining enough to do what the oppressor wants done but, at the same time, not be free, strong, or willful enough to resist or escape the exploitation (Frye, 1983). Their will and intelligence must be disengaged from resistance, but not completely broken or destroyed, so they can still work.

Exploitation of women means that women are in the service of men and men's interests, as defined by men. Although the details of service vary by race and class, women's service to men always includes personal service (e.g., cooking and cleaning), sexual service (e.g., being an attractive sexual partner and child-bearer), and ego service (e.g., providing support and encouragement) (Frye, 1983). As an example of exploitation in capitalist patriarchy, housework (the vast majority of which is performed by women) is unpaid work and thus is not included in the Gross National Product.

Language. One of the most common ways through which patriarchy and male dominance are both reflected and maintained is language. Language is a reinforcement of power relationships and an enforcement of cultural norms. A major way that male dominance in language is seen is the use of the generic masculine.

The "generic" or "neutral" masculine refers to the use of the word "man," its compound form "-man," and its pronoun form "he," as a generic for human beings or people (i.e., both men and women). One of the outcomes of male usage is to keep men constantly in mind; for example, when "mailman" is said, people do think of a man.

But male dominance in language is also more subtle and is an implicit assumption in many words that are not generically masculine. For example, when people talk about "sex," what is meant is sexual intercourse. Sexual intercourse is defined as a male penis in a female vagina with the man having an orgasm. "Foreplay" is a term that refers to sexual activities prior to sexual intercourse. What is important is the penis and the male orgasm. Regardless of how pleasurable any foreplay activities may be, they can never be the most important part of sex. Of equal importance to male dominance in this example is compulsory heterosexuality.

Knowledge. Knowledge is power. Indeed, knowledge is men's power. What is considered authoritative knowledge is that created by men, in science as well as in art. What is known, how we know, and who can know are all part of male dominance. Historically, religious and academic institutions were the only places where knowledge could be obtained, and these were the exclusive prerogative of men. Women had no place in producing ideas or knowledge. It should not be surprising that many women today still believe that they cannot produce knowledge.

Male Identification

Another core value of patriarchy is male identification. Objects, characteristics, or behaviors that are considered valuable, good, desirable, preferred, or normal are associated with men and masculinity (Johnson, 1997). Characteristics of the ideal man—control, strength, efficiency, competitiveness, logic, decisiveness, autonomy—are also associated with the work most valued in society, i.e., law and medicine.

Departures from this male norm are inevitably defined as deviant and wrong. Qualities such as cooperation, intuition, nonlinear thinking, vulnerability, and emotional expressiveness are culturally associated with women and femininity, and then are devalued. Women are made invisible.

A classic research study (Broverman, Broverman, Clarkson, Rosenkrantz, & Vogel, 1970) is still cited as representing the double standard of mental health. Mental health clinicians rated healthy, mature, socially competent women as less independent, less aggressive, less competitive, less objective, more emotional, and more unhealthy than healthy, mature, socially competent men. More importantly (and reflecting male dominance through language), mental health clinicians rated a healthy, mature, socially competent adult (sex unspecified) at similar to men and different from women. Women could be healthy and masculine or less healthy and feminine.

Little has changed. Women today are still in the double bind. A good political candidate has the characteristics of men and masculinity (e.g., autonomous, competitive, strong). Women who want to be political candidates must either accept being labeled masculine or risk being feminine.

Male Centeredness

The value of male centeredness means that the focus of attention in society is on men and what men do (Johnson, 1997). Men are important, women are not. Male centeredness is reflected in everything. The newspaper has the news, and then the women's pages. Both women and men want sons, especially firstborn sons. Two women who enter a restaurant without a man are asked by the person at the door, "Are you ladies alone?" The assumption is that women are not complete unless they are with a man.

Male centeredness also assumes that women want to be married. If married women and men have different styles or goals, it is women who are told to change (Tannen, 1990).

Effects of Patriarchy

By definition, patriarchy benefits men because it organizes society for men's benefit. Similarly, patriarchy harms women because it organizes society to the detriment of women. Women are second-class citizens. All of the institutions of society—the family, government, business, religion, medicine, and others—make men's lives easier and women's lives more difficult. For example, marriage laws protect men's interests; or women who are ill can be told "it's all in your head," given a pill, and be dismissed by physicians. Ultimately, patriarchy harms women through their oppression.

Oppression

The most significant result of patriarchy is oppression. *Oppression* is a system of interrelated forces, relationships, and barriers between groups or categories of people. These forces reduce, immobilize, and mold people who belong to one group and affect their subordination to another group (Frye, 1983). Not surprisingly, it is the group with power that creates and exaggerates differences between the groups. The group with power identifies some characteristics or attributes that they have and which the other group does not have, and these characteristics are valued and rewarded. Persons who have the characteristics are accorded privileges.

Lack of the characteristics results in stigmatization. Persons who do not have the characteristics are devalued and denied privileges. The perceived differences between groups are used both to justify discrimination against one group by the other group and also to increase the value of one group at the expense of the other group.

Oppression is self-serving. According to the theory of oppressive action (Friere, 1970), the purpose of oppression is to perpetuate and preserve the reality of the oppressors.

Oppression must be differentiated from other related concepts. Prejudice, or bias, usually involves an unreasonable dislike, which may reflect ignorance or lack of experience with another group. Discrimination is action based on bias (Adelman, 1995). But oppression is systematic subjugation that keeps persons under control.

Oppression can be identified in the actions of both the oppressor and the oppressed. Actions of oppressors include systematic overt and covert mistreatment of the oppressed group. Oppressors believe that they themselves are better than the oppressed and that the oppressed deserve the treatment meted at them by the oppressors. This can be called *internalized domination* (Pheterson, 1986)

Oppressed group behavior is a term for the individual and collective actions of a group that is oppressed. Oppressed group behavior consists of feelings of self-hatred, inferiority, powerlessness, and isolation. Self-deprecation results as the oppressed group internalizes the opinion that the oppressors hold of them. Oppressed group members accept a very limited view of what it means to be a member of their own group. They learn to recognize their "minority" status even if the group is a numerical majority, as women are.

In individuals, oppressed group behavior is sometimes called *internalized oppression.* In this process the individuals in an oppressed group incorporate and accept the dominant group's prejudices against them (Friere, 1970). It is the chief mechanism for maintaining domination because it reinforces the external control of the oppressor at the same time that it perpetuates the individual's subservience (Pheterson, 1986).

Internalized oppression causes individuals to agree with the oppressor's belief that they are deserving of discrimination and that the system should not change. Moreover, because the oppressed individual wants to be like the ideal, they identify with the oppressor, try to become like the oppressor, and, in so doing, learn to hate themselves more (Friere, 1970). Individuals eventually blame themselves for their problems instead of directing their anger and frustration at the appropriate source—the oppressor.

The results of oppressed group behavior include submissive-aggressive behavior and "horizontal violence" (Roberts, 1983). Horizontal violence refers to acts of aggression within the oppressed group. Because the oppressed are powerless to challenge the oppressor, they begin to find fault, criticize, and invalidate each other. They may ridicule or humiliate their peers, both for what they do and for what they do not do. They act defensively, with fear and mistrust. Eventually they develop unrealistic expectations of their own leaders and withdraw from their own group members. They may become aggressive toward each other because that is safer than acting aggressively against the oppressor. Unfortunately, the oppressed also learn to tolerate and perpetuate other forms of oppression, such as anti-Semitism or homophobia (Gainor, 1992).

The oppressed live in the world of the dominant culture, but they cannot completely inhabit that world. They educate themselves completely about the oppressor so that they can live in that world, but they have a good idea about the parts of the oppressor's world that they cannot inhabit. On the other hand, the oppressors have no interest in the world of the oppressed; they think it is inferior.

Although oppressed people work hard to be like the oppressor, they cannot become the oppressor. But some of the oppressed will inhabit more of the oppressor's world than others. Eventually they may find that even though they are not the oppressor, they no longer resemble the members of their oppressed group either. They do not belong to either group and may be excluded from both, a phenomenon called *marginalization.* Some feminist theorists (e.g., Anzaldua, 1987) use "borders" or "borderlands" as a metaphor for marginalized people.

For oppression to continue, persons who are oppressed must participate in and support their own oppression. Complicity happens both voluntarily and involuntarily as the oppressed accept the demands of the oppressor, including their own self-devaluation. The oppressed, too, have an unconscious need to maintain the status quo. Change is uncomfortable; there is comfort in sameness, even when it is dangerous and unhealthy.

Although the oppressed are the most seriously affected by the system of oppression, everyone is affected. Oppressive acts prevent men from being more fully human (Friere, 1970). The oppressors' lives are limited by their conscious lack of knowledge about the history of the oppressed people, by being taught to fear them, and by being kept separate from them. Division and estrangement support the system that oppresses the majority of both groups, for the benefit of the relative few (Adelman, 1995).

Nonetheless, oppressors are always afraid that the oppressed will "rise up" against them and the oppressor will cease to exist. Their fear causes them to continually suppress the oppressed. They must be simultaneously offensive and defensive.

In patriarchy, the oppressors are men. But the system of patriarchy is impossible for men to sustain alone, and they constantly feel like they could lose it at any time. So patriarchy supports the oppression known as *sexism*, i.e., valuing of one sex (male) over the other sex (female).

But patriarchy also supports the oppressions of racism, classism, and many others. And privilege coexists with oppression. One can be both an oppressor and oppressed, on the basis of certain characteristics or identities. Being oppressed as a member of one group (e.g., women) does not prevent one from being an oppressor of another group (e.g., African-Americans).

Women as an Oppressed Group

Women are an oppressed group. Women are subordinated through power relationships that exist because of patriarchy. Examples of the oppression of women as a group abound. Men's control of work and government limits women's opportunities. Women did not have the right to vote in the United States until 1920. Men generally have jobs with greater responsibility, flexibility, and income. Men are principals; women, schoolteachers. Men are administrators, women, secretaries.

Separation between private and public spheres of life remains, with women primarily identified with the private sphere and men with the public sphere. Work is a large part of that, but so is childcare, which women continually report as among their most serious concerns. Although women are increasingly employed in the paid work force, their responsibilities in the private sphere—cooking, cleaning, and childcare—have not changed substantially.

Women are objectified and commodified; women's bodies are used in advertising to sell virtually every product. Women also sell their own bodies and body parts. Prostitutes sell their bodies, but so do surrogate mothers. Young women become egg donors as a way to make money but place their own bodies in danger by doing so. Few women feel able to refuse objectification (Gadow, 1994).

Women also experience higher rates of depression than men in every culture. Depression is a logical outcome of internalized oppression for women (Steen, 1991), but depression is not equivalent to oppression.

Nurses as an Oppressed Group

Nurses are also an oppressed group. The vast majority of nurses are women, and nursing is recognized as a gendered occupation. Society believes that nurses (women) exist to serve physicians (men). Nurses are oppressed by society (culturally male) and by both physicians and hospital administrators (primarily men). Female nurses experience the same oppression as all women in society. In addition, female nurses are exploited as sex objects in greeting cards and in the mass media.

Nurses have internalized that they as a group are less educated, skilled, and competent than physicians. Physicians control much of nursing practice; they give orders to nurses, often for actions that nurses could perform independently.

Moreover, the history of nursing in the United States demonstrates the attempts of medicine as a profession to keep nurses uneducated (Ashley, 1976). Until the 1960s, rather than being educated in academic institutions (as physicians were), most nursing students received on-the-job training in hospitals and were paid (however meagerly) to be students. Physicians limited nursing's potential in health care by keeping themselves dominant.

Physicians often taught classes for nursing students and may still do today. That, too, is a form of maintaining control over what nurses are allowed to learn. Nursing students give evidence of internalized oppression when they report a preference for physicians as teachers. They believe that physicians are better qualified than nurse teachers.

Nursing students are socialized to female roles as nurses. They should be quiet and wait for (and on) doctors. Not that long ago, nurses were required to give up their chairs and pens if a physician wanted (needed) them.

The majority of nurses still practice in hospitals, where the patriarchal order of the household is replayed. Physicians are the husband/fathers, nurses the wife/mothers, and patients the children. A similar situation exists with nursing administrators, who often play a subservient, wifely role to hospital administrators. This situation, as well as the fact that most nurses were educated in hospitals, keeps nurses loyal to hospitals and physicians.

Lovell (1992) describes the effects of patriarchy on nurses as *paternalism*. In the strictest sense, paternalism is simply the caring for a person in a fatherly way, but it can also mean making decisions without the consent of the person affected. The paternalistic caregiver is usually said to operate "in the best interests" of another, but often the caregiver is functioning that way because he or she thinks the person cannot act independently or is (acting like) a child. Physicians who write orders for duties that nurses can perform independently are acting paternalistically.

Lovell (1992) describes historical evidence of physicians generally treating nurses like little girls. The power and control physicians wield over nurses is explicitly to keep them subservient and "in their place." Some physicians expect nurses to literally fear them.

In Susan Reverby's (1987) historical study of nursing, she concluded that nurses were "ordered to care." She explained both metaphors of orders and caring. Lewenson (1996) coined the term *nursism* for the oppression of nurses. She defines nursism as a form of sexism that focuses on the caring role in society. Lewenson indicates that nurses themselves suffer from nursism, by devaluing the role of caring in nursing. Nursism is thus an example of horizontal violence.

Another example of the oppression of nurses is called *the doctor-nurse game*. Even when nurses make their own judgments about patient care, they have been socialized to seek the approval of the physician. In the doctor-nurse game, nurses make a decision, but present it to the physician in such a way that the physician believes it was his idea. Then he orders the nurse to do it. The doctor-nurse game keeps nurses subservient and allows physicians to maintain their power and authority. It maintains the patriarchal system.

Nurse Practitioners as an Oppressed Group

Nurse practitioners (NPs) are also an oppressed group. The nurse practitioner role developed at a time when there was a shortage of physicians. Pediatricians, who had the greatest manpower shortage, conceived the idea of the pediatric nurse associate, a registered nurse without any advanced education (Fiorino, 1980). Using nurses was a cheap, acceptable, and quick way to accomplish medical tasks.

The first NPs were educated by physicians (who were viewed as the knowledgeable, more experienced experts). But male physicians systematically used nurses for their benefit. For example, using nurses to provide well childcare reinforced the belief that childcare is women's work; pediatricians could then manage sick children. Many physicians still view NPs as physician extenders, rather than as independent practitioners.

Roberts (1996) describes NPs as marginalized. She lists the signs of oppressed group behavior that she sees in NPs: the wish to look like physicians, the rejection of nursing identity, the feeling of superiority over other nurses, the nonsupport of nurses and nursing organizations, and the search for support from medicine. These behaviors are examples of identification with the oppressor and horizontal violence against the peer group.

SEX AND GENDER: OPPRESSION OF WOMEN AS A CLASS

The oppression of women as a group is called *sexism*; that is, women are different from men and are oppressed because of their sex (i.e., female). This assumes that women are alike and that women are different from men in fixed and predetermined ways. However, the concept of sex (and thus sexism) is not simple; gender must also be considered.

Sex is a biological definition. Sex is binary; a person can (and must) be either (and only) a woman or a man. The female genotype is 46 XX and the male genotype is 46 XY. Sex is determined simply on the basis of genitals and genetics; the presence of ovaries or testes is the predetermined biological marker of sex. Ultrasound identification of a penis tells parents that the sex of their fetus is male, but absence of a penis does not ensure that the fetus is female.

Gender is the social organization of sexual difference; it is everything other than biology that identifies a woman as female and a man as male. The meanings of gender vary across cultures and history. Gender does not imply fixed or essential differences but, rather, the knowledge that establishes meanings for bodily differences (Scott, 1988)

Gender is established at the moment of birth, and today often before birth, when the sex of the fetus is identified. If the baby is identified as a girl, a pink blanket will be used and the baby will be spoken to and held more gently and sweetly than if it is identified as a boy. That is gender.

A person appears to be female by the trappings of gender. People think that what they respond to in a person is sex, but that may be inaccurate. Very little information about biological differences (i.e., genitals) is visible; what can be seen is an individual's self-presentation (i.e., gender). People infer sex from gender and they also infer gender from sex. Thus oppression and discrimination of women involves both sex and gender.

Like sex, gender has been defined in a binary way: femininity and masculinity. Femininity is considered a constellation of characteristics or behaviors associated with being female, including passivity, quietness, and gentleness. However, the definitions of femininity and feminine are circular. Femininity means having characteristics that are considered feminine or being feminine. Feminine is an adjective that means gentle or passive.

Masculinity is the opposite of femininity. Characteristics associated with maleness include authority, rationality, aggression, assertiveness, and competitiveness. There is great consistency and societal recognition about which personal characteristics are feminine and which are masculine. One can easily see that the characteristics of masculinity are those of the ideal man, which shows the institutionalization of gender and patriarchy.

Women's Worldview

In addition to the gender characteristics just described, certain attitudes and behaviors are thought to differ between women and men. Some of those differences have been supported with research, although the differences tend to be small. However, to keep women identified as a unitary group, these characteristics and behaviors have been constructed as women's worldview. A worldview functions as a guide for life, and the concept of women's worldview—like all other components of society—is a patriarchal way of molding women. Women's worldview includes values about people, life, nature, and how women should live in the world.

Connection and Relationships

The basic component of a woman's worldview is women's emphasis on relationships with people and on the connections among people and the natural world. Women approach the world through a network of connections, and the essential element of connections is symmetry—how people are the same (Tannen, 1990).

In contrast, men are independent in a world of status, thus an asymmetrical hierarchy appears. Women are interested in achieving status and avoiding failure, but it is not the focus of their lives as it is for men (Tannen, 1990).

Because women's lives are based on symmetry, they think about equality and sharing; they willingly negotiate and compromise. They are also the caregivers. Because of their concern for people and relationships women are said to be more concerned than men about values and ethics, peace and justice.

Women try to maintain closeness and intimacy with others. One of the ways in which they do that is by being authentic and honest in relationships and expecting authenticity in return (Borysenko, 1996). Women tend to have many friends.

Erikson's (1963) theory of psychosocial development consists of eight stages and the conflict or crisis inherent in each stage. The crisis of adolescence is identity versus identity confusion. The adolescent must resolve this conflict to become an adult; usually this is done by the selection of a career. The conflict of young adulthood is intimacy versus isolation. The person must establish deep and enduring personal relationships to avoid self-absorption.

Erikson's theory has been criticized as being male-oriented, because he based it on his own life experiences. These two stages just mentioned are experienced differently by women and men and may be fused (Gilligan, 1982) or reversed. That is, women learn intimacy and establish enduring relationships, and it is through those relationships that identity develops and a career can be chosen (see Chapter 6).

Men seek independence and domination; they are competitive. Men think in hierarchies and spend their lives trying to climb the hierarchical ladder. Their relationships are those that help them to climb. Although men may have "buddies," these relationships are quite different from women's friendships.

Communication

Both what is said and the way it is said are affected by gender (Tannen, 1990). Male patterns of communication are taken as the norm and are evaluated positively. Women's communication is compared to men's.

Women's verbal and nonverbal communication styles are consistent with their emphasis on connection. Women are socialized to have a quiet voice and to wait for men to speak first. Women also make more adjustments in conversation than men; they talk about what men want to discuss. Women frequently raise their voices at the end of a statement, almost making what they say into a question, which asks, "Am I good enough?" Although there are also cultural variations, men are much more likely to interrupt women's speech than women to interrupt men's.

Power and dominance are important in nonverbal communication as well as in speech. The typical postures, gestures, and movements of men are those of dominance: they take up space and they use more nonreciprocal touch, i.e., touching but not being touched in return. Nonreciprocal touching indicates power.

Women's nonverbal communication typically indicates submission: they sit in a "ladylike" way (i.e., using only a small space), lower their eyes, turn their heads sideways, and smile. Although these behaviors are usually unconscious, they not only reflect male supremacy, they also maintain it.

Emotions

Women are thought to be emotional, men rational; that is, women are feelers, men are thinkers. Being emotional is being irrational. Being emotional is unacceptable in society; it means that women need not be taken seriously and can be dismissed (Campbell, 1994). When women are labeled as emotional, they are thought to lack self-control. Emotionality is described as involuntary behavior.

Being emotional is never positive, even though some say that women are allowed to have emotions, while men are not. For example, women are allowed to cry, but, they are also called "overemotional," implying that men's more restricted emotional expression is preferable.

Intuition and Nonlinearity

Women often engage in nonlinear thinking, which is considered indirect and inefficient. However, women describe nonlinear thinking as taking into consideration multiple factors and reflecting on outcomes ("if this, then that") before forming a conclusion or decision. Women are also said to be prone to "changing their minds."

Intuition is so gender-specific that it is often been referred to as "women's intuition." Intuition is having an immediate understanding or knowledge without formal reasoning (Rew, 1986). Intuition is not valued because it is not scientific. Intuition involves the use of multiple senses and is sometimes referred to as a "sixth" sense.

Adolescent girls learn to stop sharing their intuitions because they are not valued. However, older women may regain and nurture their intuitiveness, perhaps because they realize that they have nothing lose, and they can use their intuition in a positive way.

Spirituality

Women are considered to be more spiritual than men, and spirituality is associated with femininity. Spirituality concerns the human search for fulfillment and transcendence (King, 1989). It is a dynamic part of human development and life.

Spirituality should not be confused with religion, or, more specifically, Christianity, although it often is. Spirituality is found within oneself; whereas, religion generally directs energies outside the self. Spirituality can be considered greater than any particular religion, at the same time that it is a part of some religious practices.

It is the connection of spirituality with nature that causes spirituality to be associated with femininity and women. Women recognize the interdependence of all living things on earth. The struggle to understand the world and all that is in it, and to incorporate that into oneself, is recognized as both what women do and as what spirituality is.

Love and Sex

Women are said to be interested in love, and men in sex. This patriarchal assumption results from the double standard that allowed women to be sexual only within the confines of marriage. Although women were expected to be "virgins" when they were married, men were not. Although many people laugh at that assertion today, there are groups of people who still accept it.

Love is nearly impossible to define because the word is used to describe everything from clothing to food to the deepest, most caring feeling about a person with whom one has an intense emotional and physical relationship (i.e., a spouse or life partner). But love requires a surrender of oneself to another; it is this loss of control that makes love a feminine characteristic. Men are supposed to want and need—not give up—control.

But love need not be viewed only as a passive surrender; it is also an active giving of oneself to another. Some say it is easier to give love (i.e., unconditional caring) to another than to receive or accept love because that implies submission.

The belief that women are not interested in sex is based on the biological explanation that men are focused (on the penis) in their sexuality, while women's experience of sexuality is more diffused throughout the body. But desire is the real issue in sexuality. Men are said to have a high sex drive, and passive women wait to receive men's overtures. Women have been socialized to believe that they (should) have no sex drive. This is both sexist and heterosexist.

Many women enjoy sex for its own sake (just as men do), and at the same time sex can be an important part of love. Brown (1982) described five types of sex engaged in by women: magic sex when the woman is falling in love; intimate, comfortable sex with a well-known and adored partner; friendly sex with a known, but not that special, partner; casual sex including one-night stands or brief affairs; and scruffy sex with a new or old partner that is later regretted.

But there is another aspect of sex with regard to women. Women know that they are judged (by both men and other women) on the way they look—their sexual desirability and appearance. Thus sexuality becomes an important form of women's oppression. Cultural stereotypes actively suppress women as they try to live up to a patriarchal standard.

All of these examples demonstrate sexism and the oppression of women as a class, but one must ask: are any of these characteristics and behaviors, labeled feminine or masculine, exclusive to either gender? Or are these characteristics more closely related to culture, time, or generation? Women (and men) exhibit great variation in these characteristics, but both similarities and differences are socially constructed.

Gender Variations

Gender is more than femininity and masculinity. In the past, many researchers tried, unsuccessfully, to define characteristics as exclusively feminine or masculine and to demonstrate that people were either feminine or masculine.

"Butch" and "femme" were recognized forms of gender for lesbians in the 1950s and 1960s. Butches were women who dressed like men and accepted masculine gender roles. Femmes looked very much like feminine heterosexual women of the time, but chose butch (lesbian) women for their sexual partners.

In 1974, Sandra Bem suggested that masculinity and femininity are separate concepts, rather than opposite poles of the same concept. She categorized people who were rated high on both femininity and masculinity as being androgynous. Androgyny was thus constructed as positive, and gender was no longer simply dualistic.

Today, a new generation of young adults views gender as something with which they can play, in their dress and hairstyles, as well as in their behaviors (Weston, 1996) Lesbians, in particular, use gender to alter their self-presentations in ways that make people question who and what they are. Loulan (1996) concludes from her formal and informal research with lesbians that there are "thousands, maybe millions" of genders.

But there are other forms of gender variation as well. An entire community of persons now identify themselves as transgendered. Transsexuals, transvestites or cross-dressers, and gay male drag queens have been considered transgendered for many years, but other persons now identify themselves as transgendered too. However, whereas the three just-mentioned categories of transgendered persons ultimately align themselves with the dualities of masculinity and femininity, many people who now identify as transgendered do not. These newly proclaimed transgendered individuals do not accept being classified as either feminine or masculine, nor do they accept being labeled androgynous (both feminine and masculine). Instead they define themselves as individuals (Boswell, 1997). Transgendered persons are "freely gendered" as more fully human because they do not feel compelled to identify themselves as either masculine or feminine.

Transsexuals

Transsexual persons are people whose biological sex and emotional and cognitive feelings are incongruent. Transsexual persons are referred to as male-to-female (MTF) or female-to-male (FTM), based on the biological sex and gender they believe they are. Many transsexuals undergo hormone therapy and radical surgery, so that they can change their physical bodies as well as their gender.

Transvestites

Transvestites are individuals who derive sexual pleasure from dressing in the clothing of the opposite gender. Most transvestites are heterosexual married men. Although some involve their wives in their cross-dressing (e.g., she helps him shop for female clothing), most engage in their activities without the company of their wives.

Hermaphrodites

Hermaphrodites are individuals who do not have a binary sex. True hermaphrodites are persons who are born with both testes and ovaries and with external genitalia that may appear "ambiguous." In the past, physicians and/or parents of these infants selected one "sex" for their child, and physicians performed the "necessary" surgical procedures so that the hermaphrodite could live as either a woman or man. Other persons, sometimes called pseudohermaphrodites, are born with a discrepancy between their apparent sex based on the external genitalia and their chromosomally determined sex.

Some people today, primarily hermaphrodites (i.e., persons with ambiguous genitals), including both those who have and have not been surgically treated, advocate for the rights of these transgendered persons. A new activism for "intersexuality" has developed, and these activists encourage a nonsurgical approach, allowing the person to be an intersexual rather than gendered as either masculine or feminine.

Differences Among Women

Biological women are also not a single group. The difficulty is that classification as a group, such as women, usually implies that members of the group share a common identity. Although the presenting problems (e.g., sexism) may be similar, factors contributing to women's oppression are different (Rivers, 1995) Because of race, class, sexual orientation, age, and a myriad of other characteristics, women do not have a common identity.

The emphasis of feminists at the beginning of the second wave of feminism in the United States was to make women equal to men and, to do that, women had to be the same as men. But claiming that women are the same as (or equal to) men leads to a reluctance to acknowledge differences among women because differences can be used to justify unequal treatment and opportunity.

Classification of women as a biological group obscures differences among women, and results in normalization and exclusion. And there are huge differences among women and among men, as well as similarities between women and men, all of which cannot be appreciated when only similarities among women are addressed. All individuals are unique.

When feminists viewed women as a class, differences emerged that resulted in frustration and exclusion. Some women felt devalued and marginalized because their issues and presence were not central to the issues of feminist debate. Women of color and lesbians began to seek recognition for themselves and their issues.

Women cannot compartmentalize themselves into specific identities or characteristics; all of their identities intersect. Gender cannot be separated from race, class, and sexual orientation. Although some women may try to hide certain aspects of themselves at one time or another, doing so demonstrates oppression and harms women's health.

However, simply listing a woman's characteristics, which represent forms of oppression, tends to make the oppressions appear equal. Certain types of oppression are more culturally powerful than others, and experiencing multiple forms of oppression not only adds another level of oppression but is a case where one plus one equals more than two.

Consideration of eating disorders demonstrates differences among women and the intersection of multiple forms of oppression. White feminists suggest that eating disorders begin because of issues about appearance. They report that it is not surprising that appetites and food take on metaphorical significance in a patriarchal society where women are typically responsible for food preparation, yet are taught to deny themselves the pleasures of eating. But Thompson (1994) argues that eating disorders do not begin with appearance but rather are survival strategies and self-preservation tactics that appear in response to racism, sexism, homophobia, classism, acculturation, and abuse. Women turn to food to cope. She considers eating disorders as logical, creative responses to trauma that, nonetheless, require healing. In her research, women of various races and cultures linked their eating problems to many forms of trauma. Thompson's racial analysis does not discount the white feminist argument, but amplifies it.

Women are not all alike; they have different experiences and perspectives that inform both the meaning of and the ways in which women come to know their social and political worlds. Differences should enrich the lives of all women. But recognizing difference is not an end in itself; doing so only objectifies and oppresses those defined as "different," separates rather than unifies women, and maintains the status quo (Hurtado, 1989). Women's lives must be evaluated from their own contexts and reality and not be based on comparisons with any one group (Hurtado, 1989)

However, women can still be classified as a group. Young (1994) says that feminism depends on it. To avoid the criticisms of essentialism, Young used Sartre's concept of seriality to describe women as a collective. In this approach, all women are not assumed to have common attributes or to share a common identity, but they can be described as a social series. A social series exists when its members are passively unified by objects around which their actions are oriented or by the objectified results of the material effects of the actions of others. Women as a series or group belong to that group through the objects and practices that they use to achieve their individual purposes.

Young (1994) describes people waiting for a bus as an example of a series. The members of the group are unknown to each other, and each has a purpose (to get somewhere). The objects that make the individuals a group are the bus, its route and schedule, and perhaps a bench or shelter. The people share a passive unity because their only connection is riding the bus.

Gender has a set of structures and objects (which might be called patriarchy). Women are the individuals who are positioned as feminine by those structures and objects. Physical bodies may be objects that define gender, but enforced heterosexuality defines what bodies should do. Clothes are also objects that define gender. Individuals in this series called women have different experiences and perceptions from others in the series, yet they share a passive unity, which develops from how they are positioned in social relations (Young, 1994) Classifying women as a group in this way avoids the problems of claiming that women have a unitary identity.

EFFECTS OF PATRIARCHY AND OPPRESSION ON WOMEN'S HEALTH

Many people consider women's differential access to health care as the greatest effect of patriarchy on women's health (Benderly, 1997). Access to care simply means the ability to obtain health care in terms of time, money, and geography. Many women lack access to health care at places and times convenient to them; perhaps more women lack health care because they cannot afford it.

But access to health care is meaningful only when the care is appropriate and acceptable to the women being served (Timyan, Brechiri, Measham, & Ogunley, 1993). Appropriateness and acceptability are highly individualistic concepts but include such things as the types of providers (e.g., allopathic) and services (e.g., alcohol and drug treatment) as well as the cultural competence of the staff. This means that care must be examined from women's perspectives, not only from the provider and health system (i.e., patriarchal) view point, as is usually the case. However, patriarchy and oppression affect women's health in many other areas besides access. Some of the most important are research and technology, medicalization, and marketing.

Research

The effects of patriarchy on health research are immense. Research results are used as the basis for delivering health care; consequently, research is highly valued. What is studied, by whom, using what methods, and with what type of funding are the principal issues.

Until recently, research on health and illness concerned only men and their health, in large part because the male body was viewed as the prototype for humans, and men were considered normal. Women's bodies were considered in relation to, and deviant from, male bodies, and were studied only from that perspective.

Research began with questions about males—their anatomy, physiology, and physical or mental illnesses. Research might eventually study how women differed from that male standard that had been established. In addition, there was a tendency to label diseases, such as heart disease, as men's diseases, even though heart disease is also the number one cause of death for women in the United States. This could be used to further justify a lack of research on women. Women's illnesses were of only secondary interest to most researchers. Now that research into breast cancer (defined as a women's illness) is increasing, it is frequently noted that men also develop breast cancer, and increasing attention is being paid to prostate cancer.

Some women may have been included in research in the past, but, when results were published (the most important way for the scientific and clinical community to learn the latest developments in health care), who the participants were was not included. This may have been intentional suppression of the fact that no women were included, or it may have been an unintentional omission because research results were not analyzed by gender. Nonetheless, research results have systematically been applied to women and women's health, whether or not it was appropriate to do so.

Women were excluded as topics of research and as "subjects" in research primarily because they have monthly hormonal cycles that make control of research conditions difficult and because of the risk of pregnancy. Because hormonal variations can alter the results of research, investigators believed it was easier to use men than to try to account for the hormonal variations in women. Even studies on animals used male animals. Researchers did not acknowledge that men also have hormonal variations, even if they are less dramatic than those in women.

The paternalistic concern about protecting women and their potential children from harm caused stringent restrictions to be placed on participation of reproductive-age women in research studies. Unfortunately, this concern for women denied many the right, granted to competent men, to make their own decisions. There was also more concern about (potential) fetuses than about women. It was the risk of pregnancy that prevented women from participating; women could not be trusted not to become pregnant. For researchers who wanted to study women, it was also difficult to obtain sufficient numbers of women for studies because women of reproductive age comprise most available women. Unfortunately and ironically, lack of women's participation in testing of drugs and products, such as thalidomide and diethylstilbestrol (DES), resulted in serious harm to women and children. Today, women must be included in clinical trials if what is being tested (e.g., drugs) will be used on women.

Who conducts health research determines to a large extent the topics of study. Scientists study questions and problems of interest to themselves or providers of health care, rather than questions about the real needs of women, as defined by women. Male domination and male centeredness result in studies about problems related to men.

Historically, few women have been scientists, and it is this fact that is also used to explain the lack of research on women's health. The presumption is that female scientists would be more likely to study women's health. But female scientists also study the research questions that are deemed important by the majority of scientists, who are men. Today there are many National Institutes of Health (NIH) initiatives to increase the numbers of female scientists.

Although there are many kinds of research, it is the experimental method, and specifically in health research the controlled clinical trial, that is most highly valued. The basis of experimentation is the scientific method, which is classically a male-oriented strategy. The goal of research is to find truth, which is achieved through objectivity and control. Scientists develop hypotheses and test them, but there is a danger that scientists may begin to think of their hypotheses as facts, rather than guesses (Ketner, 1996). That is, they may stop seeking answers (e.g., about women's health) because they believe they already have the facts.

The scientific method is a reductionistic process, in which a problem is broken down into smaller and smaller parts. In health, this is referred to as *biological reductionism*, and the belief is that truth will be found in the smallest bit of life. Biological reductionism is most clearly seen in the Human Genome Project where scientists believe they will find the ultimate truth of human life as they understand and map the human genetic code. But, as noted earlier, women live in connection, so attempts to reduce answers to the most basic level are not consistent with how women live.

Finally, funding for research plays an extremely large part in determining what research is conducted. Pharmaceutical and medical equipment companies fund studies that will support the use of their drugs and products. Their motivation is profit, not women's (or even men's) health.

But the major source of money for health research is the National Institutes of Health (NIH), which receives its funding from Congress. Congressional and executive governmental interests determine the amount of money directed to NIH and to each of its institutes. Compared to other areas of federal funding, the budget for NIH is small, and the amount spent on women's health is very small.

In 1986, after urging by the Congressional Women's Caucus, the Government Accounting Office conducted an audit that showed that only 13.5% of the NIH budget was spent on women's health research. Although certain policies were established that led the NIH to increase its attention to women's health, a subsequent report in 1990 showed very little change in the overall spending for women's health. As a result, more NIH initiatives now focus specifically on women's health.

Technology, the application of scientific findings to life, is viewed as masculine and thus not of interest to women. However, much technology is used on or against women and endangers women's health. Nonetheless, many technologies are helpful to women, and technology itself is not inherently negative. It is the application of technology by male supremacists that is problematic.

Analysis of technology includes questioning both the motivation of scientists and what success means in technology. Some technologies are developed simply because it can be done, not because it will help or serve any human interests (e.g., human cloning). Eggs needed for cloning embryos must come from women's bodies, and thus women's health can be put at risk in the name of science.

Ketner (1996) argues that making scientists into the new "high priests" is dangerous because it can result in uncritical commitment to technology. That frame of mind can result in the development of technologies that are used in the United States only until a problem is recognized. For example, after the Dalkon shield resulted in significant health problems and even deaths, many women in the United States were skeptical about using any intrauterine device (IUD). Consequently, IUDs that had been produced and could no longer be sold in the United States were shipped to Third World countries for use by poor and uneducated women because capitalist men were not willing to lose money.

Other technologies (e.g., male contraceptives) are not developed because of patriarchal assumptions. In the case of male contraception, the rationale may be that since men do not become pregnant, it is not necessary for them to use contraception, or that men should make women pregnant.

Medicalization

Medicalization is the process through which physicians change a normal life process, such as menstruation or childbirth, into a disease or clinical problem. When something normal becomes abnormal, physicians find ways to treat it, and they establish standards. Then women seek care for the problem, so that physicians can manage it. Of course, more frequent medical visits from women enhance physician income, and more frequent prescriptions by physicians enhance pharmaceutical manufacturers' income.

For example, menstrual cycles "should" be 28 days, with ovulation occurring on day 14. Bleeding "should" last 3 or 4 days. Young girls "should" begin menstruation no later than age 16. Physicians manage women so that these "shoulds" occur. There are drugs to treat menstruation—to make it start, to make it stop, and to relieve the symptoms of this "disease." This is patriarchy at work so invisibly that women incorporate these standards and seek medical help for a normal process that women have self-managed for millenia.

Medicalization is disabling and disempowering for women because it makes women dependent on physicians to manage their lives and health. Medicalization systematically makes women think they are unable to take care of themselves.

Marketing Women's Health

Another effect of patriarchy and capitalism on women's health is the marketing or selling of women's health. "Women's health" is now a commodity that is bought and sold; there are both products and services. Unfortunately, the commodity of women's health is beyond the reach of many women who need it.

Women's health as an idea developed simultaneously on both coasts in the late 1960s and 1970s, before abortion was legal. On the East coast the Boston Women's Health Book Collective started with education. They taught each other about women's health and produced *Our Bodies, Ourselves*, which would become one of the most important self-help books for women in the twentieth century.

In Los Angeles, women were more concerned about health care, and specifically about reproductive rights. They believed that women could not only learn about their bodies but also could examine their bodies and control reproduction. They challenged the control of physicians over women's bodies. They started the Feminist Women's Health Centers as an antiprofessional alternative to standard medical care, a radical feminist ideal of women taking charge of their own bodies.

Although it could be argued that the women in Boston and Los Angeles commodified women's health first, when male physicians and hospital administrators recognized that women's health was a potential source of income (because huge numbers of women read the books and participated in the Feminist Women's Health Centers) they co-opted women's health and began to sell it themselves. Hospitals, and then individual physicians, moved quickly to take control of women's health. Although a national network of Feminist Women's Health Centers developed, these were freestanding and focused almost exclusively on reproductive freedom. The first "women's health center" that provided "full service" clinical care for women began in 1982; it was called Women's Health Resources.

Women's Health Resources was owned by Illinois Masonic Hospital in Chicago, but it was not physically part of the hospital. Women's Health Resources provided both education and clinical services to women by women. Providers emphasized spending sufficient time and meeting women's needs. They provided a model for alternative care of women, and women came because they were looking for something different to meet their health care needs. But the model also served to bring women to Illinois Masonic Hospital for needed services. Soon, the newest thing in hospitals was to have a women's health center.

Individual and group practices of physicians (mostly gynecologists) realized that they had been providing "women's health" care too, and suddenly the names of medical practices began to change. "John Smith, MD" became "Women's Health Services." Unfortunately, little or nothing else about the practice changed.

A similar process is happening today with "alternative" methods of health care. Medical doctors realized that many people use alternative providers; thus, doctors were losing money. Today, there is an Office of Alternative Medicine in the NIH and medical doctors are learning "alternative" health care strategies to incorporate into their own practices. Men recognize that there is money to be made, and so they take over.

Unfortunately, much of women's health has been co-opted. When something is co-opted it can mean that the dominant group is paying attention to the oppressed. But if mainstream medicine only takes the ideas and does not make real changes, women lose again. For example, with significant restructuring and downsizing of many hospitals today, women's health centers are disappearing because they do not generate sufficient income. Even though those centers probably did not serve all women, the ones who were served now must find another source for the kind of health care they want.

STRATEGIES FOR RESISTANCE AND CHANGE

Patriarchy and oppression harm women and damage women's health. Many women and some supportive men are working hard to make real change and create a new reality in the world. Liberation requires understanding oppression, practicing self-acceptance, and then taking action. Two principal strategies for resistance against patriarchy and oppression are feminism and multiculturalism.

Feminism(s) and Feminist Theory

Feminism has no universally accepted definition. In fact, there are many feminisms. Feminism is thought variously to be a political theory, an ideology, a world view, or a form of activism, but in all cases it is the oppressive structures of society that feminism aims to change. Feminists are persons who subscribe to feminism. Feminists generally want to improve the situation of women in the world.

There are also many theories of feminism because feminists come from a great variety of backgrounds and have different interests. Feminist theory has four components: description of the situation requiring change; analysis of why the situation exists as it does; a vision of what should exist; and strategies for how to change the situation (Bunch, 1987). Feminist theory is dynamic, always in flux, and often contradictory because of the unique ways that feminists interpret these four components. That is, feminists define the situation differently, explain the causes differently, have different visions and goals for the future, and use different strategies to achieve their goals.

Feminism is a challenge to the predominant ideology (i.e., patriarchy). Because the existing patriarchal structure of society is so pervasive, one strategy of feminist analysis is to challenge everything about the world so that it can be changed. Feminists challenge structures as they exist at both micro and macro levels (i.e., personal and social) as well as the historical roots of those structures.

Keddy (1995) argued that feminism "is the most effective vehicle for bringing about desired change" in nursing as well as society. But feminism is not easy or painless. Keddy noted that when women who have not been exposed to feminist thought begin to examine their lives from a feminist perspective and realize their oppression, they may experience feelings of anger, despair, and helplessness. Female nurses experience those feelings about themselves both as women and as nurses.

Keddy (1995) described "older" nurses learning about feminism in her classroom as going through a process of resistance, anger, and hope. Most of the nurses she taught were skeptical about feminism when they were introduced to it, but, when they reflected on their own experiences of oppression, they became angry. Then they moved to an unwillingness to accept the status quo and a hope that feminism could be used to change themselves (which had already happened) and nursing.

Feminist Principles

Many principles guide feminist action, and one of the most basic is *praxis*. Praxis is a dynamic interplay between theory and practice, reflection and action; it is a process (Friere, 1970). The goal of praxis is to understand and transform the world with labor. Praxis includes using feminist thought to critique social actions and integrating feminist thought into academic disciplines to revise ideas and create new knowledge.

One example of praxis is how a discussion among women who share some common experiences moves to a comparison of those experiences with extant theories about women, then creates new theories, especially when discrepancies and biases are recognized, and finally generates new research questions (Reed & Garvin, 1996). The process can then begin again.

Another principle of feminist analysis is the importance of *agency*. Agency means a woman being subject rather than object, and it can also mean identifying oneself as an individual, rather than as like everyone else, or as someone who makes her own decisions and takes responsibility for her choices. Agency can also refer to the cultivation of oneself as marginal (Gadow, 1994).

Empowerment of women is central to feminism. Empowerment means sharing power with others or assisting others to realize their own power (Mason, Backer, & Georges, 1991). In patriarchy men have power, but women also have power; feminists want women to accept and use their power. According to feminist therapy, for women to be empowered, someone (e.g., feminist therapists) must listen to and understand women's individual and collective experiences of disempowerment (Prilleltensky, 1996). That is, women must recognize their oppression and disempowerment before they can become empowered. Roberts (2000) urges nurses to understand their oppression so that they can develop more positive images of both themselves and other nurses.

One way that women can recognize their oppression is by listening to themselves and each other. By sharing and validating each other's experiences, women can regain their voice. Research shows that many adolescent women lose their voice as they are socialized to be female and to have the women's worldview. Their desire to please others and to fit in causes them to lose the identity they were developing. Many women do not regain their voice until midlife; some never do (Borysenko, 1996).

Consciousness Raising

Consciousness raising (CR) groups proliferated in the 1970s with the second wave of feminism in the United States. CR is a self-help process. Initially, women began to learn that the personal is political—that individual women's experiences were shared by other women and that women have power to change their lives. CR can be described as the first step in feminist theory (King, 1989); women cannot do anything about their oppression until they realize they are oppressed.

CR is a process through which women can regain their voices (Cheek & Rudge, 1994). CR is cost effective; it takes only women, time, and a location. In CR groups, women bond and build rapport; they listen to themselves and realize that the only authority is themselves. The only concern related to CR is that women do not generalize beyond their own identities; their experiences are their own, but other women's experiences may differ.

Writing is a strategy that can be used alone or with groups. Writing allows a woman to examine her experiences and, if she shares that with a group, to receive validation. Groups of women in prison or homeless shelters, as well as individual women in their own homes, reflect on their lives and achieve self-awareness through writing.

Coalitions and Alliances

Feminist praxis also occurs when women come together to work on issues of importance to all. Coalitions are groups of individuals who work together on a single political issue, such as violence against women. The individuals may represent themselves, an identity group, or an organization, but the goal or issue is the primary purpose of the coalition. Coalition work is difficult and dangerous (Reagon, 1983) but doing it achieves feminist goals.

Molina (1990) argues that alliances are more productive than coalitions because in coalitions individual needs are sacrificed for the cause. She says the rewards of coalition may be successful marches or actions, but that individuals get hurt, angry, and demoralized because they allow the cause to be primary and ignore their own needs. She believes that coalitions are needed but that they should be formed for very specific goals only, and, when the goal is achieved, the coalition should be disbanded.

Molina (1990) encourages feminists instead to create alliances, which she says are about individuals, love, commitment, responsibility, justice, and shared visions of a better society for all people. To be allies, people must accept and celebrate their differences. Individuals are as important as the cause, and, if individuals are valued, the cause can also be achieved. Her perspective is similar to what has been called *multiculturalism*.

Multiculturalism

Like feminism, *multiculturalism* is difficult to define, and some individuals and groups today prefer the term *diversity*. Like feminism, multiculturalism can be considered a political theory, an ideology, a worldview, or a form of activism that aims to change the oppressive structures in society. Many feminists include multiculturalism in their theories.

Multiculturalism is an approach to viewing every person as an individual in her or his own context and to embracing all people. Multiculturalism attempts to demonstrate complex relationships among all cultures, broadly defined, not only racial or ethnic pluralism.

Unfortunately, multiculturalism suffers from misunderstanding, antagonism, and oppression by persons who would rather maintain the status quo. When a group or community is trying to become multicultural, they may be criticized as being simply politically correct (PC). Antagonists think multiculturalism means reverse discrimination or being anti-white, but multiculturalism actually strives for cultural interaction among people of all backgrounds. Multiculturalism assumes no central group, and, as such, it is a radical change. Valuing differences among cultural groups and learning how all groups can live together in peace should enhance theory and political practices of all persons in society.

TRANSFORMATION OF WOMEN'S HEALTH

It is the task of the oppressed to liberate both themselves and their oppressors. Only power that comes from the weakness of the oppressed can become sufficiently strong to free both (Friere, 1970). The liberation of women has the power to liberate society from patriarchy. Transformation of women's health is one phase in the liberation of women and nurses.

Transformation requires a vision beyond what exists. Although women's health today includes much more than reproductive health, examining women's health from a lifespan perspective is common (Writing Group, 1997). But not all women's health problems have been identified (Caplan, 1992), and likewise not every avenue for improving women's health has been explored. Real transformation involves thinking outside the limits.

Nonetheless, to transform women's health care, it must be accessible to all women and of the highest quality. Women want alternatives and choices in health care, and diverse groups of women have varying needs. Thus women's health care must be eclectic and appropriate to the needs of all women. Both allopathic and complementary health providers are needed, and a health care system that provides affordable and accessible care for all persons (i.e., universal health care) is required. Oppression comes from the system, so the system must be changed.

Both individual and collective action is needed (Mason & Leavitt, 1995). Individuals serve as role models, but much more can be achieved when women (and men) work together in coalitions and alliances.

As both women's health providers and recipients of women's health care, nurses have a special mission to transform women's health, and incorporation of feminism into nursing is a way to do that. The power of feminism as a force for liberation and transformation lies in its recognition of the structures of oppression and the connections among the many forms of oppression, including sexism, racism, classism, and heterosexism.

Resistance to feminism occurs because nurses do not recognize their oppression or do not wish to change their situation. Individual nurses have always supported feminist ideals, and, since the second wave of feminism, they have also written about the application of feminism to nursing.

Nurses are increasingly calling for the integration of feminist ideas into nursing practice (Hawkins & Thibodeau, 2000), including the challenge to existing patriarchal models used in nursing practice (Roberts, 1998). Nurses are including feminism in nursing curricula (e.g., Andrist, 1997), and feminist nursing research is proliferating (Chinn, 1995). Nurses are also encouraging application of feminism to health policy and politics (Backer et al., 1993).

SUMMARY

Patriarchy results in oppression of women and of women's health. However, patriarchy is so much a part of life that many women do not realize their oppression. Until women acknowledge oppression, change cannot occur. But as an oppressed group, women have the potential to change the world. This chapter has provided numerous example of negative effects of patriarchy and oppression on women, nurses, and women's health. Hopefully, some examples will resonate with the experiences of readers, and they will become motivated to transform women's health for themselves and their clients. Feminism and multiculturalism are two vehicles that will carry women on the journey out of oppression and into a new world of women's health.

REFERENCES

Adelman, J. (1995). Raising white children in a racist society. In J. Adelman & G. Enguidanos (Eds.), *Racism in the lives of women*. New York: Harrington Park Press.

Andrist, L. C. (1997). Integrating feminist theory and women's studies into the women's health nursing curriculum: Special topics in women's health. *Women's Health Issues, 7*(2), 76–83.

Anzaldua, G. (1987). *Borderlands*. San Francisco: Spinsters/Aunt Lute.

Ashley, J. (1976). *Hospitals, paternalism, and the role of the nurse*. New York: Teachers College Press.

Backer, B. A., Costello-Nickitas, D. M., Mason, D. J., McBride, A. B., & Vance, C. (1993). Feminist perspectives on policy and politics. In D. J. Mason, S. W. Talbot, & J. K. Leavitt (Eds.), *Policy and politics for nurses*. Philadephia: Saunders.

Bem, S. (1974). The measurement of psychological androgyny. *Journal of Consulting and Clinical Psychology, 42*, 155–162.

Benderly, B. L. (1997). *In her own right: The Institute of Medicine's guide to women's health issues*. Washington, DC: National Academy Press.

Borysenko, J. (1996). *A woman's book of life*. New York: Riverhead Books.

Boswell, H. (1997). The transgender paradigm shift toward free expression. In B. Bullough, V. L. Bullough, & J. Elias (Eds.), *Gender blending* (pp. 53–57). Amherst, NY: Prometheus Books.

Broverman, I. K., Broverman, D. M., Clarkson, F. E., Rosenkrantz, P., & Vogel, S. R. (1970). Sex-role stereotypes and clinical judgments of mental health, *Journal of Consulting Psychology, 34*, 1–7.

Brown, H. G. (1982). *Having it all: Love. success. sex. money*. New York: Simon and Schuster.

Bunch, C. (1987). *Passionate politics*. New York: St. Martin's Press.

Campbell, S. (1994). Being dismissed: The politics of emotional expression. *Hypatia, 9*(3), 46–65.

Caplan, P. J. (1992). Driving us crazy: How oppression damages women's mental health and what we can do about it. *Women & Therapy, 12*(3), 5–28.

Cheek, J., & Rudge, T. (1994). Been there, done that? Consciousness raising, critical theory, and nurses. *Contemporary Nurse, 3*(2), 58–63.

Chinn, P. L. (1995). Feminism and nursing. *Annual Review of Nursing Research, 13*, 267–289.

Eisenstein, Z. R. (1979). *Capitalist patriarchy and the case for socialist feminism*. New York: Monthly Review Press.

Ellis, P., & Murphy, B. C. (1994). The impact of misogyny and homophobia on therapy with women. In M. P. Pravkin (Ed.), *Women in context: Toward a feminist reconstruction of psychotherapy* (pp. 48–73). New York: The Guilford Press.

Erikson, E. H. (1963). *Childhood and society*. New York: Norton.

Fiorino, D. (1980). *An historical study of the National Association of Pediatric Nurse Associates/Practitioners (NAPNAP) 1973-1978*. Unpublished master's thesis. Dayton, OH: Wright State University.

Friere, P. (1970). *Pedagogy of the oppressed*, New York: Seabury Press.

Frye, M. (1983). *The politics of reality*. Trumansburg, NY: Crossing Press.

Gadow, S. (1994). Whose body? Whose story? The question about narrative in women's health care. *Soundings, 77*(3/4), 295–307.

Gainor, K. A. (1992). Internalized oppression as a barrier to effective group work with black women. *Journal for Specialists in Group Work, 17*(4), 235–242.

Gilligan, C. (1982). *In a different voice*. Cambridge, MA: Harvard University Press.

Hawkins, J. W., & Thibodeau, J. A. (1996). *The advanced practice nurse: current issues*. New York: Tiresias.

Hurtado, A. (1989). Relating to privilege: Seduction and rejection in the subordination of white women and women of color. *Signs: Journal of Women in Culture and Society, 14*(4), 833–855.

Johnson, A. G. (1997). *The gender knot: Unraveling our patriarchal legacy*. Philadelphia: Temple University Press.

Keddy, B. C. (1995). Feminist teaching and the older nurse: The journey from resistance through anger to hope. *Journal of Advanced Nursing, 21*(4), 690–694.

Ketner, K. L. (1996). An implicit world view in technology and its consequences for contemporary life. *Nursing Outlook, 44*(6), 280–283.

King, U. (1989). *Women and spirituality*. London, England: Macmillan Education.

Lewenson, S. B. (1996). *Taking charge: Nursing, suffrage, and feminism in America, 1873-1920*. New York: National League for Nursing Press.

Loulan, J. (1996). Gender jail. In V. E. Vida (Ed.), *The new our right to love* (pp. 85-89). New York: Touchstone.

Lovell, M. C. (1992). Daddy's little girl: The lethal effects of paternalism in nursing. *Revolution: The Journal of Nurse Empowerment, 2*(1), 16–23, 110–111.

Mason, D. J., & Leavitt, J. K. (1995). Political activism: The individual versus the collective. *Journal of the New York State Nurses Association, 26*(1), 46–47.

Mason, D. J., Backer, B. A., & Georges, C. A. (1991). Toward a feminist model for the political empowerment of nurses. *Image: Journal of Nursing Scholarship, 23*(2), 72–77.

Molina, P. (1990). Recognizing, accepting, and celebrating our differences. In G. Anzaldua (Ed.), *Making face, making soul,* (pp. 326–331). San Francisco: Aunt Lute Foundation Books.

Pheterson, G. (1986). Alliances between women: overcoming internalized oppression and internalized domination. *Signs: Journal of Women in Culture and Society, 12*(1), 146–160.

Prilleltensky, O. (1996). Women with disabilities and feminist therapy. *Women and Therapy, 18*(1), 87–97.

Reagon, B. J. (1983). Coalition politics: Turning the century. In B. Smith (Ed.), *Home girls: A black feminist anthology.* New York: Kitchen Table Women of Color Press.

Reed, B. G., & Garvin, C. D. (1996). Feminist thought and group psychotherapy: Feminist principles as praxis. In B. DeChant (Ed.), *Women and group psychotherapy: Theory and practice.* New York: Guilford Press.

Reverby, S. M. (1987). *Ordered to care: The dilemma of American nursing, 1850–1945,* New York, 1987, Cambridge University Press.

Rew, L. (1986). Intuition: Concept analysis of a group phenomenon. *Advances in Nursing Science, 8*(2), 21–28.

Rivers, R. Y. (1995). Clinical issues and intervention with ethnic minority women. In J. F. Aponte, R. Y. Rivers, & J. Wohl (Eds.), *Psychological interventions and cultural diversity.* Boston: Allyn & Bacon.

Roberts, S. J. (1983). Oppressed group behavior: Implications for nursing. *Advances in Nursing Science, 5,* 21–30.

Roberts, S. J. (1996). Breaking the cycle of oppression: Lessons for nurse practitioners? *Journal of the American Academy of Nurse Practitioners, 8*(5), 209–214.

Roberts, S. J. (1998). Health promotion as empowerment: Suggestions for changing the balance of power. *Clinical Excellence for Nurse Practitioners, 2*(3), 183–187.

Roberts, S. J. (2000). Development of a positive professional identity: Liberating oneself from the oppressor within. *Advances in Nursing Science, 22*(4), 71–82.

Rowbotham, S. (1981). The trouble with "patriarchy." In Feminist Anthology Collective (Eds.), *No turning back: Writings from the Women's Liberation Movement, 1975–80.* London: The Women's Press.

Schreiber, R. (2000). Wandering in the dark: Women's experiences with depression. *Health Care for Women International, 22*(1/2), 85–98.

Scott, J. W. (1988). *Gender and the politics of history.* New York: Columbia University Press.

Steen, M. (1991). Historical perspectives on women and mental illness and prevention of depression in women, using a feminist framework. *Issues in Mental Health Nursing, 12,* 359–374.

Tannen D. (1990). *You just don't understand: Women and men in conversation.* New York: William Morrow and Company.

Thomas, L. W. (1995). A critical feminist perspective of the health belief model: implications for nursing theory, research, practice, and education. *Journal of Professional Nursing, 11*(4), 246–252.

Thompson, B. W. (1994). *A hunger so wide and so deep.* Minneapolis, MN: University of Minnesota Press.

Timyan, J., Brechiri, S. J. G., Measham, D. M., & Ogunleye, B: (1993). Access to care: More than a problem of distance. In M. Koblinsky, J. Timyan, & J. Gay (Eds.), *The health of women: A global perspective* (pp. 217–234). Boulder, CO, Westview Press.

Weston, K. (1996). *Render me, gender me.* New York: Columbia University Press.

Writing Group of the 1996 American Academy of Nursing Expert Panel on Women's Health. (1997). Women's health and women's health care: Recommendations of the 1996 AAN Expert Panel on Women's Health. *Nursing Outlook, 45*(1), 7–15.

Young, I. M. (1994) Gender as seriality: Thinking about women as a social collective. *Signs: Journal of Women in Culture and Society, 19*(3), 713–738.

RESOURCES

Feminist Women's Health Center: *www.fwhc.org/*
General Women/Feminism: *www.feminist.com/resources/artspeech/genwom/index.html*
Men and Feminism: *www.feminist.com/resources/artspeech/men/index.html*
Feminism and Women's Studies: *www.eserver.org/feminism/*

Chapter 3

Women and Culture

Michele J. Upvall

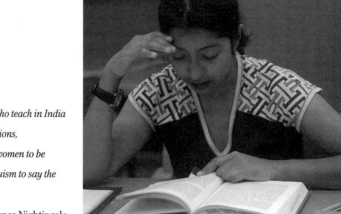

It is a truism to say that women who teach in India must know the language, the religions, superstitions and customs of the women to be taught in India. It ought to be a truism to say the very same for England.

Florence Nightingale

INTRODUCTION

Historical Perspective

The concept of culture has always influenced health care delivery, but its importance was not fully recognized in the nursing profession until the 1960s. Before this era, culture and its relationship to women's health focused upon childbearing. For example, African-American women were encouraged to give birth during the period of slavery from the 17th to the 19th century. This view changed during the early part of the 20th century, when physicians believed providing obstetrical care to African-American women would only encourage increased fertility and, ultimately, threaten the population of the perceived "superior" race (Beardsley, 1990).

Childbirth practices began to change dramatically in the 18th century as the Western, biomedical model of health supported the movement from birth at home with a midwife to physician deliveries in hospitals. This practice was restricted to upper-middle class women in America; women from other cultural backgrounds, such as African-Americans and American Indians, continued to deliver their babies at home with the help of relatives or midwives. Women with high-risk pregnancies could not afford physicians and hospital care. Many women did want to continue their traditional childbearing customs; however, Litoff (1986) noted that in the 1920s many African-American and

Mexican-American women in Texas were unsure of the skills of the midwife yet had no access to alternatives in the event of complications during pregnancy and delivery.

Racism has dominated health care service for women throughout the centuries (Bayne-Smith, 1996). Little attention was given to the health care needs of women of color; this neglect was clearly visible in morbidity and mortality statistics. Until 1940, the leading cause of death given for African-American women was "unknown causes" (Beardsley, 1990).

Change did not begin to occur until the civil rights and feminist movements of the 1960s. African-American women were the primary beneficiaries of the significant progress made in the social, political, and economic areas in the United States (Bayne-Smith, 1996). Other minorities, such as American Indians and Hispanic women, remained marginalized.

Immigration laws, especially the Hart-Cellar Immigration Act of 1965, changed the face of new arrivals to the United States. A dramatic increase in immigrants from Mexico, Asia, Central America, African countries, and the former Soviet Union into urban America occurred from 1970 through the 1990s (Bayne-Smith, 1996; U.S. Bureau of the Census, 2000). At the same time, economic forces began to impact health care policy during the Reagan-Bush administration in the 1980s. A "boot-strap" approach, which assumed that people could and should take charge of their health, was presented as empowering the individual. In the end, a "blame-the-victim" mentality evolved as individuals were expected to take responsibility for their health without consideration of socioeconomic status, cultural beliefs, and availability of health care services.

Impact of Poverty

The relationship between ethnicity, poverty, and health has been clearly established through research (Litt, 1993). Otten, Williamson, and Marks (1990) report that more than one third of excess mortality among adult African-Americans was attributable to poverty, even after taking into account chronic disease, such as hypertension, diabetes, substance use, and obesity. Kagawa-Singer (1995) has also thoroughly documented the effects of socioeconomic status among minority women with cancer who are living in poverty. These women are more likely to be diagnosed with cancer in later stages, influencing treatment choices and survival rates. However, regardless of disease, the mortality gap between low-income women of color and EuroAmerican women has been increasing. For example, death rates for African-American women with breast cancer were 17% higher than for EuroAmerican women in 1988 (Kagawa-Singer, 1995; McBarnette, 1996).

Looking ahead to the year 2003 and beyond requires careful analysis of the past and correcting inequalities in health care. Access to all health care services, from prevention to tertiary care, must be increased along with our understanding of the influence of culture on health care. As the population of women of color increases though rising birth rates and immigration, the public will also have increasing expectations of nurses who provide much-needed health care services.

The Scope of Culture

Diversity, or differences, are manifested through language, social behavior systems, styles of dress...the list goes on. Given the number of definitions of culture, it is clear that culture is not easily defined, much less understood. Definitions range from the general, such as Hall's (1988) metacommunications system with word, thoughts, and behavior encompassing meaning, to the more specific, complex definition provided by Baldwin, Cotanch, Johnson, and Williams (1996, p. 28):

> A complex, integrated system that includes knowledge, beliefs, skills, art, morals, laws, customs, and any other acquired habits and capabilities of a group of people...is learned, shaped, adapted to the environment, and subject to change. As a learned set of traits, culture is transmitted from one generation to the next by both formal education and imitation.

In essence, culture is the process of determining our reality. It is a major factor in guiding our conscious and unconscious decisions and actions for nursing care (Leininger, 1988) as we create the patterns for interactions within our world. Subcultures exist within a culture as individuals share particular traits such as language, socioeconomic status, and education. The U.S. Census Bureau (1995) classifies subcultural groups in America as African-American, Hispanic, Asian-American, and Native American. The health care system in the United States may be viewed as its own culture with nursing as a particular subculture.

All cultures and subcultures exhibit specific values, or beliefs about what is acceptable. Values influence our perception of others, guide our actions, provide meaning for our lives, and reflect our personal and professional identity (Potter & Perry, 2001). Norms for behavior are the manifestations of cultural values and provide boundaries for behavior. For example, in a particular culture children may be highly valued and desired. This value may be manifested by the behavioral norm of a woman having many children.

DEVELOPING CULTURAL COMPETENCY

In the past, nursing curricula emphasized development of cultural sensitivity in students caring for minority populations. A basic understanding of major cultural groups is necessary, but a "cookbook" approach to clients can be just as harmful as no consideration of culture and health. Developing the necessary skills to deliver culturally appropriate nursing care begins with familiarity with concepts related to culture and then utilizing this knowledge to deliver nursing care considered acceptable to the individual.

Diversity includes the cultural differences apparent in various dimensions of culture, such as physiological variations, beliefs related to time orientation, spatial behavior, social organizations, communication patterns, and value orientations (Baldwin et al., 1996).

Although *race* and *ethnicity* are often used synonymously, they are two separate concepts. Race is a biological classification of an individual as being caucasian, mongoloid, or negroid. It is based upon the physical characteristics of skin pigmentation and skeletal structure. Ethnicity is more complex and refers to one's sense of identification with a particular cultural group. The cultural heritage of an ethnic group is passed down to succeeding generations (Baldwin et al., 1996).

Racism refers to the belief in the superiority of one race over all others. It may be subtle or openly expressed through the beliefs and actions of either individuals or social organizations (Baldwin, et al., 1996).

One manifestation of racism is *ethnocentrism,* or the belief that one's own lifestyle is superior to others. The responsibility for dealing with ethnocentrism lies primarily with the nurse, who initiates therapeautic communication with a client. All individuals are ethnocentric to some extent. They are attached to their own belief systems and assume their way is desirable. Referring to other cultures as "primitive" or "superstitious" can disrupt communications with clients from that particular culture. Interactions with the client are doomed to failure before communication is even initiated.

Another common damaging ethnocentric attitude is displayed through statements such as "Those people don't want to be helped," or "Let them be sick, they always are." These biases limit nursing actions, reduce the quality of nursing care, and can result in disparities in health care services.

Biases toward certain groups of people can also be manifested through stereotyping behavior. *Stereotypes* occur when individuals are categorized into a particular group with prescribed attributes. Example of a stereotype is the belief that all Asian clients are stoic and uncomplaining or that all Americans are loud and demanding.

Values give direction to an individual's or group's actions and thoughts (Leinginger, 1978). All individuals have values but recognizing them may be difficult. However, awareness of one's personal and professional values will facilitate collaborative relationships with individuals of different cultures.

Kluckhohn and Strodtbeck (1961) provide the classic framework for assessing the values of different cultures. One of the components of the framework is *temporal orientation,* or how cultures conceptualize time. Cultures can be past, present, or future oriented. *Activity orientation* refers to either a "doing" culture or a "being" culture. Cultures that emphasize accomplishment are considered "doing" oriented, while those that value existence in the present are considered "being" oriented. *Relational orientation* refers to interpersonal patterns within a culture. Cultures can exist within a lineal mode, in which the group's welfare is of primary importance, or they can exhibit an individualistic mode, in which the individual's perspective is valued over the group's. Also, the collateral mode exists in which family or lateral groups such as siblings or peers are most important. *People-to-nature orientation* accounts for the culture's perspective on its relationship to nature. Cultures can either dominate nature, exist in harmony with nature, or be subjugated to nature. Innate *human nature orientation* characterizes the nature of human beings as either good, evil, or neutral.

The process of forming an attachment to a cultural group is known as *enculturation* (Baldwin et al., 1996). Assessing the degree to which an individual is enculturated within a particular group is necessary for planning care, as individuals may or may not believe in or manifest the value orientations of the cultural group.

Acculturation is adapting to a cultural group that is different from the one in which enculturation has taken place. Again, assessing the degree to which the individual has *assimilated*, or taken on the beliefs and values of the new group, is necessary in order to assess the level of acculturation (Baldwin et al., 1996).

Uprooting can be described as culture shock but can also have a more positive connotation. In the process of uprooting, an individual leaves the primary environment, changing relationships with family, friends, and/or country and confronts the unknown. Characteristics of uprooting include the following (Zwingmann & Gunn, 1983):

1. Uprooting is a phenomenon experienced of necessity by all individuals undergoing a social and cultural change.
2. Some biopsychosocial and spiritual discomfort will result as an individual experiences uprooting.
3. Uprooting may be associated with positive changes in the self-development and personal growth of an individual.
4. The manner in which an individual expresses discomfort from uprooting may be determined by the individual's culture.

Relationship of Health and Illness to Culture

Both health and illness are concepts that are defined by an individual's culture. What is "normal" in one society may be considered "abnormal" in another. In some societies, health may be equivalent to goodness, or absence of evil. It may also be considered a reward for "good" behavior. The perception of menopause and the interpretation of its symptoms illustrates the dialectic of health and illness. For example, EuroAmericans may expect hot flushes at this time, but women from other countries such as China, Japan, and Thailand as well as Mayan Indian women generally do not experience these symptoms (Beyenne, 1986; Kaufert, 1996; Tang, 1993). Kaufert emphasizes the need to examine the universal process of menopause within a social and cultural context instead of imposing EuroAmerican standards of what is considered "normal" menopause upon other societies.

From a cultural point of view, illness can be distinguished from disease. Disease is the biological state of illness that can be explained in pathological terms (Foster & Anderson, 1978). However, as a cultural concept, illness is "the social recognition that a person is unable to fulfill his normal roles adequately and that something must be done about the situation" (Foster & Anderson, 1978, p. 40). As societies define health, so also do they define illness. For example, malaria is prevalent among the Mano of Liberia. They do not consider this an illness but believe that everybody has experienced it, and it is a normal part of life.

Health Care Systems and Providers

There has always been some form of health care available to people of all countries, and health care systems can be found in all societies. A health care system is defined as a social institution involving, at a minimum, the interaction between a patient and healer (Foster & Anderson, 1978). The purpose of a health care system is to mobilize the resources of the patient, family, and society to resolve the patient's problem. In addition, these systems may also:

1. Provide a rationale for treatment
2. Explain why individuals become ill
3. Sanction and support cultural norms (that is, the threat of illness as retribution for unacceptable behavior maintains moral order)

Anthropologists have developed a variety of frameworks for understanding how health and illness are classified among societies. Foster and Anderson (1978) utilized a dual division to distinguish health care systems in non-Western societies. A personalistic medical system is characterized by the belief that a sensate agent, such as a deity, ghost, ancestor, evil spirit, witch, or sorcerer, causes illness. The individual afflicted with the illness is the victim of aggression or is being punished for some reason. Illness in a naturalistic medical system is explained impersonally, through the concept of equilibrium. All body elements, hot and cold, humors, the yin and yang, are in harmony with the individual's natural and social environment. Illness occurs when this equilibrium is disturbed. Major naturalistic systems include:

1. *Humoral pathology*: Common in Latin America, humoral pathology can be traced to ancient Greece and its concept of the four humors—blood (hot and moist), phlegm (cold and moist), black bile (cold and dry), and yellow bile, or choler (hot and dry). The major organs of the body (the heart, brain, and liver) are related to the qualities of dry and hot, moist and cold, and hot and moist. Healthy individuals were believed to have an excess of heat and moisture. However, individual qualities varied, and people could be described as sanguine (cheerful), phlegmatic (composed), bilious (ill-tempered), or melancholic (sad). Treatment consisted of determining which of the humors were deficient or excessive and providing a balance. Humoral pathology was brought to the New World by the Spanish conquerors. Today, in Mexico and portions of South America, illness is attributed to an excess of hot or cold, although these terms are often used metaphorically and may not necessarily indicate a specific temperature (Foster & Anderson, 1978). For example, childbearing is considered a hot experience, and so laboring women must not eat foods classified as hot, such as pork. Only foods classified as cold can restore the woman's equilibrium.

2. *Ayurvedic medicine*: Ayurvedic theory can be traced to the first millennium B.C. through historical religious documents. Its influence is felt throughout contemporary India. Similarly to humoral pathology, the human body in Ayurvedic medicine is represented by three humors, or *dosha*—phlegm, bile, and wind. Health is manifested through equilibrium among the three dosha, and illness occurs when the individual experiences an imbalance. As in humoral pathology, Ayurvedic medicine treats illness by finding the correct combination of foods and herbs to restore balance (Foster & Anderson, 1978).

3. *Traditional Chinese medicine*: Yin and yang (cloudy and sunny) are believed to be the elements from which the universe evolved, and health is manifested through their

proper balance. Foods, herbs, and curing methods are thought to have hot or cold qualities. For example, acupuncture is considered a cold treatment appropriate for diseases attributed to excessive yang, while moxibustion is a hot treatment suitable for treating disease caused by excessive yin (Helman, 1994).

Various terms have been applied to healers practicing within personalistic and naturalistic systems, including "native healer," "primitive healer," and "witch doctor," but they have often been used in a negative sense, to mean "not as good" in comparison to Western practitioners. Therefore the term "indigenous healer" should be used to refer to non-Western medical practitioners who are "of the culture" (Scrimshaw & Burleigh, 1978).

Indigenous healers are defined by the World Health Organization (1987) as: "[a] person recognized by the community in which he lives as competent to provide health care by using vegetable, animal, and mineral substances and certain other substances based on the social, cultural, and religious background as well as on the knowledge, attitudes, and beliefs that are prevalent in the community regarding physical, mental, and social well-being and the causation of disease and disability."

Indigenous healers can be classified into four major categories (Bannerman, 1983):

1. Those who have received integrated training in modern and traditional systems of medicine, such as Ayurvedic and Chinese medicine.
2. Practitioners trained mainly in traditional medicine but who also have some knowledge of modern medicine, such as a village health worker.
3. Indigenous practitioners without formal training but who obtained diplomas in some particular system, such as Ayurveda, by taking correspondence courses.
4. Those without institutional training who practice after a period of apprenticeship with an established indigenous healer.

This last category of indigenous healers can be further classified into herbalists, diviners, surgeons, bonesetters, traditional birth attendants (TBA), and spiritualists. All operate on various levels, with the simplest being the TBA and herbalist and the more complex practitioner being the diviner and spiritualist.

Developing the Concept of Culture in Nursing

In 1970, Madeleine Leininger, a nurse with a Ph.D. in anthropology, was the first to develop the concept of *transcultural nursing* in the book *Nursing and Anthropology: Two Worlds to Blend* (1970). Since its publication, transcultural nursing has emerged as a nursing specialty, complete with graduate programs.

Leininger describes transcultural nursing as "the subfield of nursing which focuses upon a comparative study and analysis of different cultures and subcultures in the world with respect to their caring behavior; nursing care; and health-illness values, beliefs, and patterns of behavior with the goal of developing a scientific and humanistic body of knowledge in order to provide culture-specific and culture-universal nursing care practices" (1970, p. 8).

Transcultural nursing, then, is both a pure and applied nursing specialty. It is considered a pure specialty because transcultural nurses investigate cultural practices to gain basic knowledge of these cultures. However, transcultural nursing can also be classified as an applied specialty because it utilizes this knowledge to provide nursing care that incorporates cultural concepts.

International nursing focuses on developing national health policies, curriculum development in nursing education, and primary health care promotion as directed by the World Health Organization and international research efforts (DeSantis, 1988). Various definitions of international nursing have been proposed. Henkle (1979) states that an international nurse "is involved in health work which concerns more than one nation." A more specific definition by Douglas and Meleis (1985) is the following:

> International nursing can be defined as any nursing care activity carried out by a nurse from a donor country to a host nation. The nurse providing the care was educated and has practiced nursing in the donor country. However, the nursing services are requested by and practiced in a host country. These services are contracted for a specific time period, and can range from a matter of days to many years (p. 84).

Terms such as *multicultural, crosscultural, transcultural,* and *transnational nursing* have been used as synonyms for international nursing. However, international nursing is a unique specialty although it is related to transcultural nursing. As a specialty, international nursing reflects the different nursing needs in other countries. It requires the nurse to work within a system in which definitions of health can differ and unique skills are necessary for blending nursing knowledge and practice from both countries.

Components of Cultural Competency

Competent nurses deliver health care services in a safe and effective manner. Competency requires knowledge, skills, and ability to meet client needs (Lendburg et al., 1995). Cultural competence implies basic role competence within a particular setting or with a specific population. Nurses must understand the concept of culture and include its implications while delivering nursing care. Culturally competent nurses not only incorporate client beliefs and practices into their nursing care but also maintain awareness of their own cultural beliefs and the effects of those beliefs on their nursing care. Such nurses are aware of stereotypes and their own potentially ethnocentric attitudes. They are committed to preventing cultural conflict by taking the time to develop a trusting relationship with clients and respecting the unique qualities of each individual client.

Stages of Cultural Competence

Attaining cultural competence begins with understanding the first stage, *cultural destructiveness,* and the effect of past attitudes and social policies upon a particular group. The second stage, *cultural incapacity,* follows successful movement from cultural destructiveness. In this stage, the dominant cultural group maintains a paternalistic attitude toward members of "the other" group. Examples of this stage include the attitude that members of the cultural group are unable to adequately solve problems themselves; they are subtly given the message that they are "less than" those from the dominant group. Movement from the second stage to the next requires elimination of such paternalistic posturing. In the third stage, *cultural blindness,* the cultural groups begin to recognize their strengths and weaknesses. However, this occurs with the attitude of "we're all human," and cultural differences are not recognized. The result of passage through this stage is acceptance of each other's identity. In the final stage, *cultural competence,* members of the group approach cultural differences with an open mind and heart, a willingness to work with others of different cultures, a flexible attitude, and application of the principles of cultural competency to the practice setting. This model of cultural competence (Baldwin et al., 1996; Giachello, 1995; Jackson & Haynes, 1992; Rorie, Paine, & Garner, 1996) identifies negative behaviors of the past and promotes individual and group growth as these behaviors are recognized. As members pass through each stage, negativity is replaced with positive attitudes in personal lifestyle and in the practice setting.

Cultural Competency in Practice

Core cultural competencies for nursing are acquired through professional education and ultimately must be put into practice. To achieve cultural competence, nurses must have the knowledge, skill, and ability to care for individuals regardless of cultural orientation. Box 3-1 lists the practice components of the three cultural competencies.

CULTURAL ASSESSMENT

Leininger defined the concept of cultural assessment for nursing as:

> A systematic appraisal or examination of individuals, groups, and communities as to their cultural beliefs, values, and practices to determine explicit nursing needs and intervention practices within the culture context of the people being evaluated (1978, pp. 85-86).

Culturally competent nurses who provide individualized nursing care will conduct a thorough, and typically ongoing, cultural assessment. Such assessments can be lengthy because of their comprehensive nature. However, they are especially helpful in understanding the meaning of a client's behavior that may be confusing to or perceived in a negative manner by a nurse.

Kleinman's (1980) Explanatory Model is one of the simplest cultural assessments and is problem focused. In this model, three sectors of health care can be utilized by the client either individually or at the same time. The *popular sector* consists of family and friends who provide advice and promote guidelines for health maintenance in the cultural group. In the *folk sector,* the client seeks outside assistance from a sacred or secular healer. These healers usually have limited formal training but have undergone an apprenticeship with a recognized healer. Western medicine, or biomedicine, comprises the *professional sector* of health care.

Box 3-1 CULTURAL COMPETENCIES

Knowledge of
- Scope of practice and legal parameters
- Impact of culture on prevention of illness, health promotion, and wellness activities
- History, values, and traditions of diverse ethnic communities
- Impact of ethnicity, socioeconomic status, gender, and age on the health beliefs of clients
- Health-seeking behaviors of diverse communities, including those of various age groups and socioeconomic status
- Language and communication patterns within diverse communities
- Impact of health policy on diverse populations
- Resources available to assist those from diverse populations and communities

Skills of
- Communication, teaching, problem-solving, and practice related to health promotion and illness prevention
- Applying health promotion strategies effectively
- Integrating health care delivery within a community
- Accepting ethnic and socioeconomic differences within diverse communities
- Techniques to understand and adapt to cultural beliefs of clients
- Working with family (immediate and extended) and caregivers in communicating health issues and prevention or treatment strategies
- Utilizing health and social policies that address disparities in health care delivery

Ability to
- Recognize one's own cultural heritage and how it influences interactions with clients
- Assess, evaluate, and use cross-cultural information and research for application to diverse populations
- Assess individual members of diverse populations with reference to ethnic and socioeconomic challenges
- Recognize barriers and develop positive strategies for clients to implement health promotion guidelines
- Communicate effectively through the use of interpretations when necessary
- Advocate on behalf of diverse populations and communities to other health care providers
- Openly acknowledge and discuss ethnic differences
- Interpret symptoms/their implications as they are uniquely expressed by clients from diverse populations

Adapted from American Nurses' Association. *Competencies for health professionals: A multicultural perspective in the promotion of breast, colorectal, and skin health.* Washington, DC: The Association.

Specific questions that account for all three sectors of health care and elicit the client's particular preferences include (Tripp-Reimer, 1984):

1. What do you think has caused your problem?
2. What do you think caused it to occur at a particular time?
3. Has your problem become better or worse since it started or has it stayed the same?
4. What kind of treatment should you receive?
5. What problems has your illness caused you?
6. What are your fears concerning this problem?
7. What have you been doing for this problem in the past and present?
8. How do you think a person with this problem should act?
9. How should a person with this problem be treated by family members?

Bloch's (Orque, Bloch, & Monrroy, 1983) Assessment Guide is one of the most comprehensive tools available and can be used in a variety of clinical settings. The guide is based on Orque's Ethnic/Cultural System Framework, which includes the cultural components of art, history, diet, religion, value orientations, healing beliefs and practices, family life processes, language and communication processes, and social group interactive patterns. To promote holistic nursing care, Orque relates the Ethnic/Cultural System Framework to the client's biological, psychological, and sociological systems.

Congruent with Orque's Framework, Bloch's Assessment Guide is divided into four major categories. Cultural data can be assessed by understanding how the client's values, beliefs, and customs influence attitudes toward health care. Sociological data include a description of the client's social background, such as economic status, education level, and social network. The client's psychological background is assessed through eliciting the client's perceptions or identity, mental and behavioral processes, and response to stress. Biological/physiological data are collected as the nurse completes a physical assessment. Identifying prevalent disease processes and susceptibility patterns are other important considerations in this category.

Leininger (1991) based her assessment tool on the Sunrise Model, which she developed, depicting diversity and universality in cultural care. Her Acculturation Health Care Assessment Tool of Cultural Patterns in Traditional and Non-Traditional Lifeways is comprehensive like Bloch's Assessment Guide. However, it is most suitable for assessing groups rather than individual clients.

Andrews and Boyle (1999) have developed the Transcultural Nursing Assessment Guide that is thorough, easy to follow, and considers the developmental phase of the client. Assessment categories with specific questions can be found in Box 3-2.

The Transcultural Assessment Model developed by Giger and Davidhizar (1991) offers another systematic approach to assessing essential cultural phenomenon. Six categories for assessment are identified in the model (Figure 3-1).

All activities exhibit these cultural phenomenon, but to varying degrees. *Communication* is the primary mode for transmitting and preserving culture. Every cultural group has its own communication patterns, which include dialects, nonverbal gestures (kineses) such as posture, eye contact, facial expressions, and gestures; context; emotional tone, such as warmth or anger; and communication style, including use of vocabulary, grammar, syntax, rhythm and rate of speech, pronunciation, and use of silence.

Principles for communicating with individuals from other cultural groups include:
1. Assessing communication patterns of the client
2. Modifying communication approaches of the nurse according to cultural needs of the client
3. Recognizing the importance of communicating respect to the client through use of active listening techniques (encouraging client to share thoughts and feelings, use of silence, clarifying, validating, and summarizing information)

Text continued on p. 63

Box 3-2 ANDREWS/BOYLE TRANSCULTURAL NURSING ASSESSMENT GUIDE

Cultural Affiliations
■ With what cultural group(s) does the client report affiliation (e.g., American, Hispanic, Navajo, or combination)? To what degree does the client identify with the cultural group (e.g., "we" concept of solidarity or as a fringe member)?

■ Where was the client born?

■ Where has the client lived (country, city) and when (during what years)? *Note:* If a recent relocation to the United States, knowledge of prevalent diseases in country of origin may be helpful. Current residence? Occupation?

Values Orientation
■ What are the client's attitudes, values, and beliefs about developmental life events such as birth and death, health, illness, and health care providers?

■ Does culture affect the manner in which the client relates to body image change resulting from illness or surgery (e.g., importance of appearance, beauty, strength, and roles in cultural group)? Is there a cultural stigma associated with the client's illness (i.e., how is the illness or client condition viewed by the larger culture)?

■ How does the client view work, leisure, education?

■ How does the client perceive change?

■ How does the client perceive changes in lifestyle relating to current illness or surgery?

■ How does the client value privacy, courtesy, touch, and relationships with individuals of different ages, social class (or caste), and gender?

■ How does the client view biomedical/scientific health care (e.g., suspiciously, fearfully, acceptingly)? How does the client relate to persons outside of his or her cultural group (e.g., withdrawal, verbally or nonverbally expressive, negatively or positively)?

Cultural Sanctions and Restrictions
■ How does the client's cultural group regard expression of emotion and feelings, spirituality, and religious beliefs? How are dying, death, and grieving expressed in a culturally appropriate manner?

■ How is modesty expressed by men and women? Are there culturally defined expectations about male-female relationships, including the nurse-client relationship?

■ Does the client have any restrictions related to sexuality, exposure of body parts, certain types of surgery (e.g., amputation, vasectomy, hysterectomy)?

■ Are there any restrictions against discussion of dead relatives or fears related to the unknown?

Communication
■ What language does the client speak at home? What other languages does the client speak or read? In what language would the client prefer to communicate with you?

■ What is the fluency level in English—both written and spoken use of the language? (Remember that stress of illness may cause clients to use a more familiar language and temporarily forget some English.)

■ Does the client need an interpreter? If so, is there a relative or a friend whom the client would like to interpret? Is there anyone whom the client would prefer did not serve as an interpreter (e.g., member of the opposite sex, a person younger/older than the client, member of a rival tribe or nation)?

■ What are the rules (linguistics) and modes (style) of communication? How does the client prefer to be addressed?

■ Is it necessary to vary the technique of communication during the interview and examination to accommodate the client's cultural background (e.g., tempo of conversation, eye contact, sensitivity to topical taboos, norms of confidentiality, and style of explanation)?

Continued

Box 3-2 ANDREWS/BOYLE TRANSCULTURAL NURSING ASSESSMENT GUIDE—Cont'd

- How does the client's nonverbal communication compare with that of individuals from other cultural backgrounds? How does it affect the client's relationship with you and with members of the health care team?
- How does the client feel about health care providers who are not of the same cultural background?
- Does the client prefer to receive care from a nurse of the same cultural background, gender, and/or age?
- What are the overall cultural characteristics of the client's language and communication processes?

Health-Related Beliefs and Practices

- To what cause(s) does the client attribute illness and disease (e.g., divine wrath, imbalance in hot/cold or yin/yang, punishment for moral transgressions, hex, soul loss, pathogenic organism)?
- What are the client's cultural beliefs about ideal body size and shape? What is the client's self-image vis-à-vis the ideal?
- What name does the client give to his or her health-related condition?
- What does the client believe promotes health (eating certain foods, wearing amulets to bring good luck, sleep, rest, good nutrition, reducing stress, exercise, prayer, rituals to ancestors, saints, or intermediate deities)?
- What is the client's religious affiliation (e.g., Judaism, Islam, Pentacostalism, West African Voodooism, Seventh-Day Adventism, Catholicism, Mormonism)? How actively involved in the practice of this religion is the client?
- Does the client rely on cultural healers (e.g., curandero, shaman, spiritualist, priest, minister, monk?) Who determines when the client is sick and when he or she is healthy?
- Who influences the choice/type of healer and treatment that should be sought?
- In what types of cultural healing practices does the client engage (use of herbal remedies, potions, massage, wearing of talismans, copper bracelets, or charms to discourage evil spirits; healing rituals; incantations; prayers)?
- How are biomedical/scientific health care providers perceived? How does the client and his or her family perceive nurses? What are the expectations of nurses and nursing care?
- What comprises appropriate "sick role" behavior? Who determines what symptoms constitute disease/illness? Who decides when the client is no longer sick? Who cares for the client at home?
- How does the client's cultural group view mental disorders? Are there differences in acceptable behaviors for physical versus psychological illnesses?

Nutrition

- What nutritional factors are influenced by the client's cultural background? What is the meaning of food and eating to the client?
- With whom does the client usually eat? What types of foods are eaten? What is the timing and sequencing of meals?
- What does the client define as food? What does the client believe comprises a "healthy" versus an "unhealthy" diet?
- Who shops for food? Where are groceries purchased (e.g., special markets or ethnic grocery stores)? Who prepares the client's meals?
- How are foods prepared at home (type of food preparation, cooking oils used, length of time foods are cooked, especially vegetables, amount and type of seasoning added to various foods during preparation)?
- Has the client chosen a particular nutritional practice such as vegetarianism or abstinence from alcoholic or fermented beverages?

Box 3-2 ANDREWS/BOYLE TRANSCULTURAL NURSING ASSESSMENT GUIDE—Cont'd

- Do religious beliefs and practices influence the client's diet (e.g., amount, type, preparation, or delineation of acceptable food combinations, such as kosher diets)? Does the client abstain from certain foods at regular intervals, on specific dates determined by the religious calendar, or at other times?
- If client's religion mandates or encourages fasting, what does the term *fast* mean (e.g. refraining from certain types or quantities of foods, eating only during certain times of the day)? For what period of time is the client expected to fast?
- During fasting, does the client refrain from liquids/beverages? Does the religion allow exemption from fasting during illness? If so, does the client believe that an exemption applies to him or her?

Socioeconomic Considerations
- Who comprises the client's social world (family, friends, peers, and cultural healers)? How do they influence the client's health or illness status? How do members of the client's social support network define caring (e.g., being continuously present, doing things for the client, providing material support, looking after the client's family)? What is the role of the various family members during health and illness?
- How does the client's family participate in the promotion of health (e.g., lifestyle changes in diet, activity level, etc.) and nursing care (e.g., bathing, feeding, touching, being present) of the client?
- Does the cultural family structure influence the client's response to health or illness (e.g., beliefs, strengths, weaknesses, and social class)? Is there a key family member whose role is significant in health-related decisions (e.g., grandmother in many African-American families or eldest adult son in Asian families)?
- Who is the principal wage earner in the client's family? What is the total annual income? (*Note*: This is a potentially sensitive question.) Is there more than one wage earner? Are the other sources of financial support (extended family, investments)?
- What insurance coverage (health, dental, vision, pregnancy) does the client have?
- What impact does economic status have on lifestyle, place of residence, living conditions, ability to obtain health care? How does the client's home environment (e.g., presence of indoor plumbing, handicap access) influence nursing care?

Organizations Providing Cultural Support
- What influence do ethnic/cultural organizations have on the client's receiving health care (e.g., Organization of Migrant Workers; National Association for the Advancement of Colored People [NAACP]; Black Political Caucus, churches such as African-American, Muslim, Jewish, and others; schools including those which are church-related; Urban League; community-based health care programs and clinics)?

Educational Background
- What is the client's highest educational level obtained?
- Does the client's educational background affect his or her knowledge level concerning the health care delivery system, how to obtain the needed care, teaching-learning, and any written material that he or she is given in the health care setting (e.g., insurance forms, educational literature, information about diagnostic procedures and laboratory tests, admission forms)?
- Can the client read and write English, or is another language preferred? If English is the client's second language, are materials available in the client's primary language?
- What learning style is most comfortable/familiar? Does the client prefer to learn through written materials, oral explanation, or demonstration?

Continued

Box 3-2 ANDREWS/BOYLE TRANSCULTURAL NURSING ASSESSMENT GUIDE—Cont'd

Religious Affiliation
- How does the client's religious affiliation affect health and illness (e.g., life events such as death, chronic illness, body image alteration, cause and effect of illness)?
- What is the role of religious beliefs and practices during health and illness? Are there special rites or blessings for those with serious or terminal illnesses?
- Are there healing rituals or practices that the client believes can promote well-being or hasten recovery from illness? If so, who performs these?
- What is the role of significant religious representatives during health and illness? Are there recognized religious healers (e.g., Islamic Imams, Christian Scientist practitioners or nurses, Catholic priests, Mormon elders, Buddhist monks)?

Cultural Aspects of Disease Incidence
- Are there any specific genetic or acquired conditions that are more prevalent for a specific cultural group (e.g., hypertension, sickle cell anemia, Tay Sachs, G6PD, lactose intolerance)?
- Are there socioenvironmental diseases more prevalent among a specific cultural group (e.g., lead poisoning, alcoholism, HIV/AIDS, drug abuse, ear infections, family violence)?
- Are there any diseases against which the client has an increased resistance (e.g., skin cancer in darkly pigmented individuals, malaria for those with sickle cell anemia)?

Biocultural Variations
- Does the client have distinctive physical features characteristic of a particular ethnic or cultural group (e.g., skin color, hair texture)? Does the client have any variations in anatomy characteristic of a particular group (e.g., body structure, height, weight, facial shape and structure [nose, eye shape, facial contour], upper and lower extremities)?
- How do anatomic and racial variations affect the physical examination?

Developmental Considerations
- Are there any distinct growth and development characteristics that vary with the client's cultural background (e.g., bone density, psychomotor patterns of development, fat folds)?
- What factors are significant in assessing children of various ages from the newborn period through adolescence (e.g., expected growth on standard grid, culturally acceptable age for toilet training, introducing types of foods, gender differences, discipline, socialization to adult roles)?
- What is the cultural perception of aging (e.g., is youthfulness or the wisdom of old age more highly valued)?
- How are elderly persons handled culturally (e.g., cared for in the home of adult children, placed in institutions for care)? What are culturally acceptable roles for the elderly?
- Does the elderly person expect family members to provide care, including nurturance and other humanistic aspects of care?
- Is the elderly person isolated from culturally relevant supportive persons or enmeshed in a caring network of relatives and friends?
- Has a culturally appropriate network replaced family members in performing some caring functions for the elderly person?

From Andrews, M. M., & Boyle, J. S. (1999). *Transcultural concepts in nursing care* (pp. 539–544). Philadelphia: Lippincott.

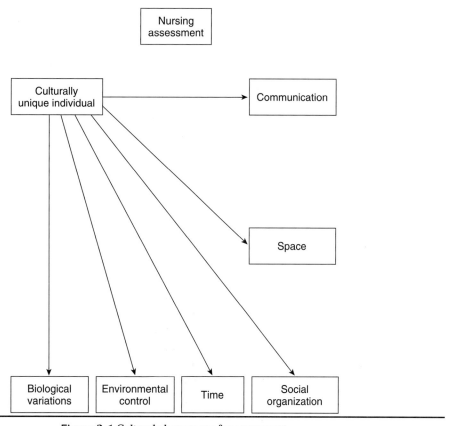

Figure 3-1 Cultural phenomena for assessment.

4. Using of nonthreatening communication patterns, giving enough time for communication to occur, proceeding from general to more specific information, and adhering to social norms of conversation
5. Avoiding health care jargon and abbreviations
6. Using interpreters when necessary for interpreting, if possible, the sensitive issues that the client may not want to share with others

   Space consists of the personal boundaries between nurse and client. This space provides privacy, a sense of security, and independence. Hall (1963) described four zones of interaction. The first, or intimate, zone is zero to one and half feet. In the personal zone, distance is maintained at one and a half to four feet. Touching by close friends and family is acceptable in this zone by EuroAmericans. The zone of social distance from four to twelve feet is used for business and social encounters. In the fourth zone, personal distance is greater then twelve feet and a more formal interaction occurs with voice projection necessary.

Social organizations teach and enforce patterns of cultural behaviors. Values are taught to children through role-modeling by family members. There are a variety of family structures: nuclear family with one man and woman and their children; nuclear dyad family with a man, woman, and no children; extended family consisting of all relatives by birth, marriage, or adoption; alternative family with individuals living together without the legal status of marriage; single-parent family; and blended family containing children from previously existing families. Religious groups are another type of social organization. Regardless of the specific religion, these groups do interact within all units of society.

Time and the perceptions of time within cultural groups can be conceptualized as more than measuring time with a clock. Social time refers to patterns for ordering the cultural group's social life. For example, cultural groups may have a past, present, or future orientation to time. Groups with a past orientation may be considered to be traditional in their action and are not concerned with setting goals. Other groups may be future oriented and delay life passages such as marriage until educational goals have been met.

Environmental control refers to both the external and the internal environment in which the cultural group interacts. In essence, it is the desired ability of the group or individual to control nature. Utilizing Kluckhohn and Strodtbeck's (1961) conceptualization of control, groups can dominate nature, exist in harmony with nature, or be controlled by nature. In addition, individuals can be classified as having either an internal locus of control, with control originating in the self, or an external locus of control whereby fate or choice influences the outcome of events. Beliefs regarding control in life and the forces of nature will impact the individual's views of health promotion, illness prevention, and choice of treatment.

Biological variations refer to the individual's body size, skin color, and physiological processes susceptible to disease. For example, mongolian spots are common in Asian and Native American infants. Sickle cell anemia is a common disorder among African-Americans (Giger & Davidhizar, 1990; 1991).

The remainder of this chapter will apply the cultural concepts of social organization and environmental control as outlined by Giger and Davidhizar to various cultural groups. These concepts can also be applied to other cultural groups for a comprehensive assessment.

THE HEALTH OF WOMEN FROM SPECIFIC CULTURAL GROUPS

The following descriptions of various cultural groups provide an overview of health care beliefs and patterns of health. However, each cultural group is composed of individuals from many different countries and/or regions. For example, one Middle Eastern American client may be of Egyptian descent while another is of Turkish ancestry. Diversity exists within cultures as well as between cultures. Native American clients come from many different tribes. Therefore general information about a specific group of people should never replace a thorough cultural assessment of the individual client.

AFRICAN-AMERICAN WOMEN

African-Americans were unwilling immigrants to the United States. As slaves, African-Americans were considered property, and both adults and children were bought and sold. However, African-Americans managed to survive despite oppression and poverty. Out of such hardships the African-American experience was born, and their cultural beliefs and values are an integral part of this historical context (Spector, 1991).

Social Organization

There are over 15 million African-American women in the United States today (U.S. Bureau of the Census, 2000). While statistics vary, it is believed that over half of all African-American households are headed by women. These women have been characterized as the foundation of the African-American family, providing strength for the family and acting as sole caretaker of the young and the elderly (Lillie-Blanton, Martinez, Taylor, & Robinson, 1993). Because circumstances have forced African-American women to work outside the home, this work role was deemed acceptable for them, unlike their EuroAmerican female counterparts. Working outside the home and being the primary caregiver became the cultural norm for a majority of African-American women, and their income has been essential to the family's survival (Greene, 1996). Such economic discrimination has fostered the negative perception of African-American women as having too much control within the home and as emasculaters of African-American men. Contradictory images of African-American women have only served to reinforce stereotypes, especially of those in poverty (Weeks, Singer, Grier, & Schensul, 1996).

Environmental Control

Health and Illness Beliefs

Traditional African-American beliefs of health and illness are rooted in those past and present in Africa. Harmony between the individual and the environment is seen to be the key to health. Illness, or disharmony, is caused by engaging in taboo behavior or it is viewed as caused by evil spirits (Spector, 1991).

Hargrove and Keller (1993) indicate that contemporary African-American women define health as avoiding disease in themselves and family members, having a balanced diet, maintaining fitness through exercise, practicing "good" habits including following positive role models and maintaining spirituality, being neither too skinny nor too fat as a younger person (older women are expected to be overweight), and reducing stress through decreased worrying.

Methods of Healing

Spiritual and religious systems are the traditional methods of healing in the African-American community. Voodoo was widely practiced in the past and it is reportedly still utilized today, but to an unknown extent. It involves the practice of white ("good") and black ("harmful") magic with clients believing that a "fix," "hex," or "spell" has caused their illness. Relics of Roman Catholic saints are also used during ceremonies to bring luck and prevent illness (Spector, 1991).

Faith healers and prayer are also used and represent the strong belief in the power of spirituality to overcome misfortune. The healers are often followers of the Pentecostal movement. However, African-Americans are also turning to the Muslim faith, considered the fastest growing religion in America today. As Black Muslims, individuals may avoid pork and pork products and alcohol and believe in a regulated, disciplined lifestyle. There are a variety of Muslim, or Islamic, sects that differ in strictness of adherence to these beliefs (Spector, 1991).

A variety of home remedies have been reported for the treatment of disease. Herb teas are used to treat cold symptoms (sassafras tea), blue stone is crushed and placed in open wounds to prevent infection, and clay is wrapped in a dark leaf and placed on a sprained ankle. Eating clay (geophagy) was a common practice among pregnant slaves. The clay was iron rich and was thought to prevent anemia. Argo starch is the modern substitute for clay. The practice of ingesting starch is known as *pica* (Spector, 1991).

Western biomedical health care providers are used by African-American women. However, these women typically do not see a provider on a regular basis but visit clinics and emergency departments for their health care (Gary, Campbell, & Serlin, 1996).

Health and Illness Patterns

Leading causes of death in African-American women include cardiovascular diseases such as hypertension, cancer (lung and breast), cerebrovascular disease including stroke, and diabetes mellitus (National Women's Health Information Center, 2000). Breast cancer in particular has been devastating as 5-year survival rates have increased for EuroAmericans (80%) but worsened for African-American women (65%). This has occurred even though the incidence of breast cancer is lower in African-American women (Leigh, 1995; McBarnette, 1996; Moormeier, 1996; NCHS, 1995; Pinn, 1995).

Rates of preterm delivery are also higher among African-American women even after accounting for socioeconomic status (Rosenberg, Adams-Campbell, & Palmer, 1995). Burks' (1992) research supported other studies that found that financial status did not affect the likelihood that African-American women received prenatal care. Rather, many of the women were unaware of the pregnancy until their fourth or fifth month.

A contributing factor to illness patterns found in African-American women include stress. Edwards (1993) reports that when asked what it is like to be a low-income African-American woman, they replied that it was stressful. Management of stress includes recognition of the stressor and developing moral courage through religious beliefs. Outside resources such as other members of the church or community were utilized as a last resort if the women were unable to solve their problem.

Camino (1989) identified "worriation and nerves" as a specific folk illness of African-American women that occurs from stress. Hargrove and Keller (1993) support Camino's findings and have further identified stress in the workplace as a major cause of "worry" and "nerves."

Biological Variations

Assessing African-American women includes inspection through use of indirect lighting. Particular signs of pathology and differences to note are (Giger & Davidhizar, 1991):

Cyanosis—Inspect lips, tongue (may be ashen gray), and plantar surfaces of hands and feet.

Erythema—Palpate skin for warmth and edema indicating inflammation.

Jaundice—Inspect sclera for yellowish discolorations; buccal mucosa may also appear yellow.

Particular skin conditions include:

Keloids—Irregular, elevated scars

Hypopigmentation or hyperpigmentation of skin

Melasma—Tan to brownish discoloration of the face during pregnancy

AMERICAN INDIAN/ALASKAN NATIVE WOMEN

As with African-American women, the health of American Indian/Alaskan Native (AI/AN) women must be appreciated within a historic context. Over 200 tribes and Indian nations exist within the United States; however, they will be discussed as one group while recognizing the potential differences that may exist.

Social Organization

Today, nearly two million individuals identify themselves as AI/AN. Their history is one of decimation and devastation upon contact with EuroAmericans. Two significant examples of forced migration and government policy were the Cherokee Trail of Tears walk of 900 miles in 1838 and the Navajo Long Walk of 1864 from Arizona to Fort Sumner, New Mexico. Cultural knowledge and languages of many tribes have been lost. Political relationships with the United States government have impacted AI/AN in many areas, including health care services. Relegation to over 50 million acres of land known as reservations has set Native Americans apart from all other cultural groups in the United States (Kauffman & Joseph-Fox, 1996). The number of AI/AN living on reservations is unknown as movement between urban and rural areas and reservations is fluid. Diversity, therefore, exists not only among tribes but also among individuals in the choice of residence and desire to follow traditional beliefs.

Women are perceived as the center of the traditional family system for AI/AN (Kauffman & Joseph-Fox, 1996). Traditionally, the Navajo, in particular, are considered matrilocal, with the husband making his home with his wife and her relatives. In addition, women have been warriors and healers and have taken leadership roles in tribal government.

Environmental Control

Health and Illness Beliefs

Maintaining balance or harmony in all aspects of life characterizes traditional AI/AN health beliefs. Balance exists between individuals as well as between individuals and the environment, animals, and all spiritual forces. Illness may occur because of a past event or an event yet to come. Regardless, disharmony and illness can occur when spiritual forces are unhappy because the environment has been harmed or ceremonies have not been conducted properly or as a direct result of evil spirits or witchcraft (Spector, 1991). Any behavior considered taboo can interfere with balance and cause illness.

Methods of Healing

A variety of indigenous healers exist within AI/AN groups. A healer who is a diagnostician may use handtrembling and stargazing. Handtremblers are able to diagnose by having spirits move their hand. The patient is first given corn pollen under the tongue, and prayers are said by the healer. The spirits then move the healer's hands so that a diagnosis can be made. During particular ceremonies a sandpainting may be completed. Stargazers pray to the star spirit for diagnosis (Plawecki, Sanchez, & Plawecki, 1994; Spector, 1991).

Treatment may take the form of herbs and/or ceremonies. A variety of ceremonies exist, both traditional and through the Native American Church. Roessel (1992) states that there are over 50 types of Navajo ceremonies today, an increase from a decade ago. The purpose of the ceremony is to restore balance or harmony within the individual. Although every ceremony is different, chanting by the singer and praying play a primary role in healing. Ceremonies differ in length from approximately one hour to nine nights. Women participate in all ceremonies unless they are menstruating. This is because women are viewed as having strong power during menses, which disrupts ceremonies. However, ceremonies are conducted that celebrate womanhood, such as the puberty ceremony of the Navajo, *Kinaaldá*, and ceremonies surrounding birth.

Use of healers and ceremonies allows AI/AN to understand why illness has occurred and to promote restoration of balance. However, biomedical providers are also used through the Indian Health Service (IHS), a part of the Department of Health and Human Services. The IHS provides direct services through clinics and hospitals on reservations. Also IHS contracts have been developed to allow tribes to provide services themselves without federal interference. Finally, IHS has developed the urban-oriented Indian Health Programs for outpatient services and health education to AI/AN living off the reservation. However, this program is limited and is a small portion of the IHS budget (Kauffman & Joseph-Fox, 1996).

Health and Illness Patterns

Major causes of death among AI/AN women are similar to those for African-American women: cardiovascular diseases, cancer (especially cervical cancer), intentional and unintentional injuries (motor vehicle accidents in particular), and diabetes mellitus (National Women's Health Information Center, 2000). HIV/AIDS was the seventh leading cause of mortality for both men and women between the ages of 25 and 44 from 1991 to 1995 (Indian Health Service, 1997; Rowell, 1997). Mortality rates are lower in AI/AN women than in the United States population in general, with the exception of motor vehicle accidents and diabetes mellitus (Kauffman & Joseph-Fox, 1996).

Health problems influencing mortality rates for AI/AN women are related to social isolation, poverty, and a history of oppression. Alcohol dependency is the primary health problem among AI/AN women and men, although their drinking patterns and health problems differ. For example, AI/AN women typically do not consume as much alcohol as men, although AI/AN women and adolescents have ever-increasing rates of alcoholism. The effects of alcohol intake are more pronounced in AI/AN women, who have three times the rate of cirrhosis of the liver seen in African-American and EuroAmerican women (Kauffman & Joseph-Fox, 1996). Watts and Gutierres (1997) have identified a cultural model of substance dependency and recovery and discuss appropriate treatment methods such as prayer, sweat lodge ceremonies, and mediating agents (influential elders, community leaders, and extended family members who have recovered). Using traditional methods for curing has also been identified as a crucial intervention in educating AI/AN women about the importance, for instance, of obtaining annual Pap tests (Strickland, Chrisman, Yallup, Powell, & Squeoch, 1996).

Domestic violence is another major health concern facing AI/AN women. Statistics documenting its prevalence are unreliable because of underreporting, but there is agreement that the incidence of domestic violence, primarily abuse of women, is increasing. Contributory factors include the history of oppression of AI/AN with resultant disintegration of traditional values and a sense of hopelessness and powerlessness (Bohn, 1993). Other factors include high rates of unemployment, inadequate support from the family and community, cultural acceptance of spouse abuse, substance use, and fear of seeking help (Tom-Orme, 1995).

Elder abuse has also been reported, but, again, statistics are unreliable and scanty. A changing social system and lack of community resources have been cited as reasons for elder abuse (Tom-Orme, 1995). In 1996, the Navajo Nation Council passed the Diné Elder Protection Act to address this issue. Regardless of the type of domestic violence, nurses have a responsibility to identify those who are being abused and approach them in a respectful manner to establish rapport. The nurse should carefully assess the severity of the abuse, explore options with the victim, and assist with planning, especially for counseling referrals and transport to attend counseling groups or shelters (Bohn, 1993).

ASIAN-AMERICAN/PACIFIC ISLANDER WOMEN

Social Organization

Immigration of the Chinese to the United States began in the early 1800s with the need for laborers to build the transcontinental railroad. Twenty percent of the immigrants returned to China before 1930 when their dreams for a new life were unrealized. However, since 1965, the rate of Asian immigration has risen 10% each year, making Asian/Pacific Islanders (A/PI) the fastest growing minority population in the United States. Countries represented by this classification include China, Korea, Japan, the Philippines, India, Vietnam, Cambodia, Tonga, Samoa, and Malaysia (Spector, 1991; Wang, 1995).

There are over 7 million A/PI in the United States today, the majority of whom are women, most of whom (74%) are at least high school graduates. Nearly 32% of these women hold a bachelor's degree or higher. A/PI women are employed primarily in technical, sales, and administrative support positions (True & Guillermo, 1996).

The family plays a central role in A/PI life, regardless of country of origin. One family member's success will reflect favorably on the other members, while failure brings dishonor to the entire family. This belief of unity within the family is in sharp contrast to the individualism so central to EuroAmerican culture (Shum, 1996).

Environmental Control

Health and Illness Beliefs

The naturalistic system of Chinese medicine with its concepts of yin and yang began as a philosophy that was later incorporated into Chinese medical practice. Taoism, the religious and philosophical foundation of Chinese medicine, originated in approximately 604 BC. It is a spiritual way of life that incorporates the individual within nature. All of creation has a purpose and nature abides by particular laws. Individuals must adapt to these laws and their actions must be in harmony with the external environment (Spector, 1991).

Yin and yang are the dualistic forces of nature. They represent the energy within the individual and the whole of creation. A healthy body maintains harmony with the yin, or female forces of nature, and the yang, or male force. Illness upsets the balance between the dualities. All parts of the body are classified as yin or yang. For example, the liver, heart, and kidneys are considered yin, and the stomach and intestines are yang. Yin forces restore life, and yang acts as a protection from harm (Giger & Davidhizar, 1991; Spector, 1991).

Traditional Chinese physicians use inspection and palpation to diagnose illness. Typically, the tongue is inspected for color, and pulses are palpated. Each hand contains six pulses, and all pulses are related to body organs. Through assessing the characteristics of the pulses, the specific illness can be determined.

The most commonly known method of Chinese healing is acupuncture. Acupuncture has been used for centuries to cure disease and eliminate pain during surgery or other procedures. In this method, a needle is placed into a particular meridian or line on the body to restore the balance between yin and yang. This practice has gained popularity throughout the United States and is used many cultural groups (Spector, 1991).

Moxibustion, or application of heat, is another method for restoring the balance between yin and yang, especially for conditions related to excess yin. This method consists of heating pulverized wormwood and placing it on a specific meridian. Moxibustion is commonly used during labor and delivery and is also used to treat cramps and convulsions (Spector, 1991).

Herbs play major role in Chinese healing. The herbalist harvests and prepares the remedy in a particular way to achieve the fullest therapeutic value possible. For example, ginseng root must be collected only during the nights of a full moon (Spector, 1991).

Health and Illness Patterns

Given the diversity of A/PI women, accurate health statistics do not exist. In fact, under-representation occurs because research instruments are usually administered only in English (e.g., National Health Interview), and random sampling techniques do not account for the high concentration of the A/PI population in only five states (California, Hawaii, New York, Texas, and Illinois). Most national research data is limited to Chinese, Japanese, Filipino, and native Hawaiians, excluding groups from India, Cambodia, Korea, Laos, Thailand, Samoa, and Tonga.

Cancer is the leading cause of death in Chinese, Japanese, and Filipino women. Sites differ according to group. For example, Chinese and Filipino women have a higher incidence of cervical cancer, and Japanese women have increased stomach cancer rates. However, incidence rates of cancer in all three groups are still lower than those in EuroAmerican women (National Women's Health Information Center, 2000; True & Guillermo, 1996).

Rates for cancer screening among A/PI women are lower than those for EuroAmericans. For example, less than half of all Chinese and Vietnamese women receive a Pap smear, 70% have never had a mammogram, and over 47% of Vietnamese women have never had a breast exam (Jenkins & Kagawa-Singer, 1994; Lee, 1992; True & Guillermo, 1996).

Cardiovascular disease is the second leading cause of death, with hypertension a contributing factor. The incidence is lower than that of EuroAmerican women. However, the success rates in controlling hypertension with medication is lower for A/PI women.

A/PI women, in particular pregnant women, have a high rate of being carriers of hepatitis B, with ranges reported from 5% to 15%. The majority of carriers are those who are recent immigrants to the United States (Hann, 1994; True & Guillermo, 1996).

The incidence of suicide increases for Chinese-American women and Japanese-American women, beginning at the age of 45. Reasons for the increased rates include death of spouses, financial difficulties, and lack of support from adult children and extended family. These women receive less support in the United States they would expect to receive in their own country (True, 1995).

As foreign-born A/PI women experience separation from family, domestic violence increases, although reliable statistics are unavailable. In New York, the Asian Women's Center receives over 3000 telephone calls each year from A/PI women who are being abused. These women typically rely economically and socially on their spouses, and they often cannot speak English. Compounding these factors, A/PI women are considered responsible for a successful marriage. A failed marriage shames the entire family (Shum, 1996; Wang, 1995).

HISPANIC/LATINO WOMEN

Hispanic/Latino women come from various countries: Mexico, Spain, Puerto Rico, Cuba, Central and South America, and some Caribbean islands. These women exhibit intraethnic similarities and differences. They are widely distributed throughout the

United States, with those of Mexican origin primarily living in the southwest, Cubans in the southeastern U.S., and Puerto Ricans in the northeast. The fastest growing segments of the Hispanic/Latino population are those from Central and South America living in Los Angeles and Washington, D.C. (Zambrana & Ellis, 1995). Reasons for their increased numbers include a higher birth rate than non-Hispanic/Latino women and increased immigration (U.S. Bureau of the Census, 1995).

Social Organization

Nearly 10% (22.3 million) of the American population is Hispanic/Latino, and women comprise half of this group. However, statistics may underrepresent this population because of illegal immigration. Hispanic/Latino women are one of the youngest cultural groups, with many in the under 21 category or in the working ages of 22 to 55 years. Social and economic characteristics of Hispanic/Latino women include high rates of unemployment, low income, low education levels, and high poverty levels. At least 26% of this group lives below the poverty line with half being families headed by women (Giachello, 1996; U.S. Bureau of the Census, 1995).

The typical Hispanic/Latino family is headed by a male in a nuclear arrangement with strong extended family ties. This strong family orientation is known as *familialism* and is demonstrated through placing family needs above those of the individual. Familialism does not seem to be affected by uprooting and its resultant acculturation effects.

Even though the majority of families are headed by men, women demonstrate a leadership role by being the primary decision makers for consulting a health care provider. Other family members often attend appointments with the ill person and remain in attendance during hospitalization.

Two other concepts related to Hispanic/Latino social interaction are *respeto* (respect) and *personalismo* (personalism). *Respeto* determines the behavior of the individual toward others according to age, gender, socioeconomic status, and perceived authority. This behavior is characterized by deference to others and use of a formal style of interaction. For example, health care providers would be perceived as having authority and the Hispanic/Latino client would agree with the provider and be hesitant to ask questions. This may lead the provider to mistakenly assume that the client understands and is willing to accept the treatment plan.

Personalismo refers to the development of interpersonal relationships. This is demonstrated by the client's asking questions about the provider's well-being and their family members. They may also bring gifts to the providers. Reciprocity, whereby the provider shows interest in the client and her family, helps to build a trusting relationship with the client (Vera, 1996).

Environmental Control

Health and Illness Beliefs

Maintaining spiritual beliefs and following the dictates of religion are part of a healthy lifestyle from the Hispanic/Latino perspective. Researchers are documenting the importance of spirituality in preventing the birth of low birth-weight babies and decreasing infant mortality despite lower socioeconomic status (Magaña & Clark, 1995).

Illness is caused by violating religious and moral codes of conduct, excessive worrying; anger, fear, or envy; evil spirits and witchcraft; and environmental conditions such as poverty, poor nutrition, germs, and bad air (Giachello, 1995). In Mexico, the hot and cold theory of disease introduced by the Spaniards is accepted. Harmony or balance must be maintained between hot and cold and wet and dry. Foods, illnesses, people, and animals are classified as hot or cold. If an individual has a hot illness it must be cured with a cold treatment. However, hot and cold do not refer to actual temperature, and classification of hot and cold may differ from individual to individual (Giger & Davidhizar, 1991; Spector, 1991).

Methods of Healing

Treatment within the context of family and religion are the initial methods of healing with Hispanic/Latino women. Advice is elicited from grandmothers, mothers, and women within the neighborhood. Home cures such as chamomile and cinnamon teas during pregnancy are commonly used. Prayers, pilgrimages to religious shrines, and lighting of religious candles are also popular. In their study of Hispanic/Latino folk healing in the eastern United States, Zapata and Shippee-Rice (1999) discovered that Western providers are consulted in addition to folk healers.

Healers such as *curandero(as)* are also consulted. These healers are strongly religious and receive the gift of healing through birth, apprenticeship, or a vision. They treat a variety of physical and psychological symptoms by using herbs, massage, prayers, and rituals such as *limpias* ("cleanings") whereby an unbroken egg or special herbs are passed over the client (Giachello, 1996; Giger & Davidhizar, 1991; Spector, 1991).

Health and Illness Patterns

Illnesses commonly treated by *curandero(as)* include:

Caida de la mollera—Sunken fontanel in an infant caused by treating the child roughly; symptoms include vomiting, diarrhea, fever, inability to grasp nipple, and restlessness; treatments are holding child upside down, applying eggs to hair then pulling hairs out, prayer, and pressing on the infant's palate.

Empacho—Inability to pass food through the stomach; food is thought to form into a ball inside the stomach cavity, causing severe abdominal cramping; stomach massage is the primary treatment.

Mal ojo—The "evil eye" is thought to be caused by witchcraft when a person admires a child but does not touch it; symptoms include fever, headache, crying, weight loss, and restlessness; onset is usually sudden and treatment consists of a placing a hen's egg mixed with water under the bed of the child; babies may wear a special charm for prevention.

Susto—The temporary loss of the spirit after a frightening experience or sudden shock; symptoms are fear, nightmares, anorexia, insomnia, crying, fever, and diarrhea;

treatment consists of *limpia* with herbs passed over the body of the patient (Giger & Davidhizar, 1991; Spector, 1991).

Leading causes of death among Hispanic/Latino women are cardiovascular disease, followed by breast and lung cancer, cerebrovascular disease, and diabetes mellitus (Giachello, 1996; Zambrana & Ellis, 1995; National Women's Health Information Center, 2000).

Menendez (1990) reports that Puerto Rican women living in New York City have the highest incidence of AIDS of any cultural group. Hispanic/Latino women in general account for 21% of all AIDS cases in women (Zambrana & Ellis, 1995). Intravenous drug use, sexual intercourse with an HIV-positive male, and blood transfusions are the primary routes of exposure (Torres & Villarruel, 1995).

Findings from the HHANES (Hispanic Health and Nutrition Examination Surveys) study identify Hispanic/Latino women as having lower rates of alcohol consumption and less illicit drug use and smoking than EuroAmerican women (Guendelman & Abrams, 1994; Torres & Villarruel, 1995). In addition, the HHANES study linked behavioral risk factors with acculturation. Acculturation is positively associated with higher alcohol consumption, multiple sex partners, less condom use, and increased prevalence of cigarette smoking (Zambrana & Ellis, 1995). The study was limited to women of Cuban, Puerto Rican, and Mexican origin.

MIDDLE EASTERN AMERICAN WOMEN

Like all other cultural groups discussed in this chapter, Middle Eastern American women come from a variety of countries, including Saudi Arabia, Egypt, Iraq, Iran, Israel, Afghanistan, Lebanon, Jordan, Kuwait, Pakistan, Yemen, Turkey, and the United Arab Emirates. These women have often been stereotyped as subordinate to males and subject to strict Islamic codes of behavior. However, these women are actually quite diverse in religious background, educational background, socioeconomic status, and profession.

Social Organization

There are over 2 million immigrants of Middle Eastern descent in the United States today. Census data are inconsistent, and this population is categorized as "other" by the U.S. Bureau of the Census. Immigration to the United States began in the late 1800s with single Christian men settling in southern states. Women and entire families followed. The most recent immigrants are mostly Islamic, or Muslim, and are highly educated and have professional status (Meleis, Omidian, & Lipson, 1993; Meleis & Hattar-Pollara, 1995).

Like women of Hispanic/Latino descent, Middle Eastern American women exhibit a strong sense of familialism. Family, including the extended family, is the first priority even if the woman is employed. Melleis and Hatter-Pollara (1995) report that this creates additional stressors for women as they try to balance the demands of family, work, and community.

Environmental Control

Health and Illness Beliefs

Humoral pathology, the belief in hot and cold, is the basis of Middle Eastern healing. The body is healthy when it is in equilibrium, and illness is the result of imbalance. The external environment in the form of drafts and winds is also believed to predispose the individual to illness. Going from one temperature extreme to another or wearing wet shoes can cause colds and fever.

The evil eye is another strong belief in Middle Eastern healing systems. In this case, illness is caused by someone who is envious of another and speaks about the person without invoking the name of God or the Cross. Children are often victims of evil eye and exhibit symptoms such as refusal to breast-feed, tremors, seizures, crying spells, and either pallor or cyanotic skin color changes. It is cured by seeking the *Raki* (indigenous healer) who uses prayers and incense for curing. It may also be prevented through wearing charms or religious amulets.

Methods of Healing

Treatment of illness may take the form of religious rites as mentioned previously. When an individual suffers from atmospheric temperature changes, the cure may consist of massaging sore muscles with oil, drinking hot lemonade for colds, and, in severe cases, use of "air cups" (*hujam*). Cotton soaked in alcohol is placed in the glass air cup and lit. The cups are placed on the afflicted areas, usually the back, for 3 to 10 minutes. The cups are thought to relieve chest congestion by increasing blood flow to the area. Fever is treated by placing the individual under many blankets to "sweat it out" (Meleis & Hattar-Pollara, 1995).

Western biomedicine is readily accepted by Middle Eastern American women. It is seen as powerful even though there still the sense that healing is in the hands of God. However, when Middle Eastern clients are hospitalized, the health care providers are expected to provide complete care to the highest degree possible. Self-care is not a value of Middle Eastern clients and may present a conflict with providers (Meleis, Omidian, & Lipson, 1993).

Statistics are unavailable regarding the incidence of disease. However, residents of the poorer countries of the Middle East suffer from infectious diseases, parasitic diseases, iron deficiency anemia, malnutrition, and a high rate of infant, child, and maternal mortality. The more affluent countries are seeing a rise in cardiovascular disease, cancer, cerebrovascular disease, and diabetes. It is not known if Middle Eastern immigrants exhibit the same patterns after residing in the United States.

There is a high rate of fertility among Middle Eastern American women as children and family are highly valued. There are a variety of rituals to celebrate the newborn's survival of the first week. Women observe a 40-day postpartum period in which they are cared for by their husbands and family. The woman is given a high-protein diet with much chicken and other meat. Breast-feeding is usually continued for the first 2 years of life.

SPECIAL CONCERNS RELATED TO GENDER AND HEALTH

Homeless Women in America

Homelessness has been increasing since the 1980s with changes in age and gender. In the past, the majority of the homeless were men over the age of 50. Today, more are women, particularly of African-American and Hispanic/Latino origin. These women may be single or the head of homeless families. Typically, the children are under 5 years of age, and the average number of children in homeless families is approximately 2.3 (Dornbusch, 1993).

Causes of homelessness range from societal problems of poverty, deindustrialization, divorce, declining employment opportunities, and low wage—earning jobs keeping individuals under the poverty limit while still being employed. Lack of affordable housing and social support also contribute to homelessness (Dornbusch, 1993).

Health and Illness Patterns

Many homeless women wait to seek health care services until the illness becomes severe. They may experience shame and ridicule from health care providers who may have a "blame-the-victim" mentality. They have no money or insurance to pay for services and lack necessary transportation to health services.

Malnutrition, substance abuse, mental health disorders (depression, anxiety, and personality disorders) are major health issues for the homeless. Other health problems include tuberculosis, impetigo, eczema, scabies, lice, diarrhea, urinary tract infections, cellulitis, dental problems, trauma (lacerations, abrasions, rape), and environmentally related problems such as hypothermia, heat stroke, and sunburn (Semien & Semien, 1995; Usatine, Gelberg, Smith, & Lesser, 1994).

There is a dearth of information regarding homelessness and its current impact on the health status of women from diverse cultures. More research targeted toward this fluid population is needed to begin addressing their social and health concerns.

Immigrants and Refugees in America

Immigrants and refugees have many similarities, but it is important to distinguish between the two groups. Immigrants may come to the United States for many reasons: marriage, employment opportunities, educational opportunities, family reunification, or they may simply seek the chance to build a new life. Refugees present a different picture. They are usually fleeing a dangerous situation in a war-torn country. They may leave their country with nothing but what they can carry. They may have experienced the death of family and friends, life in a refugee camp, and perhaps torture.

Health and Illness Patterns

The stress of relocating and acculturation produce major effects on the health of both immigrant and refugee women. Women experience conflict between the demands of being a mother and having few job skills to support the family. They may also feel isolated from members of their own cultural group for political or religious reasons. Also they may experience the stress of isolation if they too readily acculturate or completely identify with American values. Wilson (1995) suggests the need to find balance between maintaining cultural customs that are positive while adapting to the different values within the United States.

Koucharang, or "thinking too much," has been identified as a culture-bound syndrome found among Cambodian refugees now living in the United States. It is considered a direct result of stress from being a refugee and manifests itself through headaches, chest pain, palpitations, shortness of breath, excessive sleep, and general withdrawal behavior. Management of *koucharang* includes nonconfrontational methods, such as by speaking softly and actively discouraging refugees from thinking sad thoughts. Researchers have noted incongruities between reported management of *koucharang* and actual behavior. Many family members appear to withdraw from ill persons, leaving them alone to deal with their stress (Fry & D'Avanzo, 1994).

Health issues affecting Afghan refugee women, one of the largest refugee populations, include access to health care and culturally insensitive health care. For example, strict rules of modesty prevent women from removing their clothes for an examination and being examined by male providers. In Afghanistan, male physicians perform an assessment while being separated from the women by a screen. Other health concerns voiced by Afghan refugee women relate to lack of information regarding normal body processes, such as menstruation and menopause. The problem of spouse abuse is now being confronted by educated Afghan women who want to help themselves and others to find solutions to this problem (Lipson, Hosseini, Kabir, Omidian, & Edmonston, 1995).

Wilson (1995) provides suggestions for health care providers to improve the health of immigrant and refugee women. Education is the primary intervention that should be utilized. Women need information regarding routine health care schedules and available resources in the community that provide health care services at minimal or no cost.

Women in Rural America

Women in the rural United States suffer from stereotyping in the same way that women from various ethnic groups do. One perception is that these women are strong, "hard," and capable of meeting the physical demands of an agrarian lifestyle while at the same time producing numerous children and tending to domestic needs of the family. Women are not viewed apart from the context of the family and the marital relationship (LaGodna, 1981). However, Bushy (1993) emphasizes the diversity among rural women and the social context of family and the community in which they live.

Over 30 million individuals in the United States are classified as dwelling in rural areas. Characteristics of rural families include an increased number of elderly members of the family, a decreased number of children, and more females than males in the community. Economically, rural communities have more intergenerational family businesses, lower salaries, and increased rates of unemployment and underemployment (Bushy, 1993).

Women, in particular, face numerous challenges in rural areas when they lose their spouses through divorce, chronic illness, or death. Typically, these women are middle-aged to elderly and face financial crises because they may not have sufficient educational skills or employment history. Compounding this issue is the social norm among rural families to not discuss their problems, financial or otherwise, with friends or family (Bushy, 1993).

Health and Illness Patterns

Rural women often have difficulty accessing health care services. In today's world of managed care, community hospitals may be closed or offer a decreased number of services. Women may need to travel long distances to receive health care as well as having the additional worry of how to pay for it. Finances are often a greater concern than distance and transport. For example, a 100-mile trip to the clinic or hospital may not be considered an excessive distance if it can be combined with shopping and other activities that may be done on the same trip (Bushy, 1993).

Of more concern are the multiple roles and role strain women experience in rural communities. Women are expected to be nurturers of the family without having anyone to turn to *themselves*. Self-esteem may decrease as they are unable to fulfill all expectations of family and community, with depression the end result. Bushy (1993) advises health care providers to help rural women recognize their strengths and incorporate their definitions of health and illness into the plan of care. In addition, partnerships with informal and formal community leaders should be established to plan and implement services to women. These services should also be integrated with existing community activities, such as county fairs, church activities, and local cooperatives.

Female Circumcision

Female circumcision continues to be practiced throughout Africa, Asia, and the Arab world today. The World Health Organization (1994) estimates that between 85 and 114 million girls from infancy through adolescence have undergone this procedure. Types of female circumcision include.

Clitoridectomy—Removal of the clitoris; may be partial or total

Excision—Removal of the clitoris and labia minora

Infibulation—also known as *Pharaonic circumcision*; removal of clitoris, labia minora, and
    the inner surface of the labia majora; the vulva may be stitched together leaving a
    small opening for urine and menstrual fluid

The surgery is typically done without anesthesia or sterile instruments. Immediate complications, especially with infibulation include hemorrhage, infection, and tetany. Long-term complications are urinary tract infections, renal/urethral calculi formation, keloids, infertility, fistulas, and chronic pelvic infections. Episiotomy may be necessary before the first experience of sexual intercourse with infibulation or intercourse will be traumatic. Episiotomy is also necessary at labor and delivery (Calder, Brown, & Rae, 1993).

Given the traumatic circumstances and long-term sequelae of female circumcision, EuroAmerican health care providers may be surprised that the surgery continues to be performed with the consent of parents. Lane and Rubinstein (1996) provide an insightful analysis of the ethics of performing such surgeries. Reported reasons for having circumcision done include maintaining virginity until marriage, maintaining tradition (not religious tradition as female circumcision predates Christianity and Islam), increased sexual pleasure for the husband, economic security as a future husband may desire infibulation, protection of the girl against rape, and hygiene and aesthetics (Calder, Brown, & Rae, 1993; Lane & Rubinstein, 1996). Douglas (1998) reports that information related to conducting "safe" female circumcision is being sought from women who are educated and living in urban areas, dispelling the myth that female circumcision is performed only on uneducated girls of low socioeconomic status.

Health care providers in the United States are caring for women who have been circumcised. Sensitivity in caring for these women especially during labor and delivery is crucial. Women health care providers are preferred by these women. Including the family and husband in discussion of the plan of care is also important as their approval may be required before interventions are initiated (Calder, Brown, & Rae, 1993).

SUMMARY

There is no simple way to approach the inclusion of cultural concepts in health care. Differences exist among individuals of all cultural groups and these differences warrant careful consideration.

While it is critical to learn the cultural ideals in any setting, it is equally important to assess the degree to which lived behavior adheres to the stated ideal (Weeks, Singer, Grier, & Schensul, 1996, p. 357).

Recommendations for future research and development of practice guidelines include the following:
1. Development of new definitions of health based on the lives of women. Health must be considered not only from an individual perspective but also within the context of family and community norms and expectations.
2. Improvement in data collection related to demographics and health statistics and identification of cultural subgroups.
3. Consideration of the historical context of cultural groups, including slavery, policies related to American Indians/Alaskan Natives, waves of immigration, and refugee status.
4. Assessment of the effects of uprooting and acculturation among women, including stressors impacting women's perceptions of health.
5. Efforts to minimize or alleviate the impact of race, gender, and poverty on delivery of health care services.

REFERENCES

Andrews, M. M., & Boyle, J. S. (1999). *Transcultural concepts in nursing care.* Philadelphia: Lippincott.
Baldwin, D., Cotanch, P., Johnson, P., & Williams, J. (1996). *An Afrocentric approach to breast and cervical cancer early detection and screening.* Washington, DC: American Nurses Association.
Bannerman, R. H. (1983). The role of traditional medicine. In R. H. Bannerman (Ed.), *Traditional medicine and health care coverage.* Geneva: World Health Organization.
Bayne-Smith, M. (1996). Health and women of color: A contextual overview. In M. Bayne-Smith (Ed.), *Race, gender, and health* (pp. 1–42). Thousand Oaks, CA: Sage.

Beardsley, E. H. (1990). Race as a factor in health. In R. Apple (Ed.), *Women, health, and medicine in America: A historical handbook*. New York: Garland.

Beyenne, Y. (1986). *From menarche to menopause: Reproductive lives of peasant women in two cultures*. Albany: State University of New York Press.

Bohn, D. K. (1993). Nursing care of Native American battered women. *Issues in Perinatal and Women's Health Nursing, 4*, 424–436.

Brink, P. S., & Saunders, J. M. (1976). Culture shock: Theoretical and applied. In P. J. Brink (Ed.), *Transcultural nursing: A book of readings*. Englewood Cliffs, NJ: Prentice-Hall.

Burks, J. D. (1992). Factors in the utilization of prenatal services by low-income black women. *Nurse Practitioner, 17*, 34, 46–49.

Bushy, A. (1993). Rural women: Lifestyle and health status. *Nursing Clinics of North America, 28*, 187–197.

Calder, B. L., Brown, Y. M. R., & Rae, D. I. (1993). Female circumcision/genital mutilation: Culturally sensitive care. *Health Care for Women International, 14*, 227–238.

Camino, L. A. (1989). Nerves, worriation, and black women: A community study in the American South. *Health Care for Women International, 10*(2/3), 295–314.

DeSantis, L. (1988). The relevance of transcultural nursing to international nursing. *International Nursing Review, 35*, 110.

Dornbusch, S. M. (1993). Some political implications of the Stanford studies of homeless families. In S. Matteo (Ed.), *American women in the nineties* (pp. 158–172). Boston: Northeastern University Press.

Douglas, J. H. (1998). Female circumcision: Persistence and conflict. *Health Care for Women International, 19*, 477–479.

Douglas, M., & Meleis, A. (1985). International nursing: Challenges and consequences. *Mobius, 5*, 84.

Edwards, K. (1993). Low income African-American women: Expressions of their health management. *The American Black Nurses Foundation Journal, 10*, 17–19.

Eng, P. (1995). Domestic violence in Asian/Pacific Island communities. In D. L. Adams (Ed.), *Health issues for women of color* (pp. 78–99). Thousand Oaks, CA: Sage.

Foster, G. M., & Anderson, B. G., (1978). *Medical anthropology*. New York: Alfred A. Knopf.

Fry, B. A., & D'Avanzo, C. D. (1994). Cultural themes in family stress and violence among Cambodian refugee women in the inner city. *Advances in Nursing Science, 16*, 64–77.

Gary, F., Campbell, D., & Serlin, C. (1996). African American women: Disparities in health care. *Journal of the Florida Medical Association, 83*, 489–493.

Giachello, A. L. (1995). Cultural diversity and institutional inequality. In D. L. Adams (Ed.), *Health issues for women of color* (pp. 5–26). Thousand Oaks, CA: Sage.

Giachello, A. L. (1996). Latino women. In M. Bayne-Smith (Ed.), *Race, gender, and health* (pp. 121–171). Thousand Oaks, CA: Sage.

Giger, J. N., & Davidhizar, R. E. (1990). Transcultural nursing assessment: A method for advancing nursing practice. *International Nursing Review, 37*, 17–20.

Giger, J. N., & Davidhizar, R. E. (1991). *Transcultural nursing: Assessment and intervention*. St. Louis: Mosby.

Greene, B. (1996). African American women: Considering diverse identities and societal barriers in psychotherapy. *Annals of New York Academy of Sciences, 789*, 191–209.

Guendelman, S., & Abrams, B. (1994). Dietary, alcohol, and tobacco intake among Mexican-American women of childbearing age: Results of HANES study. *American Journal of Health Promotion, 8*, 363–372.

Hall, E. (1988). Introduction. In M. Matsumoto (Ed.), *The unspoken way*. Tokyo: Kodansha International.

Hall, E. (1963). Proxemics: The study of a man's spatial relations. In I. Gladston (Ed.), *Man's image in medicine and anthropology* (pp. 109–120). New York: International University Press.

Hann, H. W. L. (1994). Hepatitis B. In N. W. Zane, D. T. Takeuchi, & K. N. Young (Eds.), *Confronting critical health issues of Asian and Pacific Islander Americans* (pp. 148–172). Thousand Oaks, CA: Sage.

Hargrove, H. J., & Keller, C. (1993). Young black women: Defining health. *Journal of the National Black Nurses Association, 6*, 3–14.

Helman, C. G. (1994). *Culture, health, and illness*. Oxford: Butterworth Heinemann.

Henkle, J. (1979). International nursing: A speciality? *International Nursing Review, 26*, 170.

Indian Health Service. (1997). *Trends in Indian health*. Rockville, MD: U. S. Department of Health and Human Services.

Jackson, C., & Haynes, T. (1992). *Cultural sensitivity: A working model.* Atlanta: Southern Council on Collegiate Education for Nursing.

Jenkins, C. M., & Kagawa-Singer, M. (1994). Cancer. In N. W. Zane, D. T. Takeuchi, & K. N. Young, (Eds.), *Confronting critical health issues of Asian and Pacific Islander Americans* (pp. 105–147). Thousand Oaks, CA: Sage.

Kagawa-Singer, M. (1995). Socioeconomic and cultural influences on cancer care of women. *Seminars in Oncology Nursing, 11*(2), 109–119.

Kaufert, P. (1996). The social and cultural context of menopause. *Maturitas, 23,* 169–180.

Kauffman, J. A., & Joseph-Fox, Y. K. (1996). American Indians and Alaska Native women. In M. Bayne-Smith (Ed.), *Race, gender, and health* (pp. 68–93). Thousand Oaks, CA: Sage.

Kleinman, A. (1980). *Patients and healers in the context of culture.* Berkeley: University of California Press.

Kluckhohn, K., & Strodtbeck, F. (1961). *Variations in value orientations.* New York: Row, Peterson.

LaGodna, G. E. (1981). The single rural woman: Invisible struggles. *Advances in Nursing Science, 3,* 11–17.

Lane, S. D., & Rubinstein, R. A. (1996). Judging the other: Responding to traditional female genital surgeries. *Hastings Center Report, 26*(3), 31–40.

Lee, M. (1992). Breast and cervical cancer in Asian and Pacific Islander women. *Asian American Health Forum Focus, 3,* 2.

Leigh, W. A. (1995). The health of African American women. In D. L. Adams (Ed.), *Health issues for women of color.* Thousand Oaks, CA: Sage.

Leininger, M. (1970). *Nursing and anthropology: Two worlds to blend.* New York: John Wiley & Sons.

Leininger, M. (1978). *Transcultural nursing: Concepts, theories, and practices.* New York: John Wiley & Sons.

Leininger, M. (1988). Leininger's theory of nursing: Cultural care diversity and universality. *Nursing Science Quarterly, 1*(4), 152–160.

Leininger, M. (1991). *Culture care diversity and universality: A theory of nursing.* New York: National League for Nursing Press.

Lendburg, C. B., Lipson, J. E., Demi, A. S., Blaney, D. R., Stern, P. N., Schultz, P. R., et al. (Eds.). (1995). *Promoting cultural competence in and through nursing education.* Washington, DC: American Academy of Nursing.

Lillie-Blanton, M., Martinez, R. M., Taylor, A. K., & Robinson, B. G. (1993). Latina and African American women: Continuing disparities in health. *International Journal of Health Services, 23,* 555–583.

Lipson, J. G., Hosseini, T., Kabir, S., Omidian, P. A., & Edmonston, F. (1995). Health issues among Afghan women in California. *Health Care for Women International, 16,* 279–286.

Litoff, J. (1986). *The American midwife debate: Source book on modern origins.* Westport, CT: Greenwood.

Litt, I. F. (1993). Health issues for women in the 1990s. In S. Matteo (Ed.), *American women in the nineties.* Boston: Northeastern University Press.

Magaña, A., & Clark, N. M. (1995). Examining a paradox: Does religiosity contribute to positive birth outcomes in Mexican American populations? *Health Evaluation Quarterly, 22,* 96–109.

McBarnette, L. S. (1996). African American women. In M. Bayne-Smith (Ed.), *Race, gender, and health* (pp. 43-67). Thousand Oaks, CA: Sage.

Meleis, A. I., & Hattar-Pollara, M. (1995). Arab Middle Eastern American women. In D. L. Adams (Ed.), *Health issues for women of color* (pp. 133–163) Thousand Oaks, CA: Sage.

Meleis, A. I., Omidian, P. A., & Lipson, J. G. (1993). Women's health status in the United States: An immigrant women's project. In B. J. McElmurry, K. F. Noor, & R. S. Parker (Eds.), *Women's health and development.* Boston: Jones and Bartlett.

Menendez, B. S. (1990). AIDS-related mortality among Puerto Rican women in New York City, 1981–1987. *Puerto Rican Health Science Journal, 9,* 43–45.

Moormeier, J. (1996). Breast cancer in black women. *Annals of Internal Medicine, 124,* 897–905.

National Center of Health Statistics (NCHS) (1995). *Health, United States.* Hyattsville, MD: Public Health Service.

National Women's Health Information Center (2000). *Health information for minority women* [On-line]. *http://www.4women.gov/minority/causes.htm.*

Nightingale, F. (1894) cited in S. Dobson (1983). Bringing culture into care. *Nursing Times,* Feb. 9, 53–57.

Orque, M. S., Bloch, B., & Monrroy, S. A. (1983). *Ethnic nursing care: A multicultural approach.* St. Louis: Mosby.

Otten, M., Teutsch, S., Williamson, D., & Marks, J. (1990). The effect of known risk factors on the excess mortality of black adults in the United States, *Journal of the American Medical Association, 263,* 845–850.

Pinn, V. W. (1995). The status of women's health research: where are African American women? *Journal of the National Black Nurses Association, 10,* 8–19.

Plawecki, H. M., Sanchez, T. R., & Plawecki, J. A. (1994). Cultural aspects of caring for Navajo Indian clients. *Journal of Holistic Nursing, 12,* 291–306.

Potter, P., & Perry A. (2001). *Fundamentals of nursing* (5th ed.). St. Louis: Mosby.

Roessel, R. (1992). *Questions and answers dealing with Navajo healing.* Conference presentation, Tsaile, AZ.

Rorie, J. L., Paine, L. L., & Garner, M. K. (1996). Cultural competence in primary care services. *Journal of Nurse-Midwifery, 41,* 92–100.

Rosenburg, L., Adams-Campbell, L., & Palmer, J. R. (1995). The black women's health study: A follow-up for causes and prevention of illness, *Journal of the American Medical Women's Association, 50,* 56–58.

Rowell, R. M. (1997). Update on HIV/AIDS among American Indians and Alaskan Natives. *The IHS Primary Care Provider, 22,* 49–53.

Scrimshaw, S. L., & Burleigh, E. (1978). The potential for the integration of indigenous and western medicine in Latin American and Hispanic populations in the United States of America. In B. Velimiracoic (Ed.), *Modern medicine and medical anthropology in the United States–Mexico border population.* Washington, DC: Pan American Health Organization.

Semien, S., & Semien, S. (1995). The growth of homelessness in America: Health concerns. In D. C. Adams (Ed.), *Health issues for women of color* (pp. 188–196). Thousand Oaks, CA: Sage.

Shum, L. M. (1996). Asian-American women: Cultural and mental health issues. *Annals of the New York Academy of Sciences, 789,* 181–190.

Spector, R. (1991). *Cultural diversity in health and illness.* Norwalk, CT: Appleton & Lange.

Strickland, C. J., Chrisman, N. J., Yallup, M., Powell, K. & Squeoch, M. D. (1996). Walking the journey of womanhood: Yakama Indian women and Papanicolaou (Pap) test screening. *Public Health Nursing, 13,* 141–150.

Tang, G. (1993). *Menopause: the situation in Hong Kong Chinese women.* Paper presented at the Seventh International Congress on the Menopause, Stockholm.

Tom-Orme, L. (1995). Native American women's health concerns: Toward restoration of harmony. In D. L. Adams (Ed.), *Health issues for women of color* (pp. 27–41). Thousand Oaks, CA: Sage.

Torres, S., & Villarruel, A. M. (1995). Health risk behaviors for hispanic women. *Annual Review of Nursing Research, 13,* 293–319.

Tripp-Reimer, T. (1984). Cultural assessment: Content and process. *Nursing Outlook, 32,* 78.

True, R. H. (1995). Mental health issues of Asian/Pacific Island women. In D. L. Adams (Ed.), *Health issues for women of color* (pp. 89–111). Thousand Oaks, CA: Sage.

True, R. H., & Guillermo, T. (1996). Asian/Pacific Islander American women. In M. Bayne-Smith (Ed.), *Race, gender, and health* (pp. 94–120). Thousand Oaks, CA; Sage.

U. S. Bureau of the Census. (1995). *Statistical abstract of the United States.* Washington, DC: U. S. Government Printing Office.

U. S. Bureau of the Census. (2000). *Geographical mobility (update).* Washington, DC: U. S. Government Printing Office.

Usatine, R. P., Gelberg, G., Smith, M. H., & Lesser, J. (1994). Health care for the homeless: A family medicine perspective. *American Family Physician, 49,* 139–146.

Vera, M. (1996). Health care of Latina women. *Journal of the Florida Medical Association, 83,* 494–497.

Wang, G. M. (1995). Health issues for Asian/Pacific Island women. In D. L. Adams (Ed.), *Health issues for women of color* (pp. 71–77). Thousand Oaks, CA: Sage.

Watts, L. K. & Gutierres, S. E. (1997). A Native American–based cultural model of substance dependency and recovery. *Human Organization, 56,* 9–18.

Weeks, M. R., Singer, M., Grier, M., & Schensul, J. J. (1996). Gender relations, sexuality, and AIDS risk among African Americans and Latina women. In C. F. Sargent, & C. B. Bretthell (Eds.), *Gender and health: An international perspective* (pp. 338–370). Upper Saddle River, NJ: Prentice-Hall.

Wilson, D. (1995). Women's roles and women's health: The effect of immigration on Latina women. *Women's Health Issues, 5,* 8–14.

World Health Organization (1976). *African traditional medicine.* Brazzaville: World Health Organization.

World Health Organization (1994). WHO leads the action against female genital mutilation. *World Health Forum, 15,* 416.

Zambrana, R. E., & Ellis, B. K. (1995). Contemporary research issues in Hispanic/Latino women's health. In D. C. Adams (Ed.), *Health issues for women of color* (pp. 42–70). Thousand Oaks, CA: Sage.

Zapata, J., & Shippee-Rice, R. (1999). The use of folk healing and healers by six Latinos living in New England: A preliminary study. *Journal of Transcultural Nursing, 10*, 136–142.

Zwingmann, C. A., & Gunn, A. D. (1983). *Uprooting and health: Psychosocial problems of students from abroad.* Geneva: World Health Organization.

RESOURCES

Asian Institute on Domestic Violence: *www.apiahf.org*

National Coalition Against Domestic Violence: *www.ncadv.org*

Family Violence & Sexual Assault Institute: *www.fvsai.org*

Asian American and Pacific Islander Women's Health: *www.4woman.gov/faq/Asian-Pacific.htm*

Association of Asian Pacific Community Health Organizations: (510) 272-9536

National Asian Women's Health Organization: (415) 989-9747

Asian and Pacific Islander American Health Forum: (415) 954-9988

Latina Women's Health: *www.4woman.gov/faq/latina.htm*

Minority Women: *www.4woman.gov/faq/minority.htm*

Frequently Asked Questions about Women's Health: African-American Women's Health: *www.4women.gov/faq/african_american.htm*

Office of Minority Health Resource Center: *www.omhrc.gov/* **or (800) 444-6472**

Caribbean Women's Health Association: *www.cwha.org/* **or (718) 826-2942**

African-American Breast Cancer Alliance: *www.vmmc.org/dbBreastCancer/sec2500.htm* **or (612) 825-3675**

National Black Women's Health Project: (202) 835-0117

National Coalition of Hispanic Health and Human Services Organizations: *www.cehn.org/cehn/resourceguide/nchhso.html*

Office of Research on Minority Health: *www.louisville.edu/library/ekstrom/govpubs/federal/agencies/hhs/ormh.html*

Chapter 4

Women's Environmental Health

Maria Alvarez Amaya

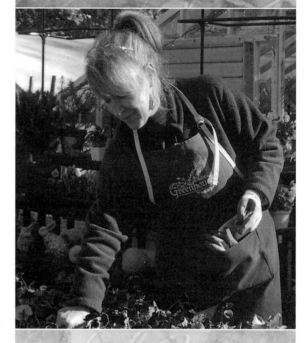

The close interaction of nurses with patients and 'on-site' aspects of nursing care provide tremendous opportunities for nurses to detect previously unrecognized health problems, including those related to environmental exposures, and to initiate appropriate interventions.

Institute of Medicine

INTRODUCTION

Environmental pollution on a global scale is perhaps the most notable unintended consequence of industrial and technological development of the twentieth century. Despite a growing body of evidence that hazardous environmental exposures impart cumulative and interactive effects on human health, the extent of the threat remains largely unknown. Hazardous environmental exposures may be the single largest unknown risk to human health that the world has ever known. During the latter half of this century more than 65,000 new chemicals were introduced into the environment. Currently, there are over 72,000 chemicals in commercial use (Institute Of Medicine, 1995), and most have never been tested for their effect on human health.

Twenty-first century women's health nurses must be adequately prepared to care for the explosive growth of clients affected by toxic exposures. The majority of cases will present not with acute toxicity but with the subtle and perplexing signs and symptoms of chronic, low-dose, and/or concomitant multiple exposures. The challenge lies, not in what is known, but in what is unknown about concomitant, chronic, low-dose toxic exposures and women's health. The first step in meeting role challenges posed by women's environmental health needs is to address education and skill gaps of women's health nurses.

Women's health nurses are key stakeholders in the interdisciplinary environmental health team. Their presence and leadership is critical to women's health outcomes. This chapter provides an overview of environmental health within a contextual framework for women's health nursing practice.

WOMEN'S ENVIRONMENTAL HEALTH AND ENVIRONMENTAL JUSTICE

Disparities in the risk of toxic exposures are based not only on race and class but also on gender. Women are disproportionately burdened by the effect of toxic exposures because more of them live in poverty. Furthermore, through the influence of childbearing, the effects of women's toxic exposures impact the entire human race.

Environmental justice refers to the socially based risk inequities of toxic exposures. Environmental injustice presumes that the poor and disenfranchised are disproportionately more likely to live near toxic sites, to eat contaminated food, and to breathe toxic fumes. In turn, toxic sites are disproportionately more likely to be found near ghettos, barrios, reservations, and in third-world-like communities. The burden is made worse by the lack of material, political, and psychological resources. The greatest toxic burden is borne by women who are racial minorities, low-income, live in substandard housing, and/or are employed in risky jobs. For example, undocumented immigrant women employed in sweat shops or agricultural fields endure overwhelming toxic exposures that are shocking to the mainstream world.

While the environmental justice movement has made great strides against environmental racism, it has utterly failed to focus attention on environmental sexism. Just as an understanding of racial context is essential to environmental justice so is an understanding of environmental sexism a key to women's environmental health.

GENES, ENVIRONMENT, AND BEHAVIOR

Disease resulting from environmental exposure is a consequence of the effect of complex interactions among a multiplicity of factors, including stressors and defenses, on the biological structure. The outcome of a particular toxic exposure is mediated by genetic makeup, the internal and external environment, and behavior. Female biological function is influenced by puberty and maintenance throughout the reproductive years of hormonal cycles that enable pregnancy, childbearing, birth, and lactation. Exposures to chemical and biological agents can disrupt and corrupt female reproductive cycles to various degrees.

Women who live in substandard housing, older homes, or in proximity to municipal waste incinerators are at risk for exposure to lead, chromium, and/or asbestos. Their income and educational level may preclude appropriate nutrition and health promotion behaviors that would ameliorate the toxic response—such as hand washing and adequate iron intake. Other individual behaviors, such as using toxic folk remedies or purchasing consumer products that contain lead, may increase vulnerability. During pregnancy, lead may cross the placental barrier. After menopause, increased osteoclast activity in bones may release sequestered lead from the bone and contribute to kidney disease.

Risk assessment and risk communication in environmental health nursing takes into account the whole client-environment interaction process. Therefore assessment of the individual or group, access to resources, inherent defenses, and external threats guide interventions designed to prevent or ameliorate the effects of hazardous environmental exposures.

Multiple factors and interactions may explain the prevalence of affected babies born to mothers who consume mercury-tainted seafood during pregnancy or account for the high rate of neural tube defects on the Texas-Mexican border. Canfield and others (1996) found an association between neural tube defects and poverty among Hispanic women. We may find that neural tube defects on the Texas-Mexico border may be explained by the interaction of a defect in folic acid metabolism (a gene-mediated factor), insufficient folic acid intake (behavior and environment), and exposure to environmental hazards.

WOMEN'S WORK AND ENVIRONMENTAL HEALTH

Women of all races and ethnic groups represent about half of the U.S. labor force at any given point in time. However, women workers are disproportionately over-represented in low-paying jobs. Gender-based pay disparity is persistent and consistent across the economic matrix as are gender-based differences in real wages, benefits, number of hours, and job security. Women remain disproportionately represented among minimum wage workers, persons in poverty, and single-parent households (United States Department of Labor, Women's Bureau, 1993; 1997). As a group, women wield less power to negotiate workplace conditions than do other groups, such as men and union members.

On the other hand, workplace regulations intended to protect women from hazardous exposures have had discriminatory effects. Historically, the prevention of such exposures in the workplace has had the unintended consequence of denying the right to work to women of childbearing age. For example, permanent sterilization was one strategy used at the beginning of the twentieth century to prevent noxious reproductive outcomes.

Of course, both men and women are at risk of exposures to human-made or natural environmental hazards in the workplace and to all the health hazards associated with such exposures. However, significant sex-based differences are known or suspected in human responses to a variety of toxic exposures. Unfortunately, research on sex-based responses to environmental exposures lags far behind other research.

Data from the Women's Bureau of the U.S. Department of Labor have shed light on the types of occupations that warrant assessment for environmental exposures among women. Hair dressers, cosmetologists, and janitors, for example, may present in the clinical setting with reactions to formaldehyde-based disinfectants, bleaching agents, detergents, and latex. These reactions are commonly manifested as dishydrotic eczema of the hands or other contact dermatoses. Acute reactive airway episodes may result from inhaling chloramine gas, produced by mixing bleach and ammonia products. Office workers may manifest the effects of exposure to organochlorine pesticides or polychlorinated biphenyls—the "sick building syndrome." Women war veterans may have been exposed to agents used in chemical and biological warfare. Finally, it is helpful to remember that housekeeping (that most universal of women's occupations) can offer a risk of hazardous exposure within a range that rivals almost any workplace.

The Nursing Profession

All nurses should initiate environmental health awareness by assessing their own risk of hazardous exposure in the workplace as well as providing prevention of health care–related pollution. Nurses may be at risk for exposure to latex, glutaraldehyde (a chemical used for disinfection of instruments), methyl methacrylate (an orthopedic surgery adhesive), powdered biological products (such as psyllium, anesthetics, chemotherapeutic agents), ionizing radiation and radiopharmaceuticals, lead, and mercury. In addition, nursing activities may also be the source of significant amounts of environmental pollution.

Nurses share a moral obligation to address the problem of pollution generated by health care delivery systems. For example, over-reliance on mercury devices poses a serious, yet needless, risk to health care workers and patients. Medical devices that contain mercury include mercury thermometers, blood pressure monitoring devices, mercury-containing Miller-Abbott tubes, cantor tubes, and fluorescent lighting tubes. It is possible to reduce this risk through alternative purchasing policies and disposal practices (Shaner, 1996; Sperrazza, 1998).

Lead exposure remains a problem as well. Battery-powered or battery-supported devices are in heavy use in nearly every hospital unit. Batteries differ in their geometry, chemical composition, and level of toxicity. Some batteries may be recycled, while others need to be disposed of as toxic waste. Improper disposal of used battery acid can result in toxic lead and cadmium exposure. Battery recovery practices significantly reduce this risk (Shaner, 1996; Sperrazza, 1998).

According to the Centers for Disease Control and Prevention only about 2% of waste that comes from hospitals in "red bags" really needs to be incinerated (Sperrazza, 1998). Although most hospital waste can be properly disposed of in landfills, "red bag" containers often become the receptacles for plastic packaging, IV bags, tubing, urine collection bags, used gloves, blood pressure cuffs, thermometers and batteries, newspapers, magazines, pizza boxes, and other trash, thereby increasing the quantity of "red bag" waste (Shaner, 1996; Sperrazza, 1998). Plastics account for approximately one third of medical waste weight. Some plastic products are chlorinated and, when incinerated, release dioxin or dioxin-like compounds (Howlett et al., 1996, Thornton, McCally, Orris, & Weinberg, 1996). Medical waste incineration is among the largest sources of dioxin emissions nation wide.

Organizations such as Health Care Without Harm (*http://www.sustain.org/hcwh)*, the Nightingale Institute for Health (*http://www.nihe.org*), and state nursing associations have useful web resources to promote nursing involvement in environmentally responsible health care as well as prevention of workplace exposures.

Hazardous Agents (Table 4-1)

Most data on the effects of chemical exposures on reproductive health, conception, pregnancy, and lactation are based on animal studies. Factors such as chemical properties, dosage, duration, timing of exposure, and genetics account for health effects of exposures. A single high dose of radiation at a critical time in development can be mutagenic, carcinogenic, or teratogenic. On the other hand, multiple exposures from thalidomide, diethylstilbestrol, folate antagonists, androgenic hormones, alcohol, anticonvulsants, warfarin, and 13-cis-retinoic acid may be required for fetal maldevelopment.

Sufficient evidence exists to suggest that exposure to one or a combination of teratogenic, genotoxic, and carcinogenic agents over time adversely affects women's reproductive health and the development of the fetus. Reproductive toxicants are agents that affect postpubertal female reproductive or sexual function. Developmental toxicants

Table 4-1	TOP HAZARDOUS SUBSTANCES	
AGENT	**SUSPECTED OR KNOWN ADVERSE EFFECT**	**EXPOSURE PATHWAY**
Lead	Miscarriage, premature birth, low birth weight, neurobehavioral disorders, multiple organ damage, anemia, encephalopathy, death	Ingestion of lead-based paint chips or contaminated foods and water; smoking; leaching from lead-soldered plumbing, ceramic pottery, and other consumer products; certain hobbies and crafts; proximity to municipal waste incinerator, smelting, and automotive industries
Arsenic	GI symptoms; anemia; impaired nerve function; "pins and needles" sensation; skin blotches and corns on palms, soles, and trunk; cancer of skin, liver, bladder, kidney, lung	Naturally occurring element; inorganic arsenic found in pesticides and wood preservatives, proximity to smelting and fossil fuel fumes; eating contaminated water, fish, shellfish
Mercury	Miscarriage, abnormal fetal growth, tremors, memory loss, kidney disease	Methylmercury bioaccumulation in fish and water; medical/dental occupations; certain face creams; proximity to chemical and metal processing; electrical, automotive, and building industries
Vinyl chloride Chloroethene Chloroethylene Ethylene monochloride	Dizziness, lack of muscle coordination, headache, unconsciousness, death; liver and lung damage; poor circulation and bone changes in fingertips; skin thickening (vinyl chloride disease); liver cancer	Used to make polyvinyl chloride (PVC) and released by burning contaminated waste; proximity to waste site, contaminated air, and water or vinyl chloride industries
Benzene	Leukemia, other cancers, birth defects, severe anemia, immune system suppression, menstrual disorders, small ovaries, death	Naturally emitted by volcanic explosions; tobacco smoke; proximity to gasoline stations, petroleum refineries, or chemical manufacturing; used in rubber, lubricants, dyes, detergents, drugs, adhesives; inhalation abuse agent (huffing); does not bioaccumulate

Table 4-1	TOP HAZARDOUS SUBSTANCES —CONT'D	
Polychlorin-ated biphenyls (PCBs) Aroclor 1260(12)* Aroclor 1254(14)*	Liver cancer, birth defects, fetal maldevelopment, acne-like lesions and rashes	Proximity to medical waste incinerators; bioaccumulation in fish; living or working in buildings with pre-1977 transformers and electrical equipment; building repair and maintenance
Cadmium	GI symptoms, kidney disease, emphysema, lung cancer	Bioaccumulation from eating contaminated food, smoking, gardening or agricultural work with phospate fertilizers; proximity to sewage sludge and smelters
Polycyclic aromatic hydro-carbons (PAHs) Benzo[a]-pyrene Benzo[b]-fluoran-thene(10)* Dibenz[a,h]-anthra-cene(17)*	Reproductive defects; skin, body fluids, immune system dysfunction in animal studies; probable carcinogen	Smoking; charcoal-grilling or charring; open burning; proximity to smoke houses; wood and coal burning; contact with creosote oil–treated wood; proximity to coal tar, coking, and asphalt production industries; proximity to municipal incinerators
Chloroform Fluoro-carbon 22 Ethylene dichloride	Fatigue, dizziness, and headache; liver and kidney damage (jaundice and burning on urination); probable carcinogen	Used in pesticide manufacturing and internal combustion engine industries, pulp and paper mills, and food processing industries; occupational exposure in paint stores; swimming in contaminated swimming pool
DDT, P' P' DDD, P' P'(19)*	Probable carcinogen; probable source of exogenous estrogens; excitability, tremors, or seizures; skin rash; eye, nose, or throat irritation	Bioaccumulation in contaminated fruits, vegetables, meat, fish, poultry, and milk (including human milk)
Tri-chloro-ethylene	Dizziness, headache, slowed reaction time, sleepiness, facial numbness; irritation of eyes, nose, and throat	Adhesive glues, paints, coatings, typewriter correction fluids, paint removers, paint strippers, spot removers, metal cleaners, air-cleaning process in waste treatment plants, burning of community and hazardous waste
Chromium (hexavalent chromium)	Acute short-term exposure results in irritation of skin and nasal mucosa, perforation of nasal septum; GI symptoms; kidney and liver effects; lung cancer	Smoking; inks; paints; paper; rubber and composition floor coverings; leather materials; magnetic tapes; stainless steel; toner powders used in copy machines; chemical industries (chromates, chrome-plated products, ferrochrome alloys, chrome pigments); leather tanning; battery, candle, dye, textile, and rubber manufacture
Chlordane	Convulsions, headaches, irritation, confusion, weakness, vision problems, GI symptoms; probable carcinogen	Living in houses treated with chlordane for termites, eating foods (e.g., corn) grown in chlordane-treated fields, fat of meat and milk from animals that eat chlordane-treated grass

*Industrial trade names or similar elements also on the priority list; their rank is given in parenthesis.

Continued

Table 4-1	TOP HAZARDOUS SUBSTANCES —CONT'D	
Hexachloro-butadiene[†]	Skin and eye irritation, kidney and liver damage; probable carcinogen	Chlorinated chemical manufacturing; solvent for organic chemicals; fire retardant for plastics, rubber, paint, paper, and electrical goods
Dieldrin Aldrin	Headache, dizziness, irritability, anorexia, nausea, muscle twitching, convulsions, loss of consciousness, death, probable carcinogen	Used in pesticides and bioaccumulates in food chain; proximity to areas treated for termites; eating food grown in treated soil; or eating products from exposed animals (fish, poultry, cows)

[†]Data from *Merck Index*. (ed. II). (1989). Rahway, NJ: Merck Publishers.
From *http://www.atsdr.cdc.gov/cxcx3.html*

affect growth, development, or function between conception and puberty. Teratogens are developmental toxicants that cause abnormal morphogenesis and result in structural malformation or birth defects. Genotoxic agents are mutagens that may affect both reproductive and developmental function. Carcinogens cause cell mutations that result in cancer (National Institute of Occupational Safety and Health, 1988).

Women's reproductive organs contain most of the body's estrogen cell receptors. Xenoestrogens (exogenous estrogens) act synergistically with natural estrogens to increase circulating estrogen levels and result in hyperestrogenic states. Reproductive toxicants that are known to have estrogenic properties include 1, 2-dibromo-3-chloropropane, hexachlorocyclohexane, lead, mercury, polycyclic aromatic hydrocarbons (benzo[a]pyrene), DDT, and polychlorinated biphenyls (PCBs).

Another significant threat to women's health emanates from those toxic agents that persist in the environment once they are released and bioaccumulate in the food chain to affect women's bodies. These include organochlorine pesticides (such as DDT), PCBs, dioxin, and heavy metals. Women's health problems thought to result from bioaccumulation of toxic agents include amenorrhea, menstrual disorders, endometriosis, breast and reproductive tract cancers, infertility, adverse pregnancy outcomes, hypertension, and dementia.

Another issue in women's environmental health is transmission of toxic agents to offspring through placental transfer or in breast milk. Organochlorine pesticides and PCBs in breast milk may become a widespread threat to infant health in coming years. Evidence suggests that currently a large proportion of the human race is born and lives with the highest toxic burdens ever known. Several studies are under way to assess the risks of breast-feeding in cohorts exposed to high levels of organochlorines and PCBs. The benefits of breast-feeding will become controversial in the new century.

DDT and Organochlorines

DDT is a type of organochlorine pesticide banned in the United States since 1972 but still used in many areas of the globe. Even in places where DDT has been banned, it is widely distributed in the soil and in the human and animal population. The body metabolizes DDT into DDE, which is stored in a woman's body fat until mobilized by physiologic processes such as pregnancy. DDT and other organochlorines are fat soluble and can, therefore, bioaccumulate in breast milk in alarming quantities. DDT and its metabolites are present in almost every human on earth (Procianoy & Schvartsman, 1981; Rogan et al., 1987).

Pesticides have been shown to cause neurotoxicity, genetic mutations (Siddiqui et al., 1983), prematurity (Procianoy & Schvartsman, 1981), and stillbirth in women with concurrent high levels of hexachlorocyclohexane and aldrin (Saxena, Siddiqui, & Kuuty, 1983). The infants of breast-feeding women with high DDT levels receive far greater doses than the 0.01 mg/kg/day thought to be safe by the World Health Organization (Siddiqui et al., 1981).

In 2000, the Environmental Protection Agency (EPA) removed Dursban (chlorpyrifos) from all over-the-counter home and garden products. About 800 consumer products contain chlorpyrifos, including Ortho Lawn Insect Spray, Real Kill Wasp & Hornet Killer II, and Spectracide Dursban Indoor & Outdoor Insect Control. The chemical was shown to cause brain damage in fetal rats. This pesticide belongs to the organophosphate family of compounds whose most potent cousins include nerve gases used as chemical weapons.

Polychlorinated Biphenyls (PCBs)

PCBs are so dangerous to human health that they were among the first twelve chemicals to be banned worldwide by the International Treaty on Persistent Organic Pollutants in 2000. PCBs were used in electrical wire insulation and lubricants beginning in the 1930s until they were banned in 1977. PCBs are stable compounds that bioaccumulate in the food chain and are absorbed in low doses that accumulate in body fat over time. PCBs are so fat soluble that they are easily passed into the breast milk from body stores. Tests have detected PCBs in virtually 100% of breast milk samples (Rogan et al., 1987). Infant toxicity is manifested by low birthweight, hyperbilirubinemia, a pigmentation syndrome, natal teeth, hypoplastic nails, scalp calcification, apathy, hypotonia, hyporeflexia, and low IQ scores (Gladen & Rogan, 1991; Rogan et al., 1986; 1987). Data suggest that the interactive effects of PCB and DDT exposure result in alteration of the normal maternal biochemistry necessary to expel the fetus after a demise (missed abortion) (Bercovici et al., 1983). PCBs are also powerful endocrine disruptors that produce aberrant estrogen metabolism.

Dioxin

Dioxin emissions emanate largely from burning plastic products. There are over 100 dioxin and dioxin-like chemical compounds. Dioxin is a known carcinogen and can also affect reproductive, endocrine, and immunologic function. Dioxin exposure may reduce a child's I.Q., even at very low doses. Nursing infants are at particular risk. Babies of exposed mothers may get 15,000 to 30,000 times the safe levels of dioxin through their mother's breast milk (Shaner, 1996). More data on long-term effects is forthcoming from studies being done in Seveso, Italy, where a massive dioxin release occurred in 1976.

Mercury
Mercury comes mainly from the burning of coal in power plants and incineration of mercury-containing waste. It finds its way into rivers, lake-beds, and oceans, converting into its most toxic form, methylmercury. The EPA estimates that 1.16 million women of childbearing age eat sufficient amounts of mercury-contaminated fish to pose a threat to childbearing outcomes. Approximately 60,000 infants are born each year with neurological damage because their mothers were poisoned with mercury (Schettler, Stein, Reich, Valenti, & Wallinga, 2000). Exposure to mercury results in central nervous system toxicity and affects kidney and liver function. Acute poisoning can result in pneumonitis, bronchitis, and bronchiolitis. Long-term low-dose exposure can result in muscle tremor, irritability, personality changes, and gingivitis.

Lead
Lead is a stable and persistant heavy metal considered a neurotoxic developmental teratogen at low doses. Disturbingly, there appears to be no threshold of safe exposure. Currently, the CDC defines the limit of acceptable exposure at less than or equal to 10 micrograms per deciliter (10 mcg/dL). However, research suggests molecular neurodevelopmental damage and neurological impairment at lower levels of exposure (Nihei, Desmond, McGlothan, Kuhlmann, & Guilarte, 2000). Fetuses, infants, and young children exposed to lead suffer the most devastating consequences. It is estimated that the prevalence rate of elevated lead levels would rise from 1.7 million to several millions if the threshold of 10 mcg/dL were updated to take account of the most current evidence on the effects of lead in children (Schettler et al., 2000). In 2000, the EPA set new lower limits for lead exposure from paint, dust, and soil and lowered the reporting threshold of industrial lead releases. This was the first time that the EPA addressed the limits of exposure in home settings.

Chronic low-level lead exposure harms a child's learning ability, memory and concentration and affects behavior. Moreover, children exposed to lead are more likely to have been exposed to other heavy metals and pesticides. Women exposed to lead as adults may develop problems during pregnancy and menopause, conditions that release stored lead into the bloodstream. Lead exposure may be the most visible environmental justice issue affecting women and children today. Lead abatement is difficult and complex, and chelation is medically risky. Fewer children are being tested, and more are being exposed. The coming years will see legal action similar to that seen against the tobacco industry. If successful, legal remedies will hold the lead industry financially responsible for residual damage stemming from over 75 years of environmental lead pollution.

Smoking
Cigarrette smoke may be the single most hazardous exposure that women experience. An emerging scientific body of evidence strongly suggests that there are devastating

effects of nicotine on women's health, including lung cancer. A number of toxins in tobacco smoke are thought to be associated with menstrual cycle aberrations, decreased fertility, osteoporosis, and cervical and vulvar cancer. Metabolic by-products of nicotine have been found in women with pre-invasive and invasive cervical disorders.

RISK ASSESSMENT

Women's health nurses prepared in environmental health can contribute significantly to women's environmental surveillance. These contributions include, but are not limited to, exposure assessments, co-management of affected women, leading multidisciplinary teams, building collaborative partnerships, and developing programs at the community level. Nursing is a holistic discipline by nature, and women's health–environmental health nursing is no exception. Women's health nurses are prepared to provide special-ized primary care to individuals and groups of women. Environmental health nurses are prepared as leaders and collaborators in risk assessment and management as well as in primary prevention and co-management of clients affected by environmentally related disease.

Exposure assessments identify actual and potential risks as well as adverse responses to actual exposures. Exposure assessments may include careful reproductive history, medical history, physical examination, lifestyle and occupational history, and a study of environmental risks in the community (Copes & Richardson, 1999). Environmental health surveillance by nurses helps to identify sentinel events that occur in women's health. These are the earliest manifestations of hazardous exposures that may be seen as atypical and suspicious patterns of occurrences. Exposure assessments also encom-pass psychological, social, and spiritual factors that contribute to risk and outcomes. The risk assessment role of the nurse further extends to a working knowledge of laboratory toxicology, specimen collection, and analysis.

RISK MANAGEMENT

Risk assessment in environmental health nursing may involve collection, analysis, and interpretation of clinical data whereas risk management may involve the application of evidence to prevent or minimize exposure, implement timely and effective interven-tions, and prevent or minimize long-term effects. In short, risk management involves the use of assessment data to identify and reduce the negative impact of toxic stressors on the health of women as much as possible through primary, secondary, and tertiary pre-vention. Primary prevention is concerned with risk abatement at the individual or aggregate level. Women's health nurses should be particularly skilled in developing and packaging education for primary prevention of toxic exposures in women. The educa-tive role extends to community-based education and outreach programs.

Primary prevention may also be furthered through activism and advocacy. Primary prevention and health promotion in women's environmental health should be first and foremost evidence-based. Research forms the conceptual foundation for clinical practice. Primary prevention models for environmental health should provide nurses with guidance to facilitate change in individual and in group behaviors and attitudes.

Secondary prevention requires an adequate background in clinical toxicology to ensure early diagnosis and treatment of toxic exposures. Clinical presentations of toxic exposures may involve skin, endocrine, urinary, reproductive or cardiorespiratory symptoms. Careful skin inspection, thyroid palpation, and respiratory and cardiac auscultation as well as assessment of hypersensitive reactions, thyroid and cardiovascular disorders, infertility, adverse obstetrical outcomes, menstrual disorders, and cancer are requisite components of the physical examination. The occupational and environmental exposure history corroborates diagnosis of exposure to a toxic agent and the probable exposure pathway. For example, knowing that a woman is a construction worker is not as useful as knowing whether she drives a construction truck or is directly involved in tearing down an old building. Recognition of the greater cumulative effect of exposure to pesticides in a woman who is a pest control worker compared to a woman who is an avid gardener is also crucial to secondary prevention. The secondary prevention role involves implementation and evaluation of the collaborative treatment plan and coordination of care.

Tertiary prevention involves accurate nursing assessment of temporary vs. permanent health outcomes and rehabilitative and restorative nursing actions. Short- and long-term follow-up needs must be identified and appropriate referrals made. For example, a woman exposed to high radiation levels or asbestos will require lifelong monitoring for cancer. A woman exposed to toxic lead levels should receive appropriate iron and/or chelation therapy and delay childbearing until lead levels return to normal. Monitoring becomes essential again during the postmenopausal years or during any bone-loss condition causing lead sequestered in the bones to be released into the circulatory system.

The environmental health nursing role also encompasses contributions to environmentally related legislation that affects women at work and in their communities as well as packaging scientific data for public consumption. The Right-to-Know Initiative, enacted by OSHA in 1983 as part of the Hazards Communication Standard, recognizes a woman's right to know about chemicals and hazardous substances to which she may be exposed at work. Women's health nurses should know where and how to access information, interpret the data for the public, and develop community-specific approaches to dissemination. Information on toxic emissions can be obtained from several reference web sites, such as the Toxic Release Inventory, a record maintained by the EPA.

Environmental health nurses may also use professional specialty organizations to further the advocacy role. Many nursing organizations advocate a woman's right to equal employment opportunities or the right to a safe birth. Several national organizations have adopted position statements against concentrating solid waste landfills, waste incinerators, chemical plants, lead smelters, or toxic waste sites near areas where the poor and powerless reside.

SUMMARY: RESEARCH DIRECTION

Clusters of cancer and birth defects have been known to appear and disappear throughout time, usually without adequate explanation. However, making the connection between environmental exposures and adverse health outcomes has been historically complicated. Much progress may be made by developing a coordinated database for cross-referencing clusters and other surveillance data. Such a database would provide an infrastructure for population-based environmental surveillance and hypotheses to guide research. Cross-disciplinary meta-analysis of environmental health research would also aid the development of an informational base that would inventory knowledge and avoid duplication and waste of research dollars. In particular, these efforts would support longitudinal studies and quasi-experimental factorial designs in women's environmental health studies.

Toxicogenomic research promises to furnish substantial data on duration, frequency, timing, and interactive effects of environmental exposures within the next decade. This technology will further the establishment of causation. Toxicogenomics is a technique that uses DNA chips to identify and monitor human responses to toxic exposures at the gene level. The use of "tox-chips" promises to reduce the need for animal experiments by determining the effect of a toxic substance on specific gene activity. For example, the distinct signature of a toxic compound may be observed. In addition, sensitivity or risk of cancer or birth defects may be observed within the pattern of gene activity. However, studies to measure total human response will continue to be needed.

Nurses can provide research leadership on total human response as well as maximize the benefits of environmental science technology for groups and communities. Investigation of psychosocial and spiritual variables, client system resources, stressors, and personal factors are relevant modifiers of research outcomes and suggest community-based approaches to implement change. A cadre of women's environmental health nurses needs to be developed in the coming years. These nurses should have graduate degrees, especially terminal degrees, in areas such as biochemistry, clinical toxicology, health education, women's health, and/or community health.

REFERENCES

Bercovici, B., Wassermann, M., Cucos, S., Ron, M., Wassermann, D., & Pines, A. (1983). Serum levels of polychlorinated biphenyl and some organochlorine insecticides in women with recent and former missed abortions. *Environmental Research, 30,* 169–174.

Canfield, M. A., Annegers, J. F., Brender, J. D., Cooper, S. P., & Greenberg, F. (1996). Hispanic origin and neural tube defects in Houston/Harris County, Texas. *American Journal of Epidemiology, 143*(1), 1–24.

Copes, M. A., & Richardson, T. C. (1999). Assessing individual, family, and community responses to toxic substances. In *Environmental Health and Nursing: Mississippi Delta Project Modular Curriculum.* Washington DC.: Minority Health Professions Foundation & Howard University.

Gladen, B. C., & Rogan, W. J. (1991, July). Effects of perinatal polychlorinated biphenyl and dichlorodiphenyl dichloroethene on later development. *Journal of Pediatrics, 119*(1), 58–63.

Howlett, C., Shaner, H., Thornton, J., McCally, M., Orris, P., & Weinberg, J. (1996). Dioxin data contested. *Public Health Reports, 111*(6), 473–475.

Institute of Medicine. (1995). *Nursing, health, & the environment.* Washington, DC.: National Academy of Sciences.

National Institute of Occupational Safety and Health. (1988). *Proposed national strategy for the prevention of disorders of reproduction* (Pub. No. 89–133). Cincinnati: NIOSH Publications.

Nehei, M. K., Desmond, N. L., McGlothan, J. L., Kuhlmann, A. C., & Guilarte, T. R. (2000). N-methyl-d-aspartate receptor subunit changes are associated with lead-induced deficits of long-term potentiation and spatial learning. *Neuroscience, 99*(2), 233–242.

Procianoy, R. S., & Schvartsman, S. (1981). Blood pesticide concentration in mothers and their newborn infants. *Acta Paediatr Scand, 70*, 925–928.

Rogan, W. J., Gladen, B. C., McKinney, J. D., Carreras, N., Hardy, P., Thullen, et al. (1986). Neonatal effects of transplacental exposure to PCBs and DDE. *Journal of Pediatrics, 109*, 335–341.

Rogan, W. J., Gladen, B. C., McKinney, J. D., Carreras, N., Hardy, P., Thullen, et al. (1987). Polychlorinated biphenyl (PCBs) and dichlorodiphenyl dichloroethene (DDE) in human milk: Effects on growth, morbidity, and duration of lactation. *American Journal of Public Health, 77*(10), 1294–1297.

Saxena, M. C., Siddiqui, M. K. J., & Kuuty, V. A. (1983). A comparison of organochlorine insecticide contents in specimens of maternal blood, placenta, and umbilical–cord blood from stillborn and live-born cases. *Journal of Toxicology and Environmental Health, 11*, 71–79.

Schettler, T., Stein, J., Reich, F., Valenti, M., & Wallinga, D. (2000). *In harm's way: Toxic threats to child development.* Cambridge, MA: Greater Boston Physicians for Social Responsibility. Available on the web: *http://www.igc.org/psr.*

Shaner, H. (1996). Pollution prevention for nurses: Minimizing the adverse environmental impact of health care delivery. *Vermont Registered Nurse, 62*(4), 1–2, 8–9.

Siddiqui, M. K. J., Saxena, M. C., Bhargava, A. K., Seth, T. D., Krishna Murti, C. R., & Kuuty, D. (1981). Agrochemicals in the maternal blood, milk, and cord blood: A source of toxicants for prenates and neonates. *Environmental Research, 24*, 24–32.

Sperrazza, K. (1998). Safe nursing: Health care without harm: Cutting down on environmental pollutants. *Massachusetts Nurse, 68*(10), 15–18.

Thornton, J., McCally, M., Orris, P., & Weinberg, J. (1996). Hospitals & plastics: Dioxin prevention and medical waste incinerators. *Public Health Reports, 111*(4), 298–313.

U. S. Department of Labor, Women's Bureau. (1993). *1993 Handbook on women workers: Trends and issues.* Washington, DC: U. S. Government Printing Office.

U. S. Department of Labor, Women's Bureau. (1997, Feb.). *Women of Hispanic origin in the labor force* (Pub. No. 97–2). Washington, DC: U. S. Government Printing Office.

U. S. Department of Labor, Women's Bureau. (1997, March). *Black women in the labor force* (Pub. No. 97–1). Washington, DC: U. S. Government Printing Office.

RESOURCES

Medscape: *www.medscape.com/Home/Topics/Womens Health*

Agency for Toxic Substances and Disease Registry (ATSDR)/HazDat: *www.atsdr.cdc.gov/hazdat.html; www.atsdr.cdc.gov/EHN*

EnviRN: *www.envirn.umaryland.edu*

National Women's Health Information Center: *www.4woman.org* **or (800) 994-woman**

American Association of Occupational Health Nursing: *www.aaohn.org/index.htm* **or (404) 262-1162**

Environmental Health Clearinghouse: *www.infoventures.com/e-hlth/* **or (800) 643-4794**

National Institute of Environmental Health Sciences: *www.niehs.nih.gov* **or (919) 541-2605**

National Institute for Occupational Safety and Health: *www.cdc.gov/niosh* **or (800) 365-4674**

EPA Office of Solid Waste and Emergency Hotline: *www.tri.us@epamila.epa.gov* **or (800) 424-9346**

Center for Biologics Evaluation and Research: *www.fda.gov/cber*

Center for Devices and Radiological Health: *www.fda.gov/cdrh*

Center for Drug Evaluation and Research: *www.fda.gov/cder*

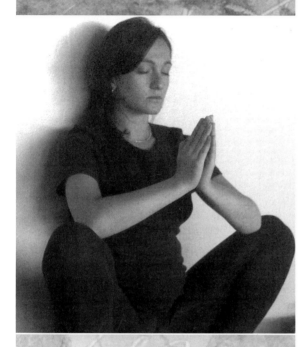

Chapter 5

Natural, Alternative, and Complementary Health Care

Roxana Huebscher

From inability to let well alone; from too much zeal for the new and contempt for what is old; from putting knowledge before wisdom, science before art, and cleverness before common sense; from treating patients as cases, and from making the cure of the disease more grievous than the endurance of the same, Good Lord, deliver us.

Sir Robert Hutchinson

INTRODUCTION

This chapter discusses natural/alternative/complementary health care (NAC) modalities and provides an overview of NAC practices for general health care and for women's common symptoms and concerns. Many NAC practices do not have a research base but are helpful in healing. Many women, throughout their lifespan and throughout time, have used NAC and have provided or been provided with comfort and healing from such measures. In addition, "Women have always been healers. Cultural myths from around the world describe a time when only women knew the secrets of life and death, and therefore they alone could practice the magical art of healing" (Achterberg, 1990, p. 1). Furthermore, researchers have found that between 1990 and 1997, the use of NAC in the United States increased from 34% to 42% (Eisenberg et al., 1993, 1998).

This chapter includes definitions, terminology, and rationale for NAC use as well as a listing of NAC practices, many of which, as mentioned, do not have a research base (Boxes 5-1 and 5-2).

Box 5-1 DEFINITIONS OF NATURAL/ALTERNATIVE/COMPLEMENTARY HEALTH CARE

- Natural/alternative/complementary health care refers to those "practices, including self-care practices, outside of the mainstream (conventional) nursing/medicine domain, including forms of care that we have not previously considered as health care" (Huebscher, 1994).
- Complementary and alternative health care and medical practices (CAM) are those health care and medical practices that are not currently an integral part of conventional medicine. The list of practices that are considered CAM changes continually as CAM practices and therapies that are proven safe and effective become accepted as "mainstream" health care practices. Today, CAM practices can be grouped in five major domains: (1) alternative medical systems, (2) mind-body interventions, (3) biologically based treatments, (4) manipulative and body-based methods, and (5) energy therapies (NCCAM, 2001).
- Complementary medical systems are characterized by a developed body of intellectual work that underlies the conceptualization of health and its precepts; that has been sustained over many generations by many practitioners in many communities; that represents an orderly, rational, conscious system of knowledge and thought about health and medicine; that relates more broadly to a way of life (or "lifestyle"); and that has been widely observed to have definable results as practiced (Micozzi, 2001, p. 7).
- From a holistic nursing can be defined as perspective, "interventions that focus on body-mind-spirit integration and evoke healing by an individual, between two individuals, or healing at a distance (e.g., relaxation, imagery, biofeedback, prayer, psychic healing) [and] may be used as complements to conventional medical treatments" (Dossey, Keegan, Guzzetta, & Kolkmeir, 1995, p. 6).

Box 5-2 TERMINOLOGY FOR NATURAL/ALTERNATIVE/COMPLEMENTARY HEALTH CARE

- *Alternative, complementary, natural, nonallopathic, unorthodox, nonconventional, nonwestern* are frequently encountered synonyms.
- *Traditional* refers to the indigenous and/or customary healing system of a culture (e.g., traditional Chinese or Native American medicine) and is often used as a synonym for NAC. However, many persons in the United States refer to allopathic medicine as traditional. Therefore, in the United States, the term *traditional* is used for both conventional and alternative forms of care and thus can be confusing.
- Another problem with terminology is the use of the prefix *un-* or *non-* with definitions. Using a term such as unconventional negates the modality.
- The term *natural* in this chapter refers to self-care practices that reflect an inner focus (e.g., physical, mental, and spiritual work by the individual) as well as to the natural nursing care so often not emphasized.

Included are self-care and provider-based practices, NAC practice resources, and a few examples of NAC practices written for women's specific concerns, including premenstrual symptoms, dysmenorrhea, and menopause/climacteric, pregnancy, and breast problems. The reader is advised to gain further information from experts in the NAC area of interest and from reputable NAC journals and organizations as well as to watch for the results of forthcoming research on NAC modalities.

RATIONALE

The rationale for NAC includes comfort and healing as well as opportunities to establish a research base for NAC modalities and explore NAC as part of various cultures. Women seek and desire health care that is compassionate, caring, comforting, and healing. Many NAC modalities provide such qualities. Conventional system providers are very reliant on pharmacological agents that treat symptoms but may not cure disease. Conversely, medications may "cure" a disease but result in new problems, such as bacterial resistance, drug interactions, or side effects (Huebscher, 1997). Most NAC practices do not involve interactions, side effects, or invasive modalities. The comfort and healing inherent in many NAC practices are key ingredients for attaining wellness. In addition, comfort and healing are goals of nursing practice.

Comfort

Comfort is a difficult term to define, yet we know when we are comfortable. Kolcabe (1991) described comfort as transcendence, relief, and ease. Transcendence refers to rising above the concern; relief is having a need met; and ease is a feeling of calm or contentment (Kolcaba, 1991). Because many NAC modalities provide transcendence, relief, and ease, comfort itself becomes a rationale for NAC use.

Healing

Curing refers to ending the pathology; *healing* relates to coming to a sense of wholeness and is not necessarily curing, although that may be an outcome also. Healing is

[the] establishment of a balance and equanimity in the midst of discomfort and agitation. We are healed when we can bring forth harmony out of the discordant strains of our life . . . . One of the most effective ways of establishing such a balance and harmony is through care . . . . To bring oneself back into the common flow, the shared culture where the mind can relate to the body with heartfulness and mercy, is one of the bases of healing (Levine, 1989, p. 197).

Extension of Research Base

Other rationales for NAC use include research opportunities. For example, the National Center for Complementary and Alternative Medicine (NCCAM) has as its purpose and mission to conduct and support "basic and applied (clinical) research and research training on CAM" and to provide "information about CAM to health care providers and the public. The Center also develops other programs to further the investigation and application of CAM treatments that show promise" (*http://nccam.nih.gov*, accessed Jan 2, 2001). Other sources of funding also are becoming available, and more nurses are doing research in NAC areas.

Cultural Opportunities

Using NAC, the provider has the privilege of practicing/witnessing or learning about modalities that other cultures have used for thousands of years. Native American practices, traditional African-American practices, East Indian (Ayurveda), and traditional

Chinese medicine are some examples of ancient healing systems. Other modalities are also rooted in ancient tradition, such as reflexology, which was practiced in ancient Egypt (Byers, 1991), and Therapeutic Touch (Krieger, 1979, 1987, 1993; Macrae, 1998), derived from the ancient practice of laying on of hands.

CLASSIFICATION

There are many NAC practices and several ways of classifying them. Box 5-3 lists various NAC practices and Table 5-1 outlines NCCAM's classification. Self-care and provider care are discussed with examples of some common symptoms and diagnoses.

SELF-CARE PRACTICES

Self-care practices are those health care practices that a person may apply on her own, such as eating vegetables, deep breathing, practicing affirmations, praying, or meditating.

Box 5-3 EXAMPLES OF NATURAL/ALTERNATIVE/COMPLEMENTARY THERAPIES

Acupressure	Homeopathy	Rebirthing
Acupuncture	Humor	Reiki
Affirmations	Hypnosis	Reflexology
Alexander		Relaxation
Aromatherapy	Imagery	Religion
Artistic expression	Iridology	Rolfing
Ayurveda		Rosen
	Laying-on-of-hands	
Bach flower	Light therapy	Shaman
Bibliotherapy		Shiatsu
Biofeedback	Macrobiotics	Social support
Bowen	Massage	Spiritual practices
	Meditation	Storytelling
Centering	Movement/dance	Support groups
Chakra balancing	Music	
Chiropractic		Tai Chi
Colonics	Naturopathy	Therapeutic Touch
Color	Neurolinguistic programming	Traditional Chinese medicine
Craniosacral	Neuromuscular	Trager
Crystals	Nutrition	
		Vitamins/minerals
Deep breathing	Pets	
	Polarity	Water therapies
Feldenkrais	Prayer	Writing/journaling
	Presence	
Healing touch		Yoga
Heller work	Qi gong	
Herbals		

Table 5-1	NCCAM CLASSIFICATION OF NAC THERAPIES
CLASSIFICATION	**DEFINITION**
Alternative medical systems	Alternative medical systems involve complete systems of theory and practice that have evolved independent of and often prior to the conventional biomedical approach. Many are traditional systems of medicine that are practiced by individual cultures throughout the world, including a number of venerable Asian approaches. Includes Ayurveda, Tibetan, Native American, traditional Chinese, African and aboriginal practices, as well as homeopathy and naturopathy.
Mind-body interventions	Techniques designed to facilitate the mind's capacity to affect bodily function and symptoms. Only a subset of mind-body interventions are considered complementary/alternative medicine. Many that have a well-documented theoretical basis; for example, patient education and cognitive-behavioral approaches are now considered "mainstream." Meditation, hypnosis, dance, music, art therapy, and prayer and mental healing are categorized as complementary and alternative.
Biologically based therapies	Natural and biologically based practices, interventions, and products, many of which overlap with conventional medicine's use of dietary supplements. Included are herbal, dietary, orthomolecular, and individual biological therapies.
Manipulative and body-based methods	Methods that are based on manipulation and/or movement of the body; for example, chiropractic, massage, and osteopathy.
Energy therapies	Energy therapies focus either on energy fields originating within the body (biofields) or those from other sources (electromagnetic fields). Qi gong, Reiki, and Therapeutic Touch; magnetic fields; alternating or direct currents are examples.

Source: *http://nccam.nih.gov.*

The primary health care of women includes psychosocial and spiritual components; therefore, this section discusses self-care in terms of NAC practices that may be helpful in the spiritual and psychosocial as well as the physical domains.

Bibliotherapy

Bibliotherapy refers to readings that can help clients through difficult times. Readings include factual information in the form of brochures and texts, self-help books, fiction, poetry, or other forms of written work that are pertinent to the patient concern. For example, *How to Survive the Loss of a Love* by Colgrove, Bloomfield, and McWilliams (a social worker, psychiatrist, and poet) (1991) has two million copies in print, is very easy to read, and can help persons through a loss, especially a relationship loss. *Final Gifts* (Callanan & Kelley, 1992), an award-winning paperback written by two nurses, deals with issues surrounding death. Many fiction works, both classic and new, present story-lines that can help patients find meaning in their situation. The health care practitioner can provide reference lists, a library shelf of books, and other resources, such as tapes and CDs.

Journaling/Writing/Storytelling/Creativity/Arts

Journaling is the writing of personal thoughts, memories, and/or experiences. Although writing need not be done on a daily basis, keeping a journal can be clarifying. To write concerns and problems, to develop solutions, and to reread one's thoughts often kindles introspection and meaning. Both formal writing, in any form such as poetry, nonfiction, fiction, and storytelling, are ways of relaxing and being creative. Breslin (1996) writes that her interest in the use of metaphor in nursing practice began with her own early nursing experience with a dying woman:

This woman taught the author the importance of storytelling as a way of creating meaning and synthesis. This interest resurfaced with the author's dissertation research, when a recovering alcoholic shared the experience of how writing a poem helped her maintain her sobriety and document her painful marriage (p. 507).

In addition, other art forms can be liberating, including painting, sculpture, photography (Soffa, 1996), and dance. Samuels (1995) writes that:

healing, art, and prayer all come from the same source, the soul. And when we travel deeply into the inner realms, we reach the insights, emotions, and transformation that are our birthright . . . . I see healing and art as one. They are the two sides of the split between rational and the intuitive; their separation historically is as profound as that between mind and body. And just as it is our task to bring mind and body together to heal the whole person, it is our task to unite healing and art to heal our bodies and the world (p. 38).

Affirmations

Affirmations are positive personal statements in the present tense that express a desirable outcome as if it has already occurred. "An affirmation is a positive thought that you consciously choose to immerse in your consciousness to produce a certain desired result" (Ray, 1980, p. 10). Examples include
Every day, in every way, I am healthy, happy, and prospering.
I am strong and full of energy.
I am clear in thought, word, and deed.
I have a meaningful job that I love.
I am happy with my relationship with___.
I say what I need to say effortlessly, honestly, and tactfully.

Affirmations include no negative words and do not involve the actions of other people. (For example, in the previous sentence there are three negative words, "no", "negative", and "not"). The premise behind affirmations is that we are what we say we are, and if we repeat affirmations enough, we will achieve what we ask for. Affirmations are good for women who have self-confidence problems or who are making changes in their lives. They are helpful in almost all health care situations but should not be relied on as the sole method of care for depressed persons or potentially violent situations.

Presence, Deep Breathing, Centering

Presence is being here now. Presence is attention with all the senses focused, no matter what the situation. When people are not present, they have accidents, get bruises, forget what is being said to them. Often they seem to "be someplace else." They may be aware of their nonpresence because they may be thinking about emotional conflicts, other activities, or be "in the wall" from a shocking situation, as happens with victims of abuse. Thus developing presence is a beginning step in awareness of the self.

Deep breathing and centering produce relaxation and are a way to become present or, conversely, to image oneself elsewhere. *Deep breathing* consists of slowly breathing from the belly: for example, taking a breath in for a count of five, holding it for a count of five, and breathing out for a count of five. The five count is a person's own personal count so it can be slow or fast. *Centering* is coming to a stabilizing point around which the chaos of the world spins. Centering may be described as an "inner reference of stability;" "a sense of self-relatedness, . . . a place of inner being, a place of quietude within oneself where one can feel truly integrated, unified, and focused" (Krieger, 1979, p. 36). Teaching affirmations and handing out 3×5 cards with instructions for being present, deep breathing, and centering are simple ways to start a plan of care for stress management.

Relaxation, Imagery, Visualization

Relaxation is defined as the absence of tension (Zahourek, 1988). Lichstein (1988) observes that the basis of modern relaxation techniques lies in the meditation heritage of the Eastern religions. Scandrett and Uecker (1985) divide relaxation techniques into two basic categories: externally oriented and internally oriented. Externally oriented examples include progressive muscle relaxation, biofeedback, and hypnosis. Internally oriented relaxation techniques are autogenics, meditation, and self-hypnosis.

Progressive relaxation is the systematic technique of tensing and releasing muscle groups while sensing the differences between tense and relaxed (Scandrett & Uecker, 1985). The goal is to sense tension that may be present. Benson (1975) popularized progressive relaxation in the 1970s (without the tensing part of the exercise). He believed that four elements are needed to elicit a relaxation response:

1. A repetitive mental device such as a word, sound, or phrase repeated silently or audibly. Examples include a chant, the rosary, the sound OM. The purpose is to free the person from logical external thought.
2. A passive attitude. Herbert Benson uses the phrase "oh well" when any distraction occurs.
3. Decreased muscle tone and a comfortable posture.
4. A quiet setting with few external stimuli.

Nurses can teach relaxation by telling clients to begin relaxation in a quiet place and in a comfortable position with hands and feet uncrossed. The client then becomes "present," takes deep breaths, and centers while practicing the repetitive mental technique or deep breathing. The client then can practice relaxing muscle groups, or a nurse trained in relaxation techniques can lead the client from foot to head with mental statements such as, "My feet and legs are feeling relaxed and tension-free," "My torso (or abdomen, chest, back) is feeling relaxed and tension-free," "My arms and hands are feeling relaxed and tension-free," "My neck and jaw are feeling relaxed and tension-free."

Another relaxation technique, *autogenics,* is derived from self-suggestion and consists of suggestions about the relaxing feelings of heaviness of the neuromuscular system, warmth in the abdominal area, a steady strong heart rate, effortless respiration, and coolness of the forehead (Scandrett & Uecker, 1985). In addition, other activities that elicit the relaxation response include walking, repetitive exercise, humor, or complete absorption in an enjoyable activity such as a hobby.

"Imagery is the deliberate formation of a mental representation while in a deeply relaxed state" (Giedt, 1997). Imagery is "the thought process that invokes and uses the senses: vision, audition, smell, taste, the senses of movement, position, and touch" (Achterberg, 1985, p. 3). In other words, imagery is a mental process that draws on the senses and consists of mental representations of external reality (Zahourek, 1988). Visualization is simply imagery using the visual sense.

To work with *imagery,* follow the general relaxation procedure including guiding the woman through relaxation of the body; then have the woman find her "safe" place. This may be the ocean, the mountains, a forest, a room in her home, or some other place she finds beautiful and safe. Here she can do mental and emotional work. In addition, she can bring a guide to help her with her concerns. Following imagery, clients need to come back or be led back to the room "safely and peacefully, fully awake, refreshed, alert, energized and full of vitality." Clients can make tapes for use at home or purchase one of the many tapes and narratives available (Gawain, 1997; Miller, 1989; Naparstek, 1994).

Practicing the relaxation response and imagery is a positive form of self-care that can help clients solve problems, enhance their self-esteem, and provide a feeling of clarity and general well-being. There are classes and training programs available for nurses to learn such techniques (see resource list).

Prayer/Religion/Spirituality/Meditation

Humans have spirituality and/or religious beliefs surrounding their health concerns. *Religious beliefs* may involve a certain religious affiliation with its inherent philosophy, whereas spirituality refers to:

values, meaning, and purpose in life. It reflects the human traits of caring, love, honesty, wisdom, and imagination. The concept of spirit implies a quality of transcendence, a guiding force, or something outside the self and beyond the individual nurse or client. It may reflect a belief in the existence of a higher power or a guiding spirit. To some, spirit may suggest a purely mystical feeling or a flowing dynamic quality of unity. It is undefinable, yet it is a vital force profoundly felt by the individual and capable of affecting life and behavior (Dossey, Keegan, Guzzetta, & Kolkmeir, 1995, p. 18).

Dossey (1993, 1997) has summarized studies and discussed the effects of prayer on health concerns, including Byrd's (1988, 1997) randomized double-blind study in which some coronary care patients were prayed for (intercessory prayer) by a prayer group while others were not. Intercessory prayer is "the idea of praying for the benefit of others" (Byrd, 1997, p. 87). The Byrd study revealed that those prayed for needed fewer antibiotics, were less likely to develop pulmonary edema, and did not need endotracheal intubation. Shuler, Gelberg, and Brown (1994) report that 92% of their sample of homeless women:

reported one or more spiritual/religious practices, such as praying, attending worship services, or reading religious materials. Forty-eight percent of the women reported the use of prayer as significantly related to less use of alcohol and/or street drugs, fewer perceived worries, and fewer depressive symptoms (p. 106).

Religion was also a factor in a study of family practice adult inpatients (King & Bushwick, 1994) that revealed that patients desired more frequent and in-depth discussions of religious issues with their physicians and that patients wished that physicians would pray with them. O'Laoire (1997) reported beneficial effects on self-esteem, anxiety, and depression with intercessory prayer. Levine (1989) reported that 250 empirical studies offered significant results of "religious indicators on morbidity and mortality" (Moore, 1996, p. 104). Finally, when Herbert Benson began teaching his patients the relaxation response, 80% chose prayer to elicit the response (Moore, 1996). In addition to prayer, there are numerous meditative techniques. Persons can use any of a variety of methods, depending on their philosophical outlook (see resource list).

Spirituality and religion are not one and the same, and health care providers need to be cognizant of differences between the two as well as their importance in patients' lives. Prayer and/or meditation may lead to positive health outcomes and should not be overlooked.

Music Therapy

Music is sound, and sound is vibration that we hear. *Music therapy* is the application of pleasant sounds to produce desired changes in behaviors, emotions, and/or physiology (Dossey et al., 1995). "The playing of appropriate music produces alpha and theta brain waves, which are known to stimulate creativity" (Guzzetta, 1995, p. 677). In addition, music aids relaxation, improves learning, and enhances audio and video tapes (including subliminal tapes) that reprogram thought patterns. Music is used for healing purposes, and, in thanatology, as a way of addressing the needs of the dying (Guzzetta, 1995).

Color Therapy

Color therapy refers to the display of colors for healing purposes. For example, certain colors enliven and others calm. Barbara Brennan, a healer, therapist, and explorer of the human energy field, gives an ethereal portrait:

All the colors of the rainbow are used in healing. Each color has its own effect in the field. Of course each color can be used to charge the chakra that metabolizes that color. Red is used to charge the field, burn out cancer and warm cold areas. Orange charges the field, increases sexual potency and immunity. Yellow is used to clear a foggy head and help the linear mind function well. Green is used as a general balancer and healer for all things. Blue cools and calms. It is also used to restructure the etheric field and in shielding. Purple helps the patient connect to his spirit, while indigo opens the third eye and enhances visualization and clears the head. White is used to charge the field, bring peace and comfort and take away pain. Gold is used to restructure the seventh layer and to strengthen and charge the field. Velvet black brings the patient into a state of grace, silence and peace with God. It is good in restructuring bones that have crumbled from cancer or other trauma. Purple-blue takes away pain when doing deep tissue work and work on bone cells. It also helps expand the patient's field in order to connect to her task (1987, p. 239).

In addition to these colors used in healing and colors associated with the chakras, certain colors create auras (meanings for color on soul-task level) (Brennan, 1987). In addition, sound is associated with color (Brennan, 1987; Dossey et al., 1995). For more information on chakras, fields, and layers, see Barbara Brennan's texts (1987, 1993).

Light Therapy

Light therapy is often used to help those who have seasonal affective disorder (SAD). This is done via phototherapy that:

consists of exposure (at a 3-foot distance) to a light source of 2500 lux for two hours daily. Light visors are an adaptation that provide greater mobility and an adjustable light intensity . . . . The dosage varies, with some patients requiring morning and night exposure. One effect is alteration of biorhythm through melatonin mechanisms (Eisendrath, 1997, p. 982).

Women with PMS or irregular menstrual cycles seem to benefit from light therapy. Several organizations have endorsed the use of light therapy for the treatment of SAD, including the American Psychiatric Association and the Society for Light Treatment and Biological Rhythms (Blanchet, 1995).

Hydrotherapy

Hydrotherapy refers to the various ways that water can be used in the healing process, including ice, hot water, steam, and cold/hot packs. Foot soaks are an especially simple therapeutic technique for general relaxation or for foot conditions. Hotpacks are helpful before a massage or other bodywork. Warm baths with essential oils or salts can also be healing (Maxwell-Hudson, 1994).

Nutrition/Ingested Substances: Food, Supplements, Herbs

Detailed discussion of nutrition, supplements, and herbs is beyond the scope of this chapter. However, there are numerous dietary options for women's health, including sensible use of macrobiotics (Kushi, 1985, 1996) and various types of vegetarian diets, including vegan and lacto-ovo diets. Messina and Messina (1996) delineate a plan for becoming vegetarian, discuss research on the health benefits, and give recipes, meal plans, and special guidelines for persons with diabetes, for athletes, and for dieters. Lemlin (1992) won the James Beard Award for Cookbook of the Year with her *Quick*

Vegetarian Pleasures. Thomas (1996) has a vegetarian epicure cookbook with over 325 recipes. Numerous other vegetarian cookbooks are now available.

Phytoestrogens are plant substances that have weak estrogenic activity. They are found in many foods, including soy, apples, carrots, garbanzo beans, garlic, green beans, peas, red clover, barley, oats, rye, citrus fruits, cherries, cranberries, blueberries, bilberries, and grapeskins (*Pharmacist's Letter/Prescriber's Letter* [*PL/PL*], 2002). Soy products are high in isoflavones, a type of phytoestrogen, and are possibly the closest natural alternative for conventional hormone replacement therapy. Approximately 20 to 60 g per day are recommended for relieving hot flashes (*PL/PL,* 2002)

Tierra (1992) provides a bibliography of herbalists; discusses the history of herbs, the Chinese and Ayurvedic classification of foods and herbs, the spiritual quality of herbs, and Western evolution of energetic herbalism; advises on preparation and processing of herbs; and includes a planetary materia medica. Amanda McQuade Crawford (1996), Subhuti Dharmananda (1987), David Hoffmann (1996), Michael Murray (1994, 1996, 1997), and Jill Stansbury (1997), among others, have authored or edited books on herbs, including therapies for women's health issues. Anne McIntyre (1995) has written *The Complete Woman's Herbal*, featuring discussions, color photographs, and diagrams of various herbs useful for "the seasons of womanhood." There is also *The Protocol Journal of Botanical Medicine*, a quarterly peer-reviewed publication (see Volume I, Number 4 on women's health [1995] and Volume II, Number 3 [1996] on anticancer therapies, including breast, colorectal, and ovarian). In addition, Mowrey (1986) has compiled a series of herbal research studies. For conventional views on herbs, *The Natural Medicines Comprehensive Database* [NMCD] (2000), *Pharmacist's Letter/Prescriber's Letter (PL/PL)* (various issues from 1999 to 2001), Fetrow and Avila's *Complementary and Alternative Medicines* (1999), *Physician's Desk Reference of Natural Medicines* (current), and the *German Commission E* (Blumenthal, 1998; translated text) are good references.

PROVIDER-ASSISTED NAC MODALITIES

Provider-assisted NAC includes numerous philosophies and therapies. Many of the NAC therapies have a very different theory base than conventional nursing/medicine. Some require regulation/licensing/certification and others do not. Thus advanced practice nurses in women's health need to use a different framework for assessing the appropriateness of provider-assisted NAC. "We can expect ethical, caring, competent, confidential, and hygienic care from NAC practitioners" (Huebscher, 1997, p. 559). However, we can not expect the same Western conventional orientation to diagnosis and treatment. Quality issues need to be assessed by checking the standard of care and other avenues for the individual therapies. Listed below are a few of the provider-assisted forms of care.

Ayurveda

Probably one of the oldest systems of health care, *Ayurveda* is the natural healing system of India, encompassing science, religion, and philosophy (Lad, 1985). The system was established by the same sages who produced yoga and meditation: "Ayurveda" means the science of life (Frawley, 1989). The concept of the five elements, ether (space), air, fire, water, and earth "lies at the heart of Ayurvedic science" (Lad, 1985, p. 21). These elements manifest in the human body as the *tridosha*, or biological humors: *vata* (wind, motion and flow); *pitta* (fire, energy, metabolism); and *kapha* (water, phlegm). Certain physical characteristics and body types are related to these humors. In addition, there are the three great cosmic forces: the energy of life (*prana*), light or radiance, and cohesion or a common unity, which is a single rhythm or love (Frawley, 1989). Frawley gives an overview of the disease process:

According to the spiritual tradition of India, diseases have two causes. First, they can arise from physical or biological causes: the imbalance of the biological humors, the elements, and prime energies of the physical body. Treatment involves mainly physical or medical methods with a naturalistic basis, including herbs, diet, body work and Yogic postures (asanas). In more extreme cases mineral and drug medicines or surgery may be required.

Second, diseases can arise from karmic causes: from the effects of wrong actions we have done in life, meaning from psychological or spiritual causes. These may be wrong occupation, problems in relationships or emotional difficulties, and treatment may require changes in life-style and attitude. Such causes include not living up to our inner purpose or spiritual will in life, what is called in Sanskrit our "dharma." Diseases can arise from wrong actions in a previous life, primarily those which brought harm to other beings or misused our power or resources.

Such karmic diseases may require some form of atonement or sacrifice, an 'inner rectification' to reestablish our well being in life. For this Ayurveda uses yoga and a system of divine or spiritual therapy (daiva cikitsa) which includes the use of gems, mantras, prayers, rituals, and meditations. These are not medieval superstition but reflect a profound understanding of the deeper levels of the mind and the means of healing the subtler aspects of our being (1989, pp. xvii-xviii).

Ayurveda practice is becoming more popular in the United States. Several schools offer training in the practices (see resources).

Biofeedback/Self-Management

Biofeedback is the use of instruments to feed back psychophysiological information to a person . . . . Instruments . . . monitor, amplify and feed back a variety of biological processes such as heart rate, blood pressure, muscle tension, blood flow in the hands and feet, and brain waves . . . . (Shellenberger & Green, 1986, pp. 2-3).

Self-management training (SMT) refers to interventions and to integrative functions of the brain that help manage the body (Nakagawa-Kogan, 1994). Biofeedback is one part of SMT. Women who know SMT strategies, including biofeedback, may be able to reduce their need for pharmaceuticals. Nakagawa-Kogan (1994) believes that the principles of SMT apply to all chronic conditions, including chronic pain, headaches, tempomandibular joint syndrome, hypertension, chronic arthritis, depression, anxiety reactions, insomnia, and somatic complaints. The SMT program begins by "defining the behaviors, cognition, emotional responses, and physical signs that are to be the targets for self-regulation . . . . Anger management, anxiety management, and depression management are the basic skills of SMT" (Nakagawa-Kogan, 1994, p. 81).

Biofeedback works through feeding back information and sensation to the subjects and allowing them to become "consciously aware of the interface between bodily status, environmental events, and internal cognitive information" (Nakagawa-Kogan, 1994, p. 81).

Thus biofeedback and self-management training are useful for many chronic disorders. Once women learn the strategies, these techniques become self-care practices.

Homeopathy

Samuel Hahnemann (1755-1843), a German physician, developed *homeopathy* in the early 1800s: It was brought to the United States around 1825 to 1830 by Hans Gram and Constantine Hering (Migodow, 1986). Homeopathy is a disease treatment system in which an ill person takes an extremely small dose of a drug that could "cause a healthy person to have the symptoms of the disease under treatment" (Alternative Medicine Editorial Board, 1986, p. 104). This process is called the *Law of Similars*, that is, "like cures like." The medicines are made through a process called *potentization* whereby the substances are serially diluted. For example, if a medicine is "diluted 1:10 three times, it is called 3x (x being the Roman numeral 10); diluted 1:100 three times, it is called 3c" (Ullman, 1993, p. 101).

Homeopathy uses "human engagement and [is] a system for approaching illness and disease which is not based on judgement or theory . . . . Homeopaths try to match up the physiological and emotional disturbances of this person at this time with a pattern of disturbance recognized with different drugs" (Reilly, 1995, p. 66).

Jacobs and Moskowitz (1996) have categorized the uses of homeopathic treatment:

■ Functional complaints with little or no tissue damage, such as headaches, insomnia, chronic fatigue, and premenstrual syndrome.
■ Conditions for which no effective conventional treatment is available, such as viral illnesses, traumatic injuries, surgical wounds, multiple sclerosis, and AIDS.
■ Conditions that require chronic use of conventional drugs, such as allergies, recurring infections, arthritis, skin conditions, and digestive problems.
■ Conditions for which elective surgery has been proposed but immediate attention is unnecessary, such as fibroid tumors, gallstones, and hemorrhoids.
■ Conditions that have not been cured by conventional treatments because of the inappropriateness of the medication, the determined nature of the disease, or the patient's noncompliance (p. 77).

Hypnosis

Hypnosis "relates to an induced, sleeplike state involving motivation, relaxation, concentration and application. In this state, the person is relaxed and the mind is directed inward" (Halo Shames, 1996, p. 38). With hypnosis, the inductee has a focus, that is, some work to do. One of the most popular forms is Eriksonian hypnosis. Hypnosis is used in psychotherapy, surgery, medical outpatient modalities such as stop-smoking programs, and in self-hypnosis, or autosuggestion. At one time, it was popular for childbirth.

Naturopathic Medicine

Naturopathy was founded in the late nineteenth century by Benedict Lust and originally focused on hydrotherapy and nature cures (Pizzorno, 1996). "Nature cure" initially referred to a vegetarian diet and the use of light and air.

Today, nutrition is the foundation of naturopathy. In addition, herbs, homeopathy, acupuncture, hydrotherapy (hot, cold, ice, steam), physical medicine (in the form of touch, heat, cold, electricity, and sound), correction of endogenous and exogenous toxicities, and counseling and lifestyle modifications are used. Cervical dysplasia, migraine headache, and hypertension are three conditions, among many, for which patients use naturopathic therapies (Pizzorno, 1996, p. 177).

Touch/Bodywork/Energywork

These modalities include the therapeutic application of *touch* or *energy work* to the body. Modalities include Swedish massage, deep tissue and neuromuscular work, Eastern massage techniques such as shiatsu and acupressure, aromatherapy, Therapeutic Touch, Healing Touch, Reiki, polarity therapy, reflexology, Feldenkrais, chiropractic, and osteopathy. There are numerous other modalities.

DePaoli (1995) gives an overview of massage techniques and their application to reproductive issues, including "massage for female issues." Tappan (1988) provides information on massage techniques and application, sports massage, massage of infants and children, and massage for animals as well as acupressure, shiatsu, polarity, Bindegewebmassage, reflexology, and lymphatic drainage. Maxwell-Hudson (1994) discusses aromatherapy, including remedies for women's health. Byers (1991) and Kunz and Kunz (1993, 1995) offer detailed information on reflexology, a technique using specific pressure on points and zones in the feet, hands, and ears.

The *energy therapies* include Therapeutic Touch (which does not necessarily include physical touch) and Reiki and Healing Touch that both use hands-on therapies. Therapeutic Touch has its origins in the ancient practice of the laying-on-of-hands and was brought into nursing by Delores Krieger (1979, 1993). Therapeutic Touch can promote relaxation, reduce pain, accelerate the healing process, and alleviate psychosomatic illness (Krieger, 1993). The process includes intention, centering, assessing the energy field (scanning), clearing the field (unruffling), modulating energy (directing energy), reassessing, and ending the treatment. In addition, Healing Touch, a program of therapies, provides other hands-on processes and works with the chakras. Reiki also has hands-on placement in specific areas. All these therapies include working with energy but have differing philosophies.

Traditional Chinese Medicine

Traditional Chinese medicine (TCM) is associated with Taoism, an ancient religion. Its history is complex and can be approached from several perspectives (Ergil, 1996). Generally, TCM is a philosophy of health and of life that includes theories about yin and yang (polar aspects of a dimension, such as black/white, hot/cold, hollow/solid, female/male, interior/exterior, winter/summer); the five elements (water, wood, metal, earth, fire); *zang-fu* (referring to internal organs); channels and collaterals (meridians and points); *qi* or *ch'i* (pronounced "chee" and referring to the life force or energy that flows), blood (*xue*) and body fluid; *jing* (vital physical essence of the body); etiology; methods of diagnosis; and differentiation of the health concerns (Chang, 1986; Connelly, 1979; Ergil, 1996; Foreign Language Press, 1980; Wolfe, 1995).

Diagnosis includes a history (which can consist of dreams, childhood experiences bowel/bladder characteristics, habits/hobbies, and personal preferences) as well as diagnosis by sound of voice, emotion, facial color, temperature, pulse-taking, and tongue examination. Differentiation of syndromes refers to exterior/interior (depth of disease), hot/cold (nature of disease), and *shi* (excess)/*xu* (deficiency); all are related to the yang/yin (basic principle). Organs have pathways through which the ch'i energy flows. Ch'i energy can be characterized as yang/yin. For example, if a person has a liver/kidney yin deficiency, the therapy may be to cultivate yin and clear heat.

The path to caring for the *ch'i* is the Tao, the way. Treatment includes Chinese herbals, dietary and lifestyle modifications, and acupuncture. Different persons may have similar symptoms that would lead a conventional Western practitioner to use one standard treatment for all, but in Chinese medicine each person may be prescribed a different treatment, depending on other parameters of diagnosis and differentiation.

Flaws and Chace (1994) describe recent TCM research from China. Flaws has also written on TCM diagnosis and treatment of vaginal diseases (1993), premenstrual syndrome (1985), and endometriosis and infertility. Wolfe (1995) discusses menopause from a TCM perspective, providing basic information about TCM, the endocrine system, and the mechanism of menstruation from a Chinese perspective. Maciocia's text on obstetrics and gynecology discusses various conditions from a Chinese medicine perspective (1998).

OTHER NAC MODALITIES

Social Support and Love

Green and Shellenberger (1996) summarize information and research studies on the healing energy of love. They review several large prospective epidemiological studies that correlate love and social support with outcomes such as mortality, onset of illness, and type of illness. For example, Kiecolt-Glaser, Fisher, Ogrocki, Stout, and Glaser (1987) compare the quality of the marital relationship and immune functioning in 473 women. The more supportive the relationship, the more competent the immune system; the poorer the relationship, the less competent the immune system, as measured by natural killer cell activity.

In addition, Sosa, Kennell, Klaus, Robertson, and Urrutia (1980) correlate social support with shorter length of labor, and Nichols and Humenick (1988) discuss the influence of supportive relationships on pregnancy and parenting. Klington and O'Sullivan (2001) give an overview of the family as a protective asset in adolescent development. "Family support, both maternal and paternal, was a predictor of consistent use of oral contraceptives among teen women" (Kalagian, Loewen, Delmore, & Busca, 1998). Teens said that partner support was important with condom use but social support was also associated with consistent use (Laraque, McLean, Brown-Peterside, Ashton, & Diamond, 1997). There is also an Israeli study of 10,000 married men that showed that love and support from a wife reduces risk for angina pectoris even in those at high risk (Medalie & Goldbourt, 1976).

Nurses can inquire about and assist clients in finding support. By introducing the client to religious groups, community organizations, and support groups and increasing family/friend contact, the nurse can help clients to get the help they need. In addition, helping clients find a hobby often leads to new friends because many hobbyists belong to associations and organizations.

Support Groups

Numerous groups of like-minded persons meet on a regular basis to offer encouragement and hope to those with specific needs. These groups include Alcoholics Anonymous, Al-Anon (for friends and relatives), Alateen, Coc-Anon, and other substance recovery groups as well as Overeaters Anonymous. In addition, there are support groups for persons who suffer from arthritis, cancer (Reach for Recovery, for example), diabetes, fibromyalgia, inflammatory bowel disease, and pychological disorders. Giving this type of information is an important part of a plan of care; a resource book with phone numbers makes referral simple.

SPECIFIC WOMEN'S ISSUES AND NATURAL/ALTERNATIVE/COMPLEMENTARY HEALTH CARE

There are numerous NAC practices available for women's concerns but, as previously mentioned, very few research studies of alternative practices have been done. Nonetheless, NAC practices may bring comfort and give a feeling of control. In addition, drug side effects may be minimized if alternatives are used in place of strong medications. The following sections offer a brief overview of some specific therapies for several common women's health concerns. Remember that herbals require the same safety precautions as any other drug and that only specific parts of plants are used for medicinal purposes (roots, leaves, seeds, or dried flowers, for example). Thus to know details of herbal treatment is as important as knowing the pharmacotherapeutics of prescription drugs, and health care providers should know interactions, effects, and side effects of herbals before using them. Sources are listed in the references in this chapter and in the resources.

Premenstrual Syndrome/Symptoms and Dysmenorrhea

Although premenstural syndrome (PMS) and dysmenorrhea are two different entities in conventional Western medicine/nursing, they are often considered together in the alternative literature. Herbals include black cohosh (*Cimicifuga racemosa*) for menstrual cramps and premenstrual syndrome (Kronenberg, Murphy, & Wade, 1999; Sierpina, 2001) although "there isn't much evidence" (*PL/PL,* 2001) for its effectiveness. Other

PMS herbs include chasteberry, for which the most evidence exists, for irritability, mood alteration, anger, headache, and breast fullness (*PL/PL,* 2001). Also ginkgo appears to relieve fluid retention, breast swelling and tenderness, pelvic pain and swelling, and swollen hands and feet (*PL/PL,* 2002). Nutrients include calcium, 1200 mg elemental daily, magnesium 200 to 360 mg daily, vitamin B_6 50 to 100 mg daily, and vitamin E 400 IU daily (*PL/PL,* 2002). Little evidence exists for the effectiveness of red clover, soy, evening primrose oil, and dong quai for PMS.

According to Chinese medicine interpretation, PMS is caused by qi congestion (or stagnation) in the liver, and treatment is aimed at improving liver qi congestion or excess of energy in the liver (Flaws, 1985). In addition, the liver is a "temperamental organ" and is "easily harmed by emotional upset" (Flaws, 1985, p. 207):

> In Chinese medicine the liver is responsible for "spreading the Qi" and maintaining its smooth and unobstructed flow. This is called in the literature the patency of the Qi. This smooth and unobstructed flow implies that the right energy arrives at the right place at the right time. Energy or Qi in Chinese medicine means function. Therefore, the cyclic flow of Qi describes from the Chinese point of view the endocrine system and the rise and fall of hormones in the body (Flaws, 1985, p. 206).

Hepatic qi congestion in females manifests as obstruction of qi flow in one of three areas of the body: pelvis, chest, or throat. Lower abdominal (pelvic) symptomatology results in flatulence, bloating, menstrual irregularities, and dysmenorrhea. The chest symptomatology can take the form of chest tightness and breast pain, swelling, and lumpiness. Finally, the throat symptoms may include esophogeal complaints, such as the feeling of having something stuck in the throat, or thyroid imbalance. In addition, secondary effects on other organs may occur. Practitioners use Chinese herbs, acupuncture points, dietary alteration, stress management, deep relaxation, and exercise for treatment of PMS.

Some sources recommend acupressure points (i.e., finger pressure instead of needles) (Figure 5-1). (See references and resources for detailed points.) The Natural Medicine Collective (Fradet et al., 1995) suggests the Liver 3 and Large Intestine 4 acupressure points for irritability and recommends the Stomach 34, Liver 3, Conception Vessel 17, Pericardium 6, and Stomach 18 points for breast tenderness. For fluid retention, pressure on Conception Vessel 9 and Kidney 3 are recommended.

Gach (1990) suggests several acupressure point areas to treat both PMS and dysmenorrhea. These include points along the Spleen Meridian 4, 6, 12, and 13 at the lower lateral abdominal area and lower leg/foot areas; Bladder Meridian 27 to 34 and 48 on the low back and buttocks area; and Conception Vessel Meridian 4 and 6 along the lower midline abdominal area meridians. Acupuncture charts are available for locating the points.

Helms (1987) reports positive findings from acupuncture treatment in a small group of women who had dysmenorrhea. Forty- three women participated in the controlled prospective year-long study; results showed decreased analgesic use in the Real Acupuncture group. Points used included Spleen 4, Kidney 3 (medial aspects of the

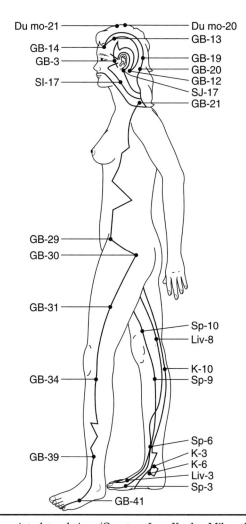

Figure 5-1 Acupressure points, lateral view. (Courtesy Jane Keuler, Milwankee, WI.)

feet), Stomach 36 (lateral aspects of the knees), Stomach 30, Conception Vessel 2 and 4 (suprapubic region), and Pericardium 6 (ventral forearms).

In addition, Oleson and Flocco (1993) reported a significant difference in PMS in a group of women who were treated with ear, hand, and foot reflexology when compared to a placebo group who were treated with inappropriate reflex points. Foot reflexology, although time intensive, may be an appropriate treatment for PMS. Figure 5-2 shows reflexology points.

Lichstein (1988) gives an overview of research on the use of progressive relaxation, imagery, autogenics, and biofeedback for dysmenorrhea. The final comment was that "symptomatic women have exhibited positive relaxation treatment responses, but significant ambiguity persists" (p. 259).

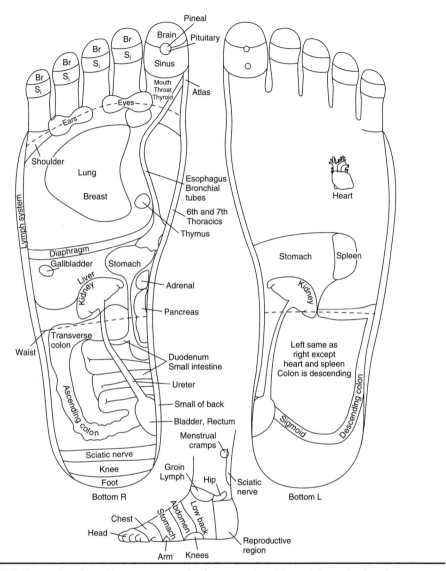

Figure 5-2 Foot reflexology. These are general reference points. The opinions of reflexology experts vary slightly on organ/system placement.

The Complete Woman's Herbal written by McIntyre (1995), a practicing medical herbalist and a director of the National Institute of Medical Herbalists of the United Kingdom at the time of the book's publication, lists self-help practices for PMS, including:

1. Discontinuing or reducing consumption of sugar, alcohol, salt, coffee, tea, and chocolate and avoiding additives and preservatives in food.
2. Discontinuing smoking.

3. Following diet rich in fresh fruits, vegetables, whole grains, nuts, seeds, beans and pulses; using unrefined cold-pressed vegetable or seed oils; solving constipation problems by increasing fiber intake; and avoiding fatty meats, processed foods, and deep-fried foods.

4. Avoiding low blood sugar (evidenced by sugar cravings, increased appetite, faintness, irritability, headaches). Eating every 2 hours may help but refined carbohydrates should be avoided.

5. Treating systemic problems such as food allergies or *Candida* infections and avoiding steroids and oral contraceptives.

6. Exercise, fresh air, and relaxation methods, including music, meditation, T'ai chi, yoga, psychotherapy, relaxation exercises, massage, and aromatherapy. McIntyre (1995) suggests massage or a relaxing bath using essential oils such as lavender, rosemary, melissa, rose, and bergamot.

7. Supplements to correct nutritional deficiencies. McIntyre (1995) recommends a daily regimen of vitamin B_6, 50 mg; evening primrose oil, 500 mg; vitamin E, 100 to 300 mg; and magnesium, 200 mg. A multivitamin is also suggested to provide supplemental chromium and zinc (pp. 89-90).

Chaste tree, false unicorn, wild yam, black haw, sage, motherwort, hops, or black cohosh are used for various hormonal imbalances (McIntyre, 1995). For tension, anxiety, or depression, skullcap, wild oats, wood betony, vervain, and chamomile are suggested. For "extreme tension," valerian and passionflower are useful. Diuretics for fluid retention, bloating, or breast tenderness include corn silk, burdock, and dandelion leaf. In addition, cleavers, poke root, and calendula are listed specifically for breast swelling and tenderness. To "lift the spirits," McIntyre suggests rosemary, cinnamon, oats, St. John's wort, ginger, and lemon balm. For constipation or digestive problems associated with PMS, herbs include yellow dock, burdock root, or licorice; chamomile, lemon balm, cinnamon, ginger, or peppermint can relieve nausea. Licorice supposedly minimizes the effects of stress on the body (McIntyre, 1995). Nurses who desire more information about herbs should contact a knowledgeable herbalist.

Homeopathic remedies for premenstrual symptoms (Fradet et al., 1995) include Bach flower remedies, Schuessler tissue salts, hydrotherapy, autosuggestion, and hypnotherapy (Olshevsky, Noy, Zwang, & Burger, 1993).

For aromatherapy, Maxwell-Hudson (1994) suggests essential oils such as clary sage, geranium, jasmine, marjoram, melissa, Roman chamomile, and rose. These oils are used as a massage blend, as a compress, and as bath oils for both PMS and dysmenorrhea.

NAC Ayurvedic treatment includes yoga, herbs, and foods that promote *sattva* (harmony of mind). Pearls or moonstone gems are suggested to "calm the mind and heart and strengthen the female reproductive system" (Frawley, 1989, p. 201).

Pregnancy

The most natural treatment in pregnancy is no substances and no medications; the best treatment is good food, good air, good exercise, good company and support, good feelings, and routine prenatal care. The best thing a woman can do for herself and her baby is to begin readying herself before pregnancy, being sure she is getting the appropriate nutrients, minerals, and vitamins and staying away from chemicals, preservatives, artificial sweeteners, and toxic environments. Although certain comfort measures are useful, other NAC measures are not recommended.

Certain herbs are *contraindicated* in pregnancy. Herbs that have emmenogogue, oxytocic, or purgative properties should not be used because they could cause abortion (Tierra, 1988). These include rue, golden seal, juniper, autumn crocus, mistletoe, bearberry, pennyroyal, poke root, southernwood, wormwood, mugwort, tansy, nutmeg, cotton root, male fern, thuja, calendula, beth root, feverfew, and sage (McIntyre, 1995). Many other herbs are considered unsafe and are thus contraindicated; for others there are insufficient data on their effects in pregnancy and lactation, and thus their safety cannot be guaranteed. These include black cohosh (Fetrow & Avila, 1999; *PL/PL,* 1999), dong quai (Fetrow & Avila, 1999; *PL/PL,* 1999), echinacea (Natural Medicines Comprehensive Database [NMCD], 2000), evening primrose (Fetrow & Avila, 1999), ginkgo (NMCD, 2000), ginseng (NMCD, 2000), kava (NMCD, 2000), red clover (NMCD, 2000), St. John's wort (NMCD, 2000), and valerian (Fetrow & Avila, 1999; NMCD, 2000). In addition, use of raspberry is cautioned because it may initiate labor (Fetrow & Avila, 1999): it is "possibly safe when the leaf is used as a food flavoring" but "likely unsafe when the leaf is used orally during pregnancy because it can cause uterine contractions" (NMCD, 2000).

Ginger and cinnamon are often recommended for nausea. The pregnant woman can chew on a cinnamon stick or suck on crystallized ginger. Or she may choose to make tea or use the ingredients in cooking. Fetrow and Avila (1999) caution against using ginger in pregnancy because its effects are unknown; however, they report a study (Fisher-Rasmussen, Ksaer, Dahl, & Asping, 1990) of its use for nausea in pregnancy. The NMCD (2000) says ginger is likely safe when used in amounts common in foods. Cinnamon beyond the amount commonly found in food should be avoided (Fetrow & Avila, 1999). In her lay book on herbs, McIntyre (1995) lists raspberry leaves, lemon balm, lavender, and chamomile as good for nausea that is accompanied by anxiety (p. 124); however, the NMCD (2000) considers chamomile possibly unsafe and advises against using lemon balm and lavender because there is insufficient reliable information. Tiran (2000) conversely recommends chamomile tea for anxiety in pregnancy. Obviously controversy exists surrounding the use of herbs in pregnancy. Prudence and current research should guide the practitioner.

Maxwell-Hudson (1994) believes that essential oils should not be used during the first 3 months of pregnancy; De Paoli (1995), an osteopath, aromatherapist, and practitioner of Chinese medicine, states that they should be avoided throughout pregnancy. Tiran (2000), a British midwife and lecturer, recommends that aromatherapy not be used before the second trimester. Buckle (1997), an experienced British nurse with an MA in clinical aromatherapy, does not recommend essential oils for the first 24 weeks of pregnancy:

The use of essential oils in pregnancy is a contentious area, especially during the vital first 3 month period. Many aromatherapists will not treat expectant mothers, as we know that essential oils cross the placenta and we do not know what effect they have on the unborn child. Whilst some midwives are happy to use essential oils during labour, to promote contractions, and for their analgesic properties, and some essential oils have been used in water births, it is generally agreed that for the first 24 weeks of pregnancy essential oils should be avoided. Too little is known about how essential oils can affect the unborn child (p. 87).

After 3 months, Maxwell-Hudson recommends use of only "low dilutions (1% or less) of gentle oils such as chamomile, citrus oils, frankincense, geranium, lavender, sandalwood, and rose" (1994, p. 16). Fradet and others (1995) warn against the use of clary sage, rosemary, and melissa because these essential oils promote the onset of menstruation. However, for hemorrhoids, they do recommend 3 drops of geranium oil to 1 ounce of vegetable oil to be massaged into the rectal area when symptoms occur. They also recommend 4 drops of rose oil to 2 teaspoons of vegetable oil massaged into the solar plexus for nausea; however, this recommendation goes against the warning against using essential oils during the first few months of pregnancy because it is usually in the early months that nausea occurs. Finally, lavendar oil has been used to relieve perineal discomfort following childbirth (Dale & Cornwell, 1994).

For massage during the first 3 months, only almond oil is used. Pillows are used to position the mother in a posture of comfort during pregnancy. Massage is *not* used for morning sickness but otherwise may provide comfort throughout pregnancy. Tiran (2000) discusses aromatherapy, accupoints, and massage for numerous conditions, including backache, breast problems, constipation, colic, depression, headaches, hemorrhoids, heartburn, insomnia, edema, tiredness, infertility, perineal discomfort, stress, anxiety, varicosities (contraindicated directly over them), and vaginal and urinary tract problems.

Reflexology has been found to be helpful during pregnancy, although the author has heard that the gynecologic points on the foot should be avoided. "It will help for some of the associative problems of pregnancy including edema and morning sickness. It is also very helpful in relaxing the entire body during the actual delivery period" (Byers, 1991, p. 191). Kuhn (1999) reports a study from the Association of Reflexologists (Motha & McGrath, 1994) performed on 64 pregnant women to determine the effects of reflexology on labor. Results suggested decreased physical symptoms and labor time; there was no control group.

Therapeutic Touch is another alternative modality that is useful during pregnancy, labor, and delivery. It is used by nurse midwives, Lamaze teachers, and nurses and usually is taught during the seventh to ninth month of pregnancy (Krieger, 1987, 1993). Therapeutic Touch is a modality that a significant other can perform on the pregnant woman. Krieger has done research with mothers and fathers-to-be and found that Therapeutic Touch increases the father's sensitivity to the mother and awareness of the growing fetus. Therapeutic Touch also may decrease discomfort in labor, can be used to decrease tenderness from episiotomy and ceasarean section, and can comfort the baby as well (Krieger, 1987, 1993).

In 1997, an NIH panel of experts issued a supporting statement that there was "clear evidence" for the use of acupuncture for nausea of pregnancy (as well as for postoperative and postchemotherapy nausea and vomiting and postoperative dental pain). In addition, acupuncture may be an effective adjunct for menstrual cramps (Villaire, 1998).

Another recommended therapy is acupressure. Acupressure points for cramps, nausea, and vomiting include:

Pericardium 5: You can find this point on either forearm, four finger-widths above the center of the inner wrist crease between the tendons.

Pericardium 6: You can locate this point about three finger-widths from the upper crease of the wrist on the inner forearm between the two tendons.

Stomach 36: This point is located on the calf, four finger-widths below the bottom of the kneecap, one finger-width outside the shinbone. The point is on a muscle; you can feel it move if you flex your foot (Fradet et al., 1995, p. 227).

For relief of hemorrhoids, Fradet and others (1995) recommend acupressure of the following points:

Governing Vessel 20: This point is situated in the center of the top of the head in line with the ears.

Bladder 57: Locate this point directly below the body of the calf muscle (p. 228).

Moxibustion, a method that uses heat generation by burning herbals to stimulate acupuncture points, has been used for fetal version. In a study by Cardini and Weixin (1998), moxibustion for primigravidas with breech presentation increased cephalic presentation after treatment at delivery. Hypnosis has been used to treat anxiety in pregnant women (Zimmer, Peretz, Eyal, & Fuchs, 1988).

In summary, many modalities are available for the comfort of the pregnant woman, including herbs, massage, reflexology, Therapeutic Touch, and acupressure. In addition, many other self-help strategies, such as deep breathing, centering, imagery, and creative endeavors, as well as playing music and reading aloud for the baby, may be helpful. It is important to note that certain herbs and aromatherapy are contraindicated during pregnancy.

Breast Conditions

For breast pain, the NMCD (2000) lists chasteberry as possibly effective. However, because chasteberries are antiandrogenic, they may interact with oral contraceptives and hormone replacement therapy (NCMD, 2000).

Breast "lumps," a frightening finding whether detected by the health care provider or by the woman herself, need professional assessment. However, the following information on NAC therapies may be of interest.

Quillin (1996) compiled Amish folk medicine remedies. For breast lumps in nonpregnant and nonnursing women, poultices are used as well as the avoidance of chocolate.

Make a poultice from equal parts of wintergreen oil, olive, and spirits of turpentine (not same as commercial type). Do not use while pregnant or nursing.

Make a poultice from equal parts of castor oil and oil of wintergreen (genuine, not synthetic). Do not use while pregnant or nursing (p. 166).

Mowrey (1986) suggests that kelp helps prevent breast cancer. (Research references include Hirayama, 1978; Nomura, Henderson, & Lee, 1978; Teas, 1983; Wynder, 1979.) This decrease is "especially [evident in] Japanese women for whom kelp is viewed as a food, not as a medicinal" (Mowrey, 1986, p. 88). The Japanese consume around 5 to 7.5 g of kelp per capita per day (Mowrey, 1986, p. 208). Mowrey also discusses the use of dandelion by the Chinese as a breast cancer treatment. Flaws and Chace (1994) discuss Chinese research studies on various breast therapies.

Fradet and others (1995) suggest the following acupressure/acupuncture points for "benign breast lumps":

Liver 14: This point is two ribs below the nipple in the sixth intercostal space.

Small Intestine 11: This point is located inside the large hollow in the middle of the shoulder blade. You may fee a slight soreness when you touch this point because it is very sensitive.

Liver 3: This point is located on the top of the foot in the depression beyond the juncture of the metatarsal bones of the big toe and the second toe (pp. 176-177).

They suggest relaxation breathing, hatha yoga, imagery (especially when combined with biofeedback or hypnosis), meditation, and massage as forms of breast "lump" treatment. The herbals suggested include milk thistle and tumeric to promote liver functioning and angelica and lady's mantle to reduce excessive estrogen levels (Fradet et al., 1995). They also recommend decreasing fats, especially saturated kinds, and eliminating coffee tea, chocolate, and other caffeine products as well as meat, sugar, and alcohol. They stress the importance of adequate levels of vitamins B, E, and A and also suggest eating liver-cleansing foods such as beets, carrots, artichokes, lemons, parsnips, and dandelion greens, which help to release the toxins from the body (1995, p. 184).

Menopause

Menopause NAC recommendations include acupuncture, exercise, behavior therapies, soy products and other phytoestrogens as well as numerous vitamins, minerals, and herbs (Bland & Ojeda, 2000; Cabot, 1999; Crawford, 1996; Dolby & Challem, 1999; Kronenberg, Murphy, & Wade, 1999; Liew, Ojeda, & Cjeda, 1999; Luchetti & Hillel, 1997; Murray, 1994; *PL/PL*, 1999; Wolfe & Flaws, 1999). Some research exists on the use of phytoestrogens, including soy, black cohosh (Kronenberg, Murphy, & Wade, 1999; *PL/PL*, 1999; Sierpina, 2001), and red clover (*PL/PL*, 1999). Other herbs that traditionally have been used but do not have a solid research base include dong quai, which probably needs to be used in combination with other herbs (*PL/PL*, 1999) and wild yam (also dehydroepiandrosterone [DHEA], a constituent of wild yam) (Fetrow & Avila, 1999; *PL/PL*, 1999). Women taking warfarin should not use dong quai; women with hypothyroidism should not use soy because it inhibits thyroid hormone synthesis; and those hypersensitive to aspirin should not use black cohosh because it has salicylate constituents (*PL/PL,* 1999).

In a more alternative vein, Farida Sharan (1994, 1995), a naturopath who specializes in herbal medicine and iridology, recommends numerous herbals and dietary aids to help a woman have a smooth transition through menopause. Her recommendations for menopausal supportive supplements and foods include antioxidants, bee pollen, calcium, evening primrose oil, iron, manganese, seaweeds, spirulina, and vitamins B_6, D, and E. In addition, she lists numerous herbal formulas and mixtures. For example, the menopause formula contains alfalfa, chickweed, dandelion, dong quai, fenugreek, horsetail, motherwort, nettles, red clover blossoms, red raspberry leaves, violet leaves, and wild yam root (Sharan, 1995, p. 151).

McIntyre (1995) recommends skullcap, wild oats, wood betony, vervain, lemon balm, and rosemary "to support the nervous system and help to buffer the effects of stress" (p. 187), and ginseng, cinnamon, ginger, huang qi, dang gui, shatavari, and sage to "improve vitality and enhance resistance to stress" (p. 187). In addition, she suggests that sage, hops, shatavari, ginseng, motherwort, wild yam, licorice, and calendula have an "estrogen action and will help smooth the transition from ovarian to adrenal production of estrogen" (p. 187).

If hot flashes are a concern, she suggests plenty of liquids (including a tea of sage and motherwort), vitamin E, selenium, vitamin B complex, calcium, evening primrose oil, and foods rich in vitamin C and flavanoids. She advocates "estrogenic hormone–balancing herbs," such as false unicorn root, chaste tree, wild yam, blue or black cohosh, hops, and licorice (p. 188). For massage or bath, McIntyre suggests essential oils of lavender, rose, geranium, rosemary, or ylang ylang.

Gach (1990) suggests several acupressure points for relieving hot flashes; these include Kidney 1 and 27, Large Intestine 4, Gallbladder 20, Governing Vessels 20 and 24.5, and Conception Vessel 17.

Byers (1991) lists the reflexology points of Diaphragm, All Glands, Reproductive System, and Chronic Uterus Area as useful points in menopause. Olshevsky and others (1993) suggest homeopathic remedies, including *Ignatia, Lachesis, Sulphuricum acidum, Fabiana imbricata, Valeriana, Pulsatilla,* and *Veratum viride* (p. 235). An appropriate homeopathic work-up is needed before initiating such therapy because numerous signs and symptoms need to be taken into account when prescribing homeopathic remedies.

The Later Years

"Old age is ten years beyond your own chronological age" (Seidell, 1985).

Natural and alternative health care for the woman in her later years relates to good diet, exercise, adequate rest, healthy elimination, enjoyable activities, and adequate social support and love, just as for a younger woman. There should be freedom from stress and time for reflection and nostalgia.

Some of the nutritive supplements McIntyre (1995) emphasizes are the antioxidants, including vitamins A, C, and E, the mineral selenium, and the amino acid cysteine (which works with magnesium in detoxification). She also suggests B vitamins, zinc, copper, and manganese. Herbs containing antioxidants are rosemary, thyme, ginger, sage, and garlic. Immunity-stimulating herbs include thyme, ginger, myrrh, sage, echinacea, garlic, rosemary, and calendula. The herbs suggested for the later years are ginkgo, hawthorn, and wood betony. Ginkgo is purported to increase circulation and improve blood flow to the brain, helping to alleviate

vertigo, tinnitus, short-term memory loss, headaches, depression, poor concentration, and other age-related disorders . . . . [It] can be used externally for hemorrhoids, varicose veins and ulcers, . . . act as a tonic to the kidney and bladder and [has] been used for incontinence and excessive urination (McIntyre, 1994, p. 201).

Fetrow and Avila (1999) report on two studies that indicate that ginkgo may be beneficial in persons with dementia. Both studies were placebo controlled (Kanowski et al., 1996; LeBars et al., 1997).

Hawthorn is beneficial for the heart and circulation—the flowers, leaves, and berries have vasodilatory effects. According to McIntyre (1994), the berries can be used for diarrhea and dysentery, have a relaxing effect on the nervous system, and a diuretic effect for relieving fluid retention (p. 204). Fetrow and Avila (1999) state that hawthorn may be "therapeutically useful in the treatment of New York Heart Association (NYHA) functional class II (mild to moderate) heart failure" (p. 325). The patient needs to be closely monitored.

If sleep is a problem, Emmett Miller's *Healing Journey* tape (1980) is relaxing (for any age) as are the tapes of Belleruth Naparstek (e.g., *Healthful Sleep*, 2000) and others. In addition, comfort measures and pain control before bedtime may help. Modalities such as foot soaks, foot rubs, back massages, and head rubs can be a comfort. Chamomile tea and valerian also may be helpful.

Healthy elimination can be enhanced by maintaining exercise even in the frailest of the elderly. Movement of the limbs while holding on to a stable railing, walking even short distances, and lifting weights (or soup cans) are easy forms of exercise. In addition, Power Pudding is helpful for constipation: 2 cups applesauce, 2 cups unprocessed bran, and 1 cup of 100% prune juice, at least 1 ounce, given daily, decreased the use of Milk of Magnesia in Behm's study (1985).

Reflection and reminiscence may be enhanced through writing or journaling. In addition, group reminiscence may increase interaction and allow the nurse to help more than one individual. Photo albums, records, maps, antiques, handiwork, and other memorabilia can stimulate group discussions, which can help women make friends and thus increase social support (Hamilton, 1985).

Books on tape or music may be helpful for those who do not see well, and relaxation or meditation tapes may also be useful for those who suffer from anxiety or depression. Spiritual and religious practices are often important to the elderly, and nurses need to encourage elderly women to continue such practices.

SUMMARY

NAC health care practices are becoming increasingly popular. Health care providers have the responsibility to remain up-to-date with NAC, including assessing the research conclusions, the standards and quality of the practices, and the comfort and healing that NAC provides to women.

REFERENCES

Achterberg, J. (1985). *Imagery in healing*. Boston: Shambhala.

Achterberg, J. (1990). *Woman as healer*. Boston: Shambhala.

Alternative Medicine Editorial Board. (1986). System of homeopathy. *Alternative Medicine, 1*(2), 104–117.

Behm, R. M. (1985). A special recipe to banish constipation. *Geriatric Nursing, 6*(4): 216–217.

Benson, H. (1975). *The relaxation response*. New York: Morrow.

Blanchet, K. (1995). Using light therapy to treat seasonal affective disorder. *Alternative and Complementary Therapies, 1*(5), 311–321.

Bland, I., & Ojeda, L. (2000). *Menopause without medicine*. Alameda, CA: Hunter House.

Blumenthal, M. (Ed.). (1998). *The complete German Commission E monographs*. Austin, TX: American Botanical Council. Boston: Integrative Medicine Communications.

Brennan, B. (1987). *Hands of light: A guide to healing through the human energy field*. New York: Bantam.

Brennan, B. (1993). *Light emerging*. New York: Bantam.

Breslin, E. T. (1996). Metaphoric communication as aesthetic method for nursing practice. *Issues in Mental Health Nursing, 17*, 507–516.

Buckle, J. (1997). *Clinical aromatherapy*. San Diego, CA: Singular.

Bulechek, G., & McCloskey, J. (1985, 1992). *Nursing interventions* (1st and 2nd eds.). Philadelphia: W. B. Saunders.

Byers, D. (1991). *Better health with foot reflexology*. St. Petersburg, FL: Ingham.

Byrd, R. C. (1988). Positive therapeutic effects of intercessory prayer in a coronary care unit population. *Southern Medical Journal, 81*(7), 826–829.

Byrd R. C. (1997). Positive therapeutic effects of intercessory prayer in a coronary care unit population (reprinted from *Southern Medical Journal*). *Alternative Therapies, 3*(6), 87–90.

Cabot, S. (1999). *Smart medicine for menopause: HRT & its natural alternatives*. Garden City Park, NY: Avery Publishing Group.

Callanan M., & Kelley P. (1992). *Final gifts*, New York: Bantam.

Cardini, F., & Weixin, H. (1998). Moxibustion for correction of breech presentation. *Journal of the American Medical Association,* 280(18), 1580–1584.

Chang, S. (1986). *The complete system of self-healing*. San Francisco: Tao.

Colgrove, M., Bloomfield, H., & McWilliams, P. (1976, 1991). *How to survive the loss of a love*. Los Angeles: Prelude.

Connelly, D. (1979). *Traditional acupuncture: The law of the five elements*. Columbia, MD: Center for Traditional Acupuncture.

Crawford A. M. (1996). *The herbal menopause book: Herbs, nutrition, & other natural therapies*. Freedom, CA: Crossing Press.

Dale, A., & Cornwell, S. (1994). The role of lavender oil in relieving perineal discomfort following childbirth: a blind, randomized clinical trial. *Journal of Advanced Nursing, 19*, 89–96.

DePaoli, C. (1995). *The healing touch of massage*. New York: Sterling.

Dharmananda, S. (Ed.). (1987). *Natural healing with herbs*. Prescott Valley, AZ: Hohm Press.

Dolby, V., & Challem, J. (Ed.). (1999). *All about soy isoflavones and women's health*. Garden City Park, NY: Avery Publishing Co.

Dossey, B., Keegan, L., Guzzetta, C., & Kolkmeir, L. (1995). *Holistic nursing: A handbook for practice*. Gaithersburg, MD: Aspen.

Dossey, L. (1993). *Healing words: The power of prayer and the practice of medicine*. San Francisco: Harper.

Dossey, L. (1997). The return of prayer. *Alternative Therapies, 3*(6), 10–17, 113–120.

Eisenberg, D. M., Davis, R. B., Ettner, S. L., Appel, S., Wilkey, S., Van Rompay, M., et al. (1998). Trends in alternative medicine use in the United States, 1990–1997. *Journal of American Medical Association, 280*(18), 1569–1575.

Eisenberg, D. M., Kessler, R. C., Foster, C., Norlock, F. E., Calkins, D. R., & Delbanco, T. L. (1993). Unconventional medicine in the United States. *New England Journal of Medicine, 328,* 246–252.

Eisendrath, S. (1997). Psychiatric disorders. In L. Tierney, S. McPhee, & M. Papadakis, *Current medical diagnosis & treatment.* Stamford, CT: Appleton & Lange.

Ergil, K. (1996). China's traditional medicine. In M. Micozzi (Ed.), *Fundamentals of complementary and alternative medicine* (pp. 185–223). New York: Churchill Livingstone.

Fetrow, C. W., & Avila, J. R. (1999). *Complementary & alternative medicines* (pp. 278–282). Springhouse, PA: Springhouse.

Fisher-Rasmussen W., Ksaer, S. K., Dahl, C., Asping, U. (1990). Ginger treatment of hyperemesis gravidarum. *European Journal of Obstetrics and Gynecology and Reproductive Biology, 38,* 19–24.

Flaws, B. (1985). Premenstrual syndrome (PMS): Its differential diagnosis & treatment. *Journal of Acupuncture, 13*(3), 205–222.

Flaws, B. (1993). *Fire in the valley: The TCM diagnosis and treatment of vaginal diseases.* Boulder, CO: Blue Poppy.

Flaws, B. & Chace, C. (1994). *Recent TCM research from China: 1991–1994.* Boulder, CO: Blue Poppy.

Foreign Language Press. (1980). *Essentials of Chinese acupuncture.* Beijing, China: Foreign Language Press.

Fradet, B., Bergman, W., Clement, B., Retholtz, E., Thomas, J., & Werness, M. (1995). *The natural way of healing: Women's health.* New York: Dell.

Frawley, D. (1989). *Ayurvedic healing.* Salt Lake City: Passage.

Gach, M. R. (1990). *Acupressure's potent points.* New York: Bantam.

Gawain, S. (1997). *Creative visualization.* New York: Bantam.

Giedt, J. (1997). A psychoneuroimmunological intervention in holistic nursing practice. *Journal of Holistic Nursing, 15*(2), 112–127.

Green, J., & Shellenberger, R. (1996). The healing energy of love. *Alternative Therapies, 2*(3), 46–56.

Guzzetta, C. (1995). Music therapy: Hearing the melody of the soul. In B. Dossey, C. Keegen, C. Guzzetta, & C. Kolkmein, *Holistic nursing.* Gaithersburg, MD: Aspen.

Halo Shames, K. (1996). *Creative imagery in nursing.* Albany: Delmar.

Hamilton, D. (1985). Reminiscence therapy. In G. Bulechek, & J. McCloskey (Eds.), *Nursing interventions* (pp. 139–151). Philadelphia: W. B. Saunders.

Hanh, T. N. (1997). *The blooming of a lotus: Guided meditation exercises for healing & transformation.* Boston: Beacon.

Helms, J. (1987). Acupuncture for the management of primary dysmenorrhea. *Obstetrics and Gynecology, 69*(1), 51–55.

Hirayama, T. (1978). Epidemiology of breast cancer with special reference to the role of diet. *Preventive Medicine, 7,* 173–195.

Hoffmann, D. (1996). *The complete illustrated holistic herbal: A safe and practical guide to making and using herbal remedies.* Rockport, MA: Element Books.

Hoffmann, D. (1996). *Herbs to relieve stress: Herbal approaches to relaxation and natural easing of depression and anxiety.* New Canaan, CT: Keats.

Huebscher, R. (1994). What is natural alternative health care? *Nurse Practitioner Forum, 5*(2).

Huebscher, R. (1997). Improving quality in natural/alternative health care practice. In C. Meisenheimer (Ed.), *Improving quality: A guide to effective programs* (pp. 559–568). Gaithersburg, MD: Aspen.

Huebscher, R. (1997). Overdrugging and undertreatment in primary health care. *Nursing Outlook, 45*(4), 161–166.

Jacobs, J., & Moskowitz, R. (1996). Homeopathy. In M. S. Micozzi (Ed.), *Fundamentals of complementary and alternative medicine* (pp. 67–77). New York: Churchill Livingstone.

Kabat-Zinn, J. (1994). *Wherever you go there you are.* New York: Hyperion.

Kalagian, W., Loewen, I., Delmore, T., & Busca, C. (1998). Adolescent oral contraceptive use: Factors predicting compliance at 3 and 12 months. *Canadian Journal of Human Sexuality, 7,* 1–8.

Kanowski, S. Hermann, W. M., Stephan, K., Wierich, W., Horr, R., et al. (1996). Proof of efficacy of the ginkgo biloba special extract EGB 761 in outpatients suffering from mild to moderate primary degenerative dementia of the Alzheimer type or multi-infarct dementia. *Pharmacopsychiatry, 29,* 47–56.

Kiecolt-Glaser, J., Fisher, L., Ogrocki, P., Stout, J., & Glaser, R. (1987). Marital quality, marital disruption, and immune function. *Psychosomatic Medicine, 49,* 13–34.

King, E. E. L., & Bushwick, B. (1994). Beliefs and attitudes of hospital inpatients about faith healing and prayer. *Journal of Family Practice, 39*, 210–213.

Klingon, Y., & O'Sullivan, A. (2001). The family as a protective asset in adolescent development. *Journal of Holistic Nursing, 19*(2), 102–121.

Kolcaba, K. Y. (1991). A taxonomic structure for the concept of comfort. *Image, 23*, 237–240.

Kornfield, J. (Speaker). (1994). *Meditations of the heart.* (Audiotape). Boulder, CO: Sounds True.

Kornfield, J. (Speaker). (1996). *The inner art of meditation.* (Videotape). Boulder, CO: Sounds True.

Krieger, D. (1979). *The Therapeutic Touch.* Englewood Cliffs, NJ: Prentice-Hall.

Krieger, D. (1987). *Living the Therapeutic Touch.* New York: Dodd, Mead & Co.

Krieger, D. (1993). *Accepting your power to heal.* Santa Fe, NM: Bear & Co.

Kronenberg, F., Murphy P., & Wade, C. (1999). Complementary/alternative therapies in select populations: Women. In J. Spencer & J. Jacobs, *Complementary/alternative medicine: an evidence-based approach* (pp. 340–362). St. Louis: Mosby.

Kuhn, M. (1999). *Complementary therapies for health care providers* (pp. 291–350). Philadelphia: Lippincott.

Kunz, K., & Kunz, B. (1993). *The complete guide to foot reflexology.* Albuquerque, NM: RRP Press.

Kunz, K., & Kunz, B. (1995). Understanding the science and art of reflexology. *Alternative and Complementary Therapies, 1*(3), 183–186.

Kushi, M. (1978). (Ninth printing, 1985). *Natural healing through macrobiotics.* New York: Japan Publications.

Kushi, M. (1996). *The standard macrobiotic diet.* Becket, MA: One Peaceful World.

Lad, V. (1985). *Ayurveda: The science of self-healing.* Wilmot, WI: Lotus Press.

Laraque, D., McLean, D., Brown-Peterside, P., Ashton, D., & Diamond, B. (1997). Predictors of reported condom use in central Harlem youth as conceptualized by the Health Belief Model. *Journal of Adolescent Health, 21*, 318–327.

LeBars, P. L., Katz, M. M., Berman, N., Ital, T., Freedman, & Schatzberg A. (1997). A placebo-controlled, double-blind randomized trial of an extract of gingko biloba for dementia. *Journal of the American Medical Association, 278*, 1327–1332.

Lemlin, J. (1992). *Quick vegetarian pleasures.* New York: Harper.

Levine, S. (1989). The healing for which we took birth. In R. Carlson & B. Shield, *Healers on healing.* Los Angeles: Tarcher.

Lichstein, K. (1988). *Clinical relaxation strategies.* New York: Wiley.

Liew, L., & Ojeda, L., (1999). *Natural estrogen diet: Health recipes for perimenopause and menopause.* Almeda, CA: Hunter House.

Luchetti, C., & Hillel, L. (1997). *The hotflash cookbook.* San Francisco: Chronicle Books.

Maciocia, G. (1998). *Obstetrics & gynecology in Chinese medicine.* New York: Churchill Livingstone.

Macrae, J. (1998). *Therapeutic Touch: A practical guide.* New York: Knopf.

Maxwell-Hudson, C. (1994). *Aromatherapy massage.* New York: Dorling Kindersley.

McIntyre, A. (1995). *The complete woman's herbal.* New York: Holt.

Medalie, J. H., & Goldbourt, U. (1976). Angina pectoris among 10,000 men: Psychosocial and other risk factors. *American Journal of Medicine, 60*, 910–921.

Messina, V., & Messina, M. (1996). *Total health for you and your family the vegetarian way.* New York: Crown.

Micozzi, M. (Ed.). (2001). *Fundamentals of complementary and alternative medicine* (2nd ed). New York: Churchill Livingstone.

Migodow, J. (1986). An introduction to homeopathic medicine and the utilization of bioenergies for healing. *Alternative Medicine, 1*(2), 163–168.

Miller, E. (Speaker). (1980). *Healing journey.* (Audiocassette). Stanford, CA: Source.

Miller, E. (Speaker). (1981). *Easing into sleep.* (Audiocassette). Stanford, CA: Source.

Miller, E. (Speaker). (1989). *I can.* (Audiocassette). Stanford, CA: Source.

Moore, N. (1996). Spirituality in medicine. *Alternative Therapies, 2*(6), 24–26, 103–105.

Motha, G., & McGrath, J. (1994). The effects of reflexology on labor outcome. In *Reflexology research report* (2nd ed). London: Association of Reflexologists.

Mowrey, D. (1986). *The scientific validation of herbal medicine.* New Canaan, CT: Keats.

Murray, M. (1994). *Chronic fatigue syndrome: How you can benefit from diet, vitamins, minerals, herbs, exercise & other natural methods.* Rocklin, CA: Prima.

Murray, M. (1996). *Encyclopedia of nutritional supplements: The essential guide for improving your health naturally.* Rocklin, CA: Prima.

Murray, M. (1997). *Heart disease and high blood pressure: How you can benefit from diet, vitamins, minerals, herbs, exercise, & other natural methods.* Rocklin, CA: Prima.

Nakagawa-Kogan, H. (1994). Self-management training: Potential for primary care. *Nurse Practitioner Forum, 5*(2), 77–84.

Naparstek, B. (1994). *Staying well with guided imagery.* New York: Warner.

Naparstek, B. (Speaker). (2000). *Healthful sleep.* (Audiotape). Akron, OH: Image Paths. *www.healthjourneys.com.*

National Center for Complementary and Alternative Medicine (NCCAM). 2001. *http://nccam.nih.gov,* (accessed 5/22/01).

Natural Medicines Comprehensive Database. (2000). (Compiled by the editors of *Pharmacist's Letter/Prescriber's Letter*). Stockton, CA: Therapeutic Research Facility.

Nichols, H., & Humenick, S. S. (1988). *Childbirth education: Practice, research, & theory.* Philadelphia: W. B. Saunders.

Nomura, A., Henderson, B. E., & Lee, J. (1978). Breast cancer and diet among the Japanese in Hawaii. *American Journal of Clinical Nutrition, 31,* 2020–2025.

Office of Alternative Medicine. (1997). *Complementary & alternative medicine at the NIH.* Bethesda, MD: DHHS.

O'Laoire, S. (1997). An experimental study of the effects of distant, intercessory prayer on self-esteem, anxiety, and depression. *Alternative Therapies, 3*(6), 38–53.

Oleson, T., & Flocco, W. (1993). Randomized controlled study of premenstrual symptoms treated with ear, hand, and foot reflexology. *Obstetrics and Gynecology, 82*(6), 906–911.

Olshevsky, M., Noy, S., Zwang, M., & Burger, R. (1993). *The manual of natural therapy.* Secaucus, NJ: Citadel.

Pharmacist's Letter/Prescriber's Letter. (1999). Menopause. *Natural Medicines in Clinical Management, 99*(4), 34–41.

Pharmacist's Letter/Prescriber's Letter. (2001). PMS. *Natural Medicines in Clinical Management, 2,* 13–20.

Pizzorno, J. (1996). Naturopathic medicine. In M. Micozzi (Ed.), *Fundamentals of complementary and alternative medicine* (pp. 163–181). New York: Churchill Livingstone.

Quillin, P. (1996). *Amish folk medicine.* Sarasota, FL: Book World Services.

Ray, S. (1980). *Loving relationships.* Berkeley, CA: Celestial Arts.

Reilly, D. (1995). Research, homeopathy, and therapeutic consultation. *Alternative Therapies, 1*(4), 65–73.

Samuels, M. (1995). Art as a healing force. *Alternative Therapies, 1*(4), 38–40.

Scandrett, S., & Uecker, S. (1985). Relaxation training. In G. Bulechek & J. McCloskey, *Nursing interventions* (pp. 22–48). Philadelphia: W. B. Saunders.

Seidell, K. M. (1985). Group support. In C. Painter, & P. Valois, *Gifts of age* (pp. 105–108). San Francisco: Chronicle.

Sharan, F. (1994). *Creative menopause.* Boulder CO: Wisdome Press.

Sharan, F. (1995). Natural treatment of menopause using herbs. *Alternative and Complementary Therapies, 1*(3), 147–153.

Shellenberger, R., & Green, J. A. (1986). *From the ghost in the box to successful biofeedback training.* Greeley, CO: Health Psychology Publications.

Shuler, P., Gelberg, L., & Brown, M. (1994). The effects of spiritual/religious practices on psychological well-being among inner city homeless women. *Nurse Practitioner Forum, 5*(2), 106–113.

Sierpina, V. (2001). Top twenty herbs for primary care. In M. Micozzi, *Fundamentals of complementary and alternative medicine* (pp. 138–145). New York: Churchill Livingstone.

Soffa, V. (1996). Artistic expressions of illness. *Alternative Therapies, 2*(3), 63–66.

Sosa, R., Kennell, J., Klaus, M., Robertson, S., & Urrutia, J. (1980). The effect of a supportive companion on perinatal problems, length of labor, and mother-infant interaction. *New England Journal of Medicine, 303,* 597–600.

Stansbury, J. (1997). *Herbs for health & healing.* Lincolnwood, IL: Publications, International.

Tappan, F. (1988). *Healing massage techniques.* Norwalk, CT: Appleton & Lange.

Teas, J. (1983). The dietary intake of *Laminaria,* a brown seaweed, and breast cancer prevention. *Nutrition and Cancer, 4*(3), 217–223.

Thomas, A. (1996). *The vegetarian epicure,* New York: Knopf.

Tierra, M. (1988, 1992). *Planetary herbology.* Twin Lakes, WI: Lotus.

Tiran, D. (2000). *Clinical aromatherapy for pregnancy and childbirth.* New York: Churchill Livingstone.

Tiran, D., & Mack, S. (2000). *Complementary therapies* (pp. 129–167). Edinburgh: Bailliere Tindall.

Ullman, D. (1993). *Homeopathic medicine: A modern view.* Sausalito, CA: Whole Earth Review.

Villaire, M. (1998). NIH consensus conference confirms acupuncture efficacy. *Alternative Therapies, 4*(1), 21.

Wolfe, H. (1995). *Menopause: A second spring.* Boulder, CO: Blue Poppy.

Wolfe, H. L., & Flaws, B. S. (1998). *Managing menopause naturally with Chinese medicine.* Boulder, CO: Blue Poppy.

Wynder, E. L. (1979). Dietary habits and cancer epidemiology. *Cancer Supplement, 43*(5) 1955–1961.

Zahourek, R. (1988). *Relaxation and imagery: Tools for therapeutic communication and intervention.* Philadelphia: W. B. Saunders.

Zimmer, E., Peretz, B., Eyal, E., & Fuchs, K. (1988). The influence of maternal hypnosis on fetal movements in anxious pregnant women. *European Journal of Obstetrics and Gynecological Reproductive Biology, 27*, 133–137.

RESOURCES

General

American Holistic Nurses Association (AHNA)
PO Box 2130
Flagstaff, AZ 86003
(800) 278-2462
AHNA-flag@flaglink.com

American Holistic Nurses' Certification Corp
AHNCC@flash.net

American Holistic Medical Association
6728 Old McClean Village Dr
McClean, VA 22101
(703) 556-9728
www.holisticmedicine.org

National Center for Complementary and Alternative Medicine
National Institutes of Health
6120 Executive Blvd, EPS Suite 450
Rockville, MD 20892-9904
(301) 402-2466
http://nccam.nih.gov

Acupuncture

American Association of Acupuncture and Oriental Medicine
433 Front St
Catasauqua, PA 18032
(610) 433-2448

Aromatherapy/Essential Oils/Oils

American Alliance of Aromatherapy
PO Box 309
Depoe Bay, OR 97341
(800) 809-9850

Aromatherapy for Health Professionals
RJ Buckle Associates, LLC
PO Box 868
Hunter, NY 12442
www.rjbuckle.com

National Association for Holistic Aromatherapy
www.nahaorg@earthlink.net

Art

American Art Therapy Association, Inc
1202 Allanson Rd
Mundelein, IL 60060
(708) 949-6064

Ayurveda
www.ayurveda.com

www.mum.edu/cmvm/mvm

www.mcvmnn.org

Biofeedback
Association for Applied Psychophysiology and Biofeedback (formerly Biofeedback Society)
10200 West 44th Ave #304
Wheatridge, CO 80033
(303) 422-8436
Stens Corporation
www.stens.com

Chiropractic
American Chiropractic Association
1701 Clarendon Blvd
Arlington, VA 22209

International Chiropractors Association
1110 Glebe Rd, Suite 1000
Arlington, VA 22201
(703) 528-5000
(800) 423-4690

National Directory of Chiropractic
PO Box 10056
Olathe, KS 66501

Energywork
Colorado Center for Healing Touch
12477 W Cedar Dr #206
Lakewood, CO 80228
(303) 989-0581
www.healingtouch.net

Nurse Healers—Professional Associates International, Inc
3760 S Highland Dr
Salt Lake City, UT 84106
nh-pai@therapeutic-touch.org

American Reiki Masters Association
(904) 755-9638
Reiki Alliance
Reikialliance@compuserve.com

Herbals
American Botanical Council
PO Box 210660
Austin, TX 78720
(800) 373-7105
(512) 331-8868
Journal *Herbalgram*

American Herb Association
PO Box 1673
Nevada City, CA 95959
(916) 265-9552

American Herbalists Guild
PO Box 1683
Soquel, CA 95073
(408) 464-2441

Gaia Herbal Research Institute
12 Lancaster County Rd
Harvard, MA 01451
(508) 772-5400

Homeopathy

American Association of Homeopathic Pharmacists
PO Box 11280
Albuquerque, NM 87192

American Institute of Homeopathy
1585 Glencoe St #44
Denver, CO 80220
(303) 370-9164

Council for Homeopathic Certification
www.homeopathicdirectory.com

Foundation for Homeopathic Research
www.indiaspace.com/homoeopathy (British spelling)

Homeopathic Nurses Association
3403 17th Ave South
Minneapolis, MN 55407

International Foundation for Homeopathy
2366 Eastlake Ave E Suite 301
Seattle, WA 98102
(206) 324-8230

National Center for Homeopathy
801 North Fairfax #306
Alexandria, VA 22314
(703) 548-7790
info@homeopathic.org

North American Society of Homeopaths
1122 East Pike St #1122
Seattle, WA 98122
(206) 720-7000
nashinfo@aol.com

Humor

American Association for Therapeutic Humor
4534 W Butler Dr
Glendale, AZ 85302
(623) 934-6068
www.aath.org
office@aath.org

Hypnosis

American Psychological Association, Division 30
750 First Suite NE
Washington, DC 20002
(202) 336-5500
www.apa.org

American Society of Clinical Hypnosis
130 East Elm Court, Suite 201
Roselle, IL 60172-2000
(630) 980-4740
info@asch.net
www.asch.net

International Medical and Dental Hypnotherapy Association
4110 Edgeland, Suite 800
Royal Oaks, MI 48073-2251
(810) 549-5594

Imagery

Nurses Certificate Program in Interactive Imagery
Beyond Ordinary Nursing
PO Box 8177
Foster City, CA 94404-3004
(650) 570-6157
NCPII@aol.com
www.imageryn.com

Light Therapy

Society for Light Treatment and Biological Rhythms
10200 West 44th Ave Suite 304
Wheatridge, CO 80033
(303) 424-3697

Massage/Bodywork

Aboutmassage.com
www.naturalhealers.com

Associated Bodywork and Massage Professionals
(303)674-8478
(800)458-2267
www.abmp.com

American Massage Therapy Association
820 Davis St
Evanston, IL 60201
www.amtamassage.org

American Society for Alexander Technique
Alexandertech.com

The Feldenkrais Guild
706 Ellsworth St SW
PO Box 489
Albany, OR 97321
(800)775-2118
www.feldenkraisschools@naturalhealers.com

Body of Knowledge/Hellerwork
406 Berry St
Mt. Shasta, CA 96067
(503)926-2500
www.hellerwork.com

International Alliance of Healthcare Practitioners (Upledger Institute—includes craniosacral manipulation,
       St. John's wort, Aston therapeutics, zero balancing, visceral manipulation)
11211 Prosperity Farms Road
Palm Beach Gardens, FL 33410

(800)233-5880 x50015
www.upledger.com

International Association of Infant Massage
www.infantmassage.org
IAIM4us@aol.com

National Association of Massage Therapy
PO Box 1400
Westminster, CO 80030

National Association of Nurse Massage Therapists
PO Box 820
Clarkdale, AZ 86324
www.aboutmassage.com/massage associations.htm

National Association of Pregnancy Massage Therapy
(888)451-4945

National Certification Board for Therapeutic Massage & Bodywork
1735 N Lyon St Suite 950
Arlington, VA 22209

North American Vodder Association of Lymphatic Therapy
www.navalt.com

The Rolf Institute of Structural Integration
205 Canyon Blvd
Boulder, CO 80302
(303)449-5903
www.rolf.org

Rosen Method Professional Association
2550 Shattuck Ave
Box 49
Berkeley, CA 94704
www.Rosenmethod.org

Trager Institute
21 Locust Ave
Mill Valley, CA 94941
www.trager.com

Worldwide Aquatic Bodywork Association
PO Box 889
Middletown, CA 95461

Meditation

Jack Kornfield produces audio and videotapes on meditation. The *Inner Art of Meditation* (1996), a videotape, and *Meditations of the Heart* (1994) are especially good for beginners. Thich Nhat Hanh (1997) has writings and tapes on the practice of mindfulness; these media present Buddhist principles for daily life.

Jon Kabat Zinn (1994) has tapes and texts on mindfulness meditation.

Music

American Music Therapy Association
info@musictherapy.org

National Association of Music Therapy
8455 Colesville Rd Suite 930
Silver Spring, MD 20910
(301)589-3300

Naturopathy

American Naturopathic Medical Association
PO Box 96273
Las Vegas, NV 89193
(702)897-7053

American Association of Naturopathic Physicians
2366 Eastlake Ave Suite 322
Seattle, WA 98102
(206)328-8510

American Naturopathic Association
1413 K St 1st Floor
Washington, DC 20005
(202)682-7352
(202)289-2027
www.Bastyr.edu

Osteopathy

American Osteopathic Association
www.aoa-net.org

Polarity

American Polarity Therapy Association
PO Box 19858
Boulder, CO 80308
(303)545-2080
www.polaritytherapy.org
hq@polaritytherapy.org

Reflexology

www.naturalhealers.com/qa/reflexology

American Reflexology Certification Board
(303)933-6921

International Institute of Reflexology
PO Box 12642
St Petersburg, FL 33733
(727)343-4811
www.reflexology-usa.net
ftreflex@concentric.net

Kunz School of Reflexology
PO Box 35820 Station D
Albuquerque, NM 87173-5829
(800)713-6711

Yoga

Yoganet@aol.com
(707)928-9898

International Association of Yoga Therapists (Division of Yoga Research & Education Center)
www.iayt.org
www.yrec.org

Yoga Alliance.org
(877)964-2255

Chapter 6

Psychosocial Development of Women

Virginia Blankenship

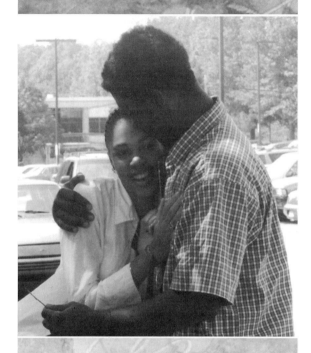

The highest form of development is to govern one's self.

Zerelda G. Wallace

INTRODUCTION

Everyone who is involved with women's health must deal effectively with women at different points in their psychosocial development. Understanding the interplay between the mind-body connection is essential. Young girls respond to information concerning their health differently from adolescents; middle-aged women are concerned with different psychological and social issues than elderly women. Knowledge of the psychosocial development of women across the lifespan helps nurses by guiding their thoughts, emotions, and behaviors as they assist women to make the best decisions possible concerning health issues.

In discussing the psychosocial development of women, three main aspects of women's personalities and motivations,—achievement, intimacy, and power—will be highlighted. These personality and motivational characteristics correspond to the three major areas of women's lives: their work, their loves, and their relationships to others and to the social realities around them. These three themes will guide the story of how women develop psychologically and socially across the lifespan.

The telling of this story will be guided by Carol Gilligan's (1982) observation that "at a time when efforts are being made to eradicate discrimination between the sexes in the search for social equality and justice, the differences between the sexes are being rediscovered in the social sciences. This discovery occurs when theories formerly considered to be sexually neutral in their scientific objectivity are found instead to reflect a consistent observational and evaluative bias" (p. 6). Gilligan noted that by adopting the male life as the norm, theorists have tried to explain the lives of women based on a masculine model. "It all goes back, of course, to Adam and Eve—a story which shows, among other things, that if you make a woman out of a man, you are bound to get into trouble. In the life cycle, as in the Garden of Eden, the woman has been the deviant" (p. 6). In her research on moral decision making, Gilligan has worked to portray women not as deviants, but as the decision makers who have had a different set of life experiences, resulting in a different "voice."

In reviewing the theories of psychosocial development, the lifespan will be divided into four major segments: childhood, adolescence, early adulthood, and late adulthood. Also discussed are the various ways in which lives are conceptualized: as a series of stages, as different paths, as ways of knowing, and as voice. Within this context, the arguments that have arisen around the issue of whether current models adequately reflect the lives of women will be outlined.

PSYCHOSOCIAL MODELS OF CHILDHOOD

In an effort to explain the development of ego identity, Erik Erikson (1963) described the eight ages of man (Table 6-1). These eight ages or stages are crises that must be successfully negotiated before the person can move on to the next crisis or stage. In general, there are four developmental stages of childhood (trust vs. distrust, autonomy vs. shame and doubt, initiative vs. guilt, and industry vs. inferiority). For example, if the child does not develop trust, her life will be characterized by distrust, which will affect the next stage and all subsequent stages. A distrustful child has trouble with autonomy

Table 6-1   ERIKSON'S PSYCHOSOCIAL STAGES

MAJOR CONFLICTS	TIME OF LIFE
Trust vs. mistrust	Infancy
Autonomy vs. shame & doubt	Early childhood
Initiative vs. guilt	Third–fifth years
Industry vs. inferiority	Sixth year – puberty
Identity vs. role confusion	Early adolescence
Intimacy vs. isolation	Late adolescence
Generativity vs. stagnation	Early adulthood
Ego integrity vs. despair	Late adulthood

Data from Erickson, E. H. (1963). *Childhood and society* (2nd ed.). New York: W. W. Norton & Company.

and will be burdened with shame and doubt. Being distrustful, shameful, and doubting, the child will not be able to develop initiative and so on. Erikson identified two stages of adolescence (identity vs. role confusion and intimacy vs. isolation) and two stages of adulthood (generativity vs. stagnation and ego integrity vs. despair).

In contrast to Freud, who focused on sexual crises in infancy and childhood, Erikson focused on social crises. For example, in the oral stage, Freud (1905) viewed the mouth as the location of sexual tension and depicted the mother's breast as a source of sexual gratification for the baby. Erikson saw the development of trust between the infant and her mother as a social interaction that built on the dependability of the mother in providing nourishment, through the breast or a bottle. The mother also had to be able to trust the child. For example, if the mother breast-fed the baby, the child had to refrain from biting the mother's breast after teething had occurred. Only when mutual trust has been established will the baby have a sense of belongingness that provides a secure foundation for the development of separateness or autonomy.

Jean Baker Miller (1991a) conceptualized the infant as a "being-in-relationship" (p. 13). For her, the important issue is whether the child feels comfortable in its emotional relationship with the caregiver. The response of others to the emotional nucleus of the infant creates a mental representation of the self. Miller believes that "this early 'interacting sense of self' is present for infants of both sexes, but the culturally induced beliefs of the caretakers about girls and boys play a role from the moment of birth" (p. 14). Girls are encouraged to develop empathy, whereas boys are treated as a lone self. Consequently, the girl's sense of self-esteem arises from her relationships to others; the boy's sense of self-esteem is tied to a sense of power resulting from individual actions.

John Bowlby (1988) developed attachment theory to explain why young children seek out close proximity to others, especially their mothers. Bowlby believed that personality development was influenced strongly by attachment behavior, the interaction between the child and her mother and the feeling of security the child gains from being encouraged and valued by her mother. Bowlby believed that attachment behavior serves the biological function of protecting the child and that infants need a committed caregiver relationship with at least one adult figure, usually the mother. Securely attached children initially stay close to the mother (the attachment figure), using her as a secure base from which they can explore the environment. Periodically, they return to her for reassurance. Children who are not securely attached have separation anxiety, a dread that they will be abandoned, and may have difficulty developing a social life outside the family. Bowlby believed that this could result from a mother who had a difficult childhood and who grew up anxiously attached to her own parents. By trying to make her child her own attachment figure, the mother is burdening the child by making it take care of her. This inversion of the usual relationship makes the child anxiously attached, guilty, and perhaps phobic.

In a study of African children and their mothers, Mary Ainsworth (1967) found that mothers who were sensitive to infant signals of happiness and distress were more likely to have children who were securely attached. Conversely, infants who were insecurely or anxiously attached had mothers who were less sensitive to their children's signals. To measure attachment, Ainsworth and Wittig (1969) devised the Strange Situation, a structured 20-minute observation period during which the child played in a laboratory. First, just the 1-year-old and its mother were present, then they were joined by a stranger (a woman), who played with the child while the mother left for a few minutes and then returned. After a few more minutes both the mother and the stranger left the child alone. Finally both the mother and stranger returned. When the mother returned, some children sought comfort from her. Others were ambivalent, seeming to want contact but hitting her when she tried to comfort them. A third group acted disinterested at their mothers' return, even though they had been upset while she was gone. These behaviors correlated with other indications that the first group of children were securely attached, the second group were ambivalent in the attachment, and the third group were avoidant.

Bretherton (1995) has summarized recent research on the measurement of attachment patterns among adults. When adults were interviewed about their childhoods, autonomous-secure adults gave a clear and coherent account of early childhood and their attachment to their parents, whether their childhood was happy or not. Preoccupied adults spoke about conflicts in childhood but couldn't bring the various memories together into a coherent picture. Dismissing adults were unable to remember childhood attachments. Bowlby (1988) believed that as children, we create an internal working model of ourselves and the world around us. If we feel secure in our families, we are able to construct a working model that is flexible and open to updating with new information. If we are insecure and anxious, we exclude information from awareness because it is threatening. Therefore our models are not coherent and do not guide us well in living our adult lives. Further, the repression of memories, which creates a lack of coherence in our lives, makes it difficult to recall our childhoods accurately.

According to Erikson (1968), at about age 2 the child is engrossed in a crisis of autonomy vs. shame and doubt. Anyone who has lived with a Terrible Two is familiar with the adamant insistence on "me, me, me" and the strident demand that "I do it myself." This crisis of separateness from the parents and caretakers coincides with muscular maturation that allows the child to "hold on" and "let go," behaviors that are particularly important in the task of toilet training and bowel control. According to Erikson, the anus is a location for holding on and letting go, rather than a site for sexual frustration and gratification, as proposed by Freud (1905). Autonomy is the result of social interaction between the child and its parents; shame and doubt result when the child exerts too much control over herself and becomes self-conscious. Erikson (1963) also proposed that shame is "rage turned against the self" (p. 252), which may be particularly apropos to the discussion of female development because many women have recently recognized an inability to express anger toward others. Shaming accentuates the smallness and vulnerability of the child and makes her aware of the relative size and greater power of the adults who control her life. Doubt arises from the part of the self that is unseen and unseeable by the child, the behind. Doubt arises when the products of the child, including bowel movements, are judged by others to be bad. Further, doubt arises when the child's attempts to control her behavior are unsuccessful or scorned. The successful achievement of autonomy, therefore, incorporates control, a necessary element for the subsequent development of initiative.

Miller's (1991a) analysis of the tasks of early childhood do not focus on autonomy and separation, but instead characterize the girl's increasing assertiveness to be the result of her increased powers and her desire to do things for others. Because she has been encouraged to continue to attune herself to others' feelings, the girl's actions are affected by their feelings. Her defiant behavior may be a reaction to her feeling that the caretaker is attempting to control her behavior, treating her like a baby. It is important for the caretaker to recognize her growing abilities and to support the girl's explorations of her expanding world.

When the tyranny of the Terrible Twos has passed, the child has a renewed sense of vigor, according to Erikson (1963). If the proper balance between trust and mistrust is providing the child with a dependable guide for deciding whom to trust and whom not to trust, and, if the child has a deep sense of control over her body and behaviors, she will be eager to discover the world and to find new ways to interact with it. A characteristic of initiative is the "free possession of a surplus of energy" which allows the child "to forget failures quickly" (p. 255). It is easy to see that this would be the opposite of depression, a condition that is more prevalent in women than in men (Beck, Steer, & Epstein, 1992). Whereas autonomy carries a sense of defiance, initiative includes planning and conquest. Erikson thought girls expressed initiative through "catching" a mate and in making themselves attractive and endearing. His contrast between boys' more active modes and girls' more receptive modes of behaving reflects the gender attitudes of his time, a practice Levinson (1996) has termed *gender-splitting*.

Gender-splitting accentuates the differences between women and men and forces them into separate worlds, the domestic world for women and the public occupational world for men. Gender-splitting ignores the coexistence of feminine and masculine qualities in both sexes and leads women to deny the masculine in themselves and men to deny the feminine in themselves. Women's work is made distinct from men's work, and girls and boys are encouraged to have different behaviors and interests (Levinson, 1996, pp. 6-7, 38-39).

During the initiative vs. guilt stage, the child comes to identify with the parent of the same sex. For a girl, identification with her mother and a dawning awareness of the incest taboo place a new restriction on her interactions with her father. The "horizon of the permissible" is narrowed but the possibility of actualizing dreams of earlier childhood is increased. Guilt arises if restrictions are transgressed, and sexual abuse is particularly damaging at this stage of a girl's life. If initiative is fully developed, the girl moves on to the next stage with a surplus of energy to take on the tasks of formal education.

Miller (1991a) challenged this interpretation of the "Oedipal" stage of development, proposing that Freud and Erikson (among others) had difficulty explaining this age for girls because girls do not go through a distinct stage at this point in their lives. Rather, Miller sees the task the girl faces is to deal with the Western culture's devaluation of the mother and the greater importance and power accorded the father. The girl is encouraged to use her energies to foster the well-being of the men around her. This does not lead to an identification with the aggressor (father), which is the outcome of the Freudian phallic stage, or with the mother, which is the outcome of the Erikson initiative stage. Miller sees the girl in a continuing struggle to gain a sense of herself and to deal with an increasingly complicated relationship with her mother.

According to Erikson, upon entering the formal education system in this country, industry vs. inferiority presents a crisis for girls, especially if they are viewed as inferior in certain school subjects, such as mathematics. In this stage, the child learns to win praise by producing something. Within her ego identity, the girl incorporates the skills and tools that she is mastering. She becomes adept on the computer and her sense of industry includes producing a story or writing a letter to an Internet pen pal. As children learn to use the tools of their society, they further prepare themselves to be productive adults. If the girl is not given adequate training or if she is made to feel clumsy or dumb, she will develop a sense of inadequacy or inferiority. She will feel distant from the productive world and be dependent on others for economic support. Her sense of identity will be dominated by negative comparisons to others and her feelings of inferiority will decrease her future options.

In her analysis of childhood, Miller (1991a) questioned the appropriateness of the concept of industry in discussing the development of girls at this age. She pointed out that the most common activity among girls at school during recess was standing around talking. She proposed that little is known about the activities of girls at this age and the meaning of their talking and emotional interactions with each other.

Childhood Development and Achievement

Achievement motivation has been defined by Atkinson (1958) as the desire to do well, a strong interest in a long-term career, or the desire to make a unique contribution such as a discovery. Achievement motivation is conceptualized as including a positive approach to succeeding and a negative avoidance of failure. Individuals are assumed to be predominantly motivated by either the hope of success or the fear of failure. Those individuals with high hopes for success will approach achievement activities and delight in doing well, being involved in a career and excited about making a unique contribution to society. Those individuals with a high fear of failure get no special pleasure from doing well; they pursue jobs and not careers and achieving a unique accomplishment does not motivate them. If given a choice, people with a high fear of failure will avoid activities with success or failure outcomes and pursue activities that do not involve such evaluations.

The application of achievement motivation theory to girls and women has always been problematic. Early studies of the choice of preferred task difficulty and of persistence at achievement tasks (Atkinson & Feather, 1966) used male subjects only. French and Lesser (1964) proposed that women did not behave according to the predictions of achievement theory because the achievement tasks were not defined within their life domains. For example, achievement theory predicted that subjects with high hope of success would persist longer at tasks of intermediate difficulty than at easy or difficult tasks. This prediction was typically tested with ring-toss games and other activities favored by boys.

Matina Horner (1987) had a different explanation for the failure of achievement motivation theory to explain women's behavior. She suggested that succeeding is not a clearly positive outcome for women and that some women have a fear of success that makes succeeding a partially negative outcome. To study fear of success, Horner had both women and men write Thematic Apperception Test (TAT) stories about Anne (for the female subjects) or John (for the male subjects). Both Anne and John were depicted as being at the top of their class in medical school. Subjects were asked to complete the story of Anne or John, to tell what had led up to this situation, what they were thinking and feeling, and what would happen to them. When the TAT stories were analyzed, it was found that 62% of the female subjects projected fear of success into their stories about Anne, while only 9% of the male subjects projected fear of success into their stories about John. The negative outcomes for Anne included being ostracized for being "uppity" and losing her boyfriend because she was not feminine enough. In one story, she proclaimed her joy over her achievement and was beaten by her fellow students and maimed for life. Fear of success was conceptualized as the fear of a loss of affiliation (or friendship) when a woman competes with someone else, a loss of femininity for achieving at a masculine activity, or the loss of family options if a woman dedicates herself to a career. All of these facets of the fear of success have an interactional element to them. That is, the feared result of succeeding is losing a friend, losing the sense of one's own gender identity, or losing out on family and love relationships.

Another element of the achievement domain that may be alien to women is the solitary nature of the achievement enterprise. The entrepreneur is the prototype of a person driven by high achievement motivation. The person who has a high need for affiliation (warm relationships with others) is viewed as being conflicted in achievement and power (leadership) domains (McClelland, 1975). Achievements that require cooperation among people differ from the individually oriented achievements that are the basis of achievement theory. These individually oriented activities include competition based on (1) a standard of excellence—called "personal best" in athletic circles; (2) long-term career involvement—climbing the corporate hierarchical ladder; and (3) unique accomplishment—the lone inventor making discoveries in an isolated laboratory. Of course, modern achievements are rarely individual accomplishments, and one of the greatest challenges business and industry face is to find (or train) people who are able to work cooperatively in groups. The childhood training of girls may make women particularly adept at cooperative forms of achievement, which have not been systematically researched.

Achievement and Developmental Crises

A secure base from which to operate is very useful in achievement tasks. The ability to discriminate between people and situations that are harmful and those that are beneficial or benign is basic to high achievement. Making judgments about reasonable risks to take in business, which educational paths to pursue, what medical research to devote one's life to—all require the ability to make distinctions about trust. If a woman does not develop a sense of trust in others or if she indiscriminatly trusts everyone, she will not be able to sort the valid information from the lies. Gullibility or cynicism will win out over accuracy. Achievement motivation is characteristic of entrepreneurship, i.e., setting up one's own business. Clearly, the fervent desire of the two-year-old to "do it myself" is the precursor to achievement motivation. The pride of succeeding reinforces achievement behavior, and failure results in the emotion of shame, a punishing state. Industry is developed through successful learning and by being good at something. However, if what the little girl is good at is devalued by parents and teachers, she will develop feelings of inferiority.

Achievement motivation research has focused recently on the attributions of success and failure, that is, the reasons we think we have succeeded or failed (Weiner, 1974). The most common attributions of success are to high ability, sustained effort, task difficulty (easy task), and good luck. The most common attributions for failure are low ability, lack of effort, task too difficult, and bad luck.

Dweck and Wortman (1982) summarized the research on gender differences in attribution styles, especially the differences among boys and girls of grade school age in their attributions of success to effort or ability. In a study of classroom interactions, Dweck, Davidson, Nelson, and Enna (1978) found that teachers socialize girls to attribute failure in school work to lack of ability but socialize boys to attribute failure to lack of effort. Erikson equated industry with productivity, and effort is closely related to productivity. With a given level of ability, effort makes the difference in whether a great deal or just a small amount is accomplished. However, Weiner (1974) pointed out that effort is an unstable attribution. If you put a lot of effort into a task now and succeed, it does not guarantee the next time you will succeed because your level of effort might not continue to be high enough. So even when girls are taught to attribute their success to effort, they still see their successes as unstable. If they ever stop trying hard, they will fail because of their underlying belief that they lack ability.

Although we have focused on the achievement motivation of girls and how that might relate to their psychosocial development, the groundwork for development in all areas of life is laid in childhood. A distrusting girl will have difficulty in her friendships, her love relationships, and her interactions with the larger society. If she lacks initiative, she will be passive and at the mercy of others in all areas of her life. As she approaches adolescence, her sense of self will be limited by feelings of inferiority.

PSYCHOSOCIAL MODELS OF ADOLESCENCE

Erikson (1963) placed two crises in adolescence: identity vs. role confusion and intimacy vs. isolation. He originally wrote that the crisis of identity must be resolved before the person is capable of establishing intimacy. In subsequent writings, Erikson (1968) acknowledged the comingling of identity and intimacy for women. However, his interpretation of that interdependence was premised on the prevalent social expectations that a woman would find her identity, as least partially, within her relationships to others, particularly her husband.

Identity

According to Erikson the crisis of identity vs. role confusion is initiated by the rapid physical changes of puberty. With sexual maturity and coming adulthood, young women are faced with transferring the roles and skills they developed in childhood to the occupational sphere. Significant people in the young woman's world, such as teachers and parents, are often forced into artificial adversarial relationships as she works to integrate the roles of childhood with the more demanding roles of adulthood. The danger in this stage is role confusion. Erikson believed that, in an attempt to keep themselves together during this confusing period, teenagers often over-identify to the point that they seem to have lost their individual identities. This over-identification is evidenced by their tendency to imitate the dress and mannerisms of rock singers and other media stars. Additionally, Erikson remarked that young people can be cruelly exclusionary of anyone who is different. They place a high value on conformity to group norms and exclude those who are different. For many, identity is determined within a love relationship. "To a considerable extent adolescent love is an attempt to arrive at a definition of one's identity by projecting one's diffused ego image on another and by seeing it thus reflected and gradually clarified. This is why so much of young love is conversation" (Erikson, 1963, p. 262). This concept of identity being determined through conversation adds importance to Carol Gilligan's (1982) concept of "voice," the ability to be heard.

Taylor, Gilligan, and Sullivan (1995) studied 26 urban girls whom they had identified as being at risk for dropping out of school and/or becoming teenage mothers. They interviewed these girls extensively from the eighth to tenth grades, focusing on the extent to which these girls kept their "voices" and became self-sufficient or gave them up to others, "learning to think, feel, and say what others want them to think, feel, and say" (p. 24). These researchers used a rigorous methodology, reading through interview materials four times in order to identify the overall shape of the narrative, use of the first person ("I"), extent to which the girls maintained a healthy resistance to being disconnected from their own thoughts and feelings, and evidence of psychological distress or loss. The majority of the girls articulated that they had trouble speaking out, that their "big mouths" got them into trouble. By tenth grade, "a number of the Latina and Portuguese girls appear to display signs of depression or self-silencing, which may be related to their efforts to comply with family restrictions, particularly sexual restriction, or to resolve the conflicts between the expectations of their cultures of origin and the dominant culture" (p. 41). A recurrent concern among these young women was protecting their reputations from rumors about their sexual activity, real or presumed. Thus a girl's identity is also a social construction that can be determined by what others say about her. The threats posed by rumors and gossip also have a striking effect on the limits of intimacy, which will be developed further in the section on intimacy vs. isolation.

Miller (1991a) believes identity or the creation of a sense of self is a life-long process that, for the adolescent girl, becomes a "being-in-relationship" (p. 21). The girl wants to use all of her capacities, including her sexuality, within relationships. She wants to be attuned to others, but this requires that others be attuned to her as well. If they exclude her perceptions and desires, she comes to exclude her own perceptions and desires. This results in her true self being excluded from the relationship. Miller believes that boys in our society are pressured to establish independent identities and are diverted from a natural path toward being-in-relationship. Levinson (1978) has termed this goal of male identity "Being Your Own Man."

Miller (1991a) holds that girls are not trying to establish an independent identity but are striving to become a person in relationship to others. Unfortunately, in today's Western culture this still leads to the "suppression of the full participation of the women's way of seeing and acting" (p. 21). Miller describes the case of Ms. D., who felt that she had no sense of self until after she recognized and dealt with the anger she felt at her mother and father. They had taught her that she had an obligation to help her brothers and father with their feelings and needs, while at the same time denying and neglecting her own. As therapy progressed, Ms. D.'s task was to recognize and value her own perceptions and desires. Although she worked on her own being-in-relationship, her sense of self was easily damaged when others did not value her feelings.

Surrey (1991) proposes a working definition of the self based on the idea of identity as self-in-relation: "a construct useful in describing the organization of a person's experience and construction of reality that illuminates the purpose and directionality of her or his behavior" (p. 52). In considering the development of self or identity, Surrey shifts the emphasis from the male focus on separateness and independence to the female mode of relational development. Both Erikson (1963) and Levinson (1978) view identity as a recurrent issue for males revolving around separation from their mother, from their family of origin, and from their teachers and other mentors. Surrey suggests that women follow a continuous developmental pathway directed toward relational competence. She assumes that the self is developed through relationships, especially mutually empathic relationships. The first example of this is the mother-daughter relationship, a prototype for the sharing of feelings that is a precursor to learning empathy. Sometimes the girl is not given mutual empathy in her relationships, and she can come to confuse the feelings of others with her own feelings. Sorting out her own perceptions from those of others can be a critical phase in her true being-in-relationship.

Distinct from the Eriksonian concept of separation, Surrey (1991) discusses the processes of differentiation and clarification that occur during the empathy process. Within the mother-daughter relationship, and increasingly in other relationships, the girl learns mutual empathy, which leads to mutual empowerment. Girls come to establish their sense of self through psychological connection to their mothers, and mothers help to empower their daughters by confirming their successes in attuning to and understanding the feelings of others. According to Surrey, "the development of a positive sense of knowing how to perceive, respond, and relate to the needs and feelings of the other person is an important aspect of woman's self-development" (p. 57). For Surrey, self-esteem relates to emotional sharing, openness, and the ability to understand one's self in relation to others. It is important to emphasize that self-in-relation is not the immersion of the self in others. Necessary to this process is the ability to recognize the differences between oneself and others. Indeed, if these differences are not established, empathy turns into projection, wherein one's needs are not recognized as belonging to one's self and are instead attributed to others. The healthy establishment of mutual empathy requires reciprocity and role flexibility. The girl must understand others and feel understood by them. She must be able to consider various perspectives, developing what Surrey terms an "oscillating self-structure" (p. 58).

Surrey (1991) suggests that the reason the identity "crisis" occurs in adolescence is that the girl may be dealing with parents who are unable or unwilling to change in their mutual relationships with the daughter. Because she is maturing physically, socially, and emotionally, she feels a need to change her relationship with them, but they are unable to make the adjustment. Her desire to set up new relationships and to give those relationships higher priority causes a strain in the parent-daughter relationships, leading to a "crisis." Another challenge at this age is that of "relationship-authenticity" (p. 60). Being honest and real at this stage in a girl's life is very risky, as Taylor, Gilligan, and Sullivan (1995) discovered in their study of urban girls. The need to be authentic often runs up against social restrictions on teenage sexuality, forcing the sexually active girl to be dishonest in her relationships with others, especially her parents.

Gilligan's (1982) focus on voice can be seen as another way of discussing identity from a female standpoint. In her study of how women decide whether or not to have an abortion Gilligan identified a "different voice" that women use to make moral judgments. First, these judgments are made in context, and they reflect an emphasis on caring and responsibility. For women deciding to terminate a pregnancy, the interest in caring and responsibility frequently creates a real-life dilemma when the woman must choose between a relationship with the father of the child, who does not want the baby, and a potential relationship with the child.

In her critique of Kohlberg's stages of moral development, Gilligan (1982) proposed that women have a different approach to moral issues, one that emphasizes caring and responsibility. Kohlberg (1981) used a moral dilemma as the basis for a hierarchical model of moral reasoning. In this hypothetical situation, a man is faced with the choice of stealing a drug that may extend the life of his wife who is dying of cancer or deciding to do nothing and witnessing her death. The drug is rare and expensive, the man cannot afford to buy it, and the druggist will not lower his price. When faced with this hypothetical dilemma, women enlarged the situation by considering the plight of the wife if her husband were caught stealing the drug and sent to prison. Not only would the woman die of cancer, but now she would die alone.

Kohlberg posits that those who extract abstract principles of justice regarding the relative value of property and human life are more highly developed morally than those who focus on getting caught or abiding by social convention. In Kohlberg's model, the women who focus on the relationship between the man and his wife, as opposed to extracting some abstract moral principle, are viewed as less highly developed. Gilligan (1982) argued that the women's way of making moral decisions was not less developed but was different in focusing on the relationships involved. She further proposed that women have been distanced from their voices because of judgments such as Kohlberg's that their ways of analyzing moral issues are deficient. Gilligan also described the development of identity in self-expression and the problem that arises when women are forced to silence their voices to protect others and preserve relationships. This places human connection up against the problem of truth, a condition not unlike Surrey's (1991) concept of relationship-authenticity. Gilligan includes the self-description of one of her subjects: "I see myself as an onion, as a block of different layers. The external layers are for people that I don't know that well, the agreeable, the social, and as you go inward, there are more sides for people I know that I show. I am not sure about the innermost, whether there is a core" (1982, pp. 67-68). If identity is seen as static and the result of separateness, this woman is left with the problem of deciding which layer is her true self. If identity is viewed as self-in-relation, she is aware of multiple selves and the one that is currently active depends upon which person she is interacting with.

Dan McAdams (1988) has conceptualized the life story as the way in which the adult defines herself through the personal myths that give her life unity and purpose. Identity formation occurs through the configuration of a plot, characters, settings, and themes that tie together the various aspects of our lives. This process of identity formation is important because it gives the person a sense of continuity across different situations and across time, which McAdams calls *identity stability.* "The story provides a coherent narrative framework within which the disparate events and the various roles of a person's life can be embedded and given meaning" (McAdams, 1988, p. 19). Identity transformation is also important, reflecting the crises and changes that made us what we are today. Story revisions can be minor or major, remembered or forgotten. The construction of a life story is an on-going process that is affected by day-to-day experiences and how we reflect those experiences back on our personal myths of who we are. In effect we construct a biography of self. Habermas and Bluck (2000) argue that the cognitive tools necessary for constructing coherence in a life story develop during adolescence.

Intimacy

Erikson's (1963) description of the intimacy vs. isolation crisis is particularly couched in male terms. "Thus, the young adult, emerging from the search for and the insistence on identity, is eager and willing to fuse his identity with that of others. He is ready for intimacy, that is, the capacity to commit himself to concrete affiliations and partnerships and to develop the ethical strength to abide by such commitments, even though they may call for significant sacrifices and compromises" (p. 263). As Miller (1991a) has pointed out, this commitment for girls starts very early. The reason it occurs so much later in males is that boys are diverted from their being-in-relationship and must find this state after an artificial detour.

Erikson believed that men fear the loss of ego identity within relationships and that this fear can lead to isolation and self-absorption. For men, sexuality relates both to identity and intimacy in that early sexual conquests are seen as part of establishing one's sexual identity. Mature sexuality renders sex less obsessive. Erikson's ideal of intimacy was also strictly heterosexual, prescribing that "the utopia of genitality should include mutuality of orgasm with a loved partner of the other sex with whom one is able and willing to share a mutual trust and with whom one is able and willing to regulate the cycles of work, procreation, recreation so as to secure to the offspring, too, all the stages of a satisfactory development" (p. 266).

It should also be noted that Erikson's emphasis on sexual intimacy minimizes the intimacy of friendship, a type of intimacy that is more important for women in our society than for men. Moore and Boldero (1991) studied 223 high school and college students to explore the relationship between friendship and Erikson's concepts of identity and intimacy. They proposed that friendship fosters the capacity for intimacy by encouraging self-disclosure, reciprocity, and mutual support. Moore and Boldero found that females rated their friendships as more important than males did, reported greater satisfaction with the closeness of their friendships, were more likely to disclose problems to their friends, and were more likely to maintain a close relationship if a friend was absent. However, when they examined the question of whether females and males differ in the order that they enter the identity and intimacy stages, as measured by the Erikson Psychosocial Stage Inventory, they found that females did not score higher on the intimacy subscale than on the identity subscale. Moore and Boldero presented this as evidence against Erikson's contention that females resolve their intimacy crises before they resolve their identity crises. For males and females combined, higher friendship quality was reported by those who scored high on both the identity and intimacy subscales and by those who scored high on the identity subscale and low on the intimacy subscale. Moore and Boldero also found that subjects scoring high on the intimacy subscale but low on the identity subscale viewed friendships as less important than other groups and were less likely to self-disclose to their friends. They interpreted this result as support for pseudointimacy as opposed to true intimacy. They also argued that this finding supports Erikson's contention that true intimacy requires the previous establishment of a personal identity.

Adolescent Development and Intimacy

For the girls in the study by Taylor, Gilligan, and Sullivan (1995), intimacy was a trust issue. Because their families emphasized female virginity, these girls lived in fear of their mothers and fathers finding out that they were sexually active. Their experiences of confiding in a friend, only to have that friend spread gossip and rumors about them, led to a shutting down and social withdrawal. After repeated betrayal of confidences, the girls described self-protective strategies that resulted in their social isolation. The different voice that Gilligan identified in her 1982 research became silenced through self-censorship because of this betrayal of intimacy (Taylor, Gilligan, & Sullivan, 1995).

Gilligan (1991) described how girls develop the social knowledge that allows them to create a sense of who they are and how they interact with other people: "Like anthropologists, they pick up the culture; like sociologists, they observe race, class and sex differences; like psychologists, they come to know what is happening beneath the surface; like naturalists, they collect their observations, laying them out, sorting them out, discussing them between themselves in an ongoing conversation about relationships and people which goes on, on and off, for much of the day, every day" (p. 16). This description differs markedly from the stage model proposed by Erikson in that the process of identity and intimacy is seen as on-going process that happens every day. Women don't live the first years of their lives without identities, waiting for that magic moment when finding it will become a crisis that they will have to attend to. Certainly, the idea that intimacy has to await the resolution of the identity crises doesn't hold up under close scrutiny. Gilligan contends that intimacy is a daily decision, the result of our culture, our race, class, and sex. Intimacy depends on our way of interpreting surface events and inferring the underlying dynamics of personality, motivation, and social interactions. We are open or closed to intimacy depending on what we observe in our work and how we come to conclusions about how the world is and how people interact. This crisis doesn't kick in at a particular age or life stage but is enmeshed in our lives from birth to death.

However, Gilligan (1991) identifies changes in intimacy that are brought about as girls mature. Specifically, she describes the change at puberty when girls can no longer be open and reveal themselves to others. " 'Cover up,' girls are told as they reach adolescence, daily, in innumerable ways. Cover your body, cover your feelings, cover your relationships, cover your knowing, cover your voice, and perhaps above all, cover desire" (p. 22). Gilligan believes that adolescence is a time of psychological risk for girls, whereas boys are more at risk in early childhood. As a working hypothesis, she proposes that adolescence precipitates a relationship crisis for girls in which they must separate from others for self-protection. Citing Miller's (1986) work, Gilligan sees women's psychology as transformational. Gilligan writes that "girls are pressed at adolescence to take on images of perfection as the model of the pure or perfectly good woman: the woman whom everyone will promote and value and want to be with" (p. 24). Gilligan sees adolescence as a time when femininity seems to be on the line for girls. She encourages older women to help girls resist the pressures to give up their own voices.

PSYCHOSOCIAL MODELS OF EARLY ADULTHOOD

For Erikson (1963) adulthood contains two crises: generativity vs. stagnation and ego integrity vs. despair. Generativity, the crisis of early adulthood, is acting on one's concern for the welfare of the next generation. Productivity and creativity are included in generativity, but they do not completely encompass it. For many people generativity is accomplished through parenting. For others, it includes teaching, nursing, and other forms of service to the public. When self-concern overpowers concern for the future, people are unable to step outside themselves and be generative. This leads to stagnation, a state in which the person is unable or unwilling to continue to develop as a person and as a professional. Stagnation is evident in the parent who cannot reach out to her child, to the doctor who does not keep up with current medical knowledge, and to the person who vegetates in front of the television every night.

McAdams and de St. Aubin (1992) have expanded on Erikson's definition of generativity, identifying seven elements of generativity that emphasize the relational aspect of this concept and the multiple contexts it operates in. They relate the concept of generativity to that of attachment, which also differs from many other psychological concepts in being relational and multifaceted. For McAdams and de St. Aubin, generativity arises from (1) cultural demands that adults live up to cultural expectations for age-appropriate activities (parenting, teaching, caring) and from (2) an inner desire to establish "symbolic immortality" and to be needed. These external and internal motivations combine to create (3) a concern for the welfare of the next generation. Additionally, cultural demands create (4) a belief system that the human species is basically worthwhile and that investment in the future of the human species is a responsible use of one's time. This belief in one's responsibility for the next generation and the concern that most people feel for the welfare of the next generation combine to form (5) a commitment to set goals and make decisions in a way that will benefit others. Generative actions (6), such as caring for children, teaching skills, promoting healthy life styles, come about because of cultural demands, inner desires, and commitment. The last element of McAdams and de St. Aubin's theory of generativity is (7) the narration or life story that the person constructs that includes a generativity script. This narration needs to reinforce generative actions, which in turn, add to the life story.

McAdams and de St. Aubin (1992) expand on their definition of generative actions, broadly outlining three categories: creating, maintaining, and offering. Creating includes parenting or any other extension of the self that results in a new conception that benefits the world. Maintaining involves nurturance, conservation, preservation, and other activities that guarantee the continuity of people, resources, traditions, and beliefs. Offering is the selfless offering up of one's time and caring to promote the further development of a child, a charitable cause, a way of life, and so on. Creating is meaningless if it is not offered up for others' benefit.

Another way to think of the narration or life story is to see it as a reflection of the identity or the self-in-relation. Constructing a life story that provides life with meaning is, according to McAdams and de St. Aubin (1992), the major psychological issue of most of one's adult life. In that, they differ from Erikson, who confined the identity crisis to late adolescence. Further, by including the narration of a life story into the generative process, McAdams and de St. Aubin step further away from a stage model of development, blurring the lines between identity and generativity. They reject the concept of a discrete stage of generativity confined to adulthood and hold out the possibility that generativity can occur in childhood and adolescence.

Epistemological Stages

In their book, *Women's Ways of Knowing*, Belenky, Clinchy, Goldberger, and Tarule (1986) outline five epistemological stages (stages of how we know about life): silence, received knowledge, subjective knowledge, procedural knowledge, and constructed knowledge. In the *silence* stage, brutalized women—victims of poverty, physical and psychological abuse, and incest—have no voice. They cannot speak for themselves. In the *received knowledge* stage, women come to trust outside sources of knowledge, experts like social workers who teach them parenting skills or nurses who advise them on birth control procedures. In the *subjective knowledge* stage, women react to "failed authority" (p. 56) and begin to listen to their own inner voices. They discover that they have opinions that are as valid as others' opinions. Their gut reactions often serve them well, leading them to end relationships that they intuit to be exploitative. However, as women move out into the world, especially the world of work and higher education, sometimes their gut instincts fail them. If they are receiving formal instruction, this can herald in the *procedural knowledge* stage, the time when analysis and formal criticism provide them with tools for examining their beliefs and expressing them to others. In the initial phase of the procedural knowledge stage they are required to analyze and critique the writings of experts. This application of analysis and criticism has an abstract and separate quality that seems foreign to many women. Especially if they have been socialized to be trusting and accepting, the doubting that is a part of separate knowing is alien to them. With practice, the separate knowing becomes connected knowing, as women learn to apply analysis to problems that concern them directly or to issues with which they have had personal experience.

For a nurse, the question of which birth control methods they should promote could be followed through the epistemological stages. In the silence stage the young woman may deny the importance of taking a stand on birth control. As she receives sex education in junior high and high school, she tends to accept what the experts tell her, perhaps going on the pill when she become sexually active. As a young woman she may begin to question the appropriateness of the pill for her, intuiting that her body is reacting negatively to the daily dose of hormones. When she becomes a nursing student, she is given principles and procedures for evaluating the usefulness of various birth control methods and their appropriateness for women of different ages and situations in life. This separate knowing becomes connected knowing when she combines her own experiences with the information she receives from the clients she deals with in her internship. The choice of a birth control method is not just the result of a formula or decision tree, but an interactive decision that includes aspects of a woman's entire life.

Finally, some women enter the *constructed knowledge* stage in which they can integrate what they have learned and produce a new synthesis and communicate their creative thoughts to others. Margaret Sanger, the mother of modern birth control, was in the stage of constructed knowledge when she took on public opinion in the early 1900s and convinced people around the world that birth control was a worthy endeavor.

Adult Development and Power

Power is concerned with having an impact, through forceful actions, persuasion, controlling the conditions of someone's life, or creating strong emotional reactions (Winter, 1973). For McClelland (1975) power is characterized by the location of its source (others or self) and its focus (self or others). He developed a quadrant of power by crossing the source and focus of power as depicted in Figure 6-1. The stages of power are intake, autonomy, assertion, and generativity.

Everyone begins life in the *intake* stage where the source of power is others and the focus is self. This is characteristic of the baby who must depend upon parents and other caregivers to provide all of its needs. Believing that power lies outside the self is appropriate for the helpless infant, but as people mature they must begin to see

Source of Power

	Others	Self
Silence		

Focus of Power

		Others	Self
Self		I. INTAKE	II. AUTONOMY
		Received Knowing	*Subjective Knowing*
Others		IV. GENERATIVITY	III. ASSERTION
		Constructed Knowing	*Procedural Knowing*

Figure 6-1 Comparison of McClelland's power quadrant (*caps*) and *Women's Ways of Knowing* epistemological stages (*italics*). (Modified from McClelland, D.C. [1975]. *Power: The inner experience.* New York: Irvington Publishers, Inc.; and Belenky, M. F., Clinchy, B. M., Goldberger, N. R., & Tarule, J. M. [1986]. *Women's ways of knowing: The development of self, voice, and mind.* New York: Basic Books, Inc.)

themselves as powerful, too. Otherwise, they continue to look outside themselves for the solutions to their problems, such as using drugs to make problems go away or seeking charismatic leaders to tell them how to live their lives.

The second power stage is the *autonomy* stage where the self is the source and the focus of power. When individuals move into the autonomy stage they depend upon themselves for power. Self-knowledge gives women power over their own lives. This stage is also exemplified when people build up their bodies through exercise or good diet and their minds through education, especially self-education. People in this stage are distrustful of institutions and depend upon themselves to solve their own problems. Using intuition and gut reactions to make decisions reflects a belief that power originates in the self and can be used for the benefit of the self. However, people who stay too long in the autonomy power stage can become narcissistic and self-centered (McClelland, 1975).

McClelland maintained that the key to achieving the third power stage, *assertion*, is the development of assertiveness, the ability to use one's personal power for the good of others. Nurses and teachers use their personal power and resources to help others. They need a degree of assertiveness to speak in public, give directions to others, and monitor their progress. Analysis and criticism are evidenced by instructors who grade term papers and determine if they are logically consistent and understandable. There are negative examples of assertiveness as well. The seducer who uses her power to manipulate others and the criminal who uses con schemes to extract money from victims are examples of people who use their power in a negative way.

McClelland proposed that *generativity*, the fourth power stage, is achieved by very few people; two notable examples are Gandhi and Mother Teresa. Ironically, when one reaches this highly developed level, the self drops away and becomes just a conduit for transmitting power from others (a religion, body of knowledge, or moral principles) to others (students, followers, patients). According to McClelland, generativity "might show itself in greater mutuality and fewer hang-ups or ego-centric attachments" (p. 69). It is difficult to distinguish between persons who are misguided in their exercise of this power stage from those who remain in the assertive stage. Jim Jones can be viewed as a con man who led his followers to their suicide in Guyana whereas the Heaven's Gate leaders may have sincerely believed that they were transmitting messages from the Hale-Bopp comet, choosing suicide when their earthly bodies had become dispensable. The line between generativity and insanity can be fine indeed.

How Power and Knowing Connect

Figure 6-1 combines the ways of knowing within the power quadrant and illustrates the relationship of power to knowing. McClelland's intake stage shares with the received knowledge stage an image of the person as the passive recipient of outside power (expert knowledge). Like the subjective knowledge stage described in *Women's Ways of Knowing*, people in the autonomy power stage see themselves as resources of knowledge, trusting their intuitions and gut reactions to make decisions. Procedural knowledge, both separate knowing and connected knowing, require the woman to demonstrate her knowledge to others. This necessitates a level of assertiveness that allows her to instruct others and to use her power for their benefit. Both generativity and constructed knowledge depend on the recognition that the individual person is unimportant compared to the contribution the person is making to the accumulated body of knowledge and wisdom in the world. A generative person is concerned about the future and sees herself as a part of a larger universe. The constructed knowledge stage also requires this mature approach to life—the integration of what one has learned and the synthesis of new material for the benefit of others.

In Figure 6-1, the stage of silence is placed outside the quadrant to emphasize that the silent woman is without power, unable to speak for herself. Responding to the criticism that women have not created their share of the world's art and literature, Tilly Olson (1978) has written eloquently about silences. "Among these, the mute inglorious Miltons: Those whose waking hours are all struggle for existence; the barely educated, the illiterate; women. Their silence the silence of centuries as to how life was, is, for most of humanity" (p. 10). Women in poverty struggle for existence. The illiterate and the barely educated do not have the tools to construct knowledge. Women who have been physically and psychologically abused may live in economic plenty but they have lapsed into silence.

Another way to think of silence is that some women have nothing to say because they have so much to say. In her book, *Conspiracy of Silence: The Trauma of Incest*, Butler

(1978) describes the tyranny experienced by the young victim of incest when a trusted family member (father, uncle, brother) violates the child's trust and then compounds the guilt for the girl by making her an accomplice in keeping it secret. If the girl tells a teacher or another family member and is not believed, further violence is done to the child's developing trust. Being silent, not having a voice, is seen in this case as being able to speak about trivial matters when the most important things must be kept secret, must go unsaid.

Miller (1991b) defines power as "the capacity to produce a change" (p. 198). Although women in most societies are expected not to have power in any domain, Miller believes that women in the traditional role of caretakers of children are extremely powerful because of their impact on others. Through their actions, women increase the capabilities and resources of others to take effective action. In this generative role, they exercise power for the benefit of others. However, according to Miller, when women think about acting powerfully, they become fearful that they will be putting down someone else or that they will reveal to themselves and to others a desire to exercise power. She outlined four problems women have with power: they see their exercise of power as being selfish; they view the exercise of power as destructive; the exercise of power threatens their feminine identity; and they fear that the use of power will lead to abandonment. When one recalls that Miller (1991a, 1991b) and Surrey (1991) have conceptualized identity as self-in-relation, one can see how the prospect of abandonment as the result of a woman using power would be threatening to her sense of identity.

Miller (1991b) gave several examples of women who had struggled with issues of power. Abby, who worked in the health care field, became self-critical when she recognized her desire to have more power in her working relationships and viewed her ambitions as selfish. As she gained more confidence in her ability to make a significant contribution to her patients' recovery, she began to fear that her desire for power would be destructive. If she insisted on more power in the medical situation, she would destroy important aspects of the institution she was working for. Although Miller does not elaborate on Abby's fear of abandonment, one can easily imagine that if she agitated for more control over her work, she might be abandoned by her supervisors and, possibly, her co-workers. However, to the extent that she viewed herself as a cooperative and caring person, this would threaten her own sense of self. And her self-in-relation would be endangered by possible ostracism. Miller and Stiver (1997) believe that women should be powerful in ways that enhance, and not diminish, the power of others. To do this, one must understand that power is a difficult concept, and it is important to distinguish between its destructive and constructive uses.

Gender and Power

Miller (1986) has written eloquently about the effects of inequality of power on dominant and subordinate groups. She recognizes several factors on which inequality is based: race, religion, class, and nationality. Miller makes an important distinction between temporary inequality and permanent inequality. The inequality between child and adult or student and teacher is considered temporary because the goal of the relationship is to bring the child or the student to the same level as the adult or the teacher. The instruction the child and the student is given is designed to eradicate the inequality. Permanent inequality, on the other hand, is not intended to change. In fact, the goal of the dominant group is to maintain the inequality, which accrues significant benefits. While acknowledging various dominant and subordinate groups, Miller is particularly interested in the inequality between men and women. Her analysis of permanent inequality and the roles of the dominant and subordinate groups translates well to the interactions of women and men in our culture.

One of Miller's most cogent insights is that the subordinate group (in this case women) always knows more about the dominant group (men) than the dominant group knows about the subordinate group. This greater knowledge accrues to the subordinate group through their greater vigilance, the necessity that they pay attention to what the dominant group wants so that they, the subordinates, don't overstep their proper roles. All dominant groups define social reality and define the inequality (their domination over the subordinate group) as legitimate. Dominant groups become the model for normal human qualities and interactions.

The proposition that dominant groups are the norm was supported by research by Broverman, Broverman, Clarkson, Rosenkrantz, and Vogel (1970). They asked practicing clinicians to fill out a sex-role stereotype questionnaire under one of three instructions; to describe a healthy, mature, and competent man, women, or adult (sex unspecified). Clinicians described men and women in ways that paralleled prevailing sex stereotypes, and their description of a healthy, mature, and competent adult matched their description of the stereotypic male. In other words, as Miller proposed, the model for the dominant group (males) is the same as the model of normal human qualities (adults, sex unspecified). Further, Broverman and others found that the stereotype of the mentally healthy female differed significantly from the characteristics of the healthy adult, leaving a woman with the uncomfortable choice of adjusting to the female stereotype and being seen as deviant from the adult model of mental health or adjusting to the male stereotype and having her femininity questioned.

According to Miller (1986), men have become the standard of mental health because they have had the power to define social reality. Women have become the deviants because they are the subordinate group and men have been able to define them so. Generally, subordinate groups are encouraged to adopt characteristics that are pleasing to the dominant group, qualities that are more characteristic of children than of adults. For example, subordinate groups are encouraged to be immature, emotional, and helpless. Submissiveness is encouraged, and any attempt on the part of subordinates to change their submissive role is seen as threatening by the dominant group (and the epitome of ingratitude). Further, dominant groups stand in the way of subordinates' increasing their range of expression and action. Indeed, subordinate groups are defined as lacking the personal characteristics necessary to expand their range of activities. Women, for years, were seen as too weak to withstand the rigors of manual labor and too unintelligent or emotional to engage in intellectual careers. Consequently, their opportunities for making a living were severely limited. Indeed, respectable women accepted their roles as daughters, wives, and mothers and worked to please the men in their lives, their fathers, husbands, and sons.

Miller has pointed out that once a group is defined as inferior, the dominant group labels many of its characteristics and activities as defective. In the sports world, one sees female athletes struggling to gain legitimacy for their sports. In professional basketball, Rebecca Lobo or Sheryl Swoopes will be unfavorably compared to Michael Jordan. Female-dominated careers are historically treated with less respect and the people in those professions are paid less. The fields of nursing and teaching are two prominent examples: activities that should be highly valued (caring for the sick and instructing the young) are undervalued because women dominate the fields. Indeed, the domestic work of women is not even included in the calculation of the gross national product of the United States.

For their part, subordinates help to maintain the inequality of the relationship by playing their roles and not agitating for change. Indeed, there are always crossover individuals who take on the characteristics of the dominant group and give legitimacy to the stereotypes by being the exception to the rule. The woman who "thinks like a man" or the queen bee who basks in the glory and power of being a token woman in a male-dominated field helps to perpetuate the inequality that she, too, will eventually suffer from. Miller is not intending to blame the victims of injustice by pointing out that some members of the subordinate group seek to imitate the dominant group. Indeed, there is a paradox that members of the subordinate group are pressured to take on the stereotypes assigned to them by the dominant group (be submissive, pleasing, and kind) or to imitate the dominate group (be assertive, abrasive, and inconsiderate). Neither choice is free because all options carry additional meaning within the context of inequality. Most women are indoctrinated to take on the roles assigned to their group, and this internalization of the dominant group's beliefs leads them to feel inferior.

Out of this background, Miller (1986) proposes a new psychology of women. She proposes that women have been discouraged from confronting their inequality. Either they manipulate the man to get their needs met (an approach illustrated in 1950s sitcoms in which father may have known best but mother got what she wanted anyway) or they deny their needs and substitute the needs of others (their fathers, their husbands, or their children) for their own. In the first case, the "smart" woman manipulates the system but ends up feeling fraudulent. In the second case, she has lost contact with herself and her lack of authenticity is unknown, even to herself. Another result of the dominant/ subordinate system is that women's concerns are viewed as unmanly. Miller detailed the different ways in which a man and a woman reacted to the offer of a promotion to a highly responsible position. The woman, who was very capable, reacted with fear, seeing herself as a little girl who was incapable of meeting the new responsibilities, an evaluation that was highly unrealistic. The man jumped at the opportunity but then developed physical symptoms that indicated a repressed fear of the new position and an inability to deal with the fear. Fear or uncertainly is generally associated with being "womanly" and must be denied by the man who must maintain his manliness. His wife offered support and nurturance, an approach that reinforces the underlying stereotypes and delays the day of reckoning when society has to face the inappropriateness and undermining effects of these stereotypes. As long as women collude to help men deny their fears, society will continue in its current path and no changes in attitudes will come about. Since Miller first analyzed male and female stereotypes, some men have worked to overcome their fear of being vulnerable and "womanly." However, these pioneers are still often seen as engaging in "touchy-feely" activities that are not deserving of serious attention.

Miller puts an interesting interpretation on the results of gender-splitting, the assignment of women and men to different domains. She describes the situation of a wife who is dependent on her husband for economic support and social position. The wife is keenly aware of her husband's limitations and cooperates in helping him deal with his anxieties without confronting his real issues—his denial of vulnerability. To maintain her sense of security, the wife begins to imagine that her husband has qualities that make him much stronger and more efficient in his job, qualities that she is not capable of acquiring. Otherwise, she cannot accommodate simultaneously her husband's weaknesses with his occupational success. This splitting of his occupational qualities from her supportive qualities allows her to make sense of her world, but it also leaves her increasingly vulnerable to a sense of inadequacy in dealing with the "real world." Miller believes that women must learn to define their own strengths in line with their experiences and not depend on definitions grounded in men's lives. Thus dependency (which has been termed a weakness) can become supportiveness (which can be termed a strength). Reevaluating behavior that has been characterized as weakness and seeing how it can be interpreted as strength will lead to a new psychology of women. Miller's new psychology of women emphasizes cooperation and creativity, concerns that she believes have been denied and devalued in the male-dominated world because they are associated with women. Miller also cautions about the dangers of objectification—the extent to which people are turned into objects. This dehumanizing process is known keenly by women who have been turned into sex objects. Once women have been objectified, it is easy to assign qualities to them that supposedly reflect their "inherent" nature. The age-old practice of equating women with evil (beginning with Eve) has had a devastating effect on women's self-concept. Recognizing these destructive processes is necessary before women can change their psychology.

Affiliation is viewed by Miller (1986) as being central to women's lives; it develops from early attachment to others. Boys are encouraged to deny their need for affiliation and become men who are free of ties to others (which, of course, is a myth that covers over a deep need to be taken care of by others). Girls are socialized to remain attached and to transfer that attachment to a male. This socialization also prepares them for their cultural role as communicators and providers of service. For men, affiliation is often viewed as a danger, and moving away from relationships is reinforced. Relationships make women feel satisfied and moving away from them is punishing. Miller believes that men need affiliation too, and that society is deeply threatened if we continue to make distinctions based on perceived manly and womanly characteristics. She does not think that women are inherently better than men or that women can clean up the mess men have made. Indeed, that analogy would perpetuate the role of women in the service (cleaning up) of others. Rather, she believes that the characteristics that have been traditionally assigned to women and then systematically devalued need to be embraced by all humans. Cooperation and service must be seen as human qualities that determine our actions toward each other.

Psychological concepts that have been developed in a male-centered society may need to be reconceptualized, too. Miller (1986) doubts that the concept of autonomy can be applied to women in the same way it is applied to men. Women do not seek separateness in the same way men do. As previously discussed, the loss of affiliation is threatening to women, and separation is to be avoided, not sought. However, women need to develop a sense of who they are, what Surrey (1991) has termed self-in-relation. Miller (1986) speaks of self-determination and authenticity. A powerful insight is that being authentic and being in a subordinate position are incompatible. Surviving in a subordinate position requires hiding one's true desires and feelings for fear of displeasing the dominant person. For women who are learning to be authentic, the first emotion that they experience is often anger. Anger has the advantage of being immediate and undeniably real, but expressing anger toward another person is extremely threatening. Arousing displeasure in another person is equated by many women with being abandoned. Taking this risk is frightening for women, but "it is only when the woman can move to thinking about the true quality of her connections and how to improve or change them rather than thinking of first pleasing another and conforming to his desires and expectations that she can even begin to know herself" (p. 110). Creativity comes into the picture when women envision who they can become and invent themselves in the context of new relationships, a continuous and on-going process.

Miller believes that women must deal with power and distinguishes between "power for oneself" and "power over others" (1986, p. 116). She sees women's use of power as differing from men's in two important ways. First, women have not historically depended on the exercise of power over others as a way of establishing self-image. Second, women are not in a position to use power to maintain a dominant-subordinate relationship. Therefore, Miller holds out the hope that women can use power for themselves, to develop a new way of living that includes authenticity, mutuality, and cooperation. However, Miller warns that the exercise of power in changing women's lives will inevitably bring them into conflict with other people and with institutions within our society. Conflict is a taboo area for women because they have traditionally been the accommodators, the ones to give in and give up. Women must learn not to fear conflict and to distinguish productive, growth-oriented conflict from "rigged conflict," which is controlled by the dominant group (men) and is designed to defeat the subordinate group (women). Women must be clear in their understanding that by changing the way they live their lives they are not creating conflict; rather, they are exposing conflict that already exists.

For Miller the key lies in learning ways to deal with conflict. Dominant groups tend to deny that conflict exists. Subordinate groups who are dependent on dominant groups for the essentials of life are in no position to approach conflict directly. So conflict is suppressed, and, if it surfaces, it is explosive in its intensity. Therefore we come to think that all conflict is dangerous and we fail to see productive conflict as a possibility. Productive conflict occurs from the moment we are born as we deal with the conflicts inherent in life. As babies we come into conflict with our parents, but the conflict is usually productive because we change, our parents change, and we adapt to each other. As we get older, however, we come to see conflict as dangerous, as the dominant and subordinate roles of child and parent become rigid. Initiating conflict is particularly threatening to women because they tend to blame themselves for any problems. However, as women dedicate themselves to living new lives, conflict is necessary on three fronts. They must work to change social institutions to respond to their needs, they must confront problems in their relationships, especially to men, and they must deal with the conflict between who they currently are and who they want to become. Miller proposes that for these conflicts to be successfully resolved women must have the support of like-minded people. This mutual support serves the dual purpose of validating one's perceptions of the conflict and assuring that women will not be abandoned in their search or a new life. The development of self can, thus, be conducted in relationship with others.

Seasons of Adulthood

Levinson (1996) has conceptualized the adult development of women as seasons, roughly divided into *early adulthood, middle adulthood,* and *late adulthood* (Table 6-2). In an interview study of 45 women, he gathered information about life structure, developmental crises, and life transitions. Drawing from multiple interviews with 15 homemakers, 15 women with corporate careers, and 15 women with academic careers, Levinson identified cycles of life transitions between successive life structures. For example, the early adult transition corresponds to the boundary between childhood and early adulthood, roughly spanning the ages from 17 to 22. This is a fundamental turning point in the life cycle during which a woman invests herself in a traditional marriage enterprise or commits herself to an anti-traditional life structure. Every woman, in the current historical period, is viewed as combining these two patterns of living, holding within herself images of both the traditional and anti-traditional choices that she must somehow balance in her own life. The homemaker who does freelance computer programming in her home has a balance that is different from the corporate executive who prides herself on her gourmet cooking.

Transitional periods involve three basic developmental tasks: termination, individuation, and initiation. For example, in *early adulthood,* a woman terminates childhood, makes life choices that serve to set herself apart from others (individuation), and initiates a new life structure that carries her to the next transitional period. Levinson believes that every life structure is provisional, being more or less useful for each woman at her particular point in life. However, a woman's life structure must be

Table **6-2**	SEASONS OF A WOMAN'S LIFE	
SEASONS		**AGE**
Early Adult Transition Boundary between childhood and adulthood. Fundamental turning point in the life cycle.		17-22
Entry Life Structure for Early Adulthood Making clear choices regarding love, marriage, family, occupation, and life style. First life structure is provisional.		22-28
Age 30 Transition Opportunity to reappraise Entry Life Structure and do further work on individuation. Time of moderate to severe developmental difficulty for most people.		28-33
Culminating Life Structure for Early Adulthood Forming a structure within which a woman can establish a more secure place for herself in society. Moving from "junior" to "senior" membership in the adult world.		33-40
Mid-Life Transition Coming to terms with the end of youth. Work of mid-life individuation forms inner framework out of which self and life evolve over the rest of this era.		40-45
Entry Life Structure for Middle Adulthood Creating a new structure for launching of middle adulthood. Establishing an initial place in a new generation and a new season of life.		45-50
Age 50 Transition Opportunity to re-appraise Entry Life Structure. Further exploration of self and world. Developmental crises are common in this stage.		50-55
Culminating Life Structure for Middle Adulthood. Structure provides the vehicle for the realization of adulthood's major aspirations and goals.		55-60
Late Adult Transition Profound reappraisal of the past and the shift to a new era.		60-65

Data from Levinson, D. J. (1996). *The seasons of a woman's life.* New York: Ballantine Books.

altered to accommodate external changes and to respond to internal changes or to correct earlier bad choices. At *age 30 transition*, it is not uncommon for a woman to divorce a partner she chose in early adulthood. The termination of the marriage forces the woman to reevaluate herself, seeing herself in ways she did not before.

The initiation of the next life structure might include returning to school to prepare herself for an anti-traditional life, now that her traditional marriage enterprise has failed.

In addition to the *early adult transition* and the *age 30 transition*, Levinson identified a *mid-life transition* (ages 40-45), an *age 50 transition,* and a *late adult transition* (ages 60-65). At the mid-life transition, one comes to terms with the end of youth. Levinson believes that developmental crises are common during the age 50 transition and that a profound reappraisal of the past occurs at the late adult transition. The women he interviewed before his death in 1994 were still in their forties, so his proposed later seasons, patterned after the lives of men he had interviewed in the 1960s and 70s, could not be compared to his female subjects' lives.

In a retrospective interview study of 60 women, Reinke, Holmes, and Harris (1985) compared the timing of psychosocial transitions to the chronological age of the women and to the family cycle phases they were involved in (no-children phase; having preschool children, school-age children, or adolescent children; launching children phase; or postparental phase). Fifteen women from each of four age groups (30, 35, 40, and 45) completed lengthy interviews about their past and current lives. Trained coders identified major psychosocial transitions in the lives of 47 of the 60 women when they were between the ages of 27 and 30. Compared to the 13 women who did not experience a transition, these 47 women reported that they had reassessed their lives and had begun seeking changes in their lives in the early part of the transition. They also reported a higher incidence of professional counseling and extramarital affairs. The middle phase of their transitions were related to setting personal goals for the first time, including educational and occupational goals. In the final phase of the transition, between ages 30 and 35, the transitional women reported greater life satisfaction and more feelings of self-confidence and personal competence. The psychosocial transitions were not reliably related to the family cycle phase that the women were involved in (whether they had children, and if so, how old the children were). Reinke and others point out that the timing of the age 30 transition differs from the reported "mid-life crisis" experienced by men at around age 40. They propose that in our society "the age 30 marker has been imbued with societal significance for women" (p. 1361).

Paths of Adulthood

Terri Apter (1995) set about to study mid-life development in women, focusing on the developmental issues that face women during their 40s. She was drawn to the paradox that women of this age exhibit increased energy and self-confidence, alongside doubt and anxiety resulting from brutal self-assessment. Apter frames this paradox as a realization by the woman at mid-life that she must continue her journey through life after having arrived at her present point with the use of a faulty map. This faulty map contains the false guidance that the adolescent girl drew from her idealism and her desire to be perfect. By mid-life the woman appreciates that it will be impossible to be perfect, that her life will be a compromise.

Apter (1995) studied 80 women over a 4-year period, combining interviews and observations. During subsequent debriefings, the observations were interpreted by the subjects themselves. Among her 80 subjects, aged 39 to 55, Apter identified four groupings: *traditional, innovative, expansive,* and *protestors.* The *traditional women* lived their lives in connection with others, performing the traditional roles of daughter, wife, and mother. *Innovative women* viewed their careers as central to their lives, becoming pioneers in the male world of work. *Expansive women* broke out of the established private and public spheres and created their own lives, expanding their horizons by returning to school. *Protestors* had been forced into early responsibilities because of pregnancy or other family demands; they approached mid-life actively protesting their past limitations and striving to establish brilliant futures.

Three different points mark mid-life crises for the first group—traditional women. These points are their identification with their husband's ambition that silenced their own needs, their lavishing time and energy on raising children, and the empty nest, when their children left home. The emptiness was initially viewed as very negative but was regularly reevaluated as a time of new direction and purpose. Almost all of the traditional women Apter interviewed expressed ambitions to accomplish goals beyond their roles as wives and mothers. Silence and alienation were common themes among these women. Although they believed that their chosen way of life had value, they felt silenced by women who had chosen other paths and who had louder voices. At mid-life, the traditional woman must shift her focus from her children, because they are leaving, and her husband, because she recognizes that his successes are not her own. Apter believes that these women had to face the regret of having put their own ambitions and desires aside as they focused on their families. To deal with this crisis, they engaged in "regret control." When these women confronted difficult feelings and integrated them into their self-awareness, they fostered mid-life development. When they denied or repressed these feelings and turned away from the confrontation, they forestalled mid-life development. At mid-life these traditional woman had to confront their suppressed visions and their stilled voices and had to get to know themselves in a new way. Only then could they embrace their new freedom and create a more flexible and confident self.

The second group in Apter's study, innovative women, devoted themselves to the pursuit of what had formerly been men's work. They chose to combine careers with family life and took on the superwoman role, much as their traditional mothers had swallowed the feminine mystique. The mid-life crises came when it became clear that work was structured around men's lives and did not allow for the care of children. To move up in the modern workplace, they had to spend long hours at work and use leisure time for networking. Because these women still desired close relationships with their children and their partners, they came to question the relentless demands that their careers imposed on their time. Twelve of the 24 innovative women in Apter's study made significant career changes in their 40s. The typical progression for these women was searching for the right career in their 20s, working hard in their chosen careers during their 30s, and identifying problems and taking measures to extricate themselves from frustrating careers in their 40s. Their mid-life crises were brought on by the stress of overwork, the conflict between professional and personal needs, the distress of discrimination, frustration with unmet ambitions, and increasing tension at work. For women who delayed marriage and/or having children, age 40 was a wake-up call that time was slipping away. When finding a partner or planning a pregnancy was precluded by demanding work schedules, these women had to reevaluate their lives and make major changes. The innovators who did stay at their high-pressure jobs during their mid-life crises did so to prove that they could perform well under stress. They dedicated themselves to changing their working conditions to make them more tolerable. Their crises were resolved by reassessing their career goals, redefining their personal roles, and transforming their workplaces to better meet their personal and professional needs.

Finding themselves in a rut because of limited education and training, the third group, expansive women, made radical changes at mid-life to create new opportunities for themselves. Spurred by internal changes, such as an awakening of ambition, or by external imperatives, such as a divorce or the death of their husbands, they set out on a pathway of self-development. Some women returned to a crossroads where they had lost their way, where they took the wrong fork. Confronting this crisis can be terrifying. As they returned to that wrong turn, many expansive women went through an early phase of "acting out," behaving impulsively and aggressively. Dealing with the anxiety they faced, these women began to take steps to change—going to school, entering training programs, taking new jobs. Once they began their journey, enormous energy was released. Some of the excitement came from meeting new people and being exposed to new perspectives. Apter found that many of the expansive women sought further education, not to gain more knowledge, but to learn how to "give voice to what they already knew" (1995, p. 155). By returning to school at mid-life, these women had to deal with the uncomfortable reality of being an older person in a younger person's domain. They felt very old and very young simultaneously, a novice in a new situation. Often they exaggerated the difficulties they would face, panicking at the thought of not being able to pass their first examination. These exaggerations served to set the scene for triumphant successes as they learned that they could cope with the new world they were entering. Paradoxically, the tension in their expanding world often surfaced at home. Their husbands and children were supportive of their new educational careers as long as it did not affect the home life. The expansive women had two choices, to share their lives (and its messiness) with their families or to hide their new lives and maintain their caregiving roles on top of their new educational demands. This double life as student and homemaker was exhausting for many of the women, but the worst part was the way their new sense of identity was undermined. At a time when they felt in charge and energetic, some of their energy was expended hiding their own personal development in order to keep their families content. When expansion was the result of divorce or when divorce was the result of expansion, the women braved economic crisis to gain a new sense of who they were. In the end they resolved their mid-life crises by becoming more flexible through self-development.

Apter's fourth group, protesting women, felt cheated of a time in adolescence to explore and to try out new things. Because of family or social crises, such as the death of a parent, an early pregnancy, or grinding poverty, they had been forced into premature adult responsibility. At mid-life these women wanted to reach back and experience the youth they had missed. Their mid-life crises were activated by a fear that this last chance for exploration would be lost. Pressured by the sense that they had to create a new self quickly, or not at all, their activities were frantic and unfocused. Apter writes of these women having been trapped by early adolescent experiences and feeling that some part of their real selves were "caught in a parallel world, which could not intersect with the one they actually lived [in]" (p. 189). They had intense desires to make a new life, but only vague ideas about how that new life should be fashioned. They somehow had to align their current lives with the person they thought they would have become if the specific setbacks (care of siblings, teenage motherhood, leaving high school to earn a living) had not intervened. Early in their lives they were responsible and dependable. Now the task they faced in mid-life was to learn to be spontaneous. Apter believes that the crisis faced by the protestors is finding the right path to change. The uncertainty about what that path might be and how to get started on it makes these women difficult to be around. They are judged by others to be "too loud, too sexual, too assertive" (p. 192). Somehow they must retrieve their past goals, refashion them, and make them functional for their current lives.

Because women's lives are so varied, Apter (1995) believes that there are no longer markers along the way for women to compare their lives to and to determine if they are on track. Several themes emerged from Apter's research. Her subjects talked of power, effectiveness, and influence as opposed to impotence, uselessness, and insignificance. Attachment, responsiveness, and commitment were desired in contrast to isolation and loneliness. They spoke of movement, direction, and freedom vs. confinement and stagnation. Other recurrent themes included time and energy well spent vs. time and energy wasted, acceptance and hope vs. anger and regret, balance vs. bias, and clear sight vs. distortion.

The emphasis on youth and beauty in our culture and the promise that the proper cosmetics will disguise the aging process or reverse it lead many women to dread aging. According to Apter (1995), at mid-life women take stock of society's definitions of beauty and put less emphasis on the reflected approval from others that once ruled their lives. As they disengage from others' expectations and assessments, they attain a new power and come to define themselves on their own terms.

Seven of Apter's subjects were mired in envy, seeing themselves as failures and as the focus of other people's contempt. They imagined other women as competitors, much more successful, attractive, and fulfilled than they were themselves. Being consumed with envy, they were unable to find a way through their mid-life crisis. Apter believes that they missed their chance for change because they were unable to face their regret. By accepting what they viewed as the rules of the game, a game that had changed during their lifetimes, they refused to take risks to form a new life. Their envy of others was the result of and a cause of recurrent depression, a state that could be viewed as stagnation.

Biological Markers

Physical and biological changes occur throughout the lifespan. During childhood the growing body brings psychological changes as the baby becomes a toddler, the toddler becomes a preschooler, the girl goes off to school and later begins to develop the secondary sex characteristics that occur with menarche. Biological changes accompanying motherhood and aging also have a psychological impact, especially in our youth-fixated culture.

In adulthood, the reality of menopause creates a psychological boundary between youth and old age. With the large number of "baby-boomers" reaching menopause, there is increased interest in and research on the topic. Apter (1995) found little evidence in her research that menopause is responsible for significant psychosocial development. Thirty-five of Apter's 80 subjects had gone through or were going through menopause by the end of the study. In analyzing the interview materials, Apter concluded that menopause accompanied, but did not cause, the mid-life crises these women confronted. In contrast to menarche, which is a single identifiable event, menopause is a process that spans several years for most women, with a wide range of "symptoms." As Zita (1997) has pointed out, "menopause is a physical event in the body, but its interpretation as the loss of true femininity, as disease, dysfunction, or functionlessness or as a natural life cycle transition with complicated political consequences determines how it is experienced and perceived" (p. 106). Apter believes that menopause is just one of the factors that can heighten a woman's concern about aging, no more important than a birthday or the image of oneself in the mirror. Apter did find that some women used menopause as a way to frame their crises. For example, some women who were struggling with their own sense of authority and control used the relative ignorance of the medical profession on health issues surrounding menopause as a means of focusing on their own self-development. By becoming more involved in their health decisions, they resolved some of their psychological issues. Apter describes the frustration that many women feel when they try to communicate with doctors, and characterizes the decision many women make to become their own authorities on menopause as their way of dealing with this mini-crisis.

PSYCHOSOCIAL MODELS OF LATE ADULTHOOD

Ego Integrity

For Erikson, the person who reaches a state of ego integrity has taken care of things and other people and has achieved a sense of accomplishment and creativity. This person has adapted to the triumphs in life and to the disappointments and has made an impact on society through the generation of new ideas or lasting material contributions. "It is the acceptance of one's one and only life cycle as something that had to be and that, by necessity, permitted of no substitutions" (Erikson, 1963, p. 268). This acceptance of one's life takes the sting out of the thought of eventual death. On the other hand, the lack of this acceptance leads to a fear of death. Despair results when a person perceives that her life has been wasted or misspent.

One reflection of ego integrity is wisdom, a form of intelligence that is associated with old age. Orwoll and Achenbaum (1993) have proposed a model of wisdom that includes intrapersonal wisdom (self-development, self-knowledge, and integrity), interpersonal wisdom (empathy, understanding, and maturity in relationships), and transpersonal wisdom (self-transcendence, recognition of the limits of knowledge and understanding, and philosophical or spiritual commitments). Intrapersonal wisdom focuses on the self and includes building one's resources to be able to impart wisdom to others. Certainly, self-development (learning more about the world) and self-knowledge (being able to acknowledge one's strengths and limitations) are necessary to the development of personal integrity. Empathy and understanding of others leads to maturity in relationships. Further, self-transcendence (the ability to go beyond personal issues to address universal concerns) and a recognition of the limits of knowledge and understanding make one's philosophical and spiritual commitments meaningful and realistic.

In a review of the literature on wisdom and its social and cultural meaning, Orwoll and Achenbaum (1993) conclude that current conceptualizations of wisdom combine masculine and feminine sensibilities. Some manifestations of wisdom, such as being a judge or a member of the clergy, have been predominantly masculine roles, whereas other reflections of wisdom, listening empathically and giving sound advice, contain elements of feminine stereotypes. They believe that any gender differences in the expression of wisdom arise from "unique challenges and opportunities associated with gendered experiences, which may themselves shift and change across the life course. Gender-specific experiences and roles also influence the opportunities and contexts for expressing wisdom" (p. 290).

In modern American society, wisdom is rare and integrity is an uncommon surprise. Aging is a threat to most people, a constant reminder of their failing physical power and ultimate mortality. For women, aging is particularly threatening. Sontag (1997) has outlined the "double standard of aging," referring to the differences between men and women in the aging process. While for men increasing age adds to their power and prestige, for women increasing age renders them sexually ineligible and socially obsolete. Especially in a society such as ours, that values youth beyond all else, aging is a relentless process. Sontag emphasizes, however, that "aging is much more a social judgment than a biological eventuality" (p. 21). Lines and scars on a man's face are judged attractive and evidence of character, a life fully lived. However, when a woman has lines or scars on her face, she is disfigured, the victim of a hard life. Women are encouraged to preserve their youth by the liberal application of cosmetics and to invent themselves through clothing. By consuming the right products, they can delay the negative consequences of time.

Aging not only undermines the psychological stamina of women, it decreases their economic power as well. In an article describing the "feminization of poverty among the elderly," Stone (1997) states that "women constitute 72.4 percent of the elderly poor although they account for only 58.7 percent of all elderly" (p. 45). Elderly women are three times as likely as elderly men to be widowed and living alone. This is because women live longer, women tend to marry men who are older and more likely to predecease them, and older women are less likely than older men to remarry following the death of their spouses. Because widowhood is related to lower economic status, poverty in old age is more prevalent among women than men. Jackson (1997) reports that black women become widows earlier than white women and are even more likely than white women to be living alone. Further, Reinharz (1997) has found that almost one-half of all women over the age of 65 feel unsafe outside their homes. To deal with this fear of the streets, many adopt a home-bound lifestyle that greatly restricts their freedom of movement. This combination of poverty and limited mobility creates a sense of powerlessness that shapes their identity, attitudes, and behavior. Reinharz believes that "powerlessness and denigration breed intimidation which has to be unlearned in new types of relationships and new institutions" (p. 75). Currently, old age is seen as a "woman's issue" because women outlive men and comprise the majority of people over 65 and the vast majority of patients in nursing homes. In our society, daughters and daughters-in-law are pressured to care for elderly relatives before they require full-time custodial care, and female workers provide the majority of care in nursing homes. Thus the majority of the elderly are women and the preponderance of care given to the elderly is provided by women.

Evers (1981) has described how submitting to the care of other women is a different experience for women than it is for men because most women are not used to being cared for by women. When they are incapacitated to the extent that others must provide for their daily needs, elderly women must surrender their own roles as care givers to others. Being helpless and dependent reinforces the idea that old age is a nonproductive phase in the lifespan. Focusing on the patient-nurse relationship within the nursing home, Evers points out that geriatric nursing is a low-status specialty. Our medical system is designed to value cures and the restoration of health. The restoration of health among the old is rare, thus robbing geriatrics of its miracle cures. Further, old people have low status in our society, so their care also has low status. Evers believes that there is a special dilemma for female geriatric nurses giving care to female patients who represent the future. That is, the elderly female patient is a constant reminder to the nurse that some day she, too, will be old and helpless.

It is difficult to see how older women can come to the end of their lives with ego integrity intact. However, Gutmann (1987), drawing on research from around the world, contends that women become more authoritative and more effective as they age. From ethnographic data, Gutmann spells out eight patterns of female striving and power in old age: *older woman as ritual leader, sexy older woman, self-sufficient older woman, the family matriarch, the mother-in-law, the woman in alliance with her oldest son, the witch,* and *the evil spirit.* Postmenopausal women are acceptable as ritual leaders because they are less sexually attractive (and less distracting to the spiritual concentration of the males), and they cannot pollute the rituals with their menstrual blood. In many societies older women are allowed to participate in rituals that younger women are barred from. Sexy older women take liberties and perform provocative acts that younger women would be censured for; for example, bawdy old women tell jokes and perform lewd dances. The Golden Girls television sitcom was an example of this phenomenon. The greater self-sufficiency of older women, in comparison to older men, comes from their domestic skills, which they need to maintain their independence. Older men lack these skills and must depend upon others to cook their food and clean their houses. Older women take on the role of matriarch when their husbands give up their dominant roles to dedicate themselves to religious or philosophical issues or just lapse into passivity. These women step into the role of making day-to-day decisions, often in collaboration with their sons. In many societies, such as India, the role of mother-in-law further consolidates the power of older women because they can direct the activities of their daughters-in-law and command respect from a large extended family. The power of the older woman is tied to the ascendancy of her oldest son. When he marries and becomes an adult, his mother's future power depends on her ability to maintain her emotional hold over her son and control over her daughter-in-law. When her husband becomes disabled or uninterested in continuing his role as head of the household, the older woman and her son share dominance over the family. One danger of older women's greater power is the fear they create in others, who may see them as witches. If she becomes angry with a family member, the older woman can be accused of sorcery. Even after she has died, the woman's evil spirit may be feared, especially if she was a powerful woman before death. To avoid the curse of a powerful woman, family members take care to treat her respectfully.

Although many anthropologists have reported greater female dominance in later life, Gutmann has identified little institutional expression or recognition of this phenomenon. In his psychological studies, he had women write stories about pictures depicting people in social relationships. He found that older women included more themes of aggression in their stories, reinforcing the interpretation that older women are more active and vital. Specifically, women over 60 wrote more stories in which they visualized direct conflict between themselves and their children. Gutmann believes that when older women realize that their nurturance is no longer needed by their adult children, they turn that nurturance inward and learn to take better care of themselves. In contrast to older men, older women are in a better position to live self-sufficient lives.

Caffarella and Olson (1993) have reviewed the literature on the psychosocial development of women, focusing on theoretical works, empirical studies that address developmental issues in all-female samples, and articles that suggest different pathways for future research. They judged the number of articles proposing alternative theories of female development to be quite small. However, they identified four major themes in this literature: *the centrality of interpersonal relationships in the self-concept of women across all ages; the importance of social roles in directing women's lives; the non-linearity of women's lives as they traverse various roles;* and *the changing development issues that women face as they mature and age.* Cohort differences, resulting from differing historical, social, and cultural experiences, make it difficult to extract any coherent developmental theory that applies to all women. From empirical studies designed to validate stage models of development for women, they concluded that key concepts include the importance of having a firm sense of self, a need for intimacy, and the alternation of stable and transitional periods within the life cycle. In addressing the development of new research methodologies for the future, Caffarella and Olson suggest that the current, almost exclusive, reliance on interviews must be augmented with standardized instruments, such as questionnaires and surveys.

SUMMARY

From this outline of the psychosocial development of women across the lifespan we can conclude that much more research is needed, especially longitudinal studies of girls and women. Whether we focus on stages of development, life paths, ways of knowing, or finding one's voice, the development of women seems to differ from the models patterned after men's lives. Of course, we must be careful to avoid what Hare-Mustin and Maracek (1988) term the *alpha bias*—the accentuation of the differences between men and women and the creation of differences that do not exist. On the other hand, ignoring differences and adopting male life patterns for women is also to be avoided. Although it is difficult, theorists and researchers need to draw meaning from women's lives that will allow them to construct theories that are not contaminated by past biases. In the process women can learn to make more sense of their lives as they continue to recognize shared life experiences.

For those in the health care professions, a knowledge of the issues that affect women at different ages will help them understand what women are telling them, better communicate the information these women need in order to live healthier lives, and deal with the challenges and frustrations that may arise in their contacts with women patients. For example, a nurse who is teaching a young girl how to deal with a chronic illness, such as diabetes, may want to consider focusing on daily medication as an achievement task, a task related to the girl's sense of industry and her ability to give herself the medication. An adolescent girl may be more concerned with how diabetes will affect her identity and her chances for intimacy. Her self-in-relation may be affected by her concern over how her friends and her lover will react to her illness. The adult woman may see the illness as undermining her ability to be generative, limiting her capacity to take care of her family. The elderly woman may see diabetes as yet another instance of her declining powers, confronting her with the reality of her aging and eventual mortality.

Further, a knowledge of psychosocial development will help women in health care deal with their own issues. By making their own thoughts, emotions, and behaviors more understandable to themselves, they can achieve their own career goals; establish intimacy with their family, friends, and co-workers; and increase their power and resources to be of service to their patients.

REFERENCES

Ainsworth, M. D. S. (1967). *Infancy in Uganda*. Baltimore, MD: Johns Hopkins University Press.

Ainsworth, M. D. S., & Wittig, B. A. (1969). Attachment and the exploratory behavior of one-year-olds in a strange situation. In B. M. Foss (Ed.), *Determinants of infant behavior* (pp. 113–136). Vol. 4. London: Methuen.

Apter, T. (1995). *Secret paths: Women in the new midlife.* New York: W. W. Norton & Company.

Atkinson, J. W. (1958). *Motives in fantasy, action, and society.* Princeton, NJ: Van Nostrand.

Atkinson, J. W., & Feather, N. T. (1966). *A theory of achievement motivation.* New York: Wiley.

Beck, A. T., Steer, R. A., & Epstein, N. (1992). Self-concept dimensions of clinically depressed and anxious out-patients. *Journal of Clinical Psychology, 48(4)*, 423–432.

Belenky, M. F., Clinchy, B. McV., Goldberger, N. R., & Tarule, J. M. (1986). *Women's ways of knowing: The development of self, voice, and mind.* New York: Basic Books, Inc.

Bowlby, J. (1988) *A secure base: Parent-child attachment and healthy human development.* New York: Basic Books, Inc.

Bretherton, I. (1995). The origins of attachment theory: John Bowlby and Mary Ainsworth. In S. Goldberg, R. Muir, & J. Kerr (Eds.), *Attachment theory: Social, developmental, and clinical perspectives* (pp. 45–84). Hillsdale, NJ: Analytic Press.

Broverman, I. K., Broverman, D. M., Clarkson, F. E., Rosenkrantz, P. S., & Vogel, S. R. (1970). Sex-role stereotypes and clinical judgments of mental health. *Journal of Consulting and Clinical Psychology, 34*, 1–7.

Butler, S. (1978). *Conspiracy of silence: The trauma of incest.* San Francisco, CA: Volcano Press, Inc.

Caffarella, R. S., & Olson, S. K. (1993). Psychosocial development of women: A critical review of the literature. *Adult Education Quarterly, 43(3)*, 125–151.

Dweck, C. S., Davidson, W., Nelson, S., & Enna, B. (1978). Sex differences in learned helplessness: II. An experimental analysis. *Developmental Psychology, 14*, 268–276.

Dweck, C. S., & Wortman, C. B. (1982). Learned helplessness, anxiety, and achievement motivation: Neglected parallels in cognition, affective, and coping responses. In H. W. Krohne & L. Laux (Eds.), *Achievement, stress, and anxiety* (pp. 93–125). New York: Hemisphere Publishing Corporation.

Erikson, E. H. (1963). *Childhood and society* (2nd ed.). New York: W. W. Norton.

Erikson, E. H. (1968). *Identity, youth, and crisis.* New York: W. W. Norton.

Evers, H. (1981). Care or custody? The experience of women patients in long-stay geriatric wards. In B. Hutter & G. Williams (Eds.), *Controlling women: The normal and the deviant* (pp. 108–130). London: Croom Helm Ltd.

French, E., & Lesser, G. S. (1964). Some characteristics of the achievement motive in women. *Journal of Abnormal Social Psychology, 68*, 119–128.

Freud, S. (1905). *Three essays on the theory of sexuality.* Leípzig: F. Dueticke.

Gilligan, C. (1982). *In a different voice: Psychological theory and women's development.* Cambridge, MA: Harvard University Press.

Gilligan, C. (1991). Women's psychological development: Implications for psychotherapy. In C. Gilligan, A. G. Rogers, & D. L. Tolman (Eds.), *Women, girls, and psychotherapy: Reframing resistance* (pp. 5–31). New York: The Haworth Press, Inc.

Gutmann, D. (1987). *Reclaimed powers: Toward a new psychology of men and women in later life.* New York: Basic Books, Inc.

Habermas, T., & Bluck, S. (2000). Getting a life: The emergence of the life story in adolescence. *Psychological Bulletin, 126,* 748–769.

Hare-Mustin, R. T., & Maracek, J. (1988). The meaning of difference: Gender theory, postmodernism, and psychology. *American Psychologist, 43,* 455–464.

Horner, M. (1987). Toward an understanding of achievement-related conflicts in women. In M R. Walsh (Ed.), *The psychology of women: Ongoing debates* (pp. 169–184). New Haven, CT: Yale University Press.

Jackson, J. J. (1997). The plight of older black women. In M. Pearsall (Ed.), *The other within us: Feminist explorations of women and aging* (pp. 37–41). Boulder, CO: Westview Press.

Levinson, D. J. (1978). *The seasons of a man's life.* New York: Alfred A. Knopf.

Levinson, D. J. (1996). *The seasons of a woman's life.* New York: Ballantine Books.

McAdams, D. P. (1988). *Power, intimacy, and the life story: Personological inquiries into identity.* New York: The Guilford Press.

McAdams, D. P., & de St. Aubin, E. (1992). A theory of generativity and its assessment through self-report, behavioral acts, and narrative themes in autobiography. *Journal of Personality and Social Psychology, 62(6),* 1003–1015.

McClelland, D. C. (1975). *Power: The inner experience.* New York: Irvington Publishers, Inc.

Miller, J. B. (1986). *Toward a new psychology of women* (2nd ed.). Boston, MA: Beacon Press.

Miller, J. B. (1991a). The development of a woman's sense of self. In J. V. Jordan, A. G. Kaplan, J. B. Miller, I P. Stiver, & J. L. Surrey (Eds.), *Women's growth in connection: Writings from the Stone Center* (pp. 11–26). New York: The Guilford Press.

Miller, J. B. (1991b). Women and power. In J. V. Jordan, A. G. Kaplan, J. B. Miller, I P. Stiver, & J. L. Surrey (Eds.), *Women's growth in connection: Writings from the Stone Center* (pp. 197–205). New York: The Guilford Press.

Miller, J. B., & Stiver, I. P. (1997). *The healing connection: How women form relationships in therapy and in life.* Boston: Beacon Press.

Moore, S., & Boldero, J. (1991). Psychosocial development and friendship functions in adolescence. *Sex Roles, 25,* 521–536.

Olson, T. (1978). *Silences.* New York: Delacorte Press.

Orwoll, L., & Achenbaum, W. A. (1993). Gender and the development of wisdom. *Human Development, 36,* 274–296.

Reinharz, S. (1997). Friends or foes: Gerontological and feminist theory. In M. Pearsall (Ed.), *The other within us: Feminist explorations of women and aging* (pp. 73–94). Boulder, CO: Westview Press.

Reinke, B. J., Holmes, D. S., & Harris, R. L. (1985). The timing of psychosocial changes in women's lives: The years 25 to 45. *Journal of Personality and Social Psychology, 48,* 1353–1364.

Sontag, S. (1997). The double standard of aging. In M. Pearsall (Ed.), *The other within us: Feminist explorations of women and aging* (pp. 19–24). Boulder, CO: Westview Press.

Stone, R. I. (1997). The feminization of poverty among the elderly. In M. Pearsall (Ed.), *The other within us: Feminist explorations of women and aging* (pp. 43–55). Boulder, CO: Westview Press.

Surrey, J. L. (1991). The self-in-relation: A theory of women's development. In J. V. Jordan, A. G. Kaplan, J. B. Miller, I P. Stiver, & J. L. Surrey (Eds.), *Women's growth in connection: Writings from the Stone Center* (pp. 51–66). New York: The Guilford Press.

Taylor, J. McL., Gilligan, C., & Sullivan, A. M. (1995). *Between voice and silence: Women and girls, race and relationship.* Cambridge, MA: Harvard University Press.

Wallace, Z. G. (1887). Quoted in S. B. Anthony & I. H. Harper (Eds.) (1969). *History of women's suffrage, Vol. 4, 1883-1900* (p. 119). New York: Arno & The New York Times. (Originally published in 1902). Quote reprinted in Biggs, M. (1996). *Women's words: The Columbia book of quotations by women* (p. 334). New York: Columbia University Press.

Weiner, B. (1974). *Achievement motivation and attribution theory.* Morristown, NF: General Learning Press.

Winter, D. G. (1973). *The power motive.* New York: The Free Press.

Zita, J. N. (1997). Heresy in the female body: The rhetorics of menopause. In M. Pearsall (Ed.), *The other within us: Feminist explorations of women and aging* (pp. 95–112). Boulder, CO: Westview Press.

RESOURCES

Centre for Development and Population Activities: *www.cedpa.org*
Institute for Women's Policy Research: *www.iwpr.org*
Society for Women's Health Research: *www.womens-health.org*
Voices of Women: *www.voicesofwomen.com*
Women's Development Council: *www.fortnet.org/WDC/*
American Psychiatric Association: *www.psych.org/*
American Psychological Association: *www.apa.org/*
National Institute of Mental Health: *www.nimh.nih.gov*
Mental Health: *www.mentalhealth.com*
National Association of Social Workers: *www.naswde.org/*
CDC Health Topic: Women's Health: *www.cdc.gov/health/womensmenu.htm*
National Women's Health Information Center (NWHIC): *www.4women.gov*

Chapter 7

Female Physical Development

Thelma Patrick

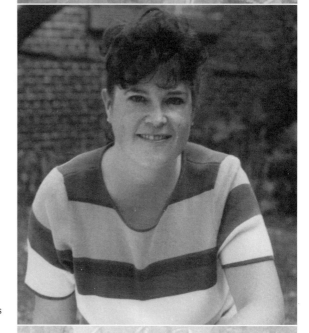

In the instinctive psyche, the body is considered a sensor, an informational network, a messenger with myriad communication systems—cardiovascular, respiratory, skeletal, autonomic, as well as emotive and intuitive. In the imaginal world, the body is a powerful vehicle, a spirit who lives with us, a prayer of life in its own right.

Clarissa Pinkola Estes

INTRODUCTION

Much progress has been made in understanding women's physiology and health. These advances have resulted from a combination of progress in scientific techniques that further our understanding of physiology and enhanced social and political awareness of the need to understand these differences. Despite this advanced understanding, there is still insufficient scientific knowledge about the unique problems of women's health and women's biology.

Historically, women's health has been described in relation to the physiological events of the reproductive cycle that are obviously unique to women, namely menarche, childbearing, and menopause (Pinn, 1995). Each of the reproductive events reflects a marked change in endocrine functioning, especially that related to the female sex hormone estrogen.

While a biological role for sex steroids was recognized in the early 1900s, estrogen was not discovered until the 1920s (Korach, 1994). Estrogen was first understood in relation to its crucial role in embryonic and fetal development and its influence on female secondary characteristics, the reproductive cycle, and fertility or maintenance of pregnancy. Researchers have sought to understand the wide-ranging effects of female hormones. Scientists have long failed to appreciate the enormous medical implications of the sexes' diverse hormonal environments (Mann, 1995).

The terms "sex" and "gender" have different meanings. *Sex* is the genetic determination of the body as male or female, while *gender* includes the social roles and behaviors attributed to a particular sex. Gender-based or gender-specific biology explores sexual differentiation at all levels of the system, including the physical and the social. Women's health involves sex and gender differences, the influences of female sex hormones on health and disease, the role of genetic-based conditions in determining women's health, and the effects of the environment in which women live, their utilization of health care, and other psychosocial and behavioral determinants (Pinn, 1998). To learn about these differences, Haseltine (1995) suggests that we "take what we know and expand on it." A study of gender differences should focus on significant gaps in our knowledge of differences across the spectrum of human development and functioning, such as genetic inheritance (both parental contributions and gene expression), in utero development, growth patterns, and hormonal influences throughout life.

This chapter examines the physical development of the female. Moving through a hierarchy from simple to complex, from the cell to the more complex physiological, processes of the human, and using the suggestions of Pinn and Haseltine cited previously, this chapter describes

■ The structure and function of the cell
■ The concept of gene expression
■ Communication within and between cells
■ Hormones as chemical messengers
■ Cellular processes involved in growth and development
■ Physical development of the female
■ Physical functioning, maturation, and aging
■ Gender-specific biology, physiology, and clinical research
■ Contributions of nursing to the health of women across the lifespan

The cell, and the molecular events in the cell, are emphasized throughout the chapter. Knowledge of molecules, signals, interactions, and responses provides a basis for understanding growth, development, and aging, as well as treatments in clinical use and those yet to be developed or implemented. Our appreciation of the molecular environment and its complexity will profoundly affect the care provided by nurses in the future in the areas of illness prevention, health promotion, and health restoration (Foley & Sommers, 1998).

THE STRUCTURE AND FUNCTION OF THE CELL

The cell is the simplest structural unit capable of the maintaining life. It is the building block of every living organism. Each cell is composed of a plasma membrane, a nucleus, and cytoplasm. The membrane is an outer border built to retain the inner contents of the cell. The cytoplasm is the region that makes up the entire interior of the cell except the nucleus and is the site of many metabolic cycles and synthetic pathways, as well as the location of protein synthesis. The two major components of the cytoplasm are the cell organelles, small structures within cells that perform dedicated functions, and the cytosol, the fluid portion that surrounds the organelles. Each organelle performs a specific function. The mitochondria, the powerhouse of the cell, are responsible for converting nutrients into energy. Other organelles include the ribosome, where amino acids are joined together to form a protein chain, the Golgi apparatus, which performs the intracellular sorting of proteins, and the peroxisome, where certain fatty acids and amino acids are degraded (Murray, 2000).

Proteins, the chief macromolecules in the cell, are essential components of all organs and chemical activities. Proteins perform many functions, such as catalyzing molecular reactions, allowing cells to move and do work, and maintaining internal cell rigidity. In addition, proteins control the genes that determine cell constitution and function, move molecules across membranes, and even direct protein synthesis (Rodwell, 2000). The proteins that comprise each cell are determined by the individual's genome.

The Concept of Gene Expression

Everything that distinguishes one cell from another, such as specification of different tissues, cellular maturity, and activation and proliferation within a single tissue, depends on selective gene expression. Regulation of gene expression is among the most fundamental processes of life and assumes increasing importance as the complexity of living organisms increases (Steel, 1996). Essentially, genes orchestrate the development of a single-celled egg into a fully formed adult. Genes influence our appearance, capabilities, and vulnerabilities. The complete set of instructions for an organism is called its *genome*.

The nucleus, the largest organelle within a cell, stores and transmits genetic information in the form of DNA. Genetic information is transferred from DNA to RNA to protein. Two sequential events, transcription and translation, constitute the central dogma of molecular biology. Transcription is the process of generating ribonucleic acid (RNA). RNA acts as a protein template in translation. There is a transfer of genetic information from the double-stranded DNA to the complementary base sequence in an RNA molecule. The product of transcription is messenger RNA (mRNA). In the second step, the mRNA is transported from the nucleus to the cytoplasm for translation. Translation is the process of converting the base sequence of mRNA into the linear sequence of amino acids in a protein. These processes are depicted in Figure 7-1 (Steel, 1996).

Somatic cells organize to form body tissues, organs, and systems. Each somatic cell nucleus contains 23 chromosome pairs, 1 sex chromosome and 22 other chromosomes, that consist of protein and deoxyribonucleic acid (DNA). Somatic cells have a pair of genes for each trait. Although both genes of a pair produce the same trait, they may carry different information about it.

Different forms of the same gene are called *alleles*. Alleles of a gene pair must occupy an identical position, known as the *locus*, on each of the identical pairs of chromosomes, referred to as *homologues*. The genetic sequence of an individual is known as its

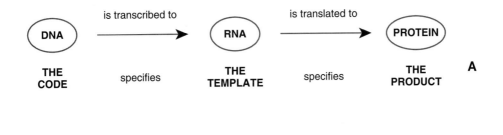

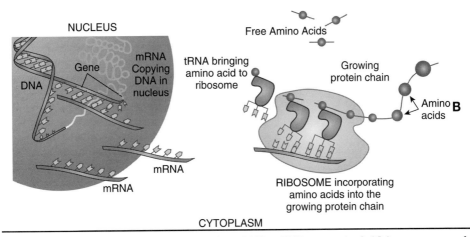

Figure 7-1 Transferring genetic information from DNA to RNA to protein. **A**, Major processes and outcomes of the central dogma. **B**, Activities of each of the processes, from DNA to protein. (**B** from the U. S. Department of Energy Office of Science, Office of Biological and Environmental Research, Human Genome Program, *http://www.ornl.gov/hgmis.*)

genotype, while the observable property (structure or function) produced by the genotype is the *phenotype.* There are many more possible phenotypic outcomes than there are genes. The phenotype expressed is a result of a complex interaction of genetic, biochemical, environmental, and behavioral factors (Scott, 2000).

For some time, we have been able to examine the chromosome pairs from somatic cells. Figure 7-2 depicts the male and female karotypes (note the difference in the appearance of the X and Y chromosomes). An idiogram (Figure 7-3) shows the location of genes on the chromosome. (The idiogram is not an all-inclusive map of the genes on all chromosomes.)

Chromosomes are often classified by the Denver system. In this nomenclature system, individual chromosomes are labeled by a number, with 1 being the largest and 22, the smallest, or the letters X or Y. Chromosomes are then grouped by appearance, and the groupings are identified by letter (A, B, C, etc.). The characteristics considered in these classifications include the size of the chromosome, the point of union of the chromosome pair, called the *centromere,* and the size or shape of the regions above and below the centromere, known as the *arms.*

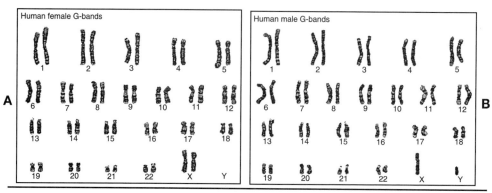

Figure 7-2 Karotypes. **A**, Female, **B**, Male. (Courtesy University of Washington, Department of Pathology, Seattle, Washington. *http://www.pathology.washington.edu.*)

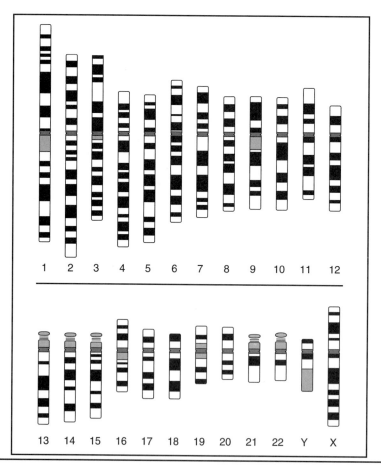

Figure 7-3 Idiogram illustrating the location of genes on the chromosomes. (From Adler, D.: *Idiogram album: Human.* Copyright 1994 David Adler.)

This standarized system of identification is also used to denote the location of genes on a chromosome. The letter *p* identifies the upper arms of the chromosome, and the letter *q* identifies the lower arms. Beginning at the centromere and extending to the end of the chromosome arm, regions are identified by number. The number 1 indicates the region closest to the centromere; thus, the greater the number of a region, the farther from the centromere. The number of regions identified per chromosome varies. Within each region and beginning at the point nearest to the centromere, bands are also numerically identified (Figure 7-4).

Chromosomes consist mainly of long chains of DNA. Genes are short segments of DNA that are separated from one another by a meaningless DNA sequence. Each set of chromosomes contains 50,000 to 100,000 genes. The number of genes on each chromosome varies. The X chromosome has an estimated 5000 genes, while the Y chromosome has only 30 (Miller & Raymond, 1999).

A gene is composed of a specific sequence of nucleotide base pairs. Nucleotides are coded by a series of letters that correspond to one of the chemical constituents of DNA, namely adenine (A), thymine (T), guanine (G), and cytosine (C). These bases form interlocking pairs of varying lengths. The base combinations, specifically A always with T and G always with C, provide the instructions for the synthesis of a specific amino acid. The genetic code also dictates the sequence of amino acids that make up specific proteins. The genes in the cell nucleus determine the function and shape of proteins. When a gene's sequence is known, the genetic code can be used to determine which amino acids make up a protein, and that protein can then be studied to determine its function (Figure 7-5).

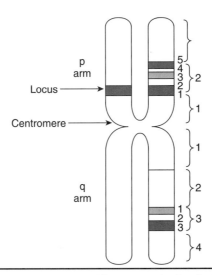

Figure **7-4** Landmarks on the chromosome used for communicating the location of genes. *p,* Arms of the chromosome above the centromere; *q,* arms below the centromere; *1,* region closest to the centromere.

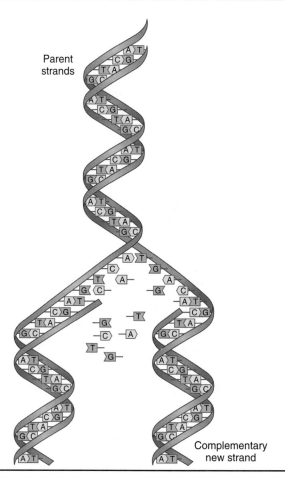

Parent strands

Complementary new strand

Figure 7-5 Each DNA molecule is a long two-stranded chain that is coiled in a double helix. (From the U. S. Department of Energy Office of Science, Office of Biological and Environmental Research, Human Genome Program, *http://www.ornl.gov/hgmis.*)

The genome is vulnerable to mutation as a result of exposure to an array of DNA-damaging agents of both endogenous and environmental origin. A gene can be disrupted by a single mutation that causes major effects. Major disruptions are usually lethal, causing embryos to die before implantation, during pregnancy, or shortly after birth. It is not likely that a gene would be mutated such that it does not produce anything. However, mutations can produce something that is nonfunctional, a protein with altered activity, (either over or under active), or a protein that is produced in the wrong amount, place, or time. The effects of the deletion of a nucleotide, a seemingly minor mutation, are depicted in Tables 7-1A and 7-1B.

Numerous fail-safe mechanisms prevent mutations from affecting the gene product. These quality control mechanisms are in place at multiple points in the transfer of information from DNA to the final protein product. One process ensures maintenance of the genome by repairing any miscoded sequences. When nucleotide alterations are detected, they are generally removed by excision repair pathways that counteract the mutagenic effects of DNA lesions. In some cases, DNA damage is not repaired, but the damaged segment is bypassed by specialized DNA proteins (Lindahl & Wood, 1999).

Translation of genetic information in messenger RNA to newly synthesized protein must be relatively error free in order to sustain homeostasis. It is speculated that an amino acid is misincorporated in about 1 in every 10,000 codons under normal growth conditions. Proofreading and editing occur following translation; these processes check the integrity of the nucleic acid substrates, namely messenger RNA (mRNA) and transfer RNA (tRNA), control the exact matching of tRNA with the appropriate amino acid, and mediate the precise pairings of transfer RNA with the corresponding mRNA codon (Ibba & Soll, 1999).

Finally, polypeptides that are formed by translation must be folded into stable protein structures. This final step occurs in the endoplasmic reticulum, the organelle that folds and assembles multiprotein complexes. Proteins can be damaged during or after assembly. Such damaged proteins have three potential fates: (1) they can be retained within the endoplasmic reticulum and degraded or reprocessed; (2) they can be retrieved by a chaperone, a protein complex that assists in protein folding and remodeling; or (3) they can be destroyed by specific enzymes called *proteases* (Ellgaard, Molinari, & Helenius, 1999).

Understanding genetic expression by sequencing the human genome is the goal of the Human Genome Project in which the exact sequences of all 3 billion nucleotide bases that make up the human genome are being decoded letter by letter. By late 1999, scientists had determined the exact order of 1 billion base pairs of DNA, about one third of the whole human genome. A major milestone achieved was the publication of the first human chromosome, chromosome 22, the second smallest chromosome, which consists of about 33 million base pairs and 500 to 1000 genes. Little (1999) describes this accomplishment as the first phase in a biological revolution. One result of this revolution, no doubt, will be a new appreciation of human individuality.

While there is much excitement about the elucidation of the sequence of the genome, interpretation of this code is ongoing and involves identifying the product that is expressed by a gene on a specific chromosome and understanding genes and their products in a physiological context. To learn anything about physiology, development, or evolution, scientists will need to convert their laundry list of genes into detailed maps of molecular pathways and interconnected networks of protein function (Pennisi, 2000). Known proteins must be linked to particular tissues or changes in cell properties. Some of what proteins do depends on interaction with other proteins, and, once scientists have identified which proteins interact, then physical disruption of their coupling can reveal why these interactions are biologically important. To date, the interactions of about 750 proteins involved in cell proliferation, development, and differentiation have been identified. An understanding of the specific factors involved in these interactions may be quite important in drug development.

Until recently, the analysis of any biochemical process (including gene expression) was laborious. In the absence of some special clues to guide discovery, scientists had to examine every chromosome to find a suspect gene. Past approaches to discovery

Table 7-1A	NORMAL SEQUENCE FOR TRANSCRIPTION AND TRANSLATION				
Template strand (No promoter; strand not copied)	TAC	CAC	GTG	GAC	TGA
Coding strand (Promoter region; strand copied)	ATG	GTG	CAC	CTG	ACT
mRNA sequence	AUG	GUG	CAC	CUG	ACU
Amino acid sequence coded	Methionine (or start)	Valine	Histidine	Leucine	Threonine

Messenger RNA (mRNA) is a sequence of nucleotides. The nucleotides are read in groups of three, called *codons*. The amino acid sequence is the order in which amino acids are linked together to form a protein. The sequence AUG, which codes for the protein methionine, is also the signal to start the translation of amino acids. Three codons, UAA, UAG, UGA, can signal the end of translation and prevent the addition of more amino acids. The newly formed protein is the gene product, or gene expression.

Table 7-1B	WHAT HAPPENS TO CODING WHEN DNA IS DAMAGED				
Template strand	No promoter; not copied	TAC	CAC	GTG	GAC
Coding strand	Promoter region; strand copied, however, DNA damage caused deletion in second sequence	ATG	G T G	CAC	CTG
Intended MRNA sequence	Does not occur	AUG	G U G	CAC	CUG
Actual mRNA sequence	All coding shifts due to deletion	AUG	GGC	ACC	UGA
Intended amino acid sequence	Does not occur	Methionine (or start)	Valine	Histidine	Leucine
Actual amino acid sequence	Protein produced may be non-functional or may cause inappropriate cellular response	Methionine (or start)	Glycine	Threonine	Stop codon

GGA	CTC	CTC	ACT
CCT	GAG	GAG	TGA
CCU	GAG	GAG	UGA
Proline	Glutamate	Glutamate	Stop Codon

TGA	CGA	CTC	CTC	ACT
ACT	CCT	GAG	GAG	TGA
ACU	CCU	GAG	GAG	UGA
CUC	CUG	AGG	AGU	GA
Threonine	Proline	Glutamate	Glutamate	Stop Codon
No new start codon; no additional protein				

included (1) hypothesizing the existence of a biochemical process or metabolic pathway from observations made at the whole-animal level; (2) analyzing of the mechanisms that control the process or pathway and their effect in specific diseases, such as cancer or inborn errors of metabolism; (3) locating the process to one or more organs, then to one or more cellular organelles or subcellular fractions; (4) delineating the number of reactions involved in it; (5) purifying individual substrates, products, enzymes, and cofactors; (6) studying the product at the gene level by recombinant DNA technology (Murray, 2000).

Unlocking the secrets of the genome in the past was hindered by the time-intensive scientific techniques that were available. Computerization and advances in biochemical techniques to locate proteins, genes, and chromosomes have contributed to expanding this body of knowledge. With the progress of the Human Genome Project, genes involved in physiological processes, as well as rare and common diseases, will be identified. Such discoveries will bring new understanding of factors that alter or damage genes and should lead to improvements in the early detection and treatment of diseases and developmental aberrations.

Communications Within and Between Cells

Cells organize to form tissues, organs, and systems. Each cell has a function to perform, and the cell must sustain its own vitality and contribute to the body system. To achieve and maintain homeostasis, the activities of cells, tissues, and organs are integrated in such a way that any change in the environment initiates a reaction to minimize the effect of the change on cellular functioning. Even when there are no environmental changes to which the cell must respond, energy must be added continuously to maintain metabolic processes at a constant, or steady, state in which there is continuous energy consumption and gain and loss of material.

Functional stability between the internal and external environments of the cell is achieved by balancing input and output. It is not the absolute magnitude of the input and output but rather the balance between them that is critical in cellular functioning.

The following concepts are important to the understanding of cellular behavior.

1. Cells are dynamic and respond to many changes in the external environment. Homeostatic control systems cannot maintain complete constancy of any given regulated variable in the internal environment; thus it is more advantageous for the cell to maintain a narrow range of normal values, dependent on the external environmental conditions, than a consistent absolute value.

2. The operating point of some variables regulated by homeostatic control systems can be reset, that is, physiologically raised or lowered.

3. Since it is not possible for all cellular functions to be maintained in relative constancy by homeostatic control systems, there is a hierarchy of importance. An activity that is of high priority will be held in relative constancy at the expense of functions that are of lesser importance.

4. When the various mechanisms that occur in cells, organs, and systems are at steady state, the body is in a state of physiological functioning.

All diseases are manifestations of abnormalities in molecules, chemical reactions, or processes. Agents that are likely to disrupt this stability include (1) physical agents, such as mechanical trauma, extremes of temperature, and radiation; (2) chemical agents, including toxic and therapeutic drugs; (3) biological agents, such as viruses, bacteria, and parasites, (4) altered oxygen supply, as in blood loss or anemia; (5) genetic disorders; (6) immunological reactions, such as anaphylaxis, (7) nutritional imbalances; and (8) endocrine imbalances, either deficiencies or excesses (Murray, 2000).

Fundamental processes performed by any single cell are carefully regulated by intracellular mechanisms. These determine, for example, which proteins a cell is to synthesizes, how large the cell will become, and when it will divide. The cell orchestrates many specific chemical transformations, including provision of sufficient energy, formation of organelles, movement of materials to the appointed place in the cell, and growth and division when new cells are needed. DNA is constantly being read out into a particular constellation of RNAs that specify a particular set of proteins. These proteins are continually being degraded and replaced by new ones, and the system is balanced so that, in the short term, neither the size nor the function of the cell changes. Cells should not be considered as unchanging, however. There are three important perspectives about cellular life that are relevant to understanding growth and aging.

■ Cells do change their functions over time. These changes may be adaptive, that is, in response to environmental stimuli or to the changes that occur with aging. These changes may also be programmed. For example, a change in protein or enzyme expression might be required only at a specific stage of development.

■ A nongrowing somatic cell can begin to grow preparatory to its division into two cells. Cell growth and division may be a response to an external regulatory signal or may result from inactivation of an internal cellular inhibitor. Cellular growth is organized into a cycle of events that has many checkpoints to determine if the various parts of the cells are duplicating in an orderly fashion. Whether a given cell will grow and divide is highly regulated, ensuring that worn out cells are replaced or more cells are created.

■ The third type of cellular change is the most dramatic and complicated. Cellular growth and differentiation that occurs during the embryonic development involves extensive cellular multiplication and change.

Knowledge of the cell cycle and its regulation is crucial to understanding the development and differentiation of normal tissues.

The Cell Cycle

To maintain body systems, cells grow, divide, and die. For somatic cells, the cell cycle is an ordered set of events culminating in cell growth and division into two identical daughter cells. It is important to make a distinction between the terms "growth" and "division." Growth refers to the buildup of new molecules and the associated increase in size and volume of a cell. Division is the actual process of mitosis, in which the parent cell divides into two daughter cells. In most exponentially growing populations, a cell must grow to two times its size between successive divisions in order to ensure that the mass of the two daughter cells (including all their constituent parts) will equal that of the parent cell prior to division.

The cell cycle phase in which the cell grows and performs its usual functions for cellular and systemic homeostasis is called the *gap 1 (G1) phase*. Normal cells must receive growth signals before they can move from a quiescent state into an active proliferative state. These signals are transmitted into the cell by transmembrane receptors that bind distinctive classes of signaling molecules, including diffusible growth factors, extracellular matrix components, and cell-to-cell adhesion molecules (Hanahan & Weinberg, 2000). Once the cell has reached a sufficient size, it enters the phase of synthesis, or the *S phase*. The S phase is the discrete period of time during which DNA replication occurs. In mammalian cells, the S phase usually lasts 6 to 8 hours and is the time when the entire complement of chromosomal DNA is replicated. The chromatin, composed of the chromosomal DNA together with associated proteins, is the most complex structure that must double in size in preparation for cell division. This process of doubling the genome must occur with extraordinary precision. If there is not an exact genomic duplication, one of the daughter cells will receive a flawed, mutant genome that can threaten its ability to survive or cause it to grow uncontrollably like a cancer cell.

Following successful completion of DNA synthesis and chromosomal replication in the S phase, the cell enters the second *gap phase* in the cycle, labeled *G2*. This gap is long, often 4 to 5 hours, and is the quiet time when the cell prepares itself for mitosis. The period of mitosis, termed *M phase,* usually takes less than an hour and encompasses the processes of chromosomal condensation, breakdown of the nuclear membrane, alignment of the condensed chromosomes in the mitotic apparatus, segregation of two sets of condensed chromosomes to opposite poles of the cell, reformation of two nuclear membranes around the two sets of recently segregated chromosomes, decondensation of the chromosomes, and pinching off and separation of the two daughter cells. The period after M but before another S phase is the first gap period, or G1 phase, of the cell cycle. Importantly, the S phase does not immediately follow the M phase. Instead, there is a period, often as long as 10 to 12 hours, after M phase when the recently divided cell prepares itself for S phase. This long preparation period allows the cell to synthesize a number of macromolecular constituents and build up mass. When cells rush too quickly into the S phase following mitosis, they will be abnormally small.

In summary, the active cell cycle is divided into four phases: G1, S, G2, and M. The time spent outside the M phase (i.e., G1, S, and G2) is sometimes known as the *interphase*. Table 7-2 summarizes the cell cycle.

Following cell division, the daughter cells confront two possible fates. They may enter immediately into another round of growth and division, which leads to repeated rounds of cell division and an increasing cell population. Conversely, the daughter cells may cease active growth, exiting the active cell cycle and entering into a state of quiescence. Most of the cells in the adult body are in this quiet state.

The tissue or organ determines the rate at which a cell becomes active and divides. In the bone marrow, skin, and gut, continual cell division balances the continual cell death; the cycle time is about 18 hours. Cells that are grown in vitro have a cell cycle

Table 7-2   THE CELL CYCLE*

PHASE	ACTIVITY	ACTIVITY ILLUSTRATED
Gap 1 (G1) *Time:* Often as long as 10–12 hours following the signal to generate a new cell	The cell synthesizes proteins and builds up mass.	Cell Cell Grows
Synthesis (S) *Time:* Approximately 6 to 8 hours	DNA replication occurs in preparation for cell division.	
Gap 2 (G2) *Time:* Approximately 4 to 5 hours	There is a gap in the activity of the cell. The cell rests in preparation for cell division.	
Mitosis (M) *Time:* Usually less than 1 hour	In mitosis each cell divides into two cells, each the same size as the original cell. Each has 23 paired chromosomes.	
Gap 1 (G1) *Time:* Often as long as 10–12 hours following the signal to generate a new cell	The process begins again. If the G1 phase is too short, resulting cells will be abnormally small.	New Cell Cell Grows

*The cell cycle is the series of events in which a nongrowing cell is stimulated to grow, its contents are replicated, and it divides into two new cells. Mitosis is the phase of the cell cycle in which cell division occurs. Approximate times for each phase are indicated; however, the length and frequency of the process are determined by the cell type.

length of about 24 hours (Leake, 1996). In other body tissues, such as the brain, cell division is a rare event.

The cellular control mechanism of programmed cell death is a part of normal development. Once cells have performed their unique developmental function, *apoptosis* or programmed cell death, occurs. Apoptosis is a complex physiological process in which individual cells initiate molecular events that eventually lead to their own death. Characteristic manifestations of programmed cell death, such as cell shrinkage, chromatin condensation, and chromosomal DNA fragmentation, are preceded or accompanied by unique changes in gene regulation (Hengartner, 2000, 2001). Those signals that influence programmed cell death are (1) regulatory signals from the extracellular matrix or specific cells that reflect the needs of tissues to maintain extant cells, (2) cell surface receptors that bind survival or death factors, and (3) intracellular sensors that monitor the cell's well-being and activate the death pathway in response to detection of abnormalities (Hanahan & Weinberg, 2000).

Apoptosis is a major source of cell attrition. Cells die either because they are damaged or because it takes less energy to kill them than to maintain them. Programmed cell death eliminates cells that are not needed or that are potentially dangerous to the rest of the organism. Cells that are not needed may have never performed a necessary function, may have lost their function, or may have competed with and lost out to other cells. Dying cells are ordinarily shed to the outside environment or eaten by specialized scavenger cells (Matzinger & Fuchs, 1996).

Signals. External stimuli, such as extracellular signals and contact with other cells, can profoundly influence cell structure and function. To appropriately respond to changes in the external environment, cells must have a means of communicating information from the external environment to induce gene expression. The response of a cell to its environment usually involves a chain of events that culminates in a change in gene expression and is highly specific, so that stimuli that affect one cell may not affect another.

To fulfill its intended purpose, a signal must be transmitted to its molecular target. The receipt of informational signals by a cell is a complex task. The cell must integrate specific combinations of signals that stimulate such complex responses as differentiation, proliferation, and programmed cell death. Specific proteins regulate and control the cell cycle, telling the cell when it is time to grow and divide and stopping the cell when the time for growth and division is not right. The absence of an intended signal or response can alter body functioning significantly. For instance, cancer cells have deficits in regulatory circuits that govern normal cell proliferation and homeostasis (Hanahan & Weinberg, 2000).

To control the products manufactured by a cell at any given time in its development or life cycle, there must be appropriate feedback mechanisms. This control can be in the form of repression of a product that is constantly produced or induction of a product that is not constantly made. Thus gene expression can be categorized as inducible or repressible. An inducible system is one in which the cell manufactures a product only when needed. In a repressible system, the cell usually manufactures a product but shuts down production when the product is not needed. This control can be exerted at the level of transcription (mRNA is not made), translation (protein is not made from the mRNA transcript), or protein or enzyme function.

Receptors. Receptors are protein molecules that read and respond to signals. Some receptors are found inside the cell, while others reside in the plasma membrane of the cell. Each receptor bears a specific structure that guides the binding of a signal to an intended receptor. This specificity, or "matching" of proteins, increases the likelihood that proteins will bind to the intended receptor. These receptors can become saturated so they are unable to take up any more chemical message. Certain similar proteins can compete for binding sites; the protein that "wins" the competition, ultimately binding successfully, will be the one that influences cellular response. An additional concept, affinity, or the tightness of the protein binding, can influence this process. When there is weak affinity, binding can easily be disrupted by subtle changes in the environment, whereas strong affinity produces a more resilient binding.

Signal transduction is a sequence of events in which information from plasma-membrane receptors are relayed to the response mechanisms within the cell. Certain of these signals bind to receptors in the plasma membrane. The movement of a signal from the membrane into the cell causes the signal to interact with proteins in the cell. These interactions result in small ion movements that propel the signal throughout the cell. Other extracellular signals bind to receptors in the plasma membrane and regulate cell proliferation, differentiation, and metabolism by activating different signaling cascades. More complex signal transduction involves the coupling of a signal molecule to a receptor that resides in the cytoplasm of the cell. This complex changes enzyme activities and protein conformations, and the eventual outcome is an alteration in cellular activity and changes in the genes expressed within the responding cells

The cell is surrounded by an insoluble noncellular material, called the *extracellular matrix (ECM),* that is composed of a complex mixture of secreted molecules. In many of the connective tissues, cells called *fibroblasts* secrete molecules that form the ECM. The ECM has three major functions: (1) it provides structural support and tensile strength, (2) it provides substrates for cell adhesion and cell migration, and (3) it regulates cellular differentiation and metabolic function, for example, by modulation of cell growth by the binding of growth factors.

The ECM is made up of two classes of macromolecules. The first class is called *glycosaminoglycans,* which are polysaccharide chains. In essence, these members of the glycosaminoglycans form a highly hydrated, gel-like substance, in which the members of the second class of *macromolecules,* the fibrous proteins, are embedded. There are two functional types of fibrous proteins: those that are mainly structural, such as collagen, and those that are mainly adhesive, such as fibronectin and laminin.

Collagen, the most abundant mammalian protein, strengthens and helps to organize the matrix. Different types of collagens provide different types of support. For example, certain collagens provide the volume-filling material between cells, while others organize into a thin, flexible, sheetlike network such as the basal lamina, which is the extracellular matrix beneath the epithelia.

Fibronectin, the first well-characterized adhesive protein, promotes the attachment of fibroblasts and other cells to the matrix in connective tissues via the extracellular parts of some members of the integrin family. Laminin has a variety of functions including the promotion of differentiation, neurite extension, and cell adhesion. Laminin promotes the attachment of epithelial cells to the basal lamina, again via the extracellular domains of some members of integrins.

Integrins, or cell adhesion receptors, are the primary means by which cells bind and respond to the ECM. As such, they are involved in cell–extracellular matrix and cell-cell interactions and promote successful binding to specific moieties of the ECM. Those that mediate cell-to cell interactions are called *cell adhesion molecules* (CAMs) and include immunoglobulins and calcium-dependent cadherin families. They link cells to substrates in the ECM and influence many cellular functions, including cell motility, resistance to cell death, entrance into the active cell cycle, wound healing, cell differentiation, and apoptosis (Hanahan & Weinberg, 2000). For signaling through the integrin receptors to occur, there must be formation of focal adhesions, which are dynamic sites where cytoskeletal and other proteins are concentrated.

Hormones as Chemical Messengers

The availability of nutrients, levels of hormones and growth factors, contact with adjacent cells or with extracellular matrix, infections, exogenous substances, and even changing temperature all evoke signals that ultimately impinge on transcription or post-transcriptional events that reflect the activity of specific genes (Steel, 1996). Within normal tissues, cells are largely instructed to grow through interactions with neighboring cells (paracrine signaling) or via systemic messengers (endocrine signals) (Hanahan & Weinberg, 2000).

Endocrine glands and the hormones secreted by them comprise one of the body's two major communication systems (the nervous system being the other). A hormone is a chemical messenger that is synthesized by a specific endocrine gland in response to certain stimuli and is secreted into the blood, which carries it to target cells (Berne & Levy, 2000). In general, minute concentrations of circulating hormones regulate cellular functioning. Normal functioning of all endocrine glands is required for good health in women and men.

Cellular response to a chemical varies among different cell types. Signal transduction is the process by which various cell types respond to a hormone. Hormones regulate cellular functioning by binding to specific receptors on the cell surface or within the cells. There are three major classes of hormones—peptides, amines, and steroids. In general, peptide hormones, such as insulin, relaxin, and prolactin, are bound by receptors residing on the plasma membrane and activate processes that release molecular signals into the cytoplasm of the cell. Amine hormones include thyroid hormones and catecholamines, such as epinephrine, norepinephrine, and dopamine. The catecholamines affect target cells in the same manner as peptide hormones; however, thyroid hormone influences cell activity by entering the cell as steroid hormones do. Protein hormones and most amine hormones act by binding to receptors on the cell's surface, then stimulating intracellular release of second messengers. Cellular reactions that must occur rapidly, on the order of seconds to minutes, involve plasma membrane receptors.

Steroid hormones diffuse into the cell and are bound by receptor proteins in the cytoplasm, nucleus, or both. Protein binding occurs in the plasma, where lipid-soluble messengers capable of penetrating the lipid membrane of the cell are formed. Once inside the cell, the messenger binds with a receptor, forming a messenger-receptor complex. This complex moves into the nucleus, where it influences the rate (increasing or decreasing) of protein synthesis by stimulating or inhibiting the production of mRNA. In some cases, the hormone combines with the receptor in the cytosol, and the complex moves into the nucleus. Once occupied by the hormone, steroid receptors undergo activation and translocation to the nucleus, where they influence gene transcription and the expression of specific proteins (Catt, 1996). This type of signal transduction, which affects transcription of genes that increase or decrease protein production, evokes a slower cellular response that affects cellular functioning over hours or days.

There are sex differences in steroid hormones. All steroid structures derive from cholesterol, a 27-carbon compound. Structurally, a base skeleton of four interconnecting steroid rings is common to all steroid hormones. Cholesterol is the precursor for steroid synthesis, a process that involves shortening of the hydrocarbon chain of cholesterol. The first reaction in this chain of events is the conversion of cholesterol to pregnenolone. Five classes of steroid hormones, glucocorticoids, mineralocorticoids, and androgens, estrogens, and progestins, which are sex hormones, are derived from pregnenolone. The synthesis and secretion of cortisone and aldosterone occur in the adrenal cortex, that of estrogens and progestins, in the ovaries and ovarian corpus luteum, and testosterone, in the testes (Zeleznik & Hillier, 1996). All sex steroids belong to three major classes, characterized by decreasing numbers of carbons: progestins, a 21-carbon series; androgens, a 19-carbon series; and estrogens, an 18-carbon series.

This process of conversion from the 27-carbon cholesterol to the 18-carbon estrogen, known as the androgen pathway, requires the presence of enzymes, which are protein biocatalysts that regulate the rates at which all physiological processes take place. A defect in enzyme activity or amount can lead to a deficiency in the synthesis of hormones or metabolites. Because all members of the pathway have potent biological activity, serious metabolic imbalances can occur if enzyme deficiencies are present (Zeleznik & Hillier, 1996). Figure 7-6 depicts the chemical structure and derivation of steroid hormones (Ferin, Jewelewicz, & Warren, 1993).

Endocrine cells in both the testes and ovaries possess a high concentration of enzymes in the androgen pathway. The cells in the testes contain a high concentration of the enzyme that converts androstenedione to testosterone, while the ovarian cells have a high concentration of the enzymes required to further transform androgens to estrogens. There are three major active forms of estrogen, identified by the site of conversion and chemical structure. Estradiol, or E2, is the primary estrogen secreted by the ovary and is the most biologically potent (Barrett-Connor & Bush, 1991; Cauley, Gutai, Kuller, LeDonne, & Powell, 1989). Estradiol is formed by the aromatization of testosterone. The primary estrogen after menopause is estrone (E1), which is derived from the aromatization of androstenedione (the substrate for testosterone production in the androgen pathway). Estrone is a less active estrogen (Barrett-Connor & Bush, 1991; Cauley et al., 1989). Estriol, or E3, is converted from estrone in the liver. The placenta secretes large amounts of estriol. Other, less potent estrogens are produced at extragonadal sites, as well as in the ovary. Low levels of estradiol that remain in the circulation when ovarian estradiol is no longer available are derived from estrone.

Steroid hormones change the rate of synthesis of specific proteins in cells targeted by the hormone. This requires the movement of the hormone from the circulating blood into the nucleus of the cell. Steroid hormones are lipid soluble, thus they readily cross the plasma membrane of target cells and combine with specific intracellular receptors. However, because they are lipophilic and hydrophobic, steroid hormones must be bound to protein to be transported from their site of synthesis to the target organ. The protein that transports a sex hormone is called a *sex-hormone-binding protein.*

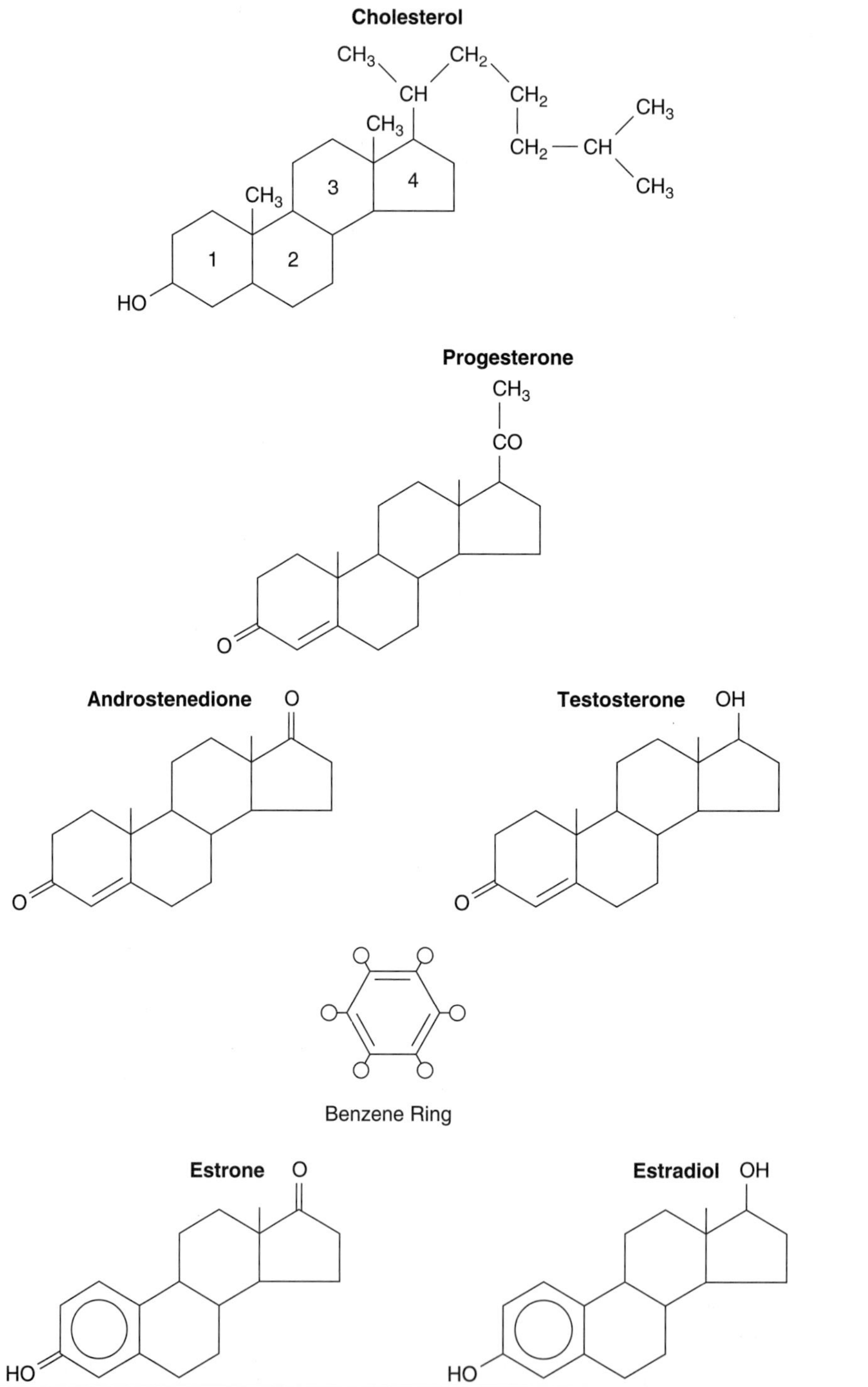

Figure **7-6** Chemical structure and derivation of steroid hormones.

Steroid hormones that bind to proteins with high affinity and specificity are transported to a target cell, where a steroid receptor must be present for the sex steroid to affect the target tissue. Estrogen thus affects only cells that make nuclear proteins called *estrogen receptors.* The bound estrogen attaches to specific genes, similar to docking sites, known as *estrogen response elements.* This attachment triggers the formation of a transcription complex, which is a cluster of coactivators necessary to activate gene transcription. The bound gene induces an enzyme to transcribe the genes into molecules of messenger RNA, a template for new proteins. The resultant proteins then induce the cell to divide or change (Jordan, 1998) (Figure 7-7).

Jensen and Jacobsen (1962) were the first to describe the intracellular receptors for steroid hormones. Following this discovery, a model was proposed that linked these receptors to the gene expression that controls physiological events. Recent advances in molecular biology have permitted the characterization of receptor structure and function at the molecular level and have revealed an extraordinary level of diversity among receptors and their associated signal transduction proteins.

Two estrogen receptors, estrogen receptor alpha (ER-α) and estrogen receptor beta (ER-β), have been described. To date, ER-α is known to be widely distributed in the body, while ER-β is found mainly in the ovary, prostate, epididymis, lung, and hypothalamus. Physiological responses attributable to each receptor are not fully known; however, the development of a knockout mouse model is advancing this work. (A knockout mouse is one that has undergone an alteration of gene such that a particular function is no longer present.) Since the mid-1990s, an estrogen receptor knockout mouse has

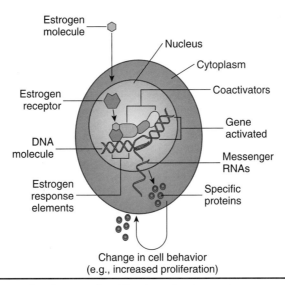

Figure 7-7 An estogen molecule enters the cell and attaches to an estrogen receptor in the nucleus. The estrogen-receptor complex attaches to an area on the DNA molecule called the *estrogen response element.* Coactivators necessary to activate gene transcription form a cluster with the estrogen-receptor complex. Gene transcription is activated, protein formed, and cellular behavior affected. (Based on artwork originally created for the National Cancer Institute; copyright 2000 Jeanne Kelly.)

been used to study estrogen function. Though early studies focused on ER-α only, the discovery of the second receptor in 1996 and the more recent generation of an ER-β knockout have allowed for comparisons of physiological differences when only one receptor type is present and when both receptors are absent. This type of study will advance our understanding of the effects of estrogen tremendously (Krege et al., 1998).

Estradiol and progesterone receptor concentrations are high in the uterus, the gut, the ovary, the breast, and the hypothalamic-pituitary unit. In some target tissues, receptors to two different but related hormones must be activated in a specific sequence. In the follicle, for instance, the receptor to follicle-stimulating hormone (FSH) is present prior to the activation of the luteinizing hormone receptors. In many ovarian steroid-sensitive organs, estradiol must activate its own receptors in order to promote the synthesis of the progesterone receptor (Ferin, Jewelewicz, & Warren, 1993).

In addition to the reproductive organs, sex steroid hormones are involved in the regulation of many glands, including sebaceous, endometrial, lactiferous, lacrimal, and salivary glands. Sex steroid hormones also play a role in maintaining epithelial tissues such as the cardiovascular endothelium, buccal mucosa, and conjunctiva. They influence collagen production, bone growth, muscle development, and liver function and modulate neural responses like auditory brainstem potentials and autonomic regulation of gastric motility. Indeed, most tissues in the human body are influenced or regulated by this sex-specific hormonal milieu (Legato, 1997a).

Estrogens are critical to the functioning and maintenance of many tissues and physiological systems (Krege et al., 1998). Estrogen triggers a broad array of tissue-and organ-specific responses by binding to a nuclear receptor protein within target cells. The estrogen receptor modulates target gene expression after binding estrogen hormone (Korach, 1994). Normal postnatal female physiology has been linked to estrogen action in several target sites in the body, most notably the reproductive tract, breast, and neuroendocrine tissues, in which it elicits a variety of tissue-specific responses, including tissue differentiation, growth, protein synthesis, and secretion. The precise role of estrogen in humans is not totally understood.

The effects of estrogen, especially on nonreproductive tissues and organs, are perhaps most evident in women who experience reduced estrogen levels due to menopause (Bryant & Dere, 1998). Before menopause, ovarian follicles produce estradiol at a controlled rate of between 60 and 600 μg per day; this amount is reduced to 20 μg per day after menopause (Rajman et al., 1996). A dramatic lowering of estrogen levels during menopause is associated with osteoporosis and cardiovascular disease and suggests a role for estrogen in bone tissue and in the cardiovascular system. It is not certain whether estrogen elicits only a direct tissue action or if indirect effects that involve other regulators or signaling systems are required.

It should not be surprising that the effects of estrogen are not entirely understood. First, it has only been in recent generations that the life expectancy of women surpassed menopause. In fact, there are few species in which longevity actually exceeds the reproductive period (Ferin, Jewelewicz, & Warren, 1993). Second, we are best able to observe the developmental and physiological effects of estrogen on the female reproductive system, and, consequently, our understanding of development, puberty, and childbearing surpasses that of other physiological processes on which estrogen has an effect.

In summary, certain concepts regarding cellular functioning are particularly important to understanding growth, development, and aging.

■ The cell is affected by multiple signals from adjacent cells, from the tissue in which the cell resides, and from the neuroendocrine systems.

■ Different cells may respond quite differently to the same chemical signal, depending on the cell type, the presence or absence of a receptor, and receptor affinity.

■ The cells that are responsive to sex steroid hormones must have receptors for those sex steroids.

■ Receptors can receive similarly structured substrates, though not usually with the same affinity as the intended substance.

■ Our knowledge of the signals, receptors, and cellular functioning is increasing rapidly as our knowledge of the human genome and molecular biology expands.

Cellular Processes in Growth and Development

Development involves groups of cells undergoing processes that alter the shape and size of cells and differentiate each cell for its specific purpose. This process begins with the union of the sperm and egg. It is the union of two X chromosomes that results in female physical development. This is known as the *genetic sex* of the individual. There are three additional major processes that occur in utero that lead to the identification of a human as female: the development of gonads, the development of organ structure, and the development of the neuroendocrine system (Andersen & Byskov, 1996). Following birth, the development of secondary sexual characteristics completes the major processes of physical development.

Each human develops and matures from a single fertilized ovum. Three distinct cellular processes—growth, differentiation, and organization—are involved in organ formation. Just as sex is determined at fertilization, so is the genetic blueprint for all events that result in a fully developed human. Events involved in the transition from cell to human are defined in Table 7-3.

Cells within the embryo are induced to develop in their specified way by cellular messages via chemical or protein substances. Thus, certain cells have the capacity to stimulate reactions, while others are programmed to respond to these messages. This process is exemplified in gonadal and somatic development as the embryo evolves from an undifferentiated sexual being to a person with unique structural differences and specific capabilities.

Most developmental processes depend upon a precisely coordinated interaction of genetic and environmental factors. Several control mechanisms guide differentiation and ensure synchronized development, such as tissue interactions, regulated migration of cells and cell colonies, controlled proliferation, and cell death. Each system of the body has its own developmental pattern, but most processes of morphogenesis are relatively similar.

Table 7-3	CELLULAR PROCESSES INVOLVED IN THE GROWTH AND DEVELOPMENT OF HUMAN LIFE	
PROCESS	**DEFINITION**	
Growth	The creation of more of a substance through an increase in cell size and number.	
Differentiation	The creation of new types of cells, tissues, and organs.	
Organization	The process by which these elements are coordinated into a functional integrated unit.	
Morphogenesis	The production of a special form, shape, or structure of a cell or group of cells that occurs by the precise organization of cell populations into distinct organs.	

There are differences in response to a particular hormonal milieu in different life forms. Invertebrates, such as insects, use their sex chromosomes to program sex differences on a cell-to-cell basis. In contrast, vertebrates, particularly mammals, employ a hormonal mechanism in which one sex becomes differentiated from the other because the gonads produce hormones that effect sex differences throughout the body. The advantage of a hormone system that affects the entire body, including the brain, is that the body is programmed to function according to the pattern of a particular sex. McEwen (1994) proposes a scheme for sex differences in brain functioning that incorporates genetic and gonadal programming, as well as hormonal and experiential influences, across the developmental continuum. In essence, sex differences arise due to the actions of hormones during early development, during puberty, and during adult life. Experience plays an important role by interacting in an epigenetic fashion with ongoing influences of hormones at various stages of development.

To form the different tissues, organs, and systems that comprise the human body, cells must differentiate, the process of transforming an unspecified cell into a specialized cell. There are 200 types of cells in the human body, identified by differences in their structure and function, all of which can be categorized into four main types: epithelial, connective tissue, nerve, and muscle cells. Cells are organized into tissues, and tissues into organ systems. Organ systems, in turn, create an environment conducive to cell functioning.

The generation of diversity must be considered the central issue of developmental biology (Andersen & Byskov, 1996). The cells that make up the tissues of very early embryos are capable, depending on circumstances, of following more than one pathway of development; in other words, the cells are *pluripotential*. This broad developmental potential becomes progressively restricted as tissues acquire specialized features necessary for structure and function. Such restriction presumes that choices must be made in order to achieve tissue diversification. Cell lineage studies can identify the range of phenotypes that arise from single cells. At present, however, most evidence indicates that these choices are determined in response to cues from the immediate surroundings, including the adjacent tissues. As a result, the architectural precision and coordination that are often required for the normal function of an organ appear to be achieved by the interaction of its constituent parts during development.

Developmental studies at the tissue, cell, or molecular level rely on knowledge of two related topics: the fate map of the embryo and the cell lineage of single precursor cells. Fate maps are depictions of what cells in various regions of an embryo will become during normal development. Construction of a fate map requires a means of following a cell (or distinct group of cells) from a defined region of the embryo. Although maps cannot by themselves tell us whether cells are committed to generate a given tissue or cell type, fate maps are the critical first step in analyzing the mechanisms of cell fate determination, embryonic induction, and tissue morphogenesis (Fraser & Harland, 2000).

To achieve differentiation, the cell is first marked in some way so that its developmental capabilities are restricted to those the cell is intended to perform. Following this phase of *determination*, a second phase of *differentiation* occurs. The regulation of differentiation is not completely understood, but it seems to occur via cellular interaction.

The interactions that lead to a change in the course of development of at least one of the cells or tissues involved is termed *induction*. The fact that one tissue can influence the developmental pathway adopted by another tissue presumes that a signal passes between these two tissues. The mechanism of signal transfer appears to vary with the specific tissues involved. Other cellular mechanisms that influence growth and development are differential cell proliferation and programmed cell death. Differential cell proliferation can yield a buildup of cells in certain areas via rapid proliferation or an invagination, wherein some cells grow more slowly than the cells that surround them. Invagination results in the development of body cavities, such as the urethra, the vagina, and the rectum.

Competence is the term used to describe time-dependent susceptibilities of tissues to inductive influences (Scott, 2000). A cell will respond only to signals it recognizes, and gene responses have similar restrictions. In terms of development, competence refers to the variety of possible developmental options available to a given cell. The actual outcome for that cell is based on the specific inducers, or signals, to which the cell is exposed (Kirschner, Gerhart, & Mitchison, 2000). Certain caveats guide this process

■ Signals will be sensed only if receptors are available.

■ If a transcription factor requires a partner to work, the time at which the partner is present determines competence. Most gene activation events during development require multiple transcription factors, so competence depends on the presence of all of them.

■ Certain signals can interfere with an inducer. Certain modifying agents that destroy or modify signals or other proteins can make a cell incompetent to respond.

■ A cell can receive signals but be unable to carry out a differentiation program due to nutritional or other environmental deficits (Scott, 2000).

It is clear that gene products function in multiple pathways, and pathways themselves are interconnected in networks. There are many more possible outcomes than there are genes. The genotype cannot be predictive of the actual phenotype but can only provide knowledge of the universe of possible phenotypes. Biological systems have evolved to restrict these phenotypes, and in self-organizing systems the phenotype might depend as much on external conditions and random events as on the genome-encoded structure of molecular components. Yet out of such a potentially nondeterminist world, the organism has fashioned a very stable physiology and embryology (Kirschner, Gerhart, & Mitchison, 2000).

PHYSICAL DEVELOPMENT OF THE FEMALE

Genetic Sex

In the early 1900s, researchers observed that somatic cells taken from female donors always contained two copies of the X chromosome, while somatic cells taken from male donors always contained one copy of the X chromosome and one copy of the Y chromosome. All of the other chromosomes in the nucleated cells of both male and female donors appeared identical. Although scientists were not sure of the mechanism, it seemed quite clear that the sex of an organism was directly related to the identity of the chromosomes in that organism's cells. Thus, sex was shown to be the direct result of a specific combination of chromosomal material, and it became the first phenotype (physical characteristic) to be assigned a chromosomal location, specifically the X and Y chromosomes.

Sex is determined when the egg and sperm unite. A female is the result of the union of one of the X chromosomes from an egg cell and the X (rather than the Y) chromosome from the sperm cell. The egg and sperm cells are specialized, generative cells called *germ cells.* Mature, fully developed sex, or germ, cells have exactly half the number of chromosomes (i.e., just one copy of each chromosome type) as are found in the somatic cells of any organism. The fertilization of a haploid egg by a haploid sperm cell produces a diploid cell called a *zygote,* which has the same number of chromosomes as the somatic cells of that organism.

Fertilization occurs when the sperm cell penetrates the egg cell. The cells each contribute 22 pairs of somatic chromosomes and one sex chromosome to this union. The nuclei of the sperm cell and the nuclei of the egg cell fuse, and the chromosomes merge to yield 22 pairs of somatic chromosomes and either an XX or an XY sex chromosome pair (Figure 7-8).

The fertilized ovum begins to divide very quickly. These mitotic divisions are called *cleavage,* and cleavage results in a rapid increase in the number of cells. In these early embryonic cell cycles, the dormant phases of the mitotic cell cycle (G1 and G2) are largely suppressed, and the cycle consists essentially of a regular alternation of extremely rapid DNA replication and division. Embryonic cell cycles are faster than somatic cell cycles. Somatic cells are small in size and must import nutrients so that they can grow and duplicate all the components of the cell. In contrast, egg cells are large and inherit from their mothers a stock of nutrients, all the structural components of the cell, and almost all of the enzymes that catalyze the processes of the cell cycle. Thus, embryonic cells synthesize and divide without the resting and growing phases needed by developed somatic cells. As a result, apart from replicating DNA, early embryonic cells have to produce only a handful of new components to proceed through a cell cycle. These

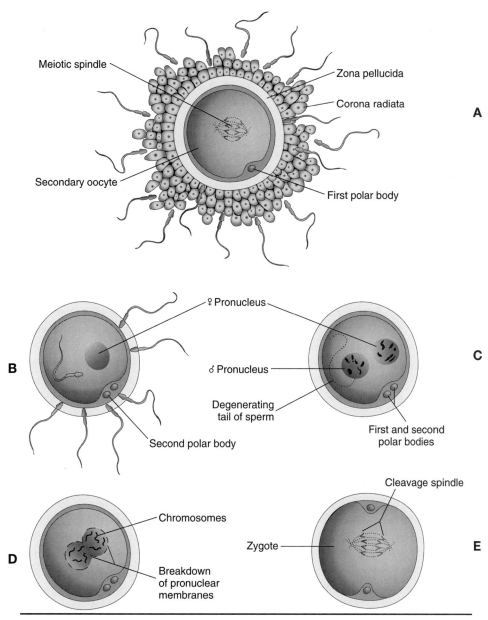

Figure **7-8** Fertilization. **A**, Secondary oocyte surrounded by several sperm. (Only four of the 23 chromosome pairs are shown.) **B**, The corona radiata has disappeared, a sperm has entered the oocyte, and the second meiotic division has occurred, forming a mature oocyte. The nucleus of the ovum is now the female pronucleus. **C**, The sperm head has enlarged to form the male pronucleus. **D**, The pronuclei are fusing. **E**, The zygote has formed; it contains 46 chromosomes, the diploid number. (From Moore, K. L., & Persaud, T. V. N. [1998]. *The developing human: Clinically oriented embryology* [6th ed.]. Philadelphia: W. B. Saunders.)

divisions convert the original solid egg into a hollow ball of identical cells, called the *blastula,* which then undergoes changes in shape that produce a recognizable embryo. This is known as the indifferent stage of sexual development. Each cell nucleus, however, includes 22 pairs of somatic chromosomes and one pair of sex chromosomes, either XX or XY (Leake, 1996; Murray & Hunt, 1993).

After the twelfth mitosis, the cell cycle slows. Until this point, each cell has been dividing in synchrony, but in the blastocyst stage, cells start aligning along three axes that shape the organism. These three axes (straight lines around which cells grow) are (1) top to bottom, (2) left to right, and (3) front to back (ventral to dorsal). From the mass of cells, three germ layers are formed, the ectoderm, the mesoderm, and the endoderm. All tissues and organs of the embryo develop from these three layers through division, migration, aggregation, and differentiation. Figure 7-9 depicts the tissues and organs that arise from each layer.

Gastrulation is the process by which cells relocate to their proper positions in the blastocyst, reorganizing the embryo to produce the ectoderm, mesoderm, and endoderm and producing dorsal-ventral organization (Fraser & Harland, 2000). This process depends on a very complex interplay of chemical signals throughout the embryo and is a result of both intracellular and extracellular signals. The genes that are expressed by the nucleus in a given cell are regulated by the molecules, mostly transcription factors, found in the cytoplasm surrounding that nucleus.

Gene expression is involved in a variety of mammalian developmental processes at the cellular, tissue, and organ levels, including cellular proliferation, differentiation, migration, apoptosis, and cell-cell interactions. These inductive processes contribute to tissue remodeling and integrity, particularly during embryonic development. Overlapping as well as unique patterns of gene expression are evident in developing tissues, including development of the lymphoid and myeloid lineages, brain and central nervous system, bone, and mammary glands (Maroulakou & Bowe, 2000).

Several recently identified genes provide critical signaling during embryonic development. The SIL gene governs formation of the left-right body axis and is believed to be important in the correct placement of organs such as the heart within the developing organism (Izraeli et al., 1999). Two types of POD (polarity and osmotic defective) genes have recently been described. In normal embryos, larger cells develop into the outer layers of an organism, such as the skin and nervous system, while smaller cells develop into the inner layers, such as the muscle, gut, and reproductive organs. When one of the POD genes is defective, cells will be of equal size, and the differentiation necessary for development will not occur (Tagawa, Rappleye, & Aroian, 2001). Sometimes the expression of one particular gene suppresses the action of another gene, and the suppression results in appropriate development at a critical stage. The Tsg (twisted gastrulation) gene acts together with another gene to suppress the action of a family of growth factors, or bone morphogenetic proteins (BMPs). The suppression of BMP activity in turn allows for the changes in the identity of cells from those associated with the belly of the embryo into cells that will become tissues associated with the embryo's back (Chang et al., 2001).

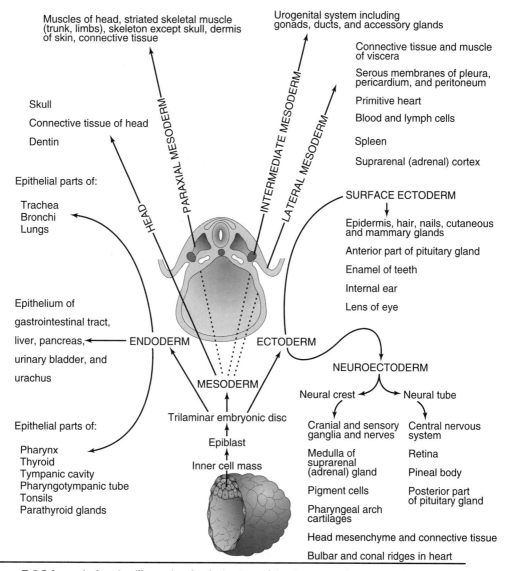

Figure 7-9 Schematic drawing illustrating the derivatives of the three germ layers: ectoderm, endoderm, and mesoderm. (From Moore, K. L., & Persaud, T. V. N. [1998]. *The developing human: Clinically oriented embryology* [6th ed.]. Philadelphia: W. B. Saunders.)

Gonadal Sex

As indicated, although genetic sex is determined at conception, morphological differences between the sexes do not become apparent until the gonads achieve sex-differentiation during fetal life (Andersen & Byskov, 1996). The structure and function of the gonads define gonadal sex. The first indication of gonadal development comes at the fifth week, yet the embryo is sexually indistinguishable through the first 6 weeks after fertilization.

Sexual differentiation in humans is genetically and hormonally controlled. The sex chromosome complex XX determines the female gonad, the ovary. The presence of a Y chromosome dictates testicular formation and results in the development of a phenotypic male. When there is no Y chromosome, the result is the formation of an ovary. Though two X chromosomes are usually essential for normal ovarian development, female differentiation of the genital ducts and external genitalia requires that only a single X chromosome be active within their constituent cells. The second X chromosome of a normal XX female is randomly inactivated in all tissues outside the gonad (Berne & Levy, 2000).

A molecular picture is beginning to emerge for mammalian sex determination, at least with respect to the known transcription factors. Our knowledge of mammalian sex determination is based on two main areas of study: first, the characterization of the biological events that determine the sexual development of the individual, including patterns of gene expression, and second, the study of genetic mutations in humans and in mice that lead to abnormal sexual phenotypes (Swain & Lovell-Badge, 1999).

The sex-determining process is set into motion during the period of organogenesis when early genital ridge development proceeds to differentiation of specific cell types in the gonads and then to organization of cells into sex-specific reproductive organs. The gonads arise as a thickening of the ventrolateral surface of each mesonephros. The genital ridges are composed of somatic cells derived from the mesonephros and primordial germ cells that have migrated, via the hindgut and mesonephros, from extraembryonic mesoderm at the base of the allantois. The first are general transcription factors, which are likely to be involved at several different stages, if not continuously, from early genital ridge development through to differentiation of specific cell types in the gonads, including factors such as LIM1, steroidogenic factor (SF1), Wilms' tumor–associated gene (WT1), and GATA4. GATA4 is present in the developing gonads, and at 11.5 days postconception (dpc), it can be found in the genital ridge of both sexes and later appears in the Sertoli and interstitial cells of the developing testis. High levels of GATA4 are present in the ovary until 16 dpc; little is known about its pattern of expression. A mouse model has been used to study this gene, and mice deficient in GATA4 die in utero between 8.5 and 10.5 dpc, before gonadal differentiation takes place (Figure 7-10).

The second group of factors, represented by the SRY and SOX9, are specific promoters of testicular development. Expression of a critical gene, SRY on the Y chromosome, results in the regression of the primordia of the female gonads and development of the male reproductive system (Ostrer, 2000). In response to a signal from a dominant-acting gene on the Y chromosome, primordial cells in the embryonic gonad ridge differentiate into Sertoli cells and affect newly migrated germ cells to differentiate as

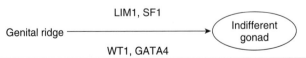

Figure **7-10** Organogenesis, a process that moves from early genital ridge development to differentiation of specific cell types in the gonads, to organization of cells into sex-specific reproductive organs.

spermatogonia, thus creating a testis. The cells of the embryonic testis secrete hormones that lead to the development of most, if not all, male secondary sexual characteristics. In addition to the SRY gene, the SOX9 gene has an identified role in testis determination. A third class of gene works against testicular development and may promote ovarian development. The only known representative of this class is DAX1 (Figure 7-11).

The pattern of expression of SF1 is complementary to that of DAX1 in the gonad and suggests that these receptors act antagonistically toward each other, consistent with in vitro studies. In the early genital ridge, SF1 expression precedes a low level of SOX9 in both sexes. The upregulation of SOX9 follows the onset of SRY expression, whereas in the XX gonad, the extinction of SOX9 is remarkably consistent with the onset of DAX1 expression. One possible role of DAX1 in females would be to prevent SOX9 transcription through repression of SF1 action (Swain & Lovell-Badge, 1999).

The process is not understood completely because of the extent of the interactions between the genes. The parts of the story that are best understood are those concerning the supporting cell lineage, and even then this is biased toward the male Sertoli cell pathway. It seems likely that critical genes are involved in establishing follicle cell fate; however, it is less clear how autonomous this process is.

Three cell lineages are present in both gonads and germ cells. Each lineage has a bipotential fate, depending on the organ in which it is found. The supporting lineage gives rise to Sertoli cells in the testis and follicle cells in the ovary. These cells surround the germ cells and provide an appropriate growth environment. The steroidogenic cell lineage produces the sexual hormones that will contribute to the development of the secondary sexual characteristics of the embryo. In the female, these are the theca cells. Organization of the ovary takes place later than that of the testis and is less structured, with the connective tissue lineage giving rise to stromal cells and with no myeloid cell equivalent.

SRY is expressed in the male genital ridge and acts to initiate testis development. Once the SRY triggers Sertoli cells, they in turn direct the differentiation of the rest of the cell types in the testis. SRY triggers Sertoli cell fate in a cell that would otherwise become a follicle cell. SOX9 is similar to SRY and is present at low levels in both male and female genital ridges when the gonad first develops. By day 11.5, it has been upreg-

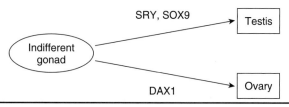

Figure 7-11 The indifferent gonad is the source of cells that develop into the ovary. The SRY gene is found on the Y chromosome and results in the development of the testes rather than the ovaries. Both SRY and SOX9 have demonstrated roles in testicular development. DAX1 promotes ovarian development and suppresses testicular development.

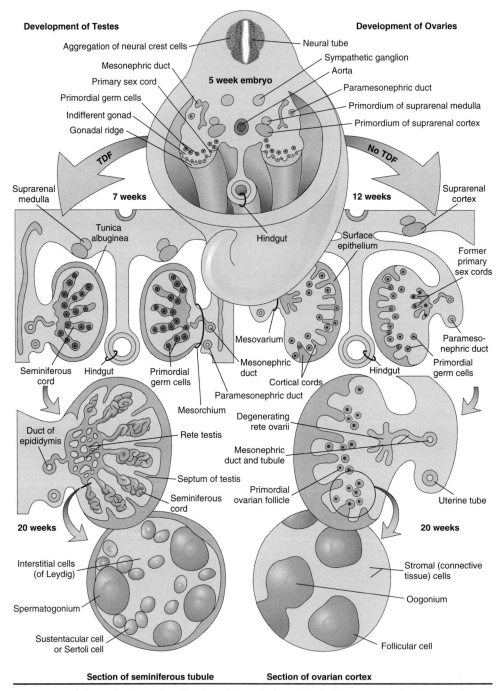

Figure **7-12** Schematic illustration showing differentiation of the indifferent gonads of a 5-week embryo (*top*) into ovaries or testes. (From Moore, K. L., & Persaud, T. V. N. [1998]. *The developing human: Clinically oriented embryology* [6th ed.]. Philadelphia: W. B. Saunders.)

ulated in the male and turned off in the female gonad. By 12.5 days postconception, SOX9 is expressed in Sertoli cells, where it persists throughout life. DAX1, an X-linked member of the nuclear hormone receptor family, is expressed in the genital ridge at the same time as SRY, but as differentiation proceeds, it is down-regulated in the testis but remains high in the ovary.

The various cell types that comprise an ovary must be organized to make a functional structure. The three unique stages in the development of the ovary, namely colonization, organization, and compartmentalization (Zamboni et al, 1980), provide an example of the process of cell division. Female ovaries are derived from three sources, the mesodermal epithelium lining the posterior abdominal wall, the mesenchyme, and the primordal germ cells (Figure 7-12). In embryos with ovaries, mesonephric ducts regress (in the male these form the epididymis, the ductus deferens, and the ejaculatory ducts), while the paramesonephric ducts are the origin of most of the female genital tract (Figure 7-13).

Colonization is the stage in which the primitive germ cells arrive from the hindgut region of the embryo and colonize the primitive gonad at the urogenital ridge. In colonization, the primordial germ cells (PGCs) migrate in an amebalike movement from the endodermic to the gonadal ridges and increase by undergoing mitosis as they travel. The PGCs are the precursors of oocytes and spermatozoa. These cells can be identified at about 3 weeks after fertilization in the human yolk sac outside the embryo proper. By five weeks' gestation, the human embryo has between 700 and 1300 migrating germ cells.

After colonizing the genital ridge, the germ cells follow two different developmental pathways, depending on the sex of the gonad. In the early differentiating testis they go into mitotic arrest, whereas in the early ovary, they go into meiotic arrest. Cells that migrate by mistake into tissues other than gonadal tissue undergo meiotic arrest, suggesting that these cells are programmed to arrest in meiosis and that the role of the embryonic testis is to produce a factor that will make them go into mitotic arrest and therefore trigger spermatogenetic fate (Swain & Lovell-Badge, 1999).

At 10 weeks' gestation, the PGCs arrive at the developing ovary, where they are known as *oogonia,* and the process of organization begins. Oogonia continue to multiply by mitosis until meiosis begins. All oogonia enter meioses early in life, often before birth, and from that point are known as *oocytes.* Meiosis begins but is arrested in the first meiotic prophase and does not resume until around the time of ovulation during adulthood (Andersen & Byskov, 1996). Approximately two million of these oogonia enlarge to become primary oocytes. When surrounded by a layer of cuboidal cells, a primary oocyte is called a *primary follicle.* These primary follicles remain quiescent until puberty. Table 7-4 depicts meiosis.

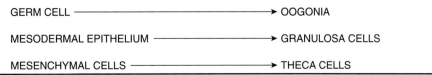

Figure **7-13** Sources of three cell types in the ovary.

Table 7-4   MEIOSIS*

ACTIVITY	ACTIVITY ILLUSTRATED	
Colonization	Primordial germ cells (PGCs) migrate from the endoderm to the genital ridge. The germ cells increase in number by mitosis as they travel.	
Organization	PGCs arrive at the developing ovary and are now known as oogonia. Mitosis continues to increase the number of oogonia.	
Meiosis	The preparation for the reduction of diploid (paired) chromosomes to haploid (single strand). The cell cycle arrests after interphase (G1, S, and G2 phases of the cell cycle).	
Meiosis I begins, then stops	DNA material is replicated and redistributed randomly into four groupings and then divides into two cells, each having two paired chromatids. The oocyte is surrounded by granulosa cells and the body is called the *primordial follicle*.	
Maturation of a recruited primordial follicle	The development of a large antral follicle takes 85 days and is *not* menstrual cycle dependent. Primordial follicles are recruited for development and become primary folllicles. The preantral follicle grows but is not competent to resume meiosis until it becomes a large antral follicle.	
Antral formation and growth	Granulosa cells have receptors for FSH. Antral growth is stimulated by FSH in the follicular portion of the cycle.	Granulosa cells
LH surge	About 8 to 10 hours before ovulation, meiosis resumes and preparation for ovulation begins. Theca cells express LH receptors in preparation for ovulation.	Granulosa cells / Theca cells

Table **7-4**	**MEIOSIS**[*]**—Cont'd**	
ACTIVITY	**ACTIVITY ILLUSTRATED**	
Ovulation	The completion of meiosis results in a secondary oocyte and the first polar body. The secondary oocyte has nearly all the cytoplasm and a haploid number of chromosomes. A breakdown of the follicle is stimulated. The oocyte is arrested at metaphase of the second meiosis.	First polar body → Secondary oocyte →
Second meiosis is completed with fertilization	The two sister chromatids separate and the germ cell nuclei form, resulting in three polar bodies and an ovum, each with a different genetic composition and a haploid number of chromosomes	Polar bodies Ovum

[*]Migration of primordial germ cells (PGCs), known as *colonization,* the organization of PGCs at the ovary, and the compartmentalization of the ovary to support follicular development are accomplished in utero. Meiosis is the specialized cell division that prepares oocytes for fertilization.

Following colonization, the primordial germ cells are transformed into oogonia and increase their mitotic activity so that by the 20th week 7 million are present. From 8 to 20 weeks' gestation, there is *organization* of the germ and somatic cells into cords, which then develop into primordial follicles. Primordial follicles characteristically contain an oocyte surrounded by flat granulosa cells.

Finally, *compartmentalization* is the development of the ovary into the outer cortex and inner medulla (Maroulis, 1997). Compartmentalization occurs as the surface epithelium, a single layer of cells that is continuous with the mesothelium of the peritoneum at the hilum of the ovary, becomes separated from the follicle in the cortex by a thin fibrous capsule.

Somatic Sex

Somatic growth is the development and maturation of organ structures. Unique organ structures for the female (i.e., the uterus, the vagina, and the external genitalia) also advance from an indifferent stage marked by mesonephric ducts and the paramesonephric ducts. Male and female external genital organs are indistinguishable until after the seventh week following fertilization and are not fully differentiated until the twelfth week. In the absence of androgens, the indifferent phallus ceases to grow and becomes the clitoris, the urogenital folds become the frenulum of the labia minora, and the phallic part of the urogenital sinus forms the vestibule of the vagina.

The mammary glands begin to develop early in embryogenesis, arising from a line of glandular tissues called the *mammary ridge,* or milk line, that extends from the axilla to the groin (Hindle, 1997). The breast and nipple buds develop from one papilla along this line; other rudimentary papillae generally atrophy later in embryonic life. In some women, remnants of this ridge may be seen in the form of supernumerary nipples and breast tissue.

The uterus and fallopian tubes develop as an expansion of the Müllerian duct. The vaginal epithelium is derived from the endoderm of the urogenital sinus, and the fibro-muscular wall of the vagina develops from the mesenchyme. Contact of the uterovaginal primordium with the urogenital sinus induces the formation of paired endodermal out-growths, the sinovaginal bulbs, that extend from the urogenital sinus to the caudal end of the uterovaginal primordium. The sinovaginal bulbs soon fuse to form a solid vaginal plate. Later, the central cells of this plate break down, forming the lumen of the vagina; its peripheral cells form the vaginal epithelium (Moore, 1988).

Neuroendocrine Sex

The mammalian brain and pituitary are clearly target organs of steroid hormone action. Several studies have demonstrated a wide distribution of receptors for all three sex steroid hormones throughout the different regions of the brain as well as in the pituitary. Neuroendocrine sex is the continuous or cyclic production of gonadotropin-releasing hormones necessary for reproductive functioning. The structures that are central to neuroendocrine sex are the hypothalamus, the anterior pituitary, and the ovary, a triad known as the *reproductive axis* (Figure 7-14).

Sexual dimorphism has been described in multiple regions of the central nervous system. Analogous to the reproductive tract, the neuroendocrine system undergoes a process of sexual differentiation and maturation that is heavily influenced by the steroid receptor signaling pathways. Sexual maturation of the neuroendocrine system may be defined as the acquisition of pituitary responsiveness to hypothalamic factors and ovari-an steroids and the onset of steroid-induced sexual behavior. In turn, differentiation of the neuroendocrine system is demonstrated by the unique ability of the female hypo-thalamus to induce a luteinizing hormone (LH) surge in response to a rise in serum estradiol. The organizational or differentiating effects of pubertal steroids are perma-

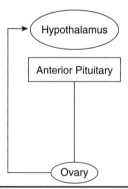

Figure 7-14 The reproductive triad includes the hypothalamus, the anterior pituitary, and the ovary. For appropriate hormonal secretion to sustain homeostasis, each of the three organs must be capable of responding to signals from the others.

nent and are manifested as measurable structural changes or as subtle fixations in the system's sensitivity to the activation effects of steroids during adulthood (Krege et al, 1998).

The hypothalamus is the interface between the central nervous system and the endocrine system. The anatomical site of the hypothalamus, forming the base of the brain and located just above the pituitary, is conducive to the translation of neuronal signals from the brain into humoral factors that stimulate appropriate actions in the anterior pituitary. The hypothalamus secretes precursor substances called *releasing factors* and *release-inhibiting factors.* Luteinizing hormone–releasing hormone (LHRH) is present by 8 weeks' gestation. This development is independent of the maternal hypothalamic-pituitary unit.

The hypothalamic-pituitary unit of the reproductive triad is complete by midgestation, but functional maturation is not complete until after birth. By 14 weeks' gestation all the hypothalamic nuclei are present, and at 14.5 weeks the hypothalamic-pituitary portal, a direct connection from the hypothalamus to the pituitary gland, is intact.

The anterior pituitary, located beneath the hypothalamus, releases stimulating hormones through the general circulation in sufficient quantity to induce function at specific target organs. The fetal pituitary secretes prolactin such that by the third fetal month levels are in the adult normal range. Cord prolactin levels are usually greater than those in maternal blood. Although the female fetus has higher follicle-stimulating hormone (FSH) levels than does the male, there is an inhibition of LH and FSH secretion in late gestation that appears to be the result of negative feedback by high levels of estrogen and progesterone in fetal circulation. Plasma levels of progesterone rise progressively during fetal life with no apparent sex difference. In contrast 17-α-hydroxyprogesterone levels are higher in the cord blood of girls than boys.

Fetal levels of estrone and estradiol rise progressively throughout gestation in both boys and girls. While in utero, the source of estrogen for the fetus is the placenta. At birth, with the separation of the placenta, and, in the presence of immature ovaries, estrogen levels decrease. During the first few days to 1 week after birth, the concentration of human chorionic gonadotropin (hCG) and placental steroids (from maternal sources) falls. This fall is followed by an increase in plasma LH and FSH. FSH rises to a peak at 3 months in both boys and girls, but reaches a much higher peak in girls and remains elevated longer, up to 2 years. LH levels increase in both sexes by the second week of life and remain elevated during the first 4 to 6 months of life in both boys and girls. Maximal levels of LH are observed in girls by the third month and then decrease by the end of the first year of life. In boys, LH levels are highest between 1 and 4 months and then decrease during the first year.

The pituitary is responsive to LHRH stimulation immediately after birth but more so after the third day of life. The response is primarily LH predominant in boys and FSH predominant in girls. FSH levels are eight to ten times higher in girls than in boys. The FSH response to LHRH is highest during the first 6 months of life.

These hormones respond primarily to negative feedback. As would be predicted in a negative feedback system, there is an increase in FSH and LH for the first several months of life. However, there is an eventual decrease in these releasing hormones due to prolonged insufficient estrogen production.

Estrone and estradiol fall rapidly during the first 5 days of life. Estrone levels remain low throughout infancy and childhood, while estradiol increases during the first 2 months in boys and the first 4 to 12 months in girls. There is a wide variation in estradiol levels, and high levels can persist for up to 2 years. Testosterone secretion begins early in gestation and reaches a peak at 10 to 18 weeks. Plasma prolactin levels remain elevated during the first day of postnatal life and then fall rapidly over the next 7 days. They continue to fall over the next 2 to 3 months until they reach normal prepubertal levels.

Following birth, plasma testosterone levels in boys peak at 6 to 15 weeks and then decrease to low levels by 6 months of age. In girls, testosterone levels decrease in the first week of life and remain low. Although wide variability is normal among girls, estradiol levels are generally elevated during the first 6 to 12 months after birth and can remain elevated for up to 2 years.

Hormonal levels fall rapidly after birth in both sexes. Between 1 and 2 years, 17-α-hydroxyprogesterone levels are at their lowest with no differences between boys and girls. The hypothalamic-pituitary-gonadal axis becomes functional during fetal development, continues during early infancy, is inhibited during childhood, and is reactivated at puberty (Klein & Cutler, 1996).

Growth

Human skeletal growth can conceptually be divided into three components—infancy growth, childhood growth, and pubertal growth. The infancy growth component can be regarded as a continuation of fetal growth that gradually wanes during the first 2 years after birth. Nutrition is the major stimulator of fetal and infant growth. The regulation of the childhood phase of human growth is dominated by growth hormone. The pubertal growth spurt is primarily due to increased secretion of estrogens and androgens. Estrogen augments growth hormone during the period of rapid growth. The mean age of maximal growth spurt is 12.4 years in girls, with a magnitude of peak height velocity of 7.3 cm per year. Estrogen stimulates growth by augmenting growth hormone and by ossifying the growth plate, a process that eventually causes cessation of growth in late puberty. There is a highly variable inter- and intraindividual growth rate from conception to adulthood in girls. The maximum growth, 8 cm per month, occurs at about 20 weeks of gestational age, and from that point, there is a gradual decrease to about 5 cm per year (0.4 cm/month) between 10 and 12 years of age. During the pubertal growth spurt, the rate of growth is about 1 cm per month or even more (Ritzen et al., 2000).

Childhood Development

During childhood, the pattern of growth is similar for both sexes. From approximately 12 months to 9 years of age, there is insufficient gonadotropin secretion from the hypothalamus to support gonadal function. In the presence of low gonadotropin levels, FSH and LH are not present in adequate quantities to stimulate ovarian secretion of estrogens in girls.

LH and FSH are secreted in a pulsatile pattern during infancy, childhood, and puberty. Before the onset of puberty, there is a low pituitary responsiveness to LHRH. This inhibitory stage is characterized by relatively high FSH levels in relation to LH levels. The amplitude and frequency of FSH pulses are greater in girls, and the amplitude and frequency of LH pulses are greater in boys. Pulsatility and nocturnal augmentation of gonadotropin secretion were previously thought to occur only after the onset of puberty, but with the increased use of sensitive and specific radioimmunoassays, pulsatile gonadotropin secretion has been observed during prepuberty as well as puberty but has not been described in infancy (Klein & Cutler, 1996).

Puberty

Puberty is a series of physiological and chemical events that leads to the development of secondary sex characteristics, increased growth, psychological changes, and fertility. There is an increase in the activity of the hypothalamic pituitary gonadal axis so that the gonads are stimulated to produce adult levels of sex steroids.

At about age 8 or 9, there is increased activity of gonadotropin-releasing hormone (GnRH), which is released in a pulsatile fashion, initially during sleep. As a result, there are detectable pulses of FSH and LH. The physiological stimulus for GnRH activity is not understood. The rate of GnRH "awakening" is assumed to be highly variable among girls, with some children experiencing a continual crescendo of activity and others, intermittent stimulation. Regardless of the pattern, even very low levels of estradiol result in the developmental changes of puberty. The first observable change related to estradiol is breast budding. In addition, proliferative changes occur in the endometrium, and maturation of the pituitary response to pulsatile release of estrogens occurs (Figure 7-15).

The increase in sex hormones results from two independent processes, gonadarche and adrenarche. Adrenarche is a maturational change in adrenal function that causes increased secretion of androgens and estrogens. Adrenarche precedes gonadarche by several years. Adrenarche causes an increase in the adrenal secretion of dehydroepiandrosterone (DHEA), DHA sulfate (DHAS) androstenedione, testosterone, estrone, pregnenolone, and 17-hydroxypregnenolone. Mean plasma DHEA increases steadily from age 5 to age 20 in both boys and girls. Estrone follows a similar pattern in boys, suggesting that it originates primarily from the adrenal gland. Androstenedione increases more rapidly once puberty starts because of its derivation from both adrenal and gonadal sources. Adrenarche is no longer thought to play a role in the control of puberty (Klein & Cutler, 1996).

Before puberty, the breasts are small with little internal glandular structure and are similar in males and females (Hindle, 1997). With the onset of puberty in females, increased estrogen causes a marked enhancement of ductal growth and branching but relatively little development of the alveoli, and much of the breast enlargement at this time is due to fat deposition. With each ovulatory cycle, the glandular tissue is prepared for lactation and then undergoes physiological regression when pregnancy does not occur. Some of the breast ductal epithelial cells proliferate, and others undergo apoptosis

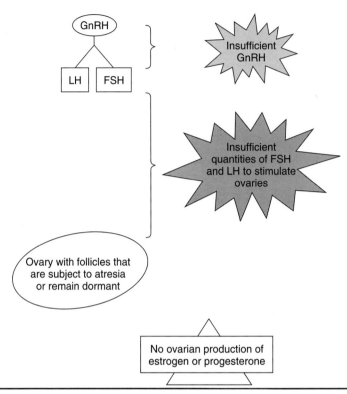

Figure 7-15 Before puberty, GnRH is not secreted in amounts adequate to stimulate activity of the releasing hormones from the anterior pituitary. With insufficient FSH to develop the support follicular growth, the ovarian cycle does not function, and there is an absence of enzyme to produce estrogen. Without a follicle, and thus a corpus luteum, the ovarian source of progesterone is also absent.

with each menstrual cycle. Complex interactions among adrenal glucocorticoids, estrogen, growth hormone, insulin, progesterone, and prolactin result in the development and maturation of the breast to full functional status, and precise cyclically variable amounts of estrogen and progesterone are essential to this process (Hindle, 1997).

The mammary gland in many respects is an embryonic organ because it undergoes its major morphological and functional maturation (differentiation) after birth. Specific developmental genes, known as Hox genes, are present in normal breast cells. Two Hox genes, Hoxa-1 and Hoxb-7, both of which are found in cultured breast epithelial cells, have provided insight into normal and abnormal cell growth in the breast. Studies in the breast in animals have shown that Hoxb-7 is present throughout mammary gland development except during lactation. However, Hoxa-1 was found only in breast tumors.

The hormone prolactin induces lobuloalveolar growth in the mammary gland. Functional differentiation of the mammary gland is a crucial step in the reproductive cycle of mammals. This developmental process, as observed in the mouse, proceeds in distinct phases. In newborn mice, a rudimentary system of small ducts is present. This ductal system grows slowly until the onset of puberty, when pronounced ductal growth occurs, leading to the formation of the ductal tree, which fills the entire mammary fat pad.

Terminal differentiation of alveolar epithelial cells is completed at the end of gestation with the onset of milk secretion at parturition. Distinct steps of cellular differentiation take place during this process, which are defined by the sequential activation of genes coding for milk proteins. The presence of lactogenic hormones is not sufficient to explain the complex development and temporal regulation of gene expression observed in the emerging gland during pregnancy. Estrogen and progesterone are required for ductal outgrowth and alveolar proliferation. In addition, growth regulators and cell cycle progression are necessary for alveolar proliferation and differentiation (Hennighausen, Robinson, Wagner, & Liu, 1997)

Other observable indicators of impending puberty include the development of pubic and axillary hair as a consequence of a shift in secretions of the adrenal gland. These observable pubertal changes are classified in a scheme known as the Tanner classification of adolescent development. This staging allows for assessment of progression of pubertal events based on assessment of breast development and body hair distribution. Breast changes are primarily estrogen dependent, while the appearance and distribution of pubic hair are primarily dependent on increased adrenal androgens (Table 7-5).

The normal sequence of pubertal changes in girls is breast budding between 8 and 13 years, appearance of pubic hair several months later, peak growth velocity between 9.5 and 14.5 years, and menarche between 10 and 16.5 years. Other physical changes include adult body odor, acne, oily skin, and vaginal discharge. The average time of ovulation is 10 months after menarche (Klein & Cutler, 1996).

The onset of menstruation, called *menarche*, is a relatively late event in development. At the time of menarche, breasts and pubic hair have often reached Tanner stage 4, and, in just about all cases, the peak height velocity has been reached and the growth rate is

Table **7-5**	**APPEARANCE OF BREAST DEVELOPMENT AND PUBIC HAIR BY TANNER STAGE**	
STAGE	**BREAST**	**BODY HAIR**
I	Elevation of papilla only	No pubic hair
II	Elevation of breast and papilla as small mound. Areola diameter enlarged. Median age 9.8 years.	Sparse, long, pigmented hair, chiefly along the labia majora. Median age 10.5 years.
III	Further enlargment without separation of breast and areola. Median age 11.2 years.	Dark, coarse, curly hair, sparsely spread over mons. Median age 11.4 years.
IV	Secondary mound of areola and papilla above breast. Median age 12.1 years.	Adult-type hair, abundant but limited to the mons. Median age 12.0 years.
V	Mature stage. Projection of papilla only, due to recession of areola to the general contour of the breast. Median age 14.6 years.	Adult hair in quantity and extent. Distribution to medial aspect of thighs. Median age 13.7 years.

slowing. The average age of menarche in the United States is 12.8 years, although it can be delayed due to malnutrition or strenuous physical exercise. There is wide variation in the age at which the Tanner stages are reached, but once puberty commences, most children complete the process of physical maturation within 2 to 3 years of the onset of Tanner stage 2 (Figure 7-16).

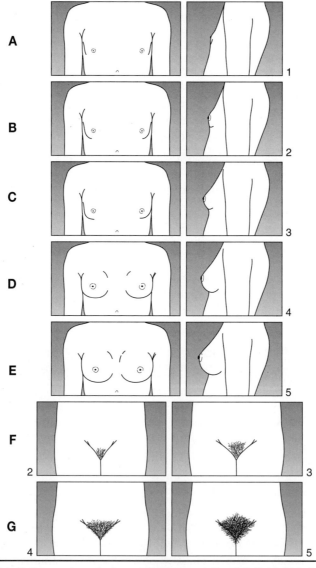

Figure 7-16 **A** to **E**, Tanner stages for breast development. **F** and **G**, Pubic hair development in the female.

Maturation of the Reproductive Axis

Menarche marks the transition to maturation of the reproductive axis. The reproductive cycle in all female primates occurs in three phases. The follicular phase, which is the time of follicular growth, is followed by the ovulatory period, when the oocyte matures and is released into the reproductive tract. In the luteal phase, a newly formed corpus luteum secretes hormones in preparation for implantation. If the egg is not fertilized and implantation does not occur, a new cycle is initiated (the phenomenon of cyclicity) as soon as the activity of the corpus luteum wanes (Ferin, Jewelewicz, & Warren, 1993). If the fertilized egg implants into the uterus, the luteal phase is prolonged and becomes the progestational phase of the pregnancy that follows. The activities of each of these phases are coordinated among the organs of the reproductive axis. The hypothalamus, pituitary, and ovary work in synchrony via an elegant communication system to control menstrual cycling and reproduction.

The Hypothalamus

Reproductive functioning is controlled by the brain through an intricate network of GnRH neurons that translate neural signals into endocrine messages by action on the pituitary gland. The hypothalamus is where systemic input, such as stress or food, is synthesized and translated into a response (Clarke, 1996).

GnRH is secreted into the hypophyseal portal blood system that runs between the hypothalamus and the pituitary gland. The hypothalamic-pituitary portal vessels originate around the base of the hypothalamus, the median eminence, where axons of the hypothalamus terminate. This area's capillary bed recombines into the portal vessels that pass down the infundibulum (stalk) of the hypothalamus, providing for the direct connection of the hypothalamus and the anterior pituitary. This direct vascular connection differs from the neural connections between the hypothalamus and the posterior pituitary.

The anterior pituitary therefore is exposed to higher plasma concentrations of hypophysiotropic hormones than those in the bloodstream because of the direct route to the anterior pituitary. The effect of hypophysiotropic hormones on the anterior pituitary is much less because the hormones are secreted into a small area and are carried via the portal system a short distance to their targets. Because hormones' short route limits the degradative effect of time/distance, low concentrations can produce secretory action in the anterior pituitary. GnRH cannot be measured in the blood because of the direct portal–anterior pituitary connection. Only the effects of the releasing hormones can be studied (Ryan, 1999).

The Pituitary

The pituitary (epithelial tissue at the base of the brain) produces, stores, and releases or halts the release of hormones in response to hypothalamic hormones. The pituitary gland is composed an anterior and a posterior lobe. The anterior pituitary secretes LH and FSH in response to GnRH. These hormones direct ovarian functioning, specifically germ cell development and secretion of hormones. LH induces ovulation in the female and stimulates estrogen and progesterone synthesis in the corpus luteum, and FSH stimulates secretion of estrogens.

The Ovary

The ovary, the target endocrine organ for stimulating hormones from the anterior pituitary, responds by releasing estrogen and progesterone in cyclic fashion. The ovary releases estrogen, the hormone that controls the menstrual cycle and promotes development of secondary sex characteristics, and progesterone, which stimulates the uterus and the mammary gland and is also involved in the implantation and maturation of the fertilized ovum (Klein & Cutler, 1996).

Estradiol and progesterone originate in the ovary (Ferin, Jewelewicz, & Warren, 1993). At the beginning of the menstrual cycle, plasma estrogen concentration is low and exerts little negative feedback. This low level of estrogen results in the release of GnRH by the hypothalamus and prods the anterior lobe of the pituitary to secrete FSH and LH. As with GnRH, LH secretion is pulsatile. However, the pattern of FSH secretion in the plasma is not completely pulsatile, possibly caused by the smoothing effect of the long half-life of FSH as compared to LH.

In response to stimulation by FSH and LH, multiple follicles within the ovary begin to enlarge and secrete estrogen. One follicle becomes dominant and secretes a very large amount of estrogen. The secretion and plasma concentration of FSH decrease, but plasma estrogen levels are high enough to have a positive feedback effect on gonadotropin secretion. Increasing blood levels of estrogen cause a midcycle surge in LH secretion that triggers ovulation, followed by the formation of the corpus luteum (Ferin, Jewelewicz, & Warren, 1993).

At birth, nearly 500,000 follicles are present in two ovaries. Follicles in their resting state are called *primordial follicles.* These follicles contain the 46 chromosomes required for reproduction; however, only a certain number of primordial follicles will be recruited for potential fertilization. Follicles can remain in the resting state for as long as 50 years. It is not yet known what factors trigger the emergence of primordial follicles from the resting state. Once a follicle begins to develop beyond the primordial state, however, it is committed to a process in which it will either be fertilized or undergo atresia. From the time of formation of the ovary in utero, follicles are moving from the resting state to the proliferating state. This process will continue until all follicles are depleted from the ovaries, which typically occurs around the age of 50 years (Ryan, 1999).

The recruitment and development of the follicle is continuous and independent of the menstrual cycle. Until recently, estimates of the number of oocytes in the ovarian follicle pool were based on autopsy and surgical specimens. These establish that the number of ovarian follicles decreases from fetal life to the menopause. During the reproductive years, the median number of follicles declined from about 104,000 in a woman's early 20s to 33,000 in her early 30s, and to 7900 in her early 40s. A decline was also seen for antral follicles that were greater than 1 mm in diameter. According to

Reuss, Kline, Santos, Levin, and Timor-Tritsch (1997) transvaginal sonography provides a noninvasive approach to studying the natural history of changes in the follicle pool. Further, the number of antral follicles may have biological consequences and may help to predict such age-related phenomena as ease of conception, trisomy conception, and time until menopause.

Atresia, which like ovulation causes follicular attrition, occurs in two settings. Monthly atresia, a gonadotropin-dependent process, occurs when a cohort of up to 50 follicles is recruited each month; eventually one dominant follicle is released from the ovary while the remainder are resorbed. This process may explain why fewer than 1% of the total endowed primordial oocyte pool is lost each month. In addition to this monthly depletion, there is a tonic, gonadotropin-independent process that allows hundreds of thousands of primordial follicles to be resolved continuously regardless of the presence or absence or oral contraceptives or pregnancy. This process is responsible for the loss of 80% of the endowed primordial oocyte pool from 6 months in utero to birth and the loss of 95% by the time puberty is reached. Follicles that begin to develop before the maturation of the reproductive axis are destined to undergo atresia. Postpubertal follicular atresia continues as a relentless underlying lifelong process upon which monthly cyclic ovulating attrition is superimposed. Although we refer to both of these processes (cyclic and tonic) as atresia, they may be fundamentally different (Seifer, 1997).

The growth of a primordial follicle to the large preantral stage takes approximately 85 days (Gougeon, 1986). In addition to increasing in size, the cells surrounding the recruited ovum proliferate and form two compartments, identified by cell types (granulosa or theca cells). An antrum (a small open space) begins to develop within the granulosa. Antral formation and growth require stimulation from FSH and thus are said to be menstrual cycle dependent. The granulosa cells form the inner envelope surrounding the oocyte and are the only cells in the body known to possess FSH receptors (Zeleznik & Hillier, 1996). Granulosa cells respond primarily to FSH and are organized to metabolize androgens to estrogens by aromatase enzyme activity and to synthesize progesterone and its metabolites. The theca cells, which surround the granulosa cell layer, are not present in the small, primary follicle, appearing only when the follicle grows. These cells synthesize androgens in response to LH stimulation. The major product of this stimulation is DHEA, which is further metabolized to androstenedione (Figure 7-17).

The theca cells express receptors for LH, while granulosa cells develop receptors for FSH (Ryan, 1999) The final maturation of the large preantral follicle to the preovulatory stage takes approximately 14 days, representing the duration of the follicular phase of the menstrual cycle (Gougeon, 1986). A follicle recruited during one menstrual cycle will actually have begun to mature at least two cycles in advance of ovulatory release. In the cycle in which a specific ovum is recruited, the follicle grows from about 0.25 mm to at least 10 mm in diameter at the midfollicular phase and at least 20 mm in diameter before ovulation. Ovulation is the end process of a series of events initiated by the gonadotropin surge, which results in the release of a mature fertilizable egg from a

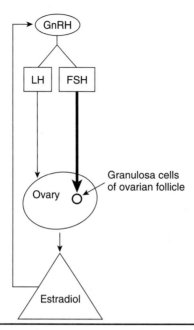

Figure 7-17 In the follicular phase, FSH stimulates the granulosa cells of the ovarian follicle. One follicle becomes dominant and secretes a large amount of estrogen. FSH secretion and plasma FSH concentration decrease, but plasma estrogen levels are high enough to exert a positive feedback on gonadotropin secretion. Increasing blood levels of estogen stimulate a surge in LH secretion.

graafian follicle. Ovulation is induced by the sudden release of large amounts of LH from the pituitary gland (the LH surge), which is triggered by the sustained high circulating level of estradiol produced by the preovulatory follicle. The gonadotropin surge terminates estradiol synthesis, and the theca cells change from androgen to progesterone-secreting tissue, yielding the preovulatory progesterone rise (Figure 7-18).

The LH surge stimulates a proteolytic cascade within the preovulatory follicle, resulting in its rupture approximately 36 hours later. The proteolytic cascade causes breakdown of collagen, fibrin, and extracellular matrix in the apical region of the follicle wall, leading to ovulation. As ovulation approaches, the ovary secretes more progesterone, while estrogen secretion temporarily declines. Progesterone levels in follicular fluid rise markedly following the LH surge or injection of hCG. It is possible that the preovulatory increase in progesterone formation is essential to follicular rupture.

Several other hormones (insulin, for example) and growth factors (the insulinlike growth factors) may play important but still poorly understood roles. The growth factors are produced by granulosa and theca cells and function as paracrine and autocrine agents. Paracrine agents are produced by a particular organ and influence another cell of the same organ by local diffusion. In autocrine control, a hormone synthesized by a cell exits the cell to bind to a membrane receptor on the same cell and reenters it to

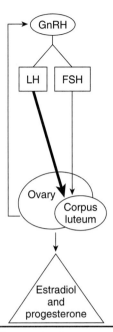

Figure 7-18 In the luteal phase, the LH surge stimulates a proteolytic cascade within the preovulato-ry follicle, causing a breakdown of collagen, fibrin, and extracellular matrix in the apical region of the follicle wall, which leads to ovulation about 36 hours later. As ovulation approaches, the ovary increasingly secretes progesterone while estrogen secretion tem-porarily declines. Progesterone levels in follicular fluid rise markedly following the LH surge.

exert its action. In intracrine control, a hormone synthesized within a cell acts without exiting the cell (Ferin, Jewelewicz, & Warren, 1993).

Certain peptide hormones control FSH synthesis and secretion; however, regulation takes place by direct action at the level of the pituitary, without any effect on the secre-tion of GnRH. Inhibins are a family of glycoproteins primarily produced by the gonads of both sexes. At least 10 different forms of inhibins are produced by ovarian follicles, and several forms block the action of FSH. Inhibin and its chemical cousin activin are named for their ability to inhibit and activate, respectively, the secretion of FSH by the pituitary gland, which helps to prepare the ovaries for ovulation. During pregnancy, inhibin prevents a woman from ovulating.

Despite their opposing functions, inhibin and activin are very similar structurally. Their subunits were first discovered in the gonads; however, they are also found in the gonadotropes themselves, which is suggestive of self- or autocrine regulatory mecha-nisms. Activin given the day before ovulation increases the percentage of cells that bind GnRH, while inhibin causes a decrease in binding. An additional polypeptide, follistatin, is thought to indirectly regulate FSH biosynthesis and secretion through its ability to bind, and therefore inhibit, activin function (Albano, Arkell, Beddington, & Smith, 1994; Bauer-Dantoin, Weiss, & Jameson, 1996).

The Corpus Luteum

After ovulation and expulsion of the unfertilized egg, a corpus luteum is formed. This new structure results from LH-induced morphological changes in both the granulosa and the theca layers of the graafian follicle after ovulation. Luteinization can be initiated once the granulosa cells have acquired receptors for LH and does not necessarily signify that ovulation has occurred. The corpus luteum is a transient endocrine organ. It has a 12- to 15-day life span, and thus its regression (i.e., luteolysis) is inevitable in the nonfertile cycle (Ryan, 1999) (Figure 7-19).

The corpus luteum attains maturation about 5 days after ovulation and when mature, is easily recognizable on the surface of the ovary. On about day 7 to 9 of the luteal phase, however, the regression of the corpus luteum begins. Progesterone values normally rise during the luteal phase of the menstrual cycle to a peak of about 7 to 9 ng/ml around the sixth day after the LH surge (Illingworth, Reddi, Smith, & Baird, 1990). In the absence of fertilization, this level of progesterone will decline over the next 12 to 15 days (Ryan, 1999). Fibrosis of the luteinized cells, a dramatic increase in the number of secretory granules with a parallel increase in lipid droplets and cytoplasmic vacuoles, and a decrease in vascularization occur with this regression. All of these phenomena result in decreased secretion of steroids. The defunct corpus luteum, referred to as the corpus albicans, becomes hyalinized within 6 months (Ferin, Jewelewicz, & Warren, 1993) (Figure 7-20).

The corpus luteum secretes progesterone and some estrogen. The granulosa cells and corpus luteum secrete inhibin, a peptide hormone. Increases in progesterone and

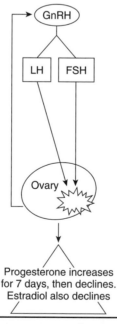

Figure **7-19** The corpus luteum sustains progesterone for approximately 7 days following ovulation. Between days 7 and 9 of the luteal phase, the corpus luteum begins to regress. Progesterone concentration will decline and menstruation will follow.

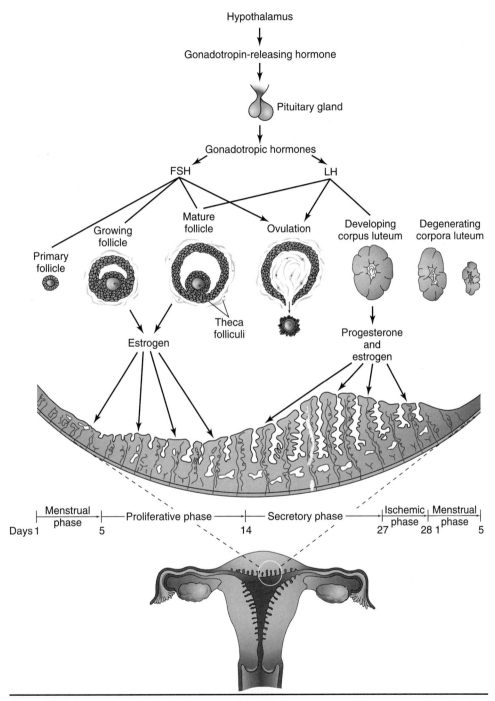

Figure 7-20 Schematic drawing illustrating the interrelations of the hypothalamus, pituitary gland, ovaries, and endometrium. One complete menstrual cycle and the beginning of another are shown. (From Moore, K. L., & Persaud, T. V. N. [1998]. *The developing human: Clinically oriented embryology* [6th ed.]. Philadelphia: W. B. Saunders.)

estrogen in the blood inhibit FSH and LH secretion during the last phase of the cycle. The corpus luteum begins to degenerate and hormone production decreases. Plasma estrogen and progesterone concentrations fall. FSH and LH secretion begins to increase, and a new cycle begins.

The Breast

During the menstrual cycle, normal breast epithelial cell proliferation is greatest during the luteal phase when both estradiol and progesterone levels are high (Popnikolov, Yang, Liu, Guzman, & Nandi, 2001). With each ovulatory cycle, the breast glandular tissue is prepared for lactational function; these changes regress when pregnancy does not occur. Some of the breast ductal epithelial cells proliferate and others undergo apoptosis (planned physiological cellular death) with each menstrual cycle. Estrogen and progesterone in precise cyclically variable amounts are essential to this process (Hindle, 1997).

The Uterus

The uterus is one of the main organs involved in reproduction and is a major anatomical component in the menstrual cycle. During each menstrual cycle, the endometrium, the glandular membrane lining of the uterus, undergoes a series of orchestrated and well-controlled changes in anticipation of the arrival of the blastocyst. The endometrium regenerates following menstruation or pregnancy to assure appropriate maturation and receptivity in each cycle. The smooth muscle of the uterine body, the myometrium, undergoes rhythmic contractions during menstrual cycling and pregnancy. At the end of pregnancy, contractions of the myometrium enable labor and delivery to take place (Critchley, 1996).

The endometrium is functionally divided into two layers: the stratum basalis and the stratum functionale. The basalis is a deeper endometrial layer from which the new endometrium matures. The stratum functionale, the superficial layer, is sensitive to estrogen and progesterone stimulation, and, consequently, its appearance varies during the different phases of the menstrual cycle.

Dramatic and well-coordinated hormone-driven changes occur in the endometrium with each uterine cycle. Estradiol plays a major role in the endometrial changes in the follicular phase, leading to repair of the glandular, stromal, and vascular elements from the previous menstrual cycle. By the late follicular phase, the endometrial glands are short, straight, and narrow and the stroma is compact. Estrogen-induced thickening of the endometrial stroma and increased number and complexity of glands characterize the proliferative phase. The luteal, or secretory, phase, which follows ovulation, is under the hormonal control of corpus luteum–derived progesterone. During this phase the glands take on a corkscrew appearance. The cells of the stroma are swollen and uniform in appearance. After ovulation, the endometrium is exposed to increasing concentrations of progesterone from the corpus luteum. In the early luteal phase, the endometrial glands elongate and coil, and their lumina fill with glycogen-rich secretions. By the late luteal phase these changes become accentuated, and the glands assume a saw tooth appearance. The stromal compartment becomes progressively more edematous because of fluid accumulation in the extracellular matrix. Three distinct layers can be identified, namely the superficial zona compacta, the intermediate zona spongiosa, and the zona basalis. The compacta and the spongiosa make up the functional endometrium, which is shed during menstruation (Cameron, Irvine, & Norman, 1996) (Figure 7-21).

Decidualization is the name given to the hormone-dependent transient formation of decidual tissue that encompasses cellular proliferation, differentiation, and death. This

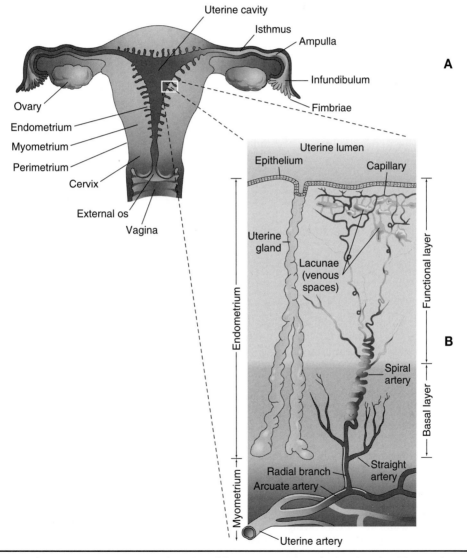

Figure 7-21 **A**, Diagrammatic coronal section of the uterus, uterine tubes, and vagina. The ovaries are also shown. **B**, Enlargement of the area outlined in *A*. The functional layer of the endometrium is sloughed off during menstruation. (From Moore, K. L., & Persaud, T. V. N. [1998]. *The developing human: Clinically oriented embryology* [6th ed.]. Philadelphia: W. B. Saunders.)

process is seen in species in which, during implantation, the trophoblast invades the uterine stroma to reach the maternal blood vessels. To prepare for implantation, there is differentiation of stromal fibroblasts into decidual cells, followed by modification of the extracellular matrix, alterations in cellular secretory function, and recruitment of precursor granulated lymphocytes. Though removal of steroid hormone support from decidualized endometrium results in menstruation, it appears that cell death is programmed once decidualization has been induced and that menstruation is an inevitable consequence unless appropriate signals are received from an implanting embryo (Cameron, Irvine, & Norman, 1996).

There is much interest in determining the molecular signals that prompt cyclic endometrial change. Three events that could stimulate gene transcription in the endometrium include (1) steroid hormone binding with subsequent target cell transcriptional activation, (2) response to nonsteroid signaling molecules such as growth factors and cytokines, and (3) cell-cell interactions. These events involve the same activities of nuclear and membrane receptors, hormones, and signaling pathways discussed earlier. As emphasized in discussions of cellular functioning, for steroid hormones to have an effect on a tissue, nuclear receptors must be present. Estrogen and progesterone receptors in the human uterus have been assessed across the menstrual cycle. An increase, or upregulation, of estrogen receptors is evident from day 5 to day 15. Progesterone receptors also peak midcycle, but the increase does not begin until day 8. During the secretory phase, both estrogen and progesterone receptors return to low levels (Critchley, 1996).

The cyclic changes in the epithelial and stromal compartments are paralleled by events in the endometrial vasculature. Angiogenesis, the growth of new blood vessels, is a rare physiological event in normal adult tissues but the female reproductive tract is an exception, with angiogenesis occurring with each cycle as the endometrium repairs, proliferates, and prepares for implantation. The spiral arteries are destined to provide the maternal side of the interface between the placental blood supply and the uterus. These spiral arteries regrow from remnant vascular fragments in the basal endometrium into markedly closed end-arterioles, each supplying 4 to 7 mm of the endometrial surface. These arterioles feed a network of superficial capillaries, which in turn drain into superficial venous lakes and larger veins near the endometrial-myometrial junction (Cameron, Irvine, & Norman, 1996).

Angiogenesis is required to support the proliferation of the human endometrium during the menstrual cycle, as well as endometrial regeneration after shedding of the functionalis layer in the absence of implantation. In addition, changes in vascular permeability throughout the menstrual cycle promote the transformation of the thin, dense endometrium into the thick, highly permeable secretory endometrium. These vascular changes are regulated by estradiol and progesterone, which induce the production of angiogenic factors. Vascularization during the female reproductive cycle and during embryogenesis has been correlated with increased expression of vascular endothelial growth factors (VEGF), and VEGF mRNA (the messenger RNA that directs protein transcription) and its resulting protein have been demonstrated in the endometrium throughout the menstrual cycle. An increase is noted in the late proliferative and luteal phases, which correspond to angiogenesis and increased vascular permeability (Meduri, Bausero, & Perrot-Applanat, 2000).

The final stage of the menstrual cycle, following luteal regression, is the menses. Menstruation is the shedding of the superficial layers of the endometrium following the withdrawal of ovarian steroids (Cameron, Irvine, & Norman, 1996). Menses occurs in the absence of fertilization. The corpus luteum undergoes the degradative process of luteolysis and, as a consequence, progesterone levels decline. In the majority of women, the menstrual cycle lasts between 25 and 30 days, with the distribution within this range skewed toward 28 to 30-day cycles. By convention, the day of menstruation is labeled day 1 of the menstrual cycle. The regular 28-day menstrual cycle is considered normal, and the average woman will have some 400 periods during her reproductive lifetime. In a typical cycle, the follicular phase lasts approximately 14 days, but this can vary; in contrast, the luteal phase is remarkably constant in duration and lasts 12 to 15 days.

Endometrial bleeding and its regulation constitute a complex process that requires participation of a diverse group of local factors (Tabibzadeh, Satyaswaroop, von Wolff, & Strowitzki, 1999). There is an aggressive effort to determine the cell types and receptors that are present in different phases of the menstrual cycle. Homeostasis events in the menstruating uterus are markedly different from the usual homeostatic mechanism. Three main mechanisms are required to control menstrual bleeding. First, there is potent vasoconstriction to check blood loss from the damaged vessels. Next, although there should be an associated deposition of platelet-fibrin plugs, there is an even greater requirement for an active fibrinolytic system to prevent clot organization for subsequent scarring and intrauterine adhesion formation. Such scarring and adhesion formation would constitute a distinct evolutionary disadvantage. Finally, the bleeding is controlled definitively by the repair of both the endometrial surface and the blood vessels themselves.

Rather than the expected platelet adhesion to control bleeding, stromal disintegration and vessel lesions are seen in the endothelium. Following this, extravasation is a prominent feature in the functional endometrium, and damaged blood vessels are sealed by intravascular thrombi consisting of various amounts of platelets and fibrin. By 20 hours after the onset of bleeding most of the functional endometrium has been shed, and hemostasis is achieved by vasoconstriction rather than by the deposition of stable platelet-fibrin plugs. Impaired platelet plug formation might be expected in the presence of potent inhibitors of platelet adhesion and aggregation in the endometrium.

With the exception of the epithelium lining's glandular stumps, most of the endometrial surface epithelium is desquamated within 24 hours of the onset of bleeding, and open-ended blood vessel segments are seen, devoid of platelet-fibrin clots. Within 24 to 48 hours, new endometrial epithelial growth is detectable, originating in the retained glandular stumps. By cycle day 4, more of the interglandular endometrial surface has been replaced by new epithelium, and by day 5 to 6 the endometrium has been completely reepithelialized, and new stromal tissue has begun to grow.

When fertilization occurs, hCG maintains the viability of the corpus luteum and hence the production of progesterone until the placenta can take over as the major source of progesterone. The developing blastocyst initially transcribes hCG mRNA around the eight-cell stage (Bonduelle et al., 1988), while initial protein production has been demonstrated in vitro at 7 days after fertilization. A significant amount of hCG, indicating implantation, is not detectable in the plasma of pregnant women until 6 to 12 days after ovulation (Wilcox, Baird, & Weinberg, 1999). The maternal plasma levels of hCG continue to double about every 2 days, peak at 10 weeks, then subsequently decline until 20 weeks; and this low level is maintained for the remainder of the pregnancy. The production of hCG during the initial 8 to 10 weeks of pregnancy stimulates the corpus luteum to sustain production of progesterone. The maintenance of the corpus luteum after fertilization is termed the "rescue of the corpus luteum." This process requires the binding of hCG to the LH receptor on the luteal cells (Braunstein, 1996) (Figures 7-22 and 7-23).

The fertilized ovum begins to undergo cell division while it is traveling down the oviduct toward the uterine cavity. Upon arrival in the uterus about 5 days after ovulation, the conceptus is a multicellular blastocyst that is capable of invading the wall of the uterus, a process called *implantation*. Within 48 hours of invading the cell layer of the uterine wall, the trophoblast begins to secrete hCG. This peptide hormone binds to LH receptors in the corpus luteum but has much greater potency and a longer half-life than

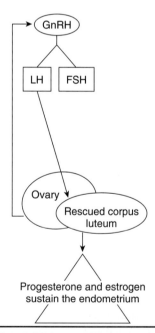

Figure 7-22 If fertilization takes place, hCG "rescues" the corpus luteum. The production of progesterone is sustained by the corpus luteum until the placenta takes over as its major source. The rescue of the corpus luteum requires the binding of hCG to LH receptors on luteal cells.

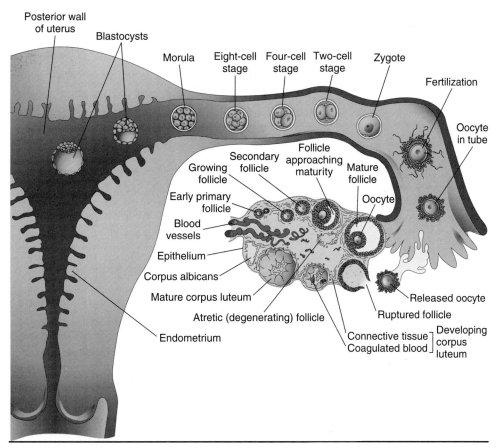

Figure 7-23 Diagrammatic summary of the ovarian cycle, fertilization, and human development during the first week. (From Moore, K. L., & Persaud T. V. N. [1998]. *The developing human: Clinically oriented embryology* [6th ed.]. Philadelphia: W. B. Saunders.)

LH. Acting in essence like a huge LH stimulus, hCG rescues the corpus luteum, thereby blocking luteal regression and supporting a steady increase in progesterone secretion. This "rescued" corpus luteum becomes the corpus luteum of pregnancy and provides the progesterone and estradiol to maintain a progestational uterine lining until the steroid secreting placenta becomes established (Ryan, 1999). In the event of fertilization, the level of progesterone remains elevated at 7 to 9 ng/ml and increases slightly over the next 10 weeks. It is not until some time after the eleventh week that the progesterone levels in a pregnancy substantially rise above the peak values seen during the luteal phase of the menstrual cycle.

There is a limited time each month when a fertilized embryo is able to implant successfully into the endometrial lining. For 2 to 3 days of each 28-day cycle, the uterine endometrium is receptive to an implanting blastocyst. This narrow window of opportunity is known as the period of uterine receptivity. To date, no single morphological or biochemical marker has been identified to indicate this period.

PREGNANCY

The numerous physiological changes of pregnancy are described in Chapter 16. Thus, information specific to pregnancy will be limited to differences in general physiological function.

The presence of a placenta, which makes a variety of hormones, and the presence of a fetus, which consumes oxygen and nutrients and produces carbon dioxide and other waste products and heat, are the two basic differences between a pregnant and a non-pregnant woman. These two differences, however, are responsible for a number of adaptive responses.

Sustained levels of progesterone and gradually increasing levels of estrogen interfere with the usual feedback mechanisms to the hypothalamus and the pituitary, thus disrupting the menstrual cycle. Vascular resistance decreases dramatically in the kidney, skin, and uterus secondary to estrogen and hCG. This change in resistance is the result of vasodilatation and structural changes in the uterine circulation at the level of the spiral arteries (Duvekot & Peeters, 1994; Gilson, Samaan, Crawford, Qualls, & Curet, 1997). The decline in vascular resistance leads to a fall in arterial blood pressure, stimulation of the renin-angiotensin-aldosterone system, and sodium and water retention. The water retention leads to an increase in plasma volume, a fall in hematocrit, and a reduction in blood oxygen capacity and venous oxygen saturation. The relative oxygen desaturation leads to an increase in erythropoetin and red blood cell production.

With the activation of the renin-angiotensin system, blood pressure should return to or exceed normal. However, blood pressure remains low in normal pregnancy because blood vessels are unresponsive to the effects of virtually all vasopressors. Were it not for this refractoriness, blood pressure would increase and plasma volume would expand.

The metabolic demands of the growing fetus require increasing quantities of oxygen and nutrients and produce increasing quantities of carbon dioxide and heat. Maternal oxygen consumption increases approximately 20%. Placental progesterone acts on the medulla, lowering the carbon dioxide threshold, and thus increasing the ventilatory drive. As a consequence of this increase in oxygen and decrease in carbon dioxide, the arterial pH during pregnancy is slightly above normal (approximately 7.42). Increased renal excretion of bicarbonate ions compensates for this respiratory alkalemia.

Placental hormones also influence renal function. Renal blood flow is increased, as is the glomerular filtration rate, and the concentration of all substances filtered by the glomerulus decreases by 30% to 50%.

The cardiovascular, respiratory, metabolic, and renal adaptations to pregnancy result in a system that is remarkably well adapted to the demands that the pregnant state creates. All of these systems gradually revert to normal when the fetus and placenta are delivered and the concentration of placental hormones decreases. By 4 to 6 weeks after delivery, virtually all of these cardiovascular, respiratory, and metabolic adaptations have disappeared.

There is variation in the length of time needed for regular ovulation and menstruation to become reestablished following delivery. In part, this time depends on the woman's choice regarding lactation. For the woman who has chosen to breastfeed her infant, menstruation and ovulation are delayed due to the systemic effects of prolactin, which reduces the sensitivity of the pituitary to the effects of GnRH, ultimately reducing the secretion of FSH and LH. The well-known effects of prolactin include serving as a luteotrophic hormone in maintaining the corpus luteum and thereby promoting blastocyst implantation (Bole-Feysot, Goffin, Edery, Binart, & Kelly, 1998).

The breast undergoes dramatic changes in size, shape, and function in association with growth, reproduction, and postmenopausal regression. The proliferation of normal human breast tissue cells in women is highest during the first trimester of pregnancy (Popnikolov, Yang, Liu, Guzman, & Nandi, 2001). Consistent with the observation that an early first full-term pregnancy exerts a protective effect on breast cancer, in vivo and in vitro studies indicate that cancer initiation requires the interaction of a carcinogen with an undifferentiated and highly proliferating mammary epithelium, whereas differentiation of the mammary gland inhibits carcinogenesis. Mammary gland differentiation is the result of complex interactions of ovarian, pituitary, and placental hormones, which in turn induce inhibition of cell proliferation, downregulation of estrogen and progesterone receptors, activation of specific genes, and expression of extracellular matrix proteins in the normal breast (Russo, Hu, Silva, & Russo, 2001).

Lactation is a complex physiological process involving integration of neuronal and endocrine mechanisms. Lactation can be divided into three phases: mammogenesis (mammary growth), lactogenesis (initiation of milk secretion) and galactopoiesis (maintenance of established milk secretion). During pregnancy, there is a marked increase in prolaction secretion due to stimulation by estrogen, yet despite elevated prolactin and enlarged, fully developed breasts, there is no secretion of milk. This is because estrogen and progesterone in large concentrations prevent milk production by inhibiting this particular action of prolactin on the breasts. Thus, while estrogen causes increased prolactin secretion and acts with prolactin in promoting growth and differentiation, estrogen and progesterone act as antagonists to prolactin during pregnancy to inhibit milk secretion. Delivery of the placenta removes the source of large amounts of sex steroids, thereby allowing milk production.

The drop in estrogen following delivery also causes a decrease in basal prolactin levels from their late-pregnancy peak and a return to prepregnancy levels after several months even though the mother continues to nurse. Superimposed upon this basal level, however, are large secretory bursts of prolactin during each nursing period. The episodic pulses of prolactin are signals for the breasts to maintain milk production, which ceases several days after the mother completely stops nursing her infant but will continue uninterrupted for years if nursing is continued. At the termination of lactation, involution occurs over a period of about 3 months. Decrease in breast size is accomplished without loss of lobular and alveolar components.

PHYSICAL FUNCTIONING, MATURATION, AND AGING

There is little documentation regarding normal physiological functioning of the female from the time of childbearing through the menopause. From a basic and clinical science perspective, there are several reasons why our understanding of this transition is limited. First, the human model for the transition from the reproductive period to menopause has been based mainly on individuals who have premature ovarian failure (POF), a diagnosis given to women under the age of 40 who present with amenorrhea and elevated circulating concentrations of LH and FSH (Rebar, Cedars, & Jiu, 1997). The study of genetic control of ovarian development has been more difficult than the analogous search for male reproductive control. The basis for this difficulty is the fact that more than one principal gene is involved in contrast to the male, in whom just one principal gene, namely the SRY, seems responsible for genetic control of reproduction (Simpson, 1997).

Perimenopause

The perimenopause is the period immediately prior to the menopause when endocrinological, biological, and clinical features of approaching menopause appear and continue for at least the first year after menopause (*Research on the menopause*, 1981). No consistent pattern of events marks the perimenopause; the onset can be indicated by irregular periods or other symptoms associated with decreasing estrogen.

There are three phases of the perimenopause. The *climacteric* is the transitional period between the years of reproductive capability and the menopause. The second phase of the perimenopause is the actual *menopause* itself, which signifies the end of reproductive capacity in women. The *postmenopause*, the third phase, begins 1 year after the cessation of menstruation. During this phase, the majority of estrogen production occurs via the conversion of estrogen from adrenal androstenedione (Purdie, 1996).

The appearance of irregular menses is often considered the hallmark of menopausal transition (Greendale & Judd, 1993). Before most women stop menstruating, the pattern of their menstrual cycles, including duration, frequency, and amount of bleeding, begins to change and becomes less predictable. Treloar and colleagues (1970) conducted a cross-sectional analysis of several hundred menstrual cycle calendars obtained from women across the reproductive years and noted that menstrual irregularity occurred with aging. The interval between menstrual periods begins to lengthen and the duration of bleeding remains unchanged. There is also evidence that the amount of flow with each menstrual period also changes, either increasing or decreasing. Excessive bleeding has been defined as greater than 80 ml of blood loss during the menstrual period, and it is estimated that between 9% and 14% of women experience menorrhagia (Archer, 1997).

It is often said that perimenopause signals a change in ovarian status in a similar but reverse sequence to puberty (Lobo, 1997). It should be emphasized, however, that although prepuberty and postmenopause are both hypoestrogenic states, the reasons for the lower concentrations of estrogen are quite different. In girls, lower concentrations of estrogen are due to an inactive GnRH system, resulting in a lack of ovarian aromatization of testosterone. In postmenopausal women, there is increased GnRH activity, but because there are no developing follicles with theca and granulosa cells, there is no ovarian response to LH and FSH (Ryan, 1999) (Figure 7-24).

Two related physiological events are involved in the transition to menopause. The first is oocyte depletion and the second is a change in endocrine functioning. Hormonal changes that signal decreased ovarian function begin to occur in the decade before development of frankly irregular cycles. Following the age of 30, the decrease in the oocyte reservoir is accompanied by a decrease in fertility potential (Maroulis, 1997). The rate of atresia of ovarian follicles increases at about 37.5 years (Faddy, Gosden, Gougeon, Richardson, & Nelson, 1992). With the gradual decline in the number of healthy, recruitable follicles, the likelihood of ovulation occurring in any one cycle decreases. As long as the follicles continue to produce any amount of estradiol, the follicular atresia will result in a drop in estradiol levels and menstrual changes.

A decrease in the reservoir below a critical point is associated with changes in ovarian function (Maroulis, 1997). Since production of ovarian hormones, especially

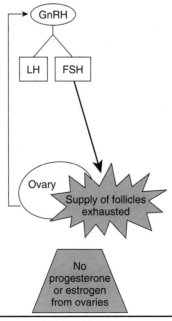

Figure 7-24 Beginning about age 30, there is a more rapid decrease in the number of follicles and a decrease in ovarian production of estradiol. Once the supply of follicles is exhausted, there is no further gonadal production of estradiol or progesterone. The decline and absence of estradiol signals the hypothalamic-pituitary unit to secret FSH. This explains the increase in FSH through the perimenopause.

estrogen, is dependent on cyclic follicular maturation, this decrease in the oocyte reserve results in a reduction in the levels of estrogen and a disruption in the cyclic balance of ovarian and endometrial cycles. Although subtle changes in endocrine and menstrual function can occur for up to 3 years before menopause, it has been shown that a major reduction in ovarian estrogen production does not occur until approximately 6 months before menopause (Lobo, 1997).

The most pronounced endocrine changes in the perimenopause are decreased ovarian production of estradiol, progesterone, testosterone, and inhibin and increased pituitary production of FSH and LH. FSH levels appear to be highest in the early follicular phase of the menstrual cycle, when estradiol levels are lower. Compared to younger women, women aged 45 to 49 have lower mean levels of inhibin while FSH levels are higher. Oocyte depletion begins in fetal life and continues until a few years following menopause, and thus can be viewed as a continuum throughout reproductive life (Maroulis, 1997). It is uncertain to what extent changes in the hypothalamic-pituitary-ovarian axis that occur in the perimenopausal years can be attributed to changes in the ovary and the depletion of oocytes (Rebar, Cedars, & Jiu, 1997).

With the increase in FSH, there is accelerated recruitment of the diminishing pool of follicles. Follicles that still respond to FSH continue to produce estradiol, so during perimenopause, estradiol is still present, although at reduced levels. The increase in FSH at this time is thought to be due to negative feedback from decreasing amounts of inhibin and estradiol in the circulation, resulting from the decrease in large antral follicles. Elevated FSH in the perimenopause results in shorter follicular phases, and accelerated recruitment of follicles by elevated FSH actually increases the rate of follicle loss.

With loss of the last follicles in the ovaries, ovarian estradiol and progesterone production cease, and, in spite of an increase in both LH and FSH, there are no follicles to convert androgens to estrogens and no corpus luteum to produce progesterone. With the loss of steroid-producing follicles in the ovary, steroid stimulation of the uterine lining ceases and menstrual periods stop. Following cessation of menses, occasional and unexpected ovarian activity can occur for a brief period of time.

These events of the perimenopause are highly variable in duration and magnitude from woman to woman. In an epidemiological survey that longitudinally assessed self-reported symptoms across a 5-year span, the mean duration of the perimenopause was 3.5 years. Nearly 10% of the 2570 participants reported no perimenopause transition at all, but rather the persistence of regular cycles until an abrupt cessation of menstruation (McKinlay, Brambilla, & Posner, 1992; Reame, 1997).

During this period of physiological waning of ovarian function, there are corresponding endocrine, somatic, and psychological changes for which estrogen withdrawal provides an explanation. The primary symptoms are seen in the vasomotor system, reproductive target tissues, and psychological/coping mechanisms. Vasomotor symptoms include hot flashes, increased perspiration, and palpitations. The target tissue symptoms include urinary frequency and dysuria and vaginal dryness and discharge (Purdie, 1996). Psychological symptoms include mood swings, irritability, depression, and insomnia. While a minority of women experience no symptoms or menstrual irregularity prior to an abrupt and complete cessation of menses, many women experience 3 years or more of changes prior to menopause and continue to have some episodic fluctuations or ovarian activity (with or without bleeding) for approximately 1 year after menopause.

The hot flash, a sensation of heat primarily felt in the upper body (chest, neck, face, and scalp) is a common experience during the perimenopause (Kronenberg, 1997). The hot flash is a response to what may best be described as a failure of the central nervous system thermostat. In the presence of low or falling plasma estrogen, the thermostat, or thermoregulatory center, located in the hypothalamus, undergoes an acute downset. In other words, the thermostat falsely signals that the body temperature is too high, which calls forth a set of adaptive responses designed to rid the body of the centrally perceived excess heat, thereby reducing core temperature to that demanded by the thermostat. The process is akin to that observed in a patient recovering from a fever. In this context, it is interesting that a diminution of menopausal flashes has been documented in febrile women.

Hot flashes are more common among women of low body weight and may begin before the menopause when ovarian estrogen output is still sufficient to maintain a menstrual cycle. Relative falls in estrogen levels rather than reduced estrogen levels appear to cause the thermoregulatory instability (Purdie, 1996).

The subjective symptoms of the hot flash often occur approximately 45 seconds before the hot flush. The hot flash and its associated flush are characterized as a sudden feeling of warmth. The flash may be followed by the flush, a visible redness of the face, neck, and upper thorax, which may be associated with profuse sweating in the same anatomical region. Hot flashes generally cease approximately 4 to 6 years after the menopause, once the alterations in estrogen production have stabilized in the postmenopausal phase (Kronenberg, 1997). No single situation or factor consistently triggers a hot flash, but hot weather, coffee, spicy food, alcohol, stress, and a hot environment have been implicated.

Some investigators have suggested that an association between mood disorders and perimenopause is purely coincidental, especially in light of the life stresses and changes that often occur during this period of a woman's life. These factors include alteration in family roles, a changing social support network, interpersonal losses, aging, and the onset of physical illness (Cook & Greene, 1981). In addition, specific somatic symptoms, such as hot flashes, may produce a secondary sleep disturbance, resulting in daytime somnolence, decreased energy, and other mood and behavioral symptoms (Schmidt, Roca & Rubinow, 1997). Finally, there is evidence suggesting that these alterations in hormonal levels can directly modulate central nervous system activity.

There does appear to be an alteration of psychobiological responses to stress. Postmenopausal women exhibited greater increases in blood pressure, heart rate, and epinephrine than premenopausal women (Matthews et al., 1986). Lindheim and others (1992) reported that women treated by estrogen replacement therapy via patch evidenced lower maximal systolic blood pressure, ACTH, noradrenalin, and androstenedione responses to psychological stress tests as compared to women treated with placebo. These results suggest that estrogen affects the autonomic nervous system response to acute stress.

The perimenopause, a complex time in which there are unpredictable and wide fluctuations in ovarian function and its physiological consequences, is associated with confusion, symptoms of estrogen deficiency and/or irregular bleeding, and concerns about getting pregnant or not being able to conceive. These experiences occur at a time when women are relatively young chronologically and many are at the peak of their careers. Physiologically at this time, altered estrogen availability leads to an increase in the risk factors for several health problems, including cardiovascular disease and osteoporosis. Although a greater understanding of this perimenopause is warranted, the events associated with the transition to menopause and those due to advancing chronological age often are so intertwined that it is difficult to distinguish among the phenomena relative to each process (Lobo, 1997).

The perimenopausal years can be a time of positive change, growth, and transition in the lives of women. As women begin to examine their perimenopausal experiences, they challenge male-biased theories that emphasize deficiency and disease. Research from the 1960s to the 1980s focused on problems such as treatment of climacteric symptoms, depression and irritability, and nonadherence to hormonal therapies. Experiences of women based on assumptions of health are documented in the literature of the 1990s and challenge the idea that a hot flash is symptomatic of disease (Hautman, 1996).

Menopause

Menopause is identified by the absence of a menstrual period for a period of 12 months; thus a definitive diagnosis of menopause is necessarily retrospective (Greendale & Judd, 1993). Although most investigators judge this absence of menstruation for more than 1 year in the appropriate age group (over 40 years) as a fairly reliable indicator of menopause, 4.5% of women over the age of 52 will have at least one more episode of menstruation following menopause (Wallace, Sherman, Bean, Treloar, & Schlabaugh, 1979). Vaginal bleeding occurring more than 1 year after the menopause is defined as postmenopausal bleeding and must be investigated because of an incidence of 10% to 20% of underlying genital tract malignancy. Nevertheless, a majority of such episodes of bleeding occur in the absence of pathology and are probably associated with growth and atresia and, rarely, even ovulation of a sporadic ovarian follicle (Fraser, 1997).

The median age for natural menopause in the United States is 51.4 years. Menopause at an earlier age has been reportedly related to lower socioeconomic class, smoking, and late onset of menarche, while menopause at a later age may occur in women who experience early onset of puberty or were relatively older at the time of the last pregnancy (Ferin, Jewelewicz, & Warren, 1993; Weel et al., 1999). Estrogen production by the postmenopausal ovary usually is minimal, and, as a result, circulating levels of estrogen decline. Even when the ovaries are removed, there is no further decrease in circulating or excreted estrogens. The source of circulating estrogens in postmenopausal women is *extragonadal aromatization.* Androgens, particularly androstenedione produced principally in the adrenal gland, are converted to estrogen outside of the ovary or the adrenals. While not all sites of this conversion have been identified, aromatization has been shown to occur in fat, liver, kidney, and specific nuclei of the hypothalamus. The estrogen end product of this conversion is estrone, the primary estrogen of the menopause (Jaffe, 1986). Low levels of estradiol that remain in the circulation are derived from estrone (Ryan, 1999). Serum estradiol levels are lower than the serum estrone concentration. Postmenopausal levels of estradiol average 15 picograms (pg) per mililiter, while serum estrone values average 30 pg/mL but may be higher in obese women as aromatization increases as a function of the mass of adipose tissue. There is also evidence that many postmenopausal women experience reduced adrenal endocrine function, evidenced by lower concentrations of circulating cortisol and androstenedione (Burger, 1999).

Developmental Concerns of Aging Women

As mentioned, it is difficult to discern which changes are directly related to the decrease in circulating estrogens and which are due specifically to the process of aging. In general, aging is associated with a decrease in the number of cells in the body, due to some combination of decreased cell division and increased cell death, and to malfunction of many of the cells that remain. The intermediate cause of these changes is probably an interference in the function of the cells' macromolecules (i.e., DNA, RNA, and cell proteins) and in the flow of information between them. One theory regarding these changes centers on the progressive accumulation of damage to the macromolecules, while another hypothesizes that cellular senescence is actually programmed in our genes; that is, certain genes responsible for the aging process become activated as one grows older.

The main physiological manifestation of aging is a gradual deterioration in the function of virtually all tissues and organ systems and in the capacity of the body's homeostatic systems to respond to environmental stresses. It is difficult to sort out the extent to which any particular age-related change is due to aging itself or is secondary to disease or lifestyle changes.

For instance, until recently it was believed that the functioning of the nervous system markedly deteriorated as a result of aging per se. It seems, however, that this conclusion was based on studies of individuals with age-related diseases. More recent studies of people without such diseases do document changes, such as loss of memory, increased difficulty in learning new tasks, slower processing by the brain, and loss of brain mass. These changes are modest, however, and most brain functions considered to underlie intelligence seem to remain relatively intact.

A similar reevaluation of changes in cardiac function with age suggests that much of the decrease in the ability of the heart to pump blood both at rest and during exercise in older people may be the result of disease and lifestyle changes (decreased physical activity) rather than the aging process itself. In contrast, a 30% to 40% decrease (somewhat less in women) in limb muscle mass and strength occurs in men between 30 and 80 years of age due to aging changes per se. Physically active individuals have greater strength at any given age compared to inactive persons, but the rate of decline with age is similar.

Finally, there is a belief that aging accelerates after menopause due to certain changes in physical functioning and in the tissues and organs of the body. To discriminate between the effects of aging and the effects of disease, one would need to study physiological trends in a population that is not diseased. By virtue of their longer lives, women are more susceptible to emerging conditions that affect the aged. Research to elucidate genetic, hormonal, and other mechanisms that affect aging and longevity in men versus women could lead to reductions in the economic burdens of illness and frailty (Pinn, 1995). Postmenopausal changes in the breast, bone, skin, and urinary bladder have been associated with changes in estrogen levels.

Breast

A decrease in the size of the breasts is common during perimenopause (Jaffe, 1986). Estrogen has a profound stimulatory influence on breast ductal epithelium (Mady, 2000). In fact, changes in ovarian endocrine functioning can significantly alter the mammographic examination by gradually changing density patterns (Hindle, 1997). Replacement of breast glandular tissue by fat begins at about age 25, and, as estrogen decreases, the process accelerates. As menopause advances, involution of the breast takes place and glandular tissue reverts toward the infantile state. Fatty tissue disappears more slowly and gradually becomes the chief tissue component (Beiler, 1990). There is marked variation in the mammographic density at a given age; however, almost all women experience a progressive decrease in density of the breast glandular tissue beginning in the early reproductive years and continuing through the perimenopausal and postmenopausal years (Hindle, 1997).

Bone Loss

Bone is dynamic and is constantly being remodeled (Legato, 1997a). The bone remodeling cycle begins with the appearance of osteoclasts at a bone surface. These marrow-derived cells excavate a cavity in the underlying bone over a period of 2 to 3 weeks, and once this excavation is complete, the cavity becomes lined with osteoblasts, or bone-forming cells, which proceed to lay down new bone and mineralize. For the bone to be in balance, the amount of bone formed must be equal to the amount previously resolved. This is generally the case in premenopausal women and in healthy men (Purdie, 1996; Spelsberg, Subramaniam, Riggs, & Khosla, 1999).

Estrogen withdrawal at menopause, whether natural or induced, is associated with a series of alterations in bone cell behavior that culminate in bone loss and increased susceptibility to fracture. The fall in ambient estradiol at the menopause results in a decoupling, or imbalance, such that the bone removed fails to be matched by subsequent bone formation, resulting in a net loss of bone and eventually a reduction in the number, thickness, and connectedness of the bone trabeculae. Key sites at which this occurs are the legs, neck, distal radius, and spine. The trabeculae confer great strength, allowing bone to fulfill its function of shock absorption and protecting against fracture. Hence, the net long-term results of estrogen deficiency are loss of bone mineral density and increased fractures.

When bone mineral density has fallen to between 1 and 2.5 standard deviations below the mean for young normal women in the population, the bone is said to be osteopenic. When bone mineral density is more than 2.5 standard deviations below the young normal mean, the bone is said to be osteoporotic. The most accelerated phase of bone loss occurs immediately after menopause and decelerates 8 to 10 years later. This phenomenon is not exclusively related to estrogen deficiency, and only 20% of women develop osteoporotic fractures within 20 years after their menses stop (Legato, 1997a).

Cells of the osteoblast lineage contain estrogen receptors that are presumably involved in the subcellular mechanisms through which estrogen deficiency uncouples bone reabsorption formation. The direct effect of estrogen on bone does not account for the full effect of menopause on the skeleton. There is evidence that calcitropic hormones are also involved. The three classic calcitropic hormones are parathyroid hormone, calcitonin, and 1-25 dihydroxyvitamin D. Slight reductions in circulatory parathyroid hormone and vitamin D occur postmenopausally, which probably reflect a homeostatic response to the increased release of calcium into the circulation as a consequence of higher bone turnover. Calcitonin has a powerful inhibitory effect on the osteoclasts and has long been thought to be a likely mediator of postmenopausal bone loss. Basal levels of calcitonin are lower in postmenopausal than in premenopausal women, and absolute values correlate with ambient estrogen concentrations.

Skin Tone

All individuals experience chronological or intrinsic aging at a variable, genetically determined rate. The associated skin changes include atrophy, wrinkling, and decreased elasticity. There is a gradual loss of dermal collagen and subcutaneous fat. Because of these changes, the skin is more susceptible to mechanical trauma. Reduction in the density of sweat ducts and sebaceous glands is reflected in a decreased perspiration and sebum production. In postmenopausal women, decreased estrogen contributes to the development of these aging phenomena (Mercurio, 1998).

Estrogen receptors have been identified in the skin, and a higher estrogen receptor content has been observed in women. The menopause related decline in skin collagen content as well as alterations in elastic fibers cause an increased laxity of the skin (Mercurio, 1998). With menopause, the skin becomes dry, the epidermis becomes thinner, and there is a gradual increase in pigmentation because of an increase in the rate of melanin production. These changes are gradual and become accentuated over the years. Estrogen administration induces dermal edema and increased epidermal proliferation (Ferin, Jewelewicz, & Warren, 1993). Biological support for a hormonal association with skin problems includes the melanin-induced pigmentary changes that arise during pregnancy and the peak incidence of melanoma coinciding with childbearing age (Mercurio, 1998).

Urinary Incontinence

It has long been understood that urinary symptoms are an integral part of the transition from the perimenopausal to the postmenopausal state. Loss of estrogen causes atrophic changes not only in the vagina but also in the bladder, urethra, and periurethral tissues.

Tissues become thin and friable due to the loss of the bulk of the periurethral tissues and the coaptation of the urethral mucosa. Such atrophic changes increase a woman's susceptibility to urinary tract infections and can cause irritative symptoms such as urethritis, urinary frequency, urgency and dysuria, vaginal dryness, and dyspareunia. Irritation in the bladder wall and urethra is believed to cause the bladder to spasm, resulting in urge incontinence. The female pelvic floor contains estrogen and progesterone receptors. Given the evidence that atrophy of these tissues can be reversed with estrogen, and that estrogen replacement reduces incontinence in many cases, it seem reasonable to propose that estrogen loss contributes to this problem (Grady et al., 2001; Hextall, 2000).

While urinary incontinence is a prevalent condition, affecting both men and women of all ages, women are more likely to develop the condition. Knowledge of female anatomy and physiology, together with epidemiological data, has provided considerable information regarding the multitude of factors that contribute to female incontinence. Women have a shorter urethra and less skeletal muscle bulk and strength. They have a posterior opening in the urogenital diaphragm that allows the bladder to descend, integrating with the urethrovesical junction, causing intrinsic urethral insufficiency and allowing bladder hypermobility. The higher prevalence of obesity in women (Foreyt & Poston, 1998; Rosenbaum, Leibel, & Hirsch, 1997) as well as the experiences of pregnancy and childbirth account for much of the damage or compromise to pelvic structures that produce incontinence (Cummings & Rodning, 2000; MacLennan, Taylor, Wilson, & Wilson, 2000; Parazzini et al., 2000). In addition, the estrogen depletion associated with menopause can alter the urethral tissues, lowering urethral coaptation and resistance and possibly making women more susceptible to urine loss (Burgio & Goode, 1997; Burgio, Locher, & Goode, 2000). Finally, the urinary and lower genital tracts share a common embryological origin, thus estrogen-sensitive changes in the urethral architecture are similar to those in the vagina (Purdie, 1996).

Atherosclerosis and Cardiovascular Disease

Several common cardiovascular diseases demonstrate gender specificity. Presenting symptoms, frequency and extent of evaluation, age of onset, treatment approaches, and outcomes differ in men and women (Hsia, 1995). The relationship between estrogens and the pathogenesis of atherosclerosis, myocardial infarction, hypertension, and stroke is still unclear. Several studies have found a possible association between decreased estrogen production and increased incidence of atherosclerosis. Changes in blood lipids probably play an important role in the genesis of atherosclerosis and cardiovascular disease (Ferin, Jewelewicz, & Warren, 1993). Estrogens have numerous actions on several physiological processes, including lipid metabolism, carbohydrate metabolism, coagulation parameters, and blood pressure, which could influence the risk of cardiovascular disease. Under the conditions of natural menopause (which occurs with increase in age and decrease in estrogen secretion), a proatherogenic state is produced, which is evidenced by increased triglyceride levels; quantitative and qualitative alterations in low-density lipoproteins (LDLs), cholesterol, and triglycerides; increased levels of intermediate-density lipoproteins (IDLs); and structural modifications in high-density lipoproteins (HDLs) that could alter their function in reverse cholesterol transport (Stevenson, 2000). The magnitude of lipid change was compared in the first 69 women in the Healthy Women Study who experienced a natural menopause. These post-menopausal women experienced a two-fold increase in LDL cholesterol and a small but significant decrease in total HDL cholesterol when compared to age-matched pre-menopausal controls (Matthews et al., 1989).

Estrogen Replacement Therapy

Estrogen replacement therapy is a prescriptive option to reduce or alleviate bothersome symptoms of menopause or to sustain the general physiological benefits of estrogen. Estrogen replacement therapy (ERT), also called *hormone replacement therapy (HRT),* is associated with maintenance of muscle and skin tone, an enhanced sense of well-being and sexual functioning, reduction in hot flashes and vaginal dryness, a preservation of bone mass. Although highly touted as a preventive therapy for multiple aging effects, there is much debate over its safety and effectiveness, and more studies are needed to resolve these questions (Santoro et al., 1999).

Risk and benefit estimates for hormone replacement vary, depending on the target tissue, the duration of effects, the nature and timing of therapy, and adherence to the prescribed regimen.

Most early studies on estrogen therapy used a conjugated equine estrogen, known as unopposed estrogen (due to lack of progestin in the therapy). In the early 1990s, the Postmenopausal Estrogen/Progestin Interventions (PEPI) Trial was conducted to assess the effects of unopposed estrogen vs. three estrogen/progestin formulations on selected cardiac risk factors in healthy postmenopausal women. It was expected that combined therapy regimens would be superior to unopposed estrogen because they mimic hormonal exposure during the menstrual cycle and thus would reduce the risk of endometrial cancer, associated with unopposed estrogen (PEPI Trial Writing Group, 1995). More than 875 women participated in this prospective randomized, double-blind, placebo-controlled trial. In contrast to the expected outcome, positive effects of unopposed estrogen therapy were greater than those of combined regimens; however, a higher rate of endometrial hyperplasia was associated with unopposed therapy.

There is extensive but inconclusive evidence regarding the use of unopposed estrogen or combined hormonal therapy and the risk of breast cancer. Current data suggest that if therapy is continued for less than 5 years, the risk for breast cancer is probably not increased. When either unopposed estrogen or combined hormonal therapy is used for a period of 10 to 20 years, a 25% increase in breast cancer risk has been reported (Grady et al., 1992). In addition, estrogen therapy has been advocated as a way to prevent urinary incontinence and osteoporosis.

Antiestrogens, which were first developed for use in the treatment of estrogen-dependent tumors, work by binding to estrogen receptors, thus blocking estrogen from binding to them. This also blocks estrogen from activating genes for specific growth-promoting proteins (Figure 7-25).

The estrogen receptor can bind with other proteins that either repress or potentiate its activity. Selective estrogen receptor modulators (SERMs), such as tamoxifen and raloxifene, have differing effects on estrogen responsive tissues. Continued research with SERMs and a greater understanding of the structure and function of the estrogen receptor should produce more therapeutic applications for SERMs (Sadovsky & Adler, 1998) (Figure 7-26).

There has been much recent interest in lifestyle and dietary factors that can influence hormonal levels and ultimately influence a woman's transition experience. Phytoestrogens are plant substances that are structurally and functionally similar to estradiol or that produce estrogenic effects. Phytoestrogens are structurally similar to tamoxifen (Horn-Ross, 1995), and it has been suggested that phytoestrogens should be considered natural SERMs. Phytoestrogens can act as either estrogen agonists or estrogen antagonists. As estrogen agonists, phytoestrogens can bind to estradiol receptors

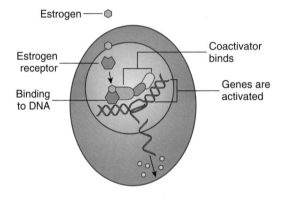

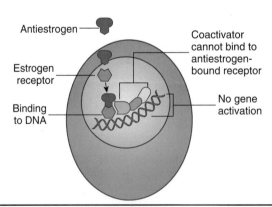

Figure 7-25 Antiestrogens bind to the estrogen receptor, preventing estrogen from binding. Although the receptor permits the binding of the alternate substance, the estrogen response element is not able to merge with the coactivators, and there is no transcription or translation of protein. The contrasting cellular responses to estrogens and antiestrogens are shown. (Based on artwork originally created for the National Cancer Institute. Copyright 2000 Jeanne Kelly.)

and produce estrogenic effects, such as relief of hot flashes. Antiestrogenic effects occur when phytoestrogens competitively bind to estrogen receptors, blocking the binding of more potent endogenous estrogens. Phytoestrogens seem to be estrogen agonists for the cardiovascular system, bone, and brain, all of which have predominantly estrogen beta

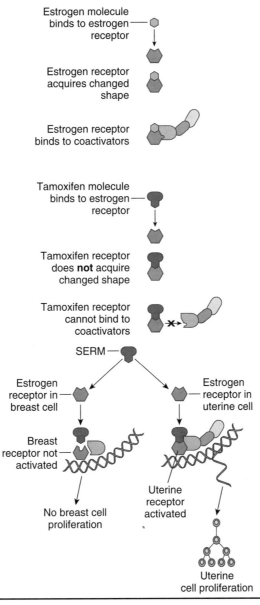

Figure 7-26 Selective estrogen receptor modulators (SERMs) were developed based on the actions of antiestrogens. The differences in response of estrogen and a SERM within a cell are depicted. (Based on artwork originally created for the National Cancer Institute. Copyright 2000 Jeanne Kelly.)

receptors, and antagonists for the breast and uterus, which contain predominantly estrogen alpha receptors (Clarkson, 2000).

GENDER-SPECIFIC BIOLOGY, PHYSIOLOGY, AND CLINICAL RESEARCH

There are many known gender differences in disease epidemiology and health outcomes. Ten specific health-related differences between men and women are found in Box 7-1.

Gender-based biology has the potential to revolutionize the way in which we understand health and disease for both women and men (Society for Women's Health Research, 2001). To study the differences in normal functioning and in disease manifestations in women and men is to take advantage of a natural experiment (Legato, 1997a). From such studies, a more accurate picture of human biology and new insights into the mechanisms of disease can emerge.

Activities in science and medicine are reflective of what is important and valued within the culture; thus a surge of interest in women's health was an inevitable outcome of the women's movement (Legato, 1997b; Pinn, 1998). In fact, three unique suffrage movements in women's history have contributed to this increased interest (Pinn, 1998). The first wave of suffrage resulted in the right to vote. This first movement was a crucial first step in women becoming full partners in shaping and influencing the home and community. Educational and economic opportunities for women were the focus of the

---

Box 7-1 10 SPECIFIC HEALTH-RELATED DIFFERENCES BETWEEN MEN AND WOMEN

- After consuming the same amount of alcohol, women have a higher blood alcohol content than men, even when allowing for body size differences.
- Women who smoke are 20% to 70% more likely to develop lung cancer than men who smoke the same amount of cigarettes.
- Women tend to wake up from anesthesia more quickly than men do—an average of 7 minutes for women and 11 minutes for men.
- Some pain medications, known as kappa-opiates, are far more effective in relieving pain in women than in men.
- Women are more likely than men to suffer a second heart attack within 1 year of their first heart attack.
- The same drug can cause different reactions and different side effects in women and men—even common drugs like antihistamines and antibiotics.
- Just as women have stronger immune systems to protect them from disease, women are more likely to get autoimmune diseases (diseases where the body attacks its own tissues), such as rheumatoid arthritis, lupus, scleroderma, and multiple sclerosis.
- During unprotected intercourse with an infected partner, women are 2 times more likely than men to contract a sexually transmitted disease and 10 times more likely to contract HIV.
- Depression is 2 to 3 times more common in women than in men, in part because women's brains make less of the hormone serotonin.
- After menopause women lose more bone than men, which is why 80% of people with osteoporosis are women.

Source: Society for Women's Health Research (2001). *10 differences between men and women that make a difference in women's health, www.womenshealth.org/insert8.HTM.*

women's movement of the late 1960s and early 1970s. The emphasis on women's health that we are witnessing now is also a suffrage movement, one that of necessity grew out of the two earlier movements, as women began to focus on their quality of life. All three movements should be seen as a continuum. Although individual health usually transcends other concerns, be they social or political, women's health all too often has been held hostage to social and political agendas.

Women's health research has evolved in response to demands that research include women in clinical studies, making women rather than men the medical model for research on conditions that affect them, and that research on conditions affecting women's health must be an integral part of contemporary scientific investigation.

There are diverse explanations for the exclusion of women from clinical trials. From a historical perspective, several events led to the exemption of women from study. The abuse of human experimental subjects during World War II in the name of science were exposed in the Doctors' Trials at Nuremburg. Civilized nations responded with legislation to protect humans from ever again being exploited as they had been by Nazi physicians. Women, particularly those of reproductive age and those who were pregnant, were excluded from clinical investigation, as were children and other vulnerable populations. Although this did not prevent researchers in underdeveloped countries from subjecting both men and women to inappropriate interventions, it did lead to mainstream American investigations being limited to men.

Clinical investigation on male subjects has been perceived as, in general, easier and cheaper. To study a population whose internal environment is changing on a cyclic basis, as is the case for premenopausal women, more subjects are required to achieve meaningful results. Many scientists warn that including women in clinical trials makes clinical research unnecessarily expensive and ultimately may limit the amount of scientific investigation that can be funded from finite resources. Women's cyclical hormonal changes confound research results. Less homogenous study populations would require gender-specific hypotheses or subgroup analyses.

Recruitment of women into studies is more difficult. There is a certain wariness due to the thalidomide tragedy and anticipation of legal and ethical problems surrounding potential harm to the fetus in a pregnant or potentially pregnant woman. In many cases, women themselves refuse to participate in clinical trials because they fear that their ability to conceive and bear healthy children will be compromised (Legato, 1998; Matthews et al. 1997).

Within the research community, some still hold the notion that women's health issues are of secondary importance, especially those that solely affect women and those that occur in men and women but have already been studied chiefly in men. However, there are four major physiological factors that explain differences in the incidence of some diseases among subgroups of women: sex steroid hormone metabolism, reproduction, anatomy, and immune responses (Ness & Kuller, 1997). In addition, lifestyle factors, environmental variables, the physical and social environment, and genetic host susceptibility interact to affect the health status of women. Women tend to take care of everyone else first, which often means that such things as regular exercise, health screenings, and adherence to medical regimens and appropriate diets do not receive proper attention.

Women have long been underrepresented in medical research. Historically, women's health research focused on diseases affecting fertility and reproduction. Research focused disproportionately on men because of the excess premature mortality in men, concerns that women's changing hormone levels could confound study results, and the possibility of pregnancy occurring during the trial (Matthews et al., 1997). Unfortunately, within the medical community, the adult woman has been classified as either premenopausal or postmenopausal. Legato (1999) states, "We have developed a restrictive and entirely regrettable tendency to pigeonhole women, as soon as they reach puberty, with one of two black-and-while labels: 'premenopausal' (read: young, sexy, viable, attractive, and healthy) and 'postmenopausal' (read: suffering from an endocrinopathy for which estrogen is the cure, no longer desirable and in sexual decline, requiring bolstering on all fronts to maintain optimal function)."

Based on these rationales for exclusion of women from study, five distinct forms of gender bias in medicine have been described, namely androcentricity, overgeneralization, gender insensitivity, double standards, and failure of identification (Wallis, 1993). Andocentricity, the use of the male frame of reference, perceives women as deviations from male physical and biochemical parameters. Overgeneralization occurs when the findings of a study of only one sex are applied to both sexes. Disregard of sex as a socially or medically important variable is labeled gender insensitivity. Such insensitivity makes it impossible to devise gender-sensitive treatments for women or men. Double standards affect evaluation and treatment or measurement of identical behaviors, traits, or situations by different means. As a result, women may not receive as aggressive a response to a complaint of chest pain or headache. Finally, a failure of identification (i.e., "If we don't experience it, it doesn't exist") is a paradigm that emphasizes the treatment of problems associated with men and has led to a lessened response to disorders that are primarily female.

Krieger and Fee (1994) emphasize the social environment as the gestalt of women's health and research. It is their contention that theories of women's inequality originated in the early 19th century when traditionalists cited scripture to prove women's inferiority. Scientists employed several measurements, such as the size of women's skulls, the length of their bones, the rate of their breathing, and the number of their blood cells, to conclude that women were the weaker sex. By the late 19th century, theories of race, gender, and class inequality were linked to the theory of Social Darwinism, which promised to provide a scientific basis for social policy. Other developments in the early 20th century encouraged biological explanations for sex differences in disease and in social roles. The discovery of the sex chromosomes in 1905 reinforced the idea that gender was a fundamental biological trait, built into the genetic constitution of the body. By the mid-1920s researchers had isolated several hormones integral to reproductive physiology and popularized the notion of sex hormones. This combination of sex chromosomes and sex hormones was imbued with almost magical powers to shape human behavior in gendered terms. Women were now at the mercy of their genetic limitations and a changing brew of hormonal imperatives. In the realm of medicine, researchers turned to sex chromosomes and hormones to understand cancers of the uterus and breast and a host of other sex-linked diseases. They no longer saw the need to worry about environmental influences. In the first few decades of the 20th century, these views were institutionalized within scientific medicine and the new field of public health. White men were used as the research subjects of choice for all health conditions other than those involving women's reproductive health, and this framework has shaped knowledge and practice to the present.

The first step in creating an alternative understanding is to recognize that the categories we traditionally treat as simply biological are in fact largely social. The second step is to realize that we need social concepts to understand these social categories, and the third is to develop social measures and appropriate strategies for a new kind of health research (Krieger & Fee, 1994).

Krieger and Fee (1994) caution that discussions of women's reproductive health that ignore social patterns of disease and focus only on endogenous factors are inadequate. We cannot assume that biology alone will provide the answers we need; instead we must reframe the issues in the context of the social shaping of our human lives as both biological creatures and historical actors. Otherwise, we will continue to mistake what is for what must be and leave unchallenged the social forces that continue to create vast inequalities in health care.

On the other hand, social policies are best based on the broadest understanding of the processes underlying them. Just as clearly, the social implications of a program designed to study social behavior cannot be ignored, no matter how "basic" the research. Social explanations have not in any sense been outflanked. Instead, both social and biological levels of explanation need to be enriched, with more attention paid to how they codevelop and interact. No one theoretical perspective can completely capture the dynamics of complex social, sexual, and cultural phenomena (Rabinowitz & Valian, 2000).

The more that is known about differences and similarities between the sexes, the more we will be able to administer efficacious prevention and therapies for everyone. While this chapter is intended to review women's physical health and functioning, opportunities to point out functional differences emerge from health problems that are unique to or more prevalent in women. Thus the following section is organized around disorders and conditions that have been the focus of gender-based research.

Depression

Epidemiological data from around the world demonstrate that major depression is approximately twice as common in women than men (Desai & Jann, 2000). The essential features of major depression are low mood and/or loss of interest or pleasure in usual activities. The disturbance is prominent, persistent, and associated with impaired functioning and a variety of other symptoms, including appetite and sleep disturbance, weight changes, psychomotor agitation or retardation, decreased energy, feelings of worthlessness or guilt, difficulty concentrating, and thoughts of death and suicide. The gender disparity in the rates of depression begins early, at around age 13 to 15, and is maintained throughout life. There is a peak of onset in the childbearing years, but no evidence of an increase during the menopausal years (Weissman & Olfson, 1995).

Depression, a multifactorial disorder influenced by numerous risk factors, is usually treated by psychotherapy and pharmacotherapy. Little information exists regarding sex differences in the effectiveness of antidepressants for patients at any age. In 1992, Jensvold published one of the first studies of the menstrual cycle's impact on psychoactive drugs like antidepressants. She discovered that for many women, a constant blood level of these drugs can be achieved only by varying the drug dose through the monthly estrogen-progesterone cycle. Some data suggest that women may be less responsive than men to tricyclic antidepressants. Differences between women and men have been described in regard to drug absorption, volume of distribution, hepatic metabolism, body weight, total blood volume, percentage of body fat, renal clearance, and a variety of other physiological variables that may affect drug availability (Weissman & Olfson, 1995).

Cognitive Functioning

The effects of estrogen and progesterone on brain structure and function have been the subject of much research. This interest is grounded in the recognition that depression and other affective disorders are more common in women and that a decline in cognitive functioning, including memory, is more prevalent in elderly women than in elderly men. An earlier assumption was that this prevalence was a phenomenon based on the greater number of women than men who survive into their 80s, which is the age when the incidence of dementia and Alzheimer's disease increases. In fact, progesterone and estrogen have physiological roles in fine motor skills and motor coordination, analgesia and pain pathways, affective state and mood, neural excitability, and declarative and episodic memory. Sex differences and estrogen effects have been documented in the serotonergic, cholinergic, dopaminergic, and noradrenergic systems that may contribute to these physiological findings (McEwen, 1998).

Numerous basic science studies point to properties of estrogen that support a biological role for the hormone in modulating mood and cognition in humans. The hippocampus is a brain region involved in memory function in humans and animals. Studies of the hippocampus show that estrogen increases the efficacy of synapses and potentiates neuronal transmission (McEwen & Woolley, 1994). Estrogen influences neurotransmitter systems relevant to Alzheimer's disease, and, in some model systems, it modulates synaptic plasticity (Pfaff et al., 2000). Estrogen also augments cholinergic function, cerebral blood flow, and cerebral glucose utilization. Additional effects that may modulate cognitive functioning include influences on antiinflammation, apolipoprotein E, and amyloid precursor protein metabolism. Estrogen may also blunt neurotoxic consequences of the stress response mediated by the hypothalamic-pituitary-adrenal axis. Central nervous system estrogen effects that can modulate mood include monoamine oxidase inhibition at high levels and tryptophan displacement from plasma albumin binding sites (Small, 1998).

Pain Sensitivity

Pain sensitivity has been examined in observational and experimental studies, and results from epidemiological studies indicate that women have higher rates of migraine and nonmigraine headaches, facial and oral pain, back pain, and musculoskeletal pain.

To understand gender differences in pain response, men and women have been subjected to painful stimuli in relation to pain tolerance or pain threshold. Analytical reviews of these studies revealed a tendency for women to be more sensitive to mechanical pressure or electrical stimuli than men. In addition, women were found to have a more enhanced sensitivity to pain (Fillingim & Ness, 2000; Riley, Robinson, Wise, Myers, & Fillingim, 1998).

Differences in physiological response to pain have also been documented. In a study of sustained forearm ischemia, women reported more intense pain, while men had a more pronounced cardiovascular response as indicated by an elevation in arterial blood pressure (Maixner & Humphrey, 1993). In addition, there are differences in response to analgesics used to treat pain, with kappa-agonist opioids producing greater analgesia in women than men (Gear et al., 1996). Nonsteroidal antiinflammatory drugs (NSAIDs) have been found to have a stronger analgesic effect in men than in women, even though similar plasma concentrations of the drug were present (Walker & Carmody, 1998).

Drug Metabolism

To understand gender differences in drug effects, there are three areas to be explored, namely pharmacokinetics, pharmacodynamics, and pharmacogenetics (Berg, 1998a). Pharmacokinetics refers to the activity of drugs in the body over time, including the processes of absorption, distribution, tissue localization, biotransformation, and excretion. Pharmacodynamics is the study of the biochemical and physiological effects of drugs and their mechanisms of action. Pharmacogenetics deals with the relationship between genetic factors and the nature of responses to drugs.

The cytochrome P450 family is the main enzyme group involved in drug metabolism and is the focus of study when hereditary variation in response to drugs is of interest. The P450 enzymes metabolize an extensive list of medications. Sex hormones, drug interactions (inhibitors and inducers), and social factors (drinking caffeine-containing beverages and smoking) affect P450 enzymes. Physiological processes that involve enzymes from this family include steroid metabolism, drug deactivation, procarcinogen activation, and xenobiotic detoxification. Two general functions of the P450 system are bioregulation and immune defense for small molecules. Health-related aspects of the P450 system include its ability to regulate salt, water, and glucose balance, reproduction, and even pain.

While a full discussion of the P450 system is beyond the scope of this chapter, there are gender-bound differences of interest. For example, women express higher levels of CYP 3A, the P450 subfamily that metabolizes such drugs as cyclosporine, diazepam, imipramine, midazolam, nifedipine, quinidine, sex hormones, tamoxifen, verapamil, and warfarin (Berg, 1998b).

Immune Function

Both clinical and experimental observations indicate that sex steroids influence the immune system in a variety of ways. Following immunization, female animals usually produce higher titers of antibodies than males. Furthermore, the prevalence of many serious clinical autoimmune diseases is several-fold higher in women than men, and many autoimmune diseases in women first appear or peak during periods of major hormonal changes (puberty, menopause). High estrogen states exacerbate systemic lupus erythematosis but often decrease the severity of autoimmune arthritis. The immune system changes dramatically with age; immune function peaks at puberty and gradually declines thereafter. The age-related decline in immune function primarily occurs in the T-cell compartment of the immune system (Anderson, 1997).

CONTRIBUTIONS OF NURSING TO THE HEALTH OF WOMEN ACROSS THE LIFESPAN

There are several actions that nurses can take to advance the understanding of women's unique health and development issues. First, the nurse can translate complex scientific information in a way that will allow meaningful choices in regard to health practices and treatment.

Consistent with the responsibility for advocacy, the nurse can advocate for access to the most advanced health care technologies for all women. In general, women must be encouraged to take action that will lead to better health. Since the 1960s, women have increasingly demanded self-determination in matters of health care, both in terms of understanding their bodies better and being informed about what is happening to them, so that they can make informed choices. Nurses have responded to consumer interest in self-help because their professional mandate has historically been expressed in terms of helping people gain independence. Because a patient's viewpoint is the starting point for considerations regarding assessment, treatment, and outcome, a person's everyday thoughts and feelings are accorded respect. This style, which is intuitive, sensitive to alternative views, personal, collaborative, and humanistic, is central to the nursing professional and to feminist methods. In both, experiential analysis is valued within situational constraints (McBride, 1997).

The nurse can utilize the expanding science base regarding sex and gender differences to inform clinical practice. In many respects, this is a difficult charge. Advances in molecular techniques and in the understanding of the genome require the nurse to think differently about health, disease, and appropriate interventions to improve health. The functional state of the cell and the response of the body, as well as the psychosocial response, will need to be a part of our working knowledge. As nurses we have been advocates of the view that women's health requires more than a biomedical view, and have called for an enhanced awareness of the context of women's lives (Writing Group of the 1996 AAN Expert Panel on Women's Health, 1997).

Finally, the nurse can contribute to this burgeoning area of science through astute clinical observations. This entails accurate reporting that includes the differences in response patterns of men and women and by subgroups of women, particularly in terms of age, race, and other meaningful demographics. In an analysis and critique of the women's health research agenda, Woods (1994) employs Haraway's (1988) concept of the "situated knower." The situated knower can have only a partial perspective on a problem based on position. The nurse is situated by profession and gender and therefore must seek multiple perspectives in planning and conducting research and in administering clinical care. Cognizant of our partial perspective, we have a need for more complex understanding when constructing studies and must regard women as legitimate sources of knowledge about their own lives and health (Woods, 1994).

SUMMARY

Recent scientific advances in the gender specificity of health and disease have great implication for clinical practice. Discoveries in the laboratory that relate to physical changes in cellular, organ, or system functioning have not been directly linked to the multiple external forces, such as lifestyle and socioeconomic status, known to influence disease. Just as male-modeled discoveries cannot be generalized to the human race, the temptation to generalize gender-related findings to all women must also be resisted. Race and age are also important factors in the overall equation for health. A clinician who is sensitive to the effects of the hormonal milieu must strive to record fully the status of a woman in terms of her cycle and physiological life stage. Research for women's health must be multidisciplinary, involving basic, clinical, behavioral, and epidemiological researchers willing to consider alternative explanations for observed events. While it is of utmost importance that women participate as subjects in research studies, researchers and clinicians have a responsibility to ensure that data will be used in a manner that will resolve gender inequalities. The ultimate objective of good science is to enhance biological understanding and inform the development of policies and medical standards that will benefit both women and men (Pinn, 1995).

REFERENCES

Albano, R. M., Arkell, R., Beddington, R. S., & Smith, J. C. (1994). Expression of inhibin subunits and follistatin during postimplantation mouse development: Decidual expression of activin and expression of follistatin in primitive streak, somites and hindbrain. *Development, 120*(4), 803–813.

Andersen, C., & Byskov, A. (1996). Gonadal differentiation. In S. Hillier, H. Kitchener, & J. Neilson (Eds.), *Scientific essentials of reproductive medicine* (pp. 105–119). London: W. B. Saunders.

Anderson, D. (1997). Interrelationship between endocrine and immunologic phenomena during the perimenopause. In R. Lobo (Ed.), *Perimenopause* (pp. 78–86). New York: Springer.

Archer, D. (1997). Medical management of menorrhagia in pre-and perimenopausal women. In R. Lobo (Ed.), *Perimenopause* (pp. 271–280). New York: Springer.

Barrett-Connor, E., & Bush, T. L. (1991). Estrogen and coronary heart disease in women. *Journal of the American Medical Association 265*(14), 1861–1867.

Bauer-Dantoin, A. C., Weiss, J., & Jameson, J. L. (1996). Gonadotropin-releasing hormone regulation of pituitary follistatin gene expression during the primary follicle-stimulating hormone surge. *Endocrinology, 137*(5), 1634–1639.

Beiler, F. (1990). Development and anatomy of the breast. In G. Mitchel & L. Bassett (Eds.), *The female breast and its disorders* (pp. 1–12). Baltimore: Williams & Wilkins.

Berg, M. J. (1998a). Drugs, vitamins, and gender. *Journal of Gender Specific Medicine, 1*(1), 10–11.

Berg, M. J. (1998b). Gender-specific prescribing: medications and the menstrual cycle. *Journal of Gender Specific Medicine, 1*(3), 17–19.

Berne, R. W., & Levy, M. N. (2000). *Principles of physiology* (3rd ed.). St. Louis: Mosby.

Bole-Feysot, C., Goffin, V., Edery, M., Binart, N., & Kelly, P. A. (1998). Prolactin (PRL) and its receptor: Actions, signal transduction pathways and phenotypes observed in PRL receptor knockout mice. *Endocrinology Review 19*(3), 225–268.

Bonduelle, M. L., Dodd, R., Liebaers, I., Van Steirteghem, A., Williamson, R., & Akhurst, R. (1988). Chorionic gonadotrophin-beta mRNA, a trophoblast marker, is expressed in human 8-cell embryos derived from tripronucleate zygotes. *Human Reproduction, 3*(7), 909–914.

Braunstein, G. D. (1996). Evidence favoring human chorionic gonadotropin as the physiological `rescuer' of the corpus luteum during early pregnancy. *Early Pregnancy, 2*(3), 183–190.

Bryant, H. U., & Dere, W. H. (1998). Selective estrogen receptor modulators: An alternative to hormone replacement therapy. *Proceedings of the Society of Experimental Biology and Medicine, 217*(1), 45–52.

Burger, H. G. (1999). The endocrinology of the menopause. *Journal of Steroid Biochemistry and Molecular Biology, 69*(1–6), 31–35.

Burgio, K. L., & Goode, P. S. (1997). Behavioral interventions for incontinence in ambulatory geriatric patients. *American Journal of Medical Science, 314*(4), 257–261.

Burgio, K. L., Locher, J. L., & Goode, P. S. (2000). Combined behavioral and drug therapy for urge incontinence in older women. *Journal of the American Geriatric Society, 48*(4), 370–374.

Cameron, I., Irvine, G., & Norman, J. (1996). Menstruation. In S. Hillier, H. Kitchener, & J. Neilson (Eds.), *Scientific essentials in reproductive medicine* (pp. 208–218). Philadelphia: W. B. Saunders.

Catt, K. (1996). Hormone receptors. In S. Hillier, H. Kitchener, & J. Neilson (Eds.), *Scientific essentials of reproductive medicine* (pp. 32–44). Philadelphia: W. B. Saunders.

Cauley, J. A., Gutai, J. P., Kuller, L. H., LeDonne, D., & Powell, J. G. (1989). The epidemiology of serum sex hormones in postmenopausal women. *American Journal of Epidemiology, 129*(6), 1120–1131.

Chang, C., Holtzman, D. A., Chau, S., Chickering, T., Woolf, E. A., Holmgren, L. M., et al. (2001). Twisted gastrulation can function as a BMP antagonist. *Nature, 410*(6827), 483–487.

Clarke, I. (1996). The hypothalamo-pituitary axis. In S. Hillier, H. Kitchener, & J. Neilson (Eds.), *Scientific essentials of reproductive medicine* (pp. 120–132). Philadelphia: W. B. Saunders.

Clarkson, T. B. (2000). Soy phytoestrogens: What will be their role in postmenopausal hormone replacement therapy? *Menopause, 7*(2), 71–75.

Cooke, D. J., & Greene, J. G. (1981). Types of life events in relation to symptoms at the climacterium. *Journal of Psychosomatic Research, 25*(1):5–11.

Critchley, D. (1996). Uterus and tubes. In S. Hillier, H. Kitchener, & J. Neilson (Eds.), *Scientific essentials of reproductive medicine* (pp. 184–195). Philadelphia: W. B. Saunders.

Cummings, J. M., & Rodning, C. B. (2000). Urinary stress incontinence among obese women: Review of pathophysiology therapy. *International Urogynecologic Journal of Pelvic Floor Dysfunction, 11*(1), 41–44.

Desai, H. D., & Jann, M. W. (2000). Major depression in women: a review of the literature. *Journal of the American Pharmacological Association (Washington, D. C.), 40*(4), 525–537.

Duvekot, J. J., & Peeters, L. L. (1994). Maternal cardiovascular hemodynamic adaptation to pregnancy. *Obstetric and Gynecologic Survey, 49*(12 Suppl) S1–14.

Ellgaard, L., Molinari, M., & Helenius, A. (1999). Setting the standards: Quality control in the secretory pathway. *Science, 286*(5446), 1882–1888.

Faddy, M. J., Gosden, R. G., Gougeon, A., Richardson, S. J., & Nelson, J. F. (1992). Accelerated disappearance of ovarian follicles in mid-life: Implications for forecasting menopause. *Human Reproduction, 7*(10), 1342–1346.

Ferin, M., Jewelewicz, R., & Warren, M. (1993). *The menstrual cycle: Physiology, reproductive disorders and infertility.* New York: Oxford University Press.

Fillingim, R. B., & Ness, T. J. (2000). Sex-related hormonal influences on pain and analgesic responses. *Neuroscience and Biobehavior Review, 24*(4), 485–501.

Foley, S., & Sommers, M. (1998). Molecular genetics: From bench to bedside. *AACN Clinical Issues, 9*(4), 491–498.

Foreyt, J. P., & Poston, W. S., II. (1998). Obesity: A never-ending cycle? *International Journal of Fertility and Women's Medicine, 43*(2), 111–116.

Fraser, I. S. (1997). Menstrual changes during the perimenopause. In R. Lobo (Ed.), *Perimenopause* (pp. 233–245). New York: Springer.

Fraser, S. E., & Harland, R. M. (2000). The molecular metamorphosis of experimental embryology. *Cell, 100*(1), 41–55.

Gear, R. W., Gordon, N. C., Heller, P. H., Paul, S., Miaskowski, C., & Levine, J. D. (1996). Gender difference in analgesic response to the kappa-opioid pentazocine. *Neuroscience Letter, 205*(3), 207–209.

Gilson, G. J., Samaan, S., Crawford, M. H., Qualls, C. R., & Curet, L. B. (1997). Changes in hemodynamics, ventricular remodeling, and ventricular contractility during normal pregnancy: A longitudinal study. *Obstetrics & Gynecology, 89*(6), 957–962.

Gougeon, A. (1986). Dynamics of follicular growth in the human: A model from preliminary results. *Human Reproduction, 1*(2), 81–87.

Grady, D., Brown, J. S., Vittinghoff, E., Applegate, W., Varner, E., & Snyder, T. (2001). Postmenopausal hormones and incontinence: The Heart and Estrogen/Progestin Replacement Study. *Obstetrics & Gynecology, 97*(1), 116–120.

Grady, D., Rubin, S. M., Petitti, D. B., Fox, C. S., Black, D., Ettinger, B., et al. (1992). Hormone therapy to prevent disease and prolong life in postmenopausal women. *Annals of Internal Medicine, 117*(12), 1016–1037.

Greendale, G., & Judd, H. (1993). The menopause: Health implications and clinical management. *Journal of the American Geriatric Society, 41*, 426–436.

Hanahan, D., & Weinberg, R. A. (2000). The hallmarks of cancer. *Cell, 100*(1), 57–70.

Haraway, D. (1988). Situated knowledges: The science question in feminism and the privilege of partial perspective. *Feminist Studies, 14*(3):575–599.

Haseltine, F. (1995). Gender-based biology—the next step. *Journal of Women's Health, 4*(3), 221–222.

Hautman, M. A. (1996). Changing womanhood: Perimenopause among Filipina-Americans. *Journal of Obsterics, Gynecology, and Neonatal Nursing, 25*(8), 667–673.

Hengartner, M. O. (2000). The biochemistry of apoptosis. *Nature, 407*(6805), 770–776.

Hengartner, M. O. (2001). Apoptosis. DNA destroyers. *Nature, 412*(6842), 27, 29.

Hennighausen, L., Robinson, G. W., Wagner, K. U., & Liu, W. (1997). Prolactin signaling in mammary gland development. *Journal of Biology and Chemistry, 272*(12), 7567–7569.

Hextall, A. (2000). Oestrogens and lower urinary tract function. *Maturitas, 36*(2), 83–92.

Hindle, W. (1997). Changes in the breast with ovarian aging: Mammography/ultrasound. In R. Lobo (Ed.), *Perimenopause.* New York: Springer.

Horn-Ross, P. L. (1995). Phytoestrogens, body composition, and breast cancer. *Cancer Causes & Control, 6*(6), 567–573.

Hsia, J. (1995). Gender and the heart. *Journal of Women's Health, 4*(4), 437–438.

Ibba, M., & Soll, D. (1999). Quality control mechanisms during translation. *Science, 286*(5446), 1893–1897.

Illingworth, P. J., Reddi, K., Smith, K., & Baird, D. T. (1990). Pharmacological `rescue' of the corpus luteum results in increased inhibin production. *Clinical Endocrinology (Oxford), 33*(3), 323–332.

Izraeli, S., Lowe, L. A., Bertness, V. L., Good, D. J., Dorward, D. W., Kirsch, I. R., et al. (1999). The SIL gene is required for mouse embryonic axial development and left-right specification. *Nature, 399*(6737), 691–694.

Jaffe, R. (1986). The menopause and perimenopausal period. In S. C. Yen & R. B. Jaffe (Eds.), *Reproductive endocrinology: Physiology, pathophysiology, and clinical management* (2nd ed.) (pp. 406–423). Philadelphia: W. B. Saunders.

Jensen, E. V., & Jacobsen, H. (1962). Basic guides to the mechanism of estrogen action. *Recent Progress in Hormone Research, 18*, 387–408.

Jordan, V. (1998). Designer estrogens. *Scientific American*, 60–67.

Kirschner, M., Gerhart, J., & Mitchison, T. (2000). Molecular "vitalism." *Cell, 100*(1), 79–88.

Klein, K., & Cutler, G. (1996). Puberty. In S. Hillier, H. Kitchener, & J. Neilson (Eds.), *Scientific essentials of reproductive medicine.* Philadelphia: W. B. Saunders.

Korach, K. (1994). Insights from the study of animals lacking functional estrogen receptor. *Science, 266*, 1524–1527.

Krege, J. H., Hodgin, J. B., Couse, J. F., Enmark, E., Warner, M., Mahler, J. F., et al. (1998). Generation and reproductive phenotypes of mice lacking estrogen receptor beta. *Proceedings of the Natural Academy of Sciences USA, 95*(26), 15677–15682.

Krieger, N., & Fee, E. (1994). Man-made medicine and women's health: The biopolitics of sex/gender and race/ethnicity. *International Journal of Health Services, 24*(2), 265–283.

Kronenberg, F. (1997). Vasomotor symptoms in the perimenopause. In R. Lobo (Ed.), *Perimenopause* (pp. 184–201). New York: Springer.

Leake, R. (1996). Cell cycle. In S. Hillier, H. Kitchener, & J. Neilson (Eds.), *Scientific essentials of reproductive medicine*. Philadelphia: W. B. Saunders.

Legato, M. J. (1997a). *Gender-specific aspects of human biology for the practicing physician*. Armonk, NY: Futura Publishing Company.

Legato, M. J. (1997b). Gender-specific physiology: How real is it? How important is it? *International Journal of Fertility and Women's Medicine, 42*(1), 19–29.

Legato, M. J. (1998). Belling the cat: Clinical investigation in vulnerable populations (a good idea, but who's going to volunteer?). *Journal of Gender Specific Medicine, 1*(2), 12–13.

Legato, M. J. (1999). Premenopausal or postmenopausal: What else is there? *Journal of Gender Specific Medicine, 2*(1), 12, 15.

Lindahl, T., & Wood, R. D. (1999). Quality control by DNA repair. *Science, 286*(5446), 1897–1905.

Little, P. (1999). The book of genes. *Nature, 402*(6761), 467–468.

Lobo, R. (1997). What is the perimenopause? In R. Lobo (Ed.), *Perimenopause* (pp. 1–3). New York: Springer.

MacLennan, A. H., Taylor, A. W., Wilson, D. H., & Wilson, D. (2000). The prevalence of pelvic floor disorders and their relationship to gender, age, parity and mode of delivery. *British Journal of Obstetrics & Gynecology, 107*(12), 1460–1470.

Mady, E. A. (2000). Association between estradiol, estrogen receptors, total lipids, triglycerides, and cholesterol in patients with benign and malignant breast tumors. *Journal of Steroid Biochemistry and Molecular Biology, 75*(4–5), 323–328.

Maixner, W., & Humphrey, C. (1993). Gender differences in pain and cardiovascular responses to forearm ischemia. *Clinical Journal of Pain, 9*(1), 16–25.

Mann, C. (1995). Women's health research blossoms. *Science, 269*(5225), 766–770.

Maroulakou, I. G., & Bowe, D. B. (2000). Expression and function of Ets transcription factors in mammalian development: A regulatory network. *Oncogene, 19*(55), 6432–6442.

Maroulis, G. (1997). Changes in oocyte number with age: Effect on fecundability. In R. Lobo (Ed.), *Perimenopause* (pp. 12–20). New York: Springer.

Matthews, K. A., Shumaker, S. A., Bowen, D. J., Langer, R. D., Hunt, J. R., Kaplan, R. M., et al. (1997). Women's health initiative. Why now? What is it? What's new? *American Psychologist 52*(2), 101–116.

Matzinger, P., & Fuchs, E. J. (1996). Beyond self and non-self: Immunity is a conversation not a war. *The Journal of NIH Research, 8*, 35–39.

McBride, A. (1997). Nursing and the women's movement: The legacy of the 1960s. *Reflections, 23*(3), 38–41.

McEwen, B. S. (1994). How do sex and stress hormones affect nerve cells? *Annals of the NY Academy of Science, 743*, 1–18.

McEwen, B. S. (1998). Multiple ovarian hormone effects on brain structure and function. *Journal of Gender Specific Medicine, 1*(1), 33–41.

McEwen, B. S., & Woolley, C. S. (1994). Estradiol and progesterone regulate neuronal structure and synaptic connectivity in adult as well as developing brain. *Experimental Gerontology, 29*(3–4), 431–436.

McKinlay, S. M., Brambilla, D. J., & Posner, J. G. (1992). The normal menopause transition. *Maturitas, 14*(2), 103–115.

Meduri, G., Bausero, P., & Perrot-Applanat, M. (2000). Expression of vascular endothelial growth factor receptors in the human endometrium: Modulation during the menstrual cycle. *Biology and Reproduction, 62*(2), 439–447.

Mercurio, M. G. (1998). Gender and dermatology. *Journal of Gender Specific Medicine, 1*(1), 16–20.

Miller, A., & Raymond. (1999). Turning point. The infertility challenge. *Newsweek, Special Edition* (Spring-Summer), 26–28.

Moore, K. L. (1988). The developing human: Clinically oriented embryology (4th ed.). Philadelphia; W. B. Saunders.

Murray, A., & Hunt, T. (1993). *The cell cycle: An introduction*. New York: W. H. Freeman.

Murray, R. (2000). Biomolecules and biochemical methods. In R. Murray, D. Granner, P. Mayes, & V. Rodwell (Eds.), *Harper's biochemistry* (25th ed.). Stamford, CT: Appleton & Lange.

Ness, R. B., & Kuller, L. H. (1997). Women's health as a paradigm for understanding factors that mediate disease. *Journal of Women's Health, 6*(3), 329–336.

Ostrer, H. (2000). Sexual differentiation. *Seminars in Reproductive Medicine, 18*(1), 41–49.

Parazzini, F., Colli, E., Origgi, G., Surace, M., Bianchi, M., Benzi, G., et al. (2000). Risk factors for urinary incontinence in women. *European Urology, 37*(6), 637–643.

Pennisi, E. (2000). Breakthrough of the year. Genomics comes of age. *Science, 290*(5500), 2220–2221.

Pfaff, D. W., Vasudevan, N., Kia, H. K., Zhu, Y. S., Chan, J., Garey, J., et al. (2000). Estrogens, brain and behavior: Studies in fundamental neurobiology and observations related to women's health. *Journal of Steroid Biochemistry and Molecular Biology, 74*(5), 365–373.

Pinn, V. W. (1995). Equity in biomedical research. *Science, 269*(5225), 739.

Pinn, V. W. (1998). An affirmation of research and health care for women in the 21st century. *Journal of Gender Specific Medicine, 1*(1), 50–53.

Popnikolov, N., Yang, J., Liu, A., Guzman, R., & Nandi, S. (2001). Reconstituted normal human breast in nude mice: Effect of host pregnancy environment and human chorionic gonadotropin on proliferation. *Journal of Endocrinology, 168*(3), 487–496.

Purdie, D. W. (1996). Menopause. In S. Hillier, H. Kitchener, & J. Neilson (Eds.), *Scientific essentials of reproductive medicine* (pp. 250–257). Philadelphia: W. B. Saunders.

Rabinowitz, V. C., & Valian, V. (2000). Sex, sex differences, and social behavior. *Annals of the New York Academy of Science, 907*, 196–207.

Rajman, I., Lip, G. Y., Cramb, R., Maxwell, S. R., Zarifis, J., Beevers, D. G., et al. (1996). Adverse change in low-density lipoprotein subfractions profile with oestrogen-only hormone replacement therapy. *Quarterly Journal of Medicine, 89*(10), 771–778.

Reame, N. E. (1997). Gonadotropin changes in the perimenopause. In R. Lobo (Ed.), *Perimenopause* (pp. 157–169). New York: Springer.

Rebar, R., Cedars, M., & Jiu, J. (1997). Premature ovarian failure: A model for the perimenopause. In R. Lobo (Ed.), *Perimenopause.* New York: Springer.

Research on the menopause. (Technical reports series 670)(1981). Geneva, Switzerland: World Health Organization.

Reuss, M., Kline, J., Santos, R., Levin, B., & Timor-Tritsch, I. (1997). Age and the ovarian follicle pool assesed with transvaginal sonography. In R. Lobo (Ed.), *Perimenopause* (pp. 255–261). New York: Springer.

Riley, J. L., III, Robinson, M. E., Wise, E. A., Myers, C. D., & Fillingim, R. B. (1998). Sex differences in the perception of noxious experimental stimuli: A meta-analysis. *Pain, 74*(2–3), 181–187.

Ritzen, E. M., Nilsson, O., Grigelioniene, G., Holst, M., Savendahl, L., & Wroblewski, J. (2000). Estrogens and human growth. *Journal of Steroid Biochemistry and Molecular Biology, 74*(5), 383–386.

Rodwell, V. (2000). Proteins: Structure and function. In R. Murray, D. Granner, P. Mayes, & V. Rodwell (Eds.), *Harper's biochemistry* (25th ed.). Stamford, CT: Appleton & Lange.

Rosenbaum, M., Leibel, R. L., & Hirsch, J. (1997). Obesity. *New England Journal of Medicine, 337*(6), 396–407.

Russo, J., Hu, Y. F., Silva, I. D., & Russo, I. H. (2001). Cancer risk related to mammary gland structure and development. *Microscopic Research Techniques, 52*(2), 204–223.

Ryan, K. (1999). Hormonal milieu and reproductive status in women. In R. B. Ness, & L. H. Kuller (Eds.), *Health and disease among women: Biological and environmental influences* (pp. 133–154). New York: Oxford University Press.

Sadovsky, Y., & Adler, S. (1998). Selective modulation of estrogen receptor action. *Journal of Clinical Endocrinology and Metabolism, 83*(1), 3–5.

Santoro, N. F., Col, N. F., Eckman, M. H., Wong, J. B., Pauker, S. G., Cauley, J. A., et al. (1999). Therapeutic controversy: Hormone replacement therapy—where are we going? *Journal of Clinical Endocrinology and Metabolism, 84*(6), 1798–1812.

Schmidt, P., Roca, C., & Rubinow, D. (1997). Perimenopausal depression. In R. Lobo (Ed.), *Perimenopause* (pp. 246–254). New York: Springer.

Scott, M. P. (2000). Development: The natural history of genes. *Cell, 100*(1), 27–40.

Seifer, D. (1997). Granulosa cell competence with aging. In R. Lobo (Ed.), *Perimenopause* (pp. 144–153). New York: Springer.

Small, G. W. (1998). Estrogen effects on the brain. *Journal of Gender Specific Medicine, 1*(2), 23–27.

Society for Women's Health Research. (2001). *10 differences between men and women that make a difference in women's health.* [on-line]. Available: *http://www.womens-health.org/insertB.htm* [2001, September 1].

Spelsberg, T. C., Subramaniam, M., Riggs, B. L., & Khosla, S. (1999). The actions and interactions of sex steroids and growth factors/cytokines on the skeleton. *Molecular Endocrinology, 13*(6), 819–828.

Steel, C. (1996). Gene expression. In S. Hillier, H. Kitchener, & J. Neilson (Eds.), *Scientific essentials of reproductive medicine.* Philadelphia: W. B. Saunders.

Stevenson, J. C. (2000). Cardiovascular effects of oestrogens. *Journal of Steroid Biochemistry and Molecular Biology, 74*(5), 387–393.

Swain, A., & Lovell-Badge, R. (1999). Mammalian sex determination: A molecular drama. *Genes and Development, 13*(7), 755–767.

Tabibzadeh, S., Satyaswaroop, P. G., von Wolff, M., & Strowitzki, T. (1999). Regulation of TNF-alpha mRNA expression in endometrial cells by TNF-alpha and by oestrogen withdrawal. *Molecular Human Reproduction, 5*(12), 1141–1149.

Tagawa, A., Rappleye, C. A., & Aroian, R. V. (2001). Pod-2, along with Pod-1, defines a new class of genes required for polarity in the early *Caenorhabditis elegans* embryo. *Developmental Biology, 233*(2), 412–424.

Treloar, A. E., Boynton, R. E., Behn, B. G., & Brown, B. W. (1970). Variation of the human menstrual cycle through reproductive life. *International Journal of Fertility, 12*(1), 77–126.

Walker, J. S., & Carmody, J. J. (1998). Experimental pain in healthy human subjects: Gender differences in nociception and in response to ibuprofen. *Anesthesia and Analgesia, 86*(6), 1257–1262.

Wallace, R. B., Sherman, B. M., Bean, J. A., Treloar, A. E., & Schlabaugh, L. (1979). Probability of menopause with increasing duration of amenorrhea in middle-aged women. *American Journal of Obstetrics and Gynecology, 135*(8), 1021–1024.

Wallis, L. (1993). Why a curriculum in women's health? *Journal of Women's Health, 2*(1), 55–60.

Weel, A. E., Uitterlinden, A. G., Westendorp, I. C., Burger, H., Schuit, S. C., Hofman, A., et al. (1999). Estrogen receptor polymorphism predicts the onset of natural and surgical menopause. *Journal of Clinical Endocrinology and Metabolism, 84*(9), 3146–3150.

Weissman, M. M., & Olfson, M. (1995). Depression in women: Implications for health care research. *Science, 269*(5225), 799–801.

Wilcox, A. J., Baird, D. D., & Weinberg, C. R. (1999). Time of implantation of the conceptus and loss of pregnancy. *New England Journal of Medicine, 340*(23), 1796–1799.

Writing Group of the 1996 American Academy of Nursing Expert Group (1997). Women's health and women's health care: Recommendations of the 1996 AAN Expert Panel on Women's Health, *Nursing Outlook 95*(1),7–15.

Woods, N. (1994). The United States women's health research agenda analysis and critique. *Western Journal of Nursing Research, 16*(5), 467–479.

Zeleznik, A. J., & Hillier, S. G. (1996). The ovary: Endocrine function. In S. Hillier, H. Kitchener, & J. Neilson (Eds.), *Scientific essentials of reproductive medicine.* Philadelphia: W. B. Saunders.

RESOURCES

Hamilton, J. A. & Jensvold, M. F. (1992), Personality, psychopathology, and depressions in women. In L. S. Brown & M. Ballou (Eds.), *Personality and psychopathology: Feminist reappraisals* (pp. 116–143). New York: Guilford Press.

Matthews, K., Weiss, S., Detre, T., Dembroski, T., Falkner, B., Manuck, S., et al. (1986). *Handbook of stress, reactivity, and cardiovascular disease.* New York: Wiley.

Simpson, E. R., Zhao, Y., Agarwal, V. R., Michael, M. D., Bulun, S. E., Hinshelwood, M. M., et al. (1997). Aromatase expression in health and disease. *Recent Progress in Hormone Research, 52,* 185–213.

Women's Health and Women's Health Care: Recommendations of the 1996 AAN Expert Panel on Women's Health. (1997). *Nursing Outlook, 45*(1), 7–15.

Wyshak, G., & Frisch, R. (1982). Evidence for a secular trend in age of menarche. *The New England Journal of Medicine, 306*(17), 1033–1035.

Zamboni, L., Upadhyay, S., Bezard, J., et al. (1980). The role of mesonephros in the development of the mammalian ovary. In R. I. Tozzini, G. Reeves, & R. I. Pineda (Eds.), *Endocrine physiopathology of the ovary* (pp. 3–42). Amsterdam: Elsevier/North Holland Biomedical Press.

Chapter 8

Health History

Susan Bragg Leight

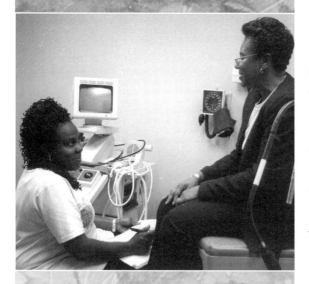

Sometimes I wish I were a physician specializing in women's medicine. I would surprise each of my patients annually with a written prescription to play hooky for a day. I would convince them that hooky is absolutely necessary for their good health: physical and psychological. Then I would give them an official note excusing them from real life. I think the crucial reason it's so difficult to be a grown-up is that there's no one to write a note for us excusing us from the job, the marriage, caring for Mom, and driving the car pool. Don't worry. I'll write your note. Will you write mine?

Sarah Ban Breathnach

INTRODUCTION

Humanistic care of women has been defined as care that is driven by compassion, empathy, and respect with the overall goal of preserving worth and dignity. An issue that is central to the provision of humanistic care is the establishment of a therapeutic relationship between the provider and woman for the purpose of health care delivery (Frank, 1996; Larson & Fanchiang, 1996; Leight, 2001). This therapeutic relationship functions to facilitate the identification of client needs and strengths within the context of personal and life events.

Satisfaction with health care services has been shown to be closely tied to the ability to communicate with providers (Brown, Boles, Mullooly, & Levinson, 1999; Grant, Cissna, & Rosenfeld, 2000; Greco, Brownlea, McGovern, & Cavanagh, 2000; Kravitz et al., 1996; Mallison, Kielhofner, & Mattingly, 1996; Walker, 1996). In a study of 80 women attending a Scottish gynecological oncology follow-up clinic, it was shown that "the ability to communicate with patients" was noted as the most important characteristic by 39% of the respondents (Walker, 1996). In an important study done during the 1980s, Cousins (1985) found that a large number of people actually terminate their relationship with their providers as a result of ineffective provider-client communication. Eighty-five percent of more than 1100 U.S. households responding

251

stated they would consider leaving their current provider and, of this number, 75% attributed their leaving to physician communication skill. Specific examples cited included the perception that the provider was not listening, did not care, and responded in language they did not understand (Cousins, 1985).

It has been shown that, in general, health care providers tend to be quite rigid in the way they collect information from clients. Brady (1987) noted a tendency by clinicians to use close-ended restricting questions with few broad opening leads when investigating a client's chief complaint. Another area noted to be problematic was clinician failure to address a client's psychosocial and emotional concerns (Badger et al., 1994; Brady, 1987; Kutner, Steiner, Corbett, Jahnigen, & Barton, 1999; Lang, Floyd, & Beine, 2000). In a study of 47 community-based practitioners, physicians who indicated a high interest in psychosocial concerns were no more likely to conduct client-centered interviews than were those who claimed little or no interest in psychosocial issues (Badger et al., 1994).

Understanding the health issues affecting women today demands more than a biomedical view of the illness; it necessitates an awareness of the individual context of each woman's life (Writing Group of the 1996 AAN Expert Panel on Women's Health, 1997). The totality of each woman's personal environment, the living conditions and home atmosphere, the cultural patterns and ethnicity, and the value placed on wellness and health care has considerable bearing on patterns of health behavior and health care outcomes (Brady, 1987; Quirk & Casey, 1995).

Meeting the unique health care needs of women across the life span is a worthy goal for advanced practice nurses. One important vehicle in this process is the establishment of a therapeutic relationship between the provider and woman. The following section discusses the art of interviewing as a critical first step in the establishment of this provider-woman alliance.

INTERVIEWING AS AN ART

Quirk and Casey (1995) speak to the notion of the "art of interviewing" as a collection of techniques, attitudes, and capabilities that not only enhances the effectiveness of subjective data acquisition but also serves as a therapeutic intervention. When a provider-woman encounter has been optimized, a woman may leave the office feeling uplifted, empowered, and satisfied, whether or not a particular solution has been found. By virtue of this process, the foundation has been set for a provider-woman relationship that will enhance the healing dynamic (Quirk & Casey, 1995).

One approach to artful interviewing is the use of a narrative. The term "narrative" refers to the relating of a story that details a life event (Boykin & Schoenhofer, 1991; Larson & Fanchiang, 1996; Leight, 2001; Polkinghorne, 1988; Sandelowski, 1991; Smith & Liehr, 1999). Through this approach, the provider is able to get an image of the woman's daily activities, family relationships, and sociocultural influences and their effects on her health (Larson & Fanchiang, 1996; Leight, 2001). Focusing on the woman's needs within the context of personal and life circumstances will provide consumer satisfaction as well as enhance the provider's knowledge base.

The way in which the women's health nurse communicates with a woman lays the foundation for all present and future health care delivery and is an essential component in the development of a trusting partnership relationship between the woman and the health care provider. The interview itself can be conceptualized as an opportunity for the woman to "tell her story" so that strengths and capabilities are identified as well as presenting concerns. It is known that 70% to 90% of the information that is needed for clinical problem solving is obtained from the client interview. The remainder of this chapter discusses strategies to enhance the interview process as well as acquire a comprehensive subjective account of health status.

THE INTERVIEW PROCESS

Environmental Factors

It is important to conduct the interview in a private setting that is free from disruption and interruptions. If the interview must take place in a setting where privacy is difficult to maintain, (e.g., an acute care setting), it is important to shut the door, close the curtains, or wait until others have left the room (Jarvis, 2000).

Although office spaces are frequently small and rather intimidating, warm colors, comfortable chairs, and an absence of furniture placed between you and the client are all helpful in promoting a productive dialogue. Arrange the equal-status seating so that the provider and the woman are facing each other at eye level. A reasonable distance between the provider and woman is usually about 4 to 5 feet, or twice one's arm length; less distance may impinge on the woman's private space while distances in excess of 5 feet communicate remoteness and detachment (Bates, 1995; Bickley, 1998; Jarvis, 2000).

It is important to avoid standing during the interview as this can communicate a superior power position as well as your haste. Remaining in a sitting position helps maintain a sense of equal power among the participants (Bates, 1995; Bickley, 1998; Jarvis, 2000). It is beneficial to place a clock on the wall behind the woman so that you can keep track of the time without needing to repeatedly check your watch. Keep the temperature of the setting comfortable and remove distracting materials from the room, such as clutter, mail, and other client records. Sufficient lighting should be provided so that the provider and woman are able to see each other clearly. Avoid having the woman face directly into the sun, since squinting is distracting and uncomfortable (Jarvis, 2000).

It is desirable for the woman to remain in her street clothes for the entirety of the interview. Provider dress should be professional and appropriate to the setting. Avoid extremes in clothing, hair, and accessories.

Nonverbal Messages

Body Posture. Body posture can be an important element in the interviewing process. Sit at a comfortable conversational distance from the client. Verify that your posture and body language convey a sense of openness and an ease of manner. Leaning slightly forward and maintaining eye contact and bodily proximity communicate emotional concern (Seidel, Ball, Dains, & Benedict, 1999).

Eye Contact. Eye contact is a way to visually express an interest in what the woman is saying. Be sure that the breaks in eye contact are natural, e.g., when the woman looks away, the provider is thinking, or the woman is contemplating the answer to a question. Constant eye contact may provoke a sense of anxiety and should be avoided.

Vocal Tone and Rate of Speech. Use a conversational tone and through both verbal and nonverbal means, convey the message that relieving the woman's worry or pain is your prime concern. It is important that vocal tone and speech rate be appropriate to the content and meaning of the discussion. In general, a slower pace with less modulation is preferable. However, appropriate variations in speech tone are a good source of stimuli and convey provider concern (Jarvis, 2000).

Speaking too quickly or too slowly may disrupt the woman's concentration. In addition, raising the voice may be inappropriate. In general, the provider should maintain a consistent approach throughout the interview.

Relationship-Centered Care

Quirk and Casey (1995) noted that while the primary goal of the interview is to formulate a diagnosis, the encounter itself may have the potential to be therapeutic in its own right. They believe that it is the provider-woman relationship itself that provides the foundation for caregiving and healing. Central to the development of this relationship-centered care are four guiding principles: respect, dialogue, eliciting and responding to feelings, and affirmation.

Respect. A respectful attitude is critical to the development of a therapeutic relationship. Respect is conveyed when each individual woman is viewed as intrinsically worthwhile. "To have respect for someone does not require acceptance of their values, beliefs, or behaviors" (Quirk & Casey, 1995, p. 101). While a provider may have different values than her clients, it is necessary to both recognize these differences and value the diversity inherent in them. Providers should strive for unconditional positive regard for women and should respect their autonomy and individuality (Kaplan, Siegel, Madill, & Epstein, 1997).

Within the context of the interview, a respectful attitude is conveyed through nonverbal communication. Respect is expressed with simple gestures such as shaking hands, attentive listening, and maintaining eye contact. Conversely, a lack of respect is demonstrated when the provider seems rushed, is inattentive, or fails to look at the client (Quirk & Casey, 1995).

Sharing of power is another way in which respect can be communicated during the interview process. While the provider draws on her medical knowledge and clinical experience, the woman also possesses information crucial to making an accurate diagnosis. This information includes knowledge of the symptoms, history of the presenting problem, and the lived experience of the illness. If one person in the relationship assumes a position of superiority it is likely that the information flow between the individuals will be impeded. Conversely, shared power is achieved by allowing the woman to participate in defining the direction of the interview (Harvard Medical School, 1997; Quirk & Casey, 1995). Provider behaviors that demonstrate a desire to share power include a willingness to discuss diagnostic and treatment decisions with women and their families, a willingness to work with persons from diverse backgrounds with varied personal styles, curiosity about the differing dimensions of the illness and its impact on the individual's life, and a willingness to explore one's own personal beliefs and values as they relate to the healing arts (Grant et al., 2000; Harvard Medical School, 1997; Kaplan et al., 1997).

Dialogue. Dialogue, defined in this context as an authentic sharing of information, is the second key component of relationship-centered care. Providers who listen patiently and carefully, who summarize the information, and encourage further interaction convey the message that the woman's perspective is important in the relationship. Attentive listening gives the provider information about the impact of the experience on the client's life, her expectations of the visit, and her overall interpretation of the problem (Lang et al., 2000; Quirk & Casey, 1995).

Eliciting and Responding to Feelings. Eliciting and acknowledging the woman's feelings conveys the sentiment that it is acceptable to discuss these matters with the provider. If the atmosphere is such that fears and concerns can be freely expressed, the provider can clarify issues and further address problem areas. Eliciting feelings also gives the provider a sense of the impact the condition is having on the woman's life. Since individuals have varying coping styles and levels of resiliency, it is important to elicit this information to enhance understanding of the woman's experience with the problem (Quirk & Casey, 1995; Swartz, 1998).

Affirmation/Providing Positive Reinforcement. Affirming the woman's problem gives her two messages: (1) the provider cares about her and her health concerns, and (2) she is being heard and understood. Positive reinforcement occurs when the provider indicates that the visit was necessary and appropriate. One of the most common fears of consumers of health care is that a problem might be seen as insignificant and not worthy of a visit. It is therefore important for the provider to compliment the individual on her health-seeking behaviors (Quirk & Casey, 1995; Swartz, 1998).

Communication Skills

Effective questioning is the secret to successful interviewing. Both the wording of questions and the tone of voice affect the quality of the responses received. Open-ended and closed-ended nonbiased questions, clarification of ambiguous information, periodic summarization of the discussion, demonstration of empathy when necessary, and consistent expression of unconditional positive regard are essential communication techniques.

The successful interview proceeds smoothly and appears effortless. There are several strategies that novice interviewers can use to improve their interviewing skills. These include understanding and practicing specific communication techniques, observing other interviews, taping (both audio and video) their own interviews, and receiving feedback on interviewing techniques (Swartz, 1998). The following sections briefly review types of questions used during interviewing as well as specific skills to enhance the provider-woman dialogue.

Open-Ended Questions. Open-ended questions are asked to obtain broad narrative information from the woman. These types of questions are generally used to begin the interview or to introduce a different area of inquiry. These questions have no provider bias and allow the woman to tell her story. Open-ended questions elicit feelings and ideas and build trust within the provider-woman relationship (Box 8-1).

It is important that as the person answers the open-ended question, the provider take cues from their story and asks appropriate follow-up questions. Changing the topic at this time may result in a loss of much of the original story.

Closed, or Direct, Questions. These questions solicit a specific answer and function to clarify and add further detail to the narrative account related by the client. They tend to elicit short answers from clients or present a forced-choice option (i.e., yes/no). These questions allow the interviewer to add detail and/or focus on a particular issue. Providers must take extreme care, however, to avoid introducing bias with the use of closed questions (Box 8-2).

In building a chronological account of the problem, questions such as "What happened next?" are helpful to sequence the events. Continue to fill in the detail with more direct questions that ask for specific information. It is also important to ask only one question at a time. A question such as, "Do you have chest pain, shortness of breath, ankle swelling or fatigue?" can be overwhelming.

Take care to choose language that is understood by the woman. Be aware of cultural patterns of usage in your community and the meaning behind these messages. A client in Appalachia might respond to the above question by saying, "Yes, I have all those problems you mentioned; I have dropsy," a term used to described the symptom complex associated with congestive heart failure.

Box 8-1 EXAMPLES OF OPEN-ENDED QUESTIONS

"Tell me how I can help you?"
"What brings you to the office today?"
"What kind of problems are you having?"
"You mentioned swelling in your legs—tell me more about it."

Box 8-2 EXAMPLES OF CLOSED (DIRECT) QUESTIONS

"Tell me where it hurts."
"When do you notice you are short of breath?"
"How would you compare your headache today with headaches you have had in the past?"

Attributes of a Symptom. There are several fundamental attributes of a symptom that should be determined during the interview. The exact questions will vary based on the nature of the complaint, but, in general, the following information needs to be elicited:

Timing. This includes mode of onset. If possible, identify date and time. When did it start? How long does it last? How often does it occur?

Location. Where is it? Does it radiate? Describe the site in terms of fixed landmarks. Have the client show you the exact site. Does it radiate or move?

Quality. What is it like? Try to use the client's descriptive terms for the pain, e.g., aching, sharp, dull, heavy, burning, cramping

Quantity. How severe is this pain? Use a reproducible scale such as 0 to 10 with 10 being the worst imaginable pain.

Setting. Where does it occur? Is there a temporal relationship with environmental factors, personal activities, emotional factors, injury, pregnancy, medications, therapeutic procedures, etc.?

Alleviating/Aggravating Factors. What brings on the pain? What makes it better? What makes it worse? Do medications, physical position, emotions affect the problem?

Associated Manifestations. What effects (or significance) does the problem have on sleep, strength, work, weight, appetite, and activities of daily living?

Attributions. To what does the client attribute the symptoms? What is she afraid of?

Provider Responses: Enhancing the Narrative

As the woman answers the open- and closed-ended questions, it is important that the provider's responses assist in the amplification and clarification of her story. There are nine types of verbal responses that can be made by the provider: silence, facilitation, clarification, confrontation, interpretation, reflection, empathy, explanation, and summary.

Silence. Silence is truly golden during the interviewing process. When the provider is silent following an open-ended question, it gives the woman time to think, collect her thoughts, and organize what she would like to say. Unfortunately, this "thinking silence" can be quite difficult for novice clinicians to employ. There is a tendency among beginning practitioners to feel responsible for keeping the dialogue going and to feel at fault if it ceases. Silence, however, has many advantages. It allows time for both parties to thoughtfully respond, as well as to observe nonverbal behavior cues (Seidel et al., 1999; Swartz, 1998).

Facilitation. These are verbal and nonverbal communication responses on the part of the provider that encourage the woman to elaborate on her story. Common verbal facilitations include *"Go on," "Tell me more," "Uh huh," "Mmmm,"* and *"And then?"*

Nonverbal facilitation techniques are also useful to encourage the woman to continue with her account of the problem. These include nodding the head, hand gestures, and moving closer to the client. These gestures demonstrate provider interest in the client and what she is saying and encourage her to continue.

Clarification. This technique is used to elucidate a woman's word choice, context, or meaning. Clarification includes responses such as, "Tell me what 'taking a spell' means to you?" Clarification serves to summarize and simplify an individual's expressions and verify that you are correctly understanding their meaning.

Confrontation. In confrontation, you communicate your observations of the woman's behavior, feelings, statements, or actions. It is used as a vehicle to provide feedback to the woman about how you are perceiving her actions or emotions. It may serve to highlight a discrepancy or verify the correctness of your assessment. Examples of confrontational statements include: "*You look upset,*" and "*You tell me that area doesn't hurt, but I notice that you grimaced when I touched you there.*" While confrontation is helpful in encouraging the women to continue her narrative, it must be used cautiously to avoid seeming overbearing.

Interpretation. Interpretive statements are based upon provider inferences or interpretations of the woman's behavior. They differ from confrontation in that they are not based upon behavioral observations but rather focus on inferences and conclusions drawn by the provider. Examples of interpretive statements include: "*Your headaches seem to be aggravated by work stress,*" and "*You sound very upset by this situation.*"

It is important that you attempt to fully understand the clues given by the woman before offering an interpretation. The client will usually tell you if your inferences are incorrect. Interpretive statements serve to demonstrate support and understanding as well as prompt further discussion of the topic.

Reflection. Reflection is a response that echoes the woman's words such that the provider in effect actually repeats part or all of what has just been said. This technique serves to mirror the woman's responses and encourages her to elaborate further. Consider the following example:

Woman: *I cannot be hospitalized during this pregnancy because I have no one to care for my children at home.*

Provider: *You are worried about your children at home in the event of a hospitalization?*

The provider may also use reflection to mirror the woman's emotional tone during the interview, which can be a stimulus for further discussion (Bates, 1995; Bickley, 1998; Jarvis, 2000).

Empathy. Empathy is a response that recognizes a feeling and puts it into words. It gives a voice and a name to the feeling and brings it to the forefront of the discussion. It is an understanding of the emotional response, not a sympathetic state on the part of the provider. In essence, empathy says, "I'm with you" (Swartz, 1998). Examples of empathetic statements include: "*I'm sure your daughter's death has been incredibly hard on you,*" "*It must be hard to feel so out of control in this situation,*" and "*This must be very hard on you.*"

Empathetic responses can be verbal or nonverbal. Examples of nonverbal responses include giving an understanding nod, placing your hand on the woman's arm, or reaching for a tissue during an emotional moment. Empathy strengthens rapport, acknowledges and accepts emotion, and allows for the safe expression of emotional concerns within the context of the interview.

Explanation. This communication technique is used to inform consumers of the availability of health care services and to disseminate factual information. It may include information on clinical entities, therapeutic modalities, or cause and effect relationships. An example of an explanatory statement includes *"This medication will help strengthen the contractility of your heart."*

Summary. This review condenses what has transpired during the interview. It presents a synopsis of the interview and should be validated by both provider and woman prior to the termination of the interview. If necessary, the woman should be given adequate time to review and elaborate on the summary data.

Facilitators to Open Communication

Better communication between providers and women leads to better outcomes and improved consumer satisfaction with services. Kaplan and colleagues (1997) have identified a core of specific skills that promote effective communication in the clinical setting, which are summarized in Box 8-3.

Barriers to Open Communication

While it has been shown that effective communication fosters better information gathering, increased motivation, and the sense that the provider is interested in the woman's well-being, poor communication has been linked to malpractice suits and decisions by women to leave provider practices (Kaplan et al., 1997). Among these barriers are a number of provider behaviors that make the interview less productive and in some way restrict the woman's responses (Jarvis, 2000). These verbal and nonverbal behaviors are summarized in Box 8-4.

At times, women present to a care setting with preexisting sensory or cognitive impairments that affect their ability to provide a good history. It is incumbent on the provider to implement measures to overcome these barriers. In the event of language differences, it may be necessary to engage the services of an interpreter if the family is unable to assist with translation. If a woman is hearing impaired, it may be necessary to raise your voice or solicit assistance from the family. Women with cognitive impairments should be interviewed along with family members. Be open to issues that surface during

---

Box 8-3 FACILITATORS TO OPEN COMMUNICATION

Verbal Behaviors
Skillfully eliciting the woman's story
Considering the impact of her present symptoms in the broader context of her lived experience
Negotiating mutual responsibility for problems

Nonverbal Behaviors
Accommodating and overcoming barriers, such as hearing/visual impairment, language, cultural differences, and anxiety
Giving attention to environmental needs, such as comfort and privacy

---

Box 8-4 PROVIDER BARRIERS TO EFFECTIVE COMMUNICATION

Verbal Behaviors
False reassurance
Unsolicited advice
Overuse of technical jargon
Paternal/domineering/authoritarian behavior
Avoidance of difficult topics
Manipulative, leading, or biased questions
Talking too much
Frequent interruptions
Asking "why" questions
Dismissing concerns

Nonverbal Behaviors
Reading or writing during the interview
Disinterested posture
Breaking eye contact
Allowing interruptions
Inattention to physical environment
Inattention to personal dress and grooming
Facial expression reflecting boredom, disgust, distraction, or criticism
Standing during the interview
Gestures such as finger-pointing, finger-tapping
High-pitched voice
Too frequent touching
Sitting behind a desk more than 5 feet from the client
Overly stiff and formal demeanor

---

the interview and validate perceptions with the woman. Be aware as well that women may present with a "hidden agenda" (Lang et al., 2000; Seidel et al., 1999).

Some women may attempt to distance themselves from a personal threat through the use of impersonal speech such as, "*She is afraid that there may be a lump in her breast.*" This technique allows the woman to deny a personal association with the disease and therefore protect herself from it (Cassell, 1989). Similar attempts by the provider will be ineffective, since such distancing will convey the message that you too are concerned about the diagnosis (Jarvis, 2000).

At times, women may not tell you the entire story, either deliberately or unconsciously. Try to neither push too hard to obtain the information nor neglect it. Allow the interview to progress and come back to the issue by saying, "You seem more concerned about this problem than you are telling me" (Seidel et al., 1999).

Cultural Considerations

The United States is culturally and ethnically heterogeneous. It is projected that by the end of the 21st century, more than 50% of the U.S. population will no longer be

Caucasian (Hodgkinson, 1992). At the present time, there are more than 100 different ethnic groups and 400 different Native American tribes in the United States (Swartz, 1998). Of the 275,844,000 people living in the United States, 226,718,000 (82.2%) are white; 35,432,000 (12.8%), African American; 2,445,000 (0.9%), Native American (American Indians, Eskimo, Aleut); and 11,249,000 (4.1%), Asian and Pacific Islander. Among these numbers are 32,734,000 persons of Hispanic origin, who represent a diverse multicultural group (U.S. Bureau of the Census, 2000).

The *Random House Webster's College Dictionary* (1999) defines *race* as "a group of persons related by common descent or heredity; a classification based on a selection of physical characteristics; and any people united by common history, language, cultural traits, etc." The term *culture* is defined as the "the sum total of ways of living built up by a group of human beings and transmitted from one generation to another; and the behaviors and beliefs characteristic of a particular social, ethnic, or age group." Culture provides the values and beliefs that are mutually shared by persons of particular social groups and is the perspective from which all personal experiences are viewed. As such, the verbal and nonverbal behaviors of both the client and the provider are influenced by their respective cultural backgrounds.

There is a greater likelihood of miscommunication when the woman and the provider come from different cultural backgrounds. Cross-cultural, or intercultural, communication takes place between a provider and woman from differing cultural backgrounds (Jarvis, 2000). It is critical that health care providers have an appreciation for the cross-cultural family values, language, health care beliefs, norms, religious ideology, and political convictions of their women clients. It has been estimated that 80% or more of all self-identified illness episodes are managed outside of our traditional health care system (Swartz, 1998). The use of traditional or folk healers, alternative therapies, self-help groups, and religious practitioners constitutes a large percentage of health care in the United States (Swartz, 1998).

Since the development of a mutually respectful relationship is of paramount importance in relationship-centered care, be sure to introduce yourself and ask the woman how she would like to be addressed. This simple step allows you to address the woman in a culturally appropriate manner and serves to set the stage for a mutually beneficial relationship.

Be aware that it is likely that both you and the woman bring cultural stereotypes to your interaction. Included among these may be sets of expectations regarding nursing versus physician functioning (Jarvis, 2000). For example, research has found that Italian-Americans tend to have very traditional expectations regarding the role of nurses, assuming that they carry out physician orders without making independent health care judgments (Jarvis, 2000). Therefore interacting with an advanced practice women's health practitioner may represent a divergence from a woman's expectations for her visit.

Practitioners must be aware of two potential problem areas in working with women from diverse backgrounds. The first of these, ethnocentrism, is defined as the "belief in the inherent superiority of one's own ethnic group or culture, and a tendency to view alien groups or cultures from the perspective of one's own" (*Random House Webster's College Dictionary*, 1999). Potential problems with ethnocentrism arise when practitioners believe that their way of life is the most desirable and acceptable. This perspective can lead to behavior that is both domineering and supercilious. In addition, providers must also be aware of the tendency toward "cultural imposition," or the dictating of personal beliefs, values, and behavior patterns to individuals from differing cultures. While the identification and awareness of ethnocentrism and cultural imposition are increasing in the United States, it remains difficult to overcome cultural biases (Jarvis, 2000).

Although it is beyond the scope of this chapter to address the diversity of cultures in the United States, it remains an imperative that practitioners provide culturally sensitive health care to their women clients. Providers who work with culturally diverse women must take the necessary steps to prepare themselves to address the health care needs of these groups.

Developmental Considerations

Adolescence. Adolescence is the period of life beginning with puberty and extending 8 to 10 years beyond that time until the individual is cognitively, emotionally, and physically ready to meet the challenges of adulthood and assume its corresponding responsibilities (Murray & Zentner, 1997). It is a time of rapid physiological, emotional, cognitive, and sexual development. The development of self-concept and body image is closely tied to the adolescent woman's cognitive appraisal of past experiences and current level of identity formation. Therefore sensitive health care delivery to the adolescent woman necessitates both a consideration of her present context as well as an understanding of her past experiences. If those previous experiences were positive ones such that the adolescent woman enters this time of life with a positive body and self-image, this developmental period tends to be easier. Conversely, the young woman with impaired body- and/or self-image may find this time of life more troubling (Murray & Zentner, 1997).

This is a time when adolescents are capable of mature behavior but may fall back on childhood patterns of coping. Especially in the face of an illness or in times of stress, do not expect an adolescent to consistently behave in an adult manner. Do not treat her as a child, but likewise do not assume that she is capable of consistently adult communication, thinking, and motivation.

Adolescent women crave acceptance by their peers and place a high value on fitting in. There is a tendency during adolescence to think that no adult could possibly understand their experiences, and, as a result, young women may act aloof or disdainful during an interview, answer in short sentences, and minimally focus on the presenting problem. Just like adults, adolescent women want to be treated with respect and honesty by their health care providers. While having attention paid to their needs is critical, they do not want to be treated in a patronizing manner by adults (Bates, 1995; Jarvis, 2000; Seidel et al., 1999).

Box 8-5 STRATEGIES FOR INTERVIEWING ADOLESCENT WOMEN

Facilitators

Initiate the interview by focusing on the person and not the problem.

Start with an informal discussion of friends, school, hobbies, social activities.

Demonstrate a genuine interest in the adolescent as a person.

Keep the atmosphere friendly and informal.

Maintain your professional demeanor; do not attempt to be a peer to the adolescent.

Validate to adolescents that they are worthy of respect and consideration.

Be totally honest in your communication and always tell them the truth.

Explain each step of the interview and physical examination and give rationales.

Keep questions short and simple.

Be prepared in the event the adolescent does not know the purpose of the visit (if the parent is seeking care for the adolescent).

Allow adolescents time to collect their thoughts.

When it is necessary to divulge confidential information, have the adolescent share in this process.

Flash cards with subjects common to adolescents may be helpful in getting a recalcitrant adolescent to communicate.

Detractors

Avoid focusing solely on the problem; adolescents respond better if the focus is on them as individuals.

Avoid use of adolescent jargon or language that is inconsistent with your age.

Refrain from asking questions about parents and family if these areas are emotionally charged for the adolescent.

Avoid the use of the reflection technique with adolescents; they will probably respond by saying "What?"

Avoid undue silences with adolescents because they may find this threatening.

Do not force conversation or confrontation.

Be aware that adolescents may not be comfortable discussing feelings with a health care provider.

Adolescents who personally seek out health care may come alone or with at least one parent. If the young woman comes to the primary care center with a parent, it is important for the provider to explain to him or her that some degree of confidentiality is needed and that some aspects of the interview and/or physical examination will entail talking with the adolescent woman individually. It is important to clarify that confidentiality is not about "keeping secrets" but is about mutual respect in the relationship. If it becomes necessary to share any of the confidential information, the adolescent must be involved in this process (Bates, 1995).

There are a number of helpful strategies to employ when interviewing adolescent women. Box 8-5 presents some helpful suggestions.

Older Adults. The population in the United States is aging. Population estimates for persons 65 years of age or older were 34.9 million in 2000, representing 12.66% of the U.S. population (U.S. Bureau of the Census , 2000). This number is expected to grow in the future, and the most rapid increase is expected between the years 2010 and

2030 when the baby boom generation reaches age 65. By the year 2030, there will between 65 and 70 million older persons, and 25% of the U.S. population will be over the age of 65 (Murray & Zentner, 1993).

Interestingly, the word "geriatrics" originates from two Greek words meaning "old age" and "healing" or "physician." Human aging is characterized by a progressive loss of each organ system's homeostatic reserve. These declines, which begin in the third decade of life, tend to be gradual, linear, variable among individuals, and not readily apparent at rest. Thus the hallmark of aging lies not in the resting performance but in the capability of the individual to respond under conditions of stress (e.g., illness states, environmental challenges, drug therapies, etc.) (Kane, Ouslander, & Abrass, 1999; Resnick, 1998).

Women who are nearing the end of the life cycle pose certain challenges as well as opportunities for health care providers. Sensory organs may be impaired and responses slower. Physical disability and chronic illnesses may be present with their accompanying discomforts and infirmity. Older women may be afraid to tell you about their symptoms because of embarrassment, fear of the diagnosis and/or diagnostic testing, or concerns about ability to pay for treatment. Others may think their symptoms are merely a normal part of aging and therefore do not need to be reported (Kane, Ouslander, & Abrass, 1999; Murray & Zentner, 1997).

In working with aging women it is paramount to avoid dismissing treatable pathology as simple aging and treating normal aging as a disease process. An abrupt decline in any body system or function is usually the hallmark of disease, while the physiological decline in homeostatic reserve that characterizes normal aging should not cause symptoms or impair functional capabilities (Resnick, 1998).

It is important to recognize that there is no homogeneity of aging; in fact, today's aged as compared to one generation ago are either healthier and more vital or more disabled and infirm (Kane, Ouslander, & Abrass, 1999). Individuals tend to become more dissimilar as they age, not stereotypically similar, as they are frequently portrayed (Resnick, 1998).

Much of our knowledge about aging comes from cross-sectional studies comparing a younger group with an older group. These data may, however, reflect differences other than age; for example, the older cohorts grew up in a very different environment with regard to diet, physical activity, occupation, and activities. Older women are largely a product of what they bring to old age, including the totality of their life's experiences (Chenitz, Stone, & Salisbury, 1991: Kane, Ouslander, & Abrass, 1999; Murray & Zentner, 1997).

It is important to understand that from middle age forward, people begin to measure their lives in terms of time left rather than years lived. It is therefore normal for aging women to reminisce about the past and discuss their joys, sorrows, triumphs, and regrets. Listening to their life's review will give the clinician important information on coping strengths and capabilities as well as areas of deficiency (Murray & Zentner, 1997).

In working with aging women, it is important to establish a baseline functional scale with which to make future comparisons. There are a number of strategies for collecting

Box 8-6 STRATEGIES FOR INTERVIEWING AGING WOMEN

Facilitators

Address aging persons by their last name, e.g., "Hello, Ms. Jones."

Allow aging individuals more time to tell their stories and to respond to provider questions.

Provide a comfortable room free of noise and distractions.

Do not try to accomplish everything in one visit. Plan for multiple visits, which may be less fatiguing and more productive.

Be patient with the life review of aging clients.

Identify priorities, goals, and adaptive patterns in your aging clients and verify your impressions with the client.

Find out how they currently perceive themselves.

Establish indices of functional capacity including ADLs: walking, getting out of bed, bathing, hair care, dressing, eating (chewing), and toileting.

Establish indices of IADLs, including driving a car, using public transportation, making phone calls, banking, obtaining groceries, preparing meals, and taking medications.

Consider safety and support issues in the home environment.

Be aware of any depressive symptomatology and/or changes in cognition; if necessary, administer mental status and depression scales.

Be attentive to the needs of hearing or visually impaired clients.

When necessary, ask short questions in simple language.

Plan ahead to meet the needs of those with physical limitations.

Obtain a comprehensive drug history with special attention to the interactions of drugs, diseases, and the aging process.

Detractors

Avoid use first names or nicknames unless this is acceptable to the client.

Avoid trying to hurry along aging clients.

Avoid stereotyping clients by assuming that they have all the so-called normal changes of aging.

Avoid shouting at hearing-impaired clients because this tends to distort the sounds of consonants and vowels.

Avoid glaring light sources.

ADLs = activities of daily living; IADLs = instrumental activities of daily living.

this baseline information as well as for making a holistic appraisal of the aging woman (Box 8-6).

Sources of Information

During the interviewing process, be aware of additional sources of information such as the woman's family and friends, the preexisting medical record, laboratory testing, and letters of referral. If one is concerned about the accuracy of a woman's responses, it may be helpful to briefly separate the woman and the family in an attempt to solicit the needed information. Some geriatric settings allow for two or more interviewers to meet with women and families in an attempt to develop a comprehensive picture of present-ing problems and capabilities, functional status, safety, and so forth; the interviewers often come away with have differing perceptions about the woman and her situation. Plotting a client's capabilities, health care needs, ADL and IADL skills, cognitive function, and depression scores on a composite scale gives you an objective baseline from which to compare all future performance.

Be sure to record the source of the historical information and a statement about how reliable you judge this material to be. Reliability is usually defined as the same answers to the same questions even if rephrased or repeated later in the interview.

Conducting the Interview

The Introductory Phase. The goals for the introductory phase include establishing rapport between the provider and woman, ensuring mutual comfort, and defining what each expects from the interview. It is important to set the tone and direction for the interview and to establish a mutual understanding of the purpose of the exchange.

Introduce yourself to the woman and clearly state your name and your role in the setting. If you are a student, do not hide this fact from the client. Be sure to address the woman properly (Miss, Ms., Mrs.) and verify correct pronunciation of her name if necessary. Avoid the use of first names or surrogate names such as "mother" or "grandmother." Be sure to ask the woman's permission to proceed with the history and physical examination; this serves to preserve and respect her autonomy.

As one begins to structure the interview and obtain the chronological and sequential data as well as probe for underlying concerns, it is important to appear unhurried. If at all possible, try to listen to the entire story and avoid asking too many questions early in the process. The woman will take her cues from you; you will need to balance the obvious time constraints with the needs of the interview (Bates, 1995). Let the woman know that time is available for her by leaning back in your chair, maintaining good eye contact, and really listening to what she is saying. Avoid interrupting and do not ask a follow-up question until you have heard the complete answer to the first question.

Ask the woman to state the reason for the visit and allow her to "spill it all out." Avoid being overly directive during this segment of the interview. Listen to the first flow of words and let that shape the direction for the remainder of the interview.

The Working Phase. This is the data collection phase of the interview. All sources of data are considered, including verbal and nonverbal responses, biographic data, health status data, family contributions, and chart and lab information. It is hoped at the end of this phase that you will be able to correctly identify and respond to the woman's health care needs.

The Focused Interview. This process may be used to collect data during the working phase of the interview. Focused or structured interviews typically use preprinted surveys consisting of varying questions. Familiarity with these tools allows the interviewer to concentrate on the woman's responses rather than be concerned about what question to ask next. In general, the structured interview proceeds from general to specific. General biographical data pertaining to health perception are discussed prior to asking about sexuality, relationships, and other intimate matters (Fuller & Schaller-Ayers, 2000).

The structured interview should be viewed as a guide to questions rather than as a rigid set of directions. As discussed previously, excessive questioning can undermine rapport; so a guided set of questions should be used cautiously (Fuller & Schaller-Ayers, 2000).

The Terminating Phase. The end of the interview is signaled by cues such as, "*We have about 5 minutes left. Is there anything else you want to tell me?*" If all areas of concern have not been addressed, this is a good time to make future appointments.

During the terminating phase, a brief summary of the most salient issues of the discussion should be made. This allows both the provider and the woman time to validate perceptions and correct any inconsistencies.

THE HEALTH HISTORY

Health history involves obtaining the following elements:

Biographic Data. Name, address, phone number, age, birth date and birthplace, sex, race, ethnicity, marital status, occupation, religion, referring agency, date and time of the interview, and the source and reliability of the history

Reason for Care. This should be a short statement in the client's own words that describes the reason for the visit. It should be put in quotation marks to indicate that these were the client's exact words. This statement is not intended to be a diagnostic entity; instead consider it the title of your story (Jarvis, 2000). It should include one or more signs and symptoms and a statement of their duration.

History of Present Illness/Illness Event. If a woman is well, this should be a short statement regarding her general health status. In the event the woman is ill, this section should be a clear, concise, chronological account of the reason for seeking care. The narrative should describe the problem from the onset of the symptom(s) until the present time. Although data are elicited from the woman, it is incumbent on the provider to give a complete yet succinct account of the problem.

It is desirable that the woman's response be in the form of a narrative summary; however, in the final written account, any symptom the person has noted should be described in terms of eight attributes: timing, location, quality, quantity, setting, alleviating/aggravating factors, associated manifestations, and attributions. In this section, it is also important to note any significant negatives (absence of symptoms) that may help in the clinical decision-making process. If a symptom is not mentioned, the reader will assume that no questions were asked. Remember that the "History of Present Illness" section is considered the best compilation of the narrative story in the health care record (Bates, 1995).

When recording this information, start a new paragraph with each new symptom or chronological period. This will help the reader understand the evolution of the symptom. Whenever possible, try to use the day, month, and year as reference points for dating events in the history. All relevant information about the problem/system should be included in the "History of Present Illness" section. This includes a statement regarding the woman's response to her symptoms and health care problems. The provider should try to determine her underlying concerns; the effects of the problem on her daily life; any changes in capabilities at home, work, or in leisure and social activities; any changes in the performance of usual roles (e.g., wife, mother, employee); and any changes in her self-concept as a result of the illness state (Bates, 1995).

Past Health History. Any previous health events may have a bearing on the present problem. In addition, the manner and style of coping with previous illness experiences may give the provider clues about how the woman may respond to the current health threat.

General State of Health. This is a general statement of health status as the woman perceives it.

Childhood Illness. Measles, mumps, rubella, whooping cough, chickenpox, rheumatic fever, scarlet fever, polio, pertussis, strep throat. Inquire about any long-term effects of rheumatic fever, scarlet fever, polio, etc. Describe age at the time and any important complications or treatment.

Accidents or Injuries. Fractures, automobile accidents, head trauma, burns, penetrating wounds. Record the woman's age at the time of the accident or date of occurrence, complications, and treatment.

Serious or Chronic Illness. Diabetes, hypertension, cancer, heart disease, sickle cell anemia, chronic obstructure pulmonary disease, seizure disorder, etc. Record age at onset, complications, treatment.

Hospitalizations. (If not previously described.) Include the name and location of the hospital, condition being treated, length of stay, health care personnel involved.

Surgery. Type of procedure, date, surgeon, name of hospital, location of hospital, recovery, complications.

Obstetric History. Note gravidity, parity, term, prematurity, abortion, and living children (these are denoted as G–P–T–P–A–L–). For each complete pregnancy, note the course of the pregnancy, type of delivery and setting, sex, weight, and general health of the infant, and postpartum course.

Transfusions. Note the date, type of product (e.g., red cells, platelets), reason, setting, and any documented reactions.

Current Health Status. Although some of the variables noted here have a past as well as present component, they tend to bear directly on current health status:

Current Medications. Include all prescription medications, nonprescription/over the counter medications, home remedies, vitamin and mineral supplements, and any borrowed medicines. For each medication, ask dosage, schedule, why taken, and length of time being taken. Try to determine "actual" usage, which may differ from prescribed usage. It may be necessary to ask the woman to bring in all the medications that she takes to get an accurate picture of her medication use.

Allergies. Include both the allergen (medication, food, contact agent, environmental agent) as well as the woman's reaction to exposure. Be specific and note such things as rash, rhinitis, difficulty breathing, ocular effects.

Tobacco Use. Include the type(s) of tobacco product, daily patterns of use, and duration of use. For cigarette smoking, record usage in pack-years format (calculated by multiplying the number of packs per day by the number of years of smoking). Thus a 20-year history of smoking 2 packs of cigarettes per day corresponds to a 40 pack-year history.

Alcohol, Drugs, and Related Substances. Attempt to provide a detailed, quantitative account of alcohol and/or nonprescription drug use. Be aware of the potential for problematic alcohol or drug use. If the woman answers yes to questions about alcohol intake, ask specific questions regarding usual amount, frequency of use, patterns of alcohol ingestion, etc. You may want to include the CAGE questions to gain insight into possible client concerns about alcohol consumption (Ewing, 1984). The CAGE questions include: (1) Have you ever thought you should *C*ut down on your drinking? (2) Have you been *A*nnoyed by criticism of your drinking? (3) Have you ever felt *G*uilty about your drinking? and (4) Do you ever have an *E*yeopener in the morning?

Include questions about history of alcohol treatment, alcohol recovery activities, and any family history of alcohol or drug problems. If the woman answers positively about the use of street drugs, ask specifically what drugs are used, how frequently this occurs, and the effect of the drug use on patterns of daily living.

Nutrition/Weight. Note weight loss or gain, usual weight, usual daily nutritional intake including caffeinated beverages such as coffee, tea, and cola. Address any dietary restrictions or the use of any diet supplements.

Screening Tests. As appropriate for the client, include Pap smears, tuberculin tests, mammograms, stool for occult blood, cholesterol levels, glucose level, etc. Include the date and results of lab tests.

Immunization Status. Include most recent boosters with dates, including tetanus, pertussis, diphtheria, polio, measles, rubella, mumps, influenza, hepatitis B, pneumococcal vaccine, and *Hemophilus influenzae* type b.

Sleep Patterns. Include usual time to retire at night and arise in the morning. Any problems falling asleep or staying asleep. Use of any aids to sleep. Sense of feeling rested after sleep and any napping during the day.

Environmental Hazards. Include those encountered at home, work, school, or during leisure activities.

Use of Safety Measures. Include questions on seat belts, smoke detectors, air bags, etc.

Personal and Social History. This section is a narrative description of the important information about the woman as a person; it includes sections on home, family, work, social adjustment, etc.

Important Life Experiences. Place of birth, places of residency and duration, early life, years of education and literacy, marriage, personal and family finances.

Significant Others or Living Partners. Inquire about age, health, occupation, relationships, previous marriages, sexual orientation/preferences. Is there an existing social support structure? Has the woman ever been injured by a partner? Is there concern that this might occur? Is there a history of violence in the home, i.e., emotional, physical, or sexual abuse? Inquire about the use and types of contraception, STD prevention.

Home Situation. Inquire about others living in the home. Ask about the home's location and condition (include stairs, heating, plumbing, water source).

Occupation. Note occupational history including duties, hazards, exposures, and retirement. Include questions on role expectations and occupational and educational goals.

Daily Life. Inquire about typical daily activities from arising to retiring.

Military Record. Include dates of service, duties, locations, and service-connected disabilities.

Foreign Travel. Include dates, locations, and whether or not any illnesses occurred.

Exercise and Leisure Activities. Include description of hobbies, exercise plan, spare-time activities.

Religious Beliefs. Inquire about those beliefs relevant to perceptions of health and illness, treatment, etc.

Stress Management/Coping. Note existing social support. What coping styles/activities are employed under stressful circumstances? How helpful are these activities?

Values History. What gives your life meaning? What is the meaning of your illness in the context of your life? What are the supporting or conflicting religious convictions?

Living Will or Advance Directives. Inquire if a living will, medical power of attorney, or other advance directive has been prepared. If so, a copy should be placed in the current health care record.

Family History. Ask about the age, health status, and cause of death of immediate family members (parents, siblings, grandparents, spouse, children). Ask specifically about the presence of the following conditions in family members: diabetes, heart disease, hypercholesterolemia, cancer, hypertension, stroke, kidney disease, tuberculosis, arthritis, anemia, allergies, asthma, headaches, seizure disorders, mental illness, alcoholism, drug addiction, sickle cell anemia, obesity, blood disorders, goiter, atherosclerosis, congenital defects, deafness, muscular disorders, and any symptoms similar to those exhibited by the client. Construct a family tree or genogram to show this information clearly and concisely (West Virginia University School of Medicine, 1997).

Review of Systems. The purpose of this section is to systematically evaluate the past and current health status of each system and to consider the necessary health promotion practices for each body system. This information is usually asked in a head-to-toe sequence and questions asked typically include only the most common presenting problems. If the system has been previously discussed in the "History of Present Illness" section, it does not need to be addressed here.

The interviewer should indicate the presence or absence of symptoms under each of these systems. Remember to collect only subjective data at this point and refrain from including objective data. This section should be limited to the symptoms the client indicates are present.

General. Current weight (gain or loss); dieting; change in appetite; weight at age 25 or a comparable time; presence of fatigue, weakness or malaise, fever, chills, sweating, or night sweats.

Skin. History of skin disease, acne, boils, shingles, rashes, eczema, psoriasis, hives, color changes, bruising, bleeding, lesions, change in a mole, itching, excessive dryness or moisture, or any change in hair or nails.

Head. Any complaints of headache, dizziness, vertigo, or head trauma.

Eyes. Change in vision, glasses or contact lenses, last eye examination, pain, redness, lacrimation, dryness, scotoma, injury, diplopia, pain, strabismus, cataract, or blurred vision.

Ears. Earaches, infections, discharge, tinnitus, vertigo, change in hearing, use of hearing aids.

Nose and Sinus. Change in olfactory sensation, discharge, obstruction, bleeding, injury, sinus drainage, frequent or severe colds, allergies, hay fever, stuffiness, or itching.

Mouth and Throat. Change in taste sensation, teeth, dentures, gums, tongue, ulcers, lesions, frequent sore throats, bleeding gums, difficulty swallowing, hoarseness, tonsillectomy, and last dental examination.

Neck. Pain, limitation of motion, lumps or swelling, masses, goiter, or "swollen glands."

Breast and Axilla. Pain, masses, nipple discharge, breast disease, surgery, breast self-examination, axillary swelling, tenderness, mass, or rash.

Respiratory System. Chest pain, pleurisy, cough, sputum (amount and appearance), history of lung disease (asthma, emphysema, bronchitis, pneumonia, tuberculosis), wheezy or noisy breathing, orthopnea, shortness of breath, hemoptysis, cyanosis, night sweats, and last chest X-ray.

Cardiovascular System. Exertional chest pain, palpitations, dyspnea on exertion (attempt to specify the amount of exertion, e.g., walking up one flight of stairs, moving from the chair to the bed), cyanosis, orthopnea, paroxysmal nocturnal dyspnea, nocturia, edema, hypertension, heart murmur, coronary artery disease, anemia, congenital lesions, last ECG or other cardiac studies.

Peripheral Vascular System. Claudication or poor circulation, varicosities, stasis dermatitis or ulcer, cold reactivity, leg cramps, previous deep vein thrombosis, coolness, numbness, or tingling.

Gastrointestinal System. Difficulty swallowing, abdominal pain, heartburn, change in appetite, nausea/vomiting, vomiting of blood, indigestion, ulcer, previous GI studies and results, jaundice, dark urine, pruritus, gallstones, gas, diarrhea, constipation, laxative use, painful defecation, rectal bleeding, black tarry stools, or hemorrhoids.

Urinary System. Frequency, urgency, infection, burning, retention, incontinence, hesitancy, dribbling, colic, groin pain, suprapubic or low back pain, kidney stone, fever, chills, oliguria, cloudy or bloody urine, stricture, or history of protein or sugar in the urine.

Female Reproductive System. Menstrual history (age at menarche, last menstrual period, cycle length, duration, amenorrhea, menorrhagia, premenstrual pain, or dysmenorrhea). Date of last Pap smear, pelvic pain, menopausal symptoms, age at menopause, postmenopausal bleeding, discharge, or itching.

Sexual Health. Inquire if presently in a relationship involving intercourse. Is there any dyspareunia? Is the sexual expression satisfactory to client and partner? Use of contraception? Is the contraceptive method satisfactory? Is client aware of contact with a partner who has been diagnosed with any STD (gonorrhea, chlamydia, genital herpes, condyloma, syphilis, HIV or AIDS) (MacLaren, 1995).

Musculoskeletal System. Muscle or joint pain, trauma and sequelae, arthritis, gout, muscle spasms, backache, intervertebral disk disease, weakness, deformity, crepitus, gait problems, or limitations in range of motion.

Nervous System. Inquire about history of seizure disorder, fainting, blackouts, stroke, loss of sensation, or "pins and needles." With regard to motor function, presence of history of tremors, involuntary movements, paralysis, or coordination problems. Regarding mental status, presence or history of memory problems, depression, hallucinations, or anxiety.

Hematological System. History or presence of anemia, easy bruising, unusual or excessive bleeding, exposure to toxic agents or radiation, or any abnormalities of blood cells.

Endocrine System. Any history or presence of thyroid problems, hot or cold intolerance, diabetes or diabetic symptoms (polyuria, polydipsia, polyphagia), abnormal hair distribution, tremors, or anxiety.

Emotional Status. Personal profile and self-evaluation. Inquire about how the woman is coping with the present illness. Inquire about insomnia, depression, crying, anxiety, history of a nervous breakdown or psychiatric treatment, problems with race, nationality, language, or legal issues.

DOCUMENTATION

Because it is not possible to remember all of the details of a comprehensive health history, most providers take abbreviated notes during the interview. The majority of women are familiar with note taking, but it is possible that some individuals may be uncomfortable with this. If this is the case, it is important that the provider explain the need to make an accurate and comprehensive record. Taking minimal notes throughout the interview and using them later to build a comprehensive account of will become easier with practice. Do not attempt to write your final version as you talk with the woman. As a caution, note taking should not unduly divert attention from the woman. When discussing sensitive or emotionally-laden topics, it is probably best not to take notes at all.

Follow the documentation requirements of your agency. It may be helpful to use a preprinted written questionnaire to prompt the categories and questions to be asked. In some progress note sheets, a guide to the history and physical examination is printed in the left-hand margin. If you need prompting to collect a complete history, be sure to carry a guide at all times.

The sooner you can write up your notes, the better. It is helpful to dictate the summary or transcribe notes in a written format. Try not to have too many additional client encounters between the interview and its documentation.

SUMMARY

Advanced practice nurses have a critical role to play in the promotion of health among American women. The use of relationship-centered care as a vehicle for humanistic health care delivery to women is a positive step in this regard. Shared responsibility among health care providers and consumers in the promotion of healthier lives will move the nation collectively and individually toward a healthier future.

REFERENCES

Aho, W. R. (1979). Participation of senior citizens in the swine flu inoculation program: An analysis of health belief model variables in preventive health behavior. *Journal of Gerontology, 34*, 201–208.

Badger, L. W., deGruy, F. V., Hartman, J., Plant, M. A., Leeper, J., Ficken, R., et al. (1994). Psychosocial interest, medical interview, and the recognition of depression. *Archives of Family Medicine, 3*, 899–907.

Bandura, A. (1977). *Social learning theory.* Englewood-Cliffs, NJ: Prentice-Hall.

Bandura, A. (1997). *Self-efficacy; the exercise of control.* New York: W. H. Freeman.

Bates, B. (1995). *A guide to physical examination and history taking* (6th ed.). Philadelphia: J. B. Lippincott.

Becker, M. H., Drachman, R. H., & Kirscht, J. P. (1972). Predicting mothers' compliance with pediatric medical regimens. *Medical Care, 81*, 843–854.

Becker, M. H., Drachman, R. H., & Kirscht, J. P. (1974). A new approach to explaining sick role behavior in low income populations. *American Journal of Public Health, 64*, 204–216.

Bickley, L. S. (1998). *Bates' guide to physical examination and history taking* (7th ed.). Philadelphia: Lippincott Williams & Wilkins.

Boykin, A., & Schoenhofer, S. O. (1991). Story as link between nursing practice, ontology, epistemology. *Image: Journal of Nursing Scholarship, 23*, 245–248.

Brady, M. L. (1987). Psychological interactions for women with breast disease. *Obstetric and Gynecologic Clinics of North America, 14*, 797–816.

Brown, J. B., Boles, M., Mullooly, J. P., & Levinson, W. (1999). Effect of clinician communication skills training on patient satisfaction. A randomized controlled trial. *Annals of Internal Medicine, 131*, 822–829.

Cassell, E. J. (1989). Making good interview skills better. *Patient Care, 23*, 145–166.

Chenitz, W. C., Stone, J. T., & Salisbury, S. A. (1991). *Clinical gerontological nursing: A guide to advanced practice.* Philadelphia: W. B. Saunders.

Cousins, N. (1985). Occasional notes: How patients appraise physicians. *New England Journal of Medicine, 313*, 1422–1425.

Ewing, J. A. (1984). Detecting alcoholism: The CAGE questionnaire. *Journal of the American Medical Association, 252*, 1905–1907.

Frank, G. (1996). Life histories in occupational therapy clinical practice. *The American Journal of Occupational Therapy, 50*, 251–264.

Fuller, J., & Schaller-Ayers, J. (2000). *Health assessment. A nursing approach* (3rd ed.). Philadelphia: J. B. Lippincott.

Grant, C. H., Cissna, K. N., & Rosenfeld, L. B. (2000). Patients' perceptions of physicians' communication and outcomes of the accrual to trial process. *Health Communication 2000, 12*, 23–39.

Greco, M., Brownlea, A., McGovern, J., & Cavanagh, M. (2000). Consumers as educators: Implementation of patient feedback in general practice training. *Health Communication 2000, 12*, 173–193.

Harvard Medical School. (1997, October). Women's health centers. *Harvard Women's Health Watch*, p.1.

Hodgkinson, H. L. (1992). *A demographic look at tomorrow.* Washington, DC: Institute for Educational Leadership.

Jarvis, C. (2000). *Physical examination and health assessment* (3rd ed.). Philadelphia: W. B. Saunders.

Kane, R. L., Ouslander, J. G., & Abrass, I. B. (1999). *Essentials of clinical geriatrics* (4th ed.). New York: McGraw-Hill Professional Publishing.

Kaplan, C. B., Siegel, B. Madill, J. M., & Epstein, R. M. (1997). Communication and the medical interview. Strategies for learning and teaching. *Journal of General Internal Medicine, 12*, (Suppl 2), S49–S55.

Kravitz, R. L., Callahan, E. J., Paterniti, D., Antonius, D., Dunham, M., & Lewis, C. E. (1996). Prevalence and sources of patients' unmet expectations for care. *Annals of Internal Medicine, 125*, 730–737.

Kutner, J. S., Steiner, J. F., Corbett, K. K., Jahnigen, D. W., & Barton, P. L. (1999). Information needs in terminal illness. *Social Science and Medicine, 48*(10), 1341–1352.

Lang, F., Floyd, M. R., & Beine, K. L. (2000). Clues to patients' explanations and concerns about their illnesses. A call for active listening. *Archives of Family Medicine, 9*, 222–227.

Larson, E. A., & Fanchiang, S. P. (1996). Life history and narrative research: Generating a humanistic knowledge base for occupational therapy. *The American Journal of Occupational Therapy, 50*, 247–250.

Leight, S. B. (2002). Starry night: Using story to inform aesthetic knowing in women's health nursing. *Journal of Advanced Nursing, 37*(1), 108–114.

MacLaren, A. (1995). Primary care for women. Comprehensive sexual health assessment. *Journal of Nurse Midwifery, 40*, 104–119.

Maiman, L. A., & Becker, M. H. (1974). The Health Belief Model: Origins and correlates in psychological theory. *Health Education Monographs, 2*, 328–335.

Mallison, T., Kielhofner, G., & Mattingly, C. (1996). Metaphor and meaning in the clinical interview. *The American Journal of Occupational Therapy, 50*, 338–346.

Murphy, P. A. (1996). Primary care for women. Health assessment, health promotion, and disease prevention services. *Journal of Nurse Midwifery, 41*, 83–90.

Murray, R. B., & Zentner, J. P. (1993). *Nursing assessment and health promotion. Strategies through the life span* (5th ed.). Norwalk, CT: Appleton & Lange.

Murray, R. B., & Zentner, J. P. (1997). *Nursing assessment and health promotion strategies through the life span* (6th ed.). Upper Saddle River, NJ: Prentice Hall.

Pender, N. J. (1996). *Health promotion in nursing practice.* Stamford, CT: Appleton & Lange.

Polkinghorne, D. E. (1988). *Narrative knowing and the human sciences.* Albany, NY: State University of New York Press.

Quirk, M., & Casey, L. (1995). Primary care for women. The art of interviewing. *Journal of Nurse Midwifery, 40*, 97–103.

Random House Webster's College Dictionary (2nd ed.). (1999). New York: Random House.

Resnick, N. M. (1998). Geriatric medicine. In L. M. Tierney, S. J. McPhee, & M. A. Papadakis (Eds.), *Current medical diagnosis and treatment* (pp. 43-64). Stamford, CT: Appleton & Lange.

Rosenstock, I. M. (1966). Why people use health services. *Milbank Memorial Fund Quarterly, 44*, 99–121.

Rosenstock, I. M., Strecher, V. J., & Becker, M. H. (1988). Social learning theory and the Health Belief Model. *Health Education Quarterly, 15*, 175–183.

Sandelowski, M. (1991). Telling stories: Narrative approaches to qualitative research. *Image: Journal of Nursing Scholarship, 23*, 161–166.

Seidel, H. M., Ball, J. W., Dains, J. E., & Benedict, G. (1999). *Mosby's guide to physical examination* (4th ed.). St. Louis: Mosby.

Smith, M. J., & Liehr, P. (1999). Attentively embracing story: A middle-range theory with practice and research implications. *Scholarly Inquiry for Nursing Practice: An International Journal, 13*, 187–210.

Swartz, M. H. (1998). *Textbook of physical diagnosis—history and examination* (3rd ed.). Philadelphia: W. B. Saunders.

U.S. Bureau of the Census. (2000). *Population estimates—2000* [On-line]. Available: *http://www.census.gov/population/estimates/nation.*

U.S. Department of Health and Human Services. (2000). *Healthy people 2010* [On-line]. Available: *http://www.health.gov/healthypeople/.*

Walker, L. G. (1996). Communication skills: When, not if, to teach. *European Journal of Medicine, 32A*, 1457–1459.

West Virginia University School of Medicine. (1997). *Clinical evaluation of patients.* [Brochure]. Morgantown, WV: Author.

Writing Group of the 1996 AAN Expert Panel on Women's Health. (1997). Women's health and women's health care: Recommendations of the 1996 AAN Expert Panel on Women's Health. *Nursing Outlook, 45*, 7–15.

RESOURCES

Journals
Health Communication
Communication Research

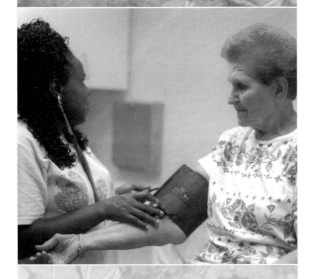

Chapter 9

Screening and Diagnostic Tests

Margaret Burns

An ounce of prevention is worth a pound of cure.

T. C. Haliburton

INTRODUCTION

As primary care providers the women's health care nurse practitioner and the nurse in ambulatory care are able to provide optimal and appropriate care through knowledge of primary care and women's health. Primary health care consists of services as well as disease prevention, health promotion, and restoration. The primary care provider's role offers the opportunity to reduce morbidity and mortality for women of all ages, not only in the diagnosis and treatment of specific symptoms but also in the prevention and early detection of illness. Screening is the search for disease in the asymptomatic individual and usually implies administration of specific diagnostic tests. However, screening can be more comprehensive and include any preliminary procedure such as a test, history, or physical examination in the evaluation of the woman's health status. This chapter gives an overview of preventive health care and screening and of specific screening and diagnostic tests and reviews diagnostic testing for specific common conditions.

Primary care is important to prevent health problems from developing. The content and frequency of primary health care visits are tailored to the woman's age and risk factors (Tables 9-1 and 9-2). Understanding women's health requires more than a biomedical view; the nurse working in women's health care needs an awareness of how health and illness are linked closely to the social, physical, community, political, and cultural environment of the woman (Expert panel, 1997). The context of the individual experience of health is assessed and managed while applying the recommended preventive health guidelines described in Box 9-1. Balancing the woman's experiences and expected norms allows the nurse to provide personal services to promote and maintain health.

OVERVIEW OF PREVENTIVE HEALTH CARE AND SCREENING

The leading causes of death in women in the United States are largely preventable. Certain diseases increasingly result from chronic and acute conditions for which associated risk factors and behaviors can be modified. The leading causes of death differ for each age group. Research has demonstrated that specific interventions by primary care providers such as screening, immunization, and counseling can dramatically reduce morbidity and premature mortality in women (Parker, Tong, Bolden, & Wing, 1997; *Put Prevention into Practice*, 1998; U.S. Preventive Services Task Force, 1996).

As with other clinical strategies the nurse practitioner can evaluate individual preventive services before incorporating them into routine practice. Recommendations by the American College of Obstetricians and Gynecologists (ACOG) Primary Care Task Force (see Box 9-1) encompass the recommendations by the U.S. Preventive Services Task Force referred to within this chapter.

Prevention can be conceptualized as intervention to prevent a morbid event from occurring in a woman's life. Preventive interventions such as screening, diagnostic tests, and immunizations typically are performed on a woman who is asymptomatic (Heudebert, 1993). Types of prevention are primary, secondary, or tertiary. Primary prevention is the prevention of a disease before it occurs, involving immunizations or health education about risk reduction. Secondary prevention is the detection and treatment of a disease in its early stages before the woman is symptomatic. Screening tests such as sphygmomanometry and Papanicolaou (Pap) smears are types of secondary prevention. Tertiary prevention is directed at the woman who has a history or diagnosis of a disease to maximize function by slowing deterioration and preventing complications caused by the disease and restoring health. Teritary intervention may be directed toward patient education to reduce further sequelae in conditions such as osteoporosis.

EVALUATION OF PREVENTIVE SERVICES

Implementation of preventive interventions varies. Certain interventions are mandated by law, such as using a seat belt, wearing a helmet, or chlorinating pool water. Other interventions are compiled from research conducted by various task forces, government agencies, and professional or specialty organizations. Review processes and strictness of evaluation methods may differ among these groups. Cost effectiveness of the different screening interventions is incorporated into the recommendations.

Preventive interventions generally should not be used unless they have been shown to be effective in evidence-based research. Many health care providers look to these

Table 9-1 RECOMMENDED SCREENING AND DIAGNOSTIC TESTS FOR WOMEN

TEST	AGE	FREQUENCY
Blood pressure	18+	At every health maintenance visit
Skin exam	20 to 39 40+	Every 3 years Yearly
Breast exam	18+ 20 to 39 40+	Self-exam of breasts done monthly Clinical breast exam every 3 years Clinical breast exam yearly
Mammogram	40 40 to 49 50+	First mammogram Every 1 to 2 years or as advised by primary care provider Annually or as advised by primary care provider
Pelvic exam	18 to 39 40+	Every 1 to 3 years; gynecological problems may necessitate greater frequency Yearly
Pap smear	18	Begin at age 18 or at onset of sexual activity. After 3 or more consecutive satisfactory, normal tests, perform less frequently based on presence of risk factors
Digital rectal examination	50+	Yearly
Colorectal examination	50+	Yearly
Sigmoidoscopy	50+	Every 3 to 5 years
Colonoscopy	35 to 40 18+	Every 3 to 5 years for women who have one or more first-degree relatives with history of colorectal disorders Recommended for those with ulcerative colitis of 10-year duration, history of colon cancer, adematous polyps, or familial polyposis syndrome
Cholesterol test	19+ 64+	Every 5 years if levels are within normal range Every 3 to 5 years if levels are within normal range
Thyroid-stimulating hormone test	>65 <65	Every 3 to 5 years For women who have autoimmune conditions or a strong family history of thyroid disorders
Glucose tolerance test	45+	Every 3 to 5 years (only for high-risk women)

groups as experts in putting forth guidelines. Recommendations may vary among the numerous preventive care authorities, and not all authorities agree about every preventive service (Maldow-Kay, 1997).

When making a decision in planning care for women, nurse practitioners are to evaluate the screening intervention and be selective in ordering tests and providing preventive services. Improvement in clinical outcomes and reduction of mortality and morbidity are important considerations. In addition to weighing evidence for effectiveness, selecting appropriate screening tests requires considering age, gender, and other individual risk factors. A screening intervention allows the discovery of a disorder in its asymptomatic state. However, screening occasionally may result in more harm than good, because of side effects from testing, false-negative or false-positive results,

Table 9-2 | HIGH-RISK FACTORS

INTERVENTION	HIGH-RISK FACTOR
STD testing	History of multiple sexual partners or a sexual partner with multiple contacts, sexual contact with persons with culture-proven STD, history of repeated episodes of STD, attendance at clinics for STDs
Skin	Increased recreational or occupational exposure to sunlight, family or personal history of skin cancer, clinical evidence of precursor lesions
Thyroid-stimulating hormone	Strong family history of thyroid disease, autoimmune disease (evidence of subclinical hypothyroidism may be related to unfavorable lipid profiles)
Tuberculosis (TB) skin test	HIV infection, close contact with persons known or suspected to have TB, medical risk factors known to increase risk of disease if infected, born in country with high TB prevalence, medically underserved, low income, alcoholism, intravenous drug use, resident of long-term care facility (e.g., correctional institutions, mental institutions, nursing homes and facilities), health professional working in high-risk health care facilities

American College of Obstetricians and Gynecologists. (1996). *Guidelines for women's health care.* Washington, DC: ACOG.

Box 9-1 RECOMMENDED PREVENTIVE GUIDELINES FOR WOMEN'S HEALTH CARE

AGES 13-18 YEARS

Screening

History
Reason for visit
Health status: medical, surgical, family
Dietary/nutritional assessment
Physical activity
Tobacco, alcohol, other drugs
Abuse/neglect
Sexual practices

Physical Examination
Height
Weight
Blood pressure
Secondary sexual characteristics (Tanner staging)
Pelvic examination (yearly when sexually active or by age 18)
Skin*

Laboratory Tests
Periodic
Pap test (yearly when sexually active or by age 18)
Cholesterol, high-density lipoprotein cholesterol (every 5 years)

*High-Risk Groups**
Hemoglobin
Bacteriuria testing
Sexually transmissible disease testing
Human immunodeficiency virus (HIV) testing
Genetic testing/counseling
Rubella titer
Tuberculosis skin test
Lipid profile
Fasting glucose

Evaluation and Counseling

Sexuality
Development
High-risk behaviors

Preventing unwanted/unintended pregnancy
Postponing sexual involvement
Contraceptive options
Sexually transmissible diseases
Partner selection
Barrier protection

Fitness
Hygiene (including dental); fluoride supplementation
Dietary/nutritional assessment (including eating disorders)
Exercise: discussion of program

Psychosocial Evaluation
Interpersonal/family relationships
Sexual identity
Personal goal development
Behavioral/learning disorders
Abuse/neglect

*See Table 9-2, *High-Risk Factors.*
From American College of Obstetricians and Gynecologists. (1996). *Guidelines for women's health care.* Washington, DC: Author.

Box 9-1 RECOMMENDED PREVENTIVE GUIDELINES FOR WOMEN'S HEALTH CARE

Cardiovascular Risk Factors
Family history
Hypertension
Dyslipidemia
Obesity
Diabetes mellitus

Health/Risk Behaviors
Injury prevention
Safety belts and helmets
Recreational hazards
Firearms
Hearing
Skin exposure to ultraviolet rays
Suicide: depressive symptoms
Tobacco, alcohol, other drugs

Screening

History
Reason for visit
Health status: medical, surgical,
    family
Dietary/nutritional assessment
Physical activity
Tobacco, alcohol, other drugs
Abuse/neglect
Sexual practices

Physical Examination
Height
Weight
Blood pressure
Neck: adenopathy, thyroid
Breasts
Abdomen
Pelvic examination
Skin*

Laboratory Tests
Periodic
Pap test (physician and patient
    discretion after 3 consecutive
    normal tests if low risk)
Cholesterol, high-density lipopro-
    tein cholesterol (every 5 years)

*High-Risk Groups**
Hemoglobin
Bacteriuria testing
Mammography

AGES 13-18 YEARS

Immunizations

Periodic
Tetanus-diphtheria booster (once
    between ages 14 and 16)

*High-Risk Groups**
Measles, mumps, rubella (MMR)
    vaccine
Hepatitis B vaccine

Leading Causes of Death

Motor vehicle accidents
Homicide
Suicide
Leukemia

AGES 19-39 YEARS

Fasting glucose test
Sexually transmissible disease
    testing
Human immunodeficiency virus
    (HIV) testing
Genetic testing/counseling
Rubella titer
Tuberculosis skin test
Lipid profile
Thyroid-stimulating hormone

Evaluation and Counseling

Sexuality
High-risk behaviors
Contraceptive options
Genetic counseling
Preventing unwanted pregnancy
Sexually transmissible diseases
Partner selection
Barrier protection
Sexual function

Fitness
Hygiene (including dental)
Dietary/nutritional assessment
Exercise: discussion of program

Psychosocial Evaluation
Interpersonal/family relationships
Domestic violence
Job satisfaction
Lifestyle/stress
Sleep disorders

Leading Causes of Morbidity

Nose, throat, and upper respirato-
    ry conditions
Viral, bacterial, and parasitic
    infections
Sexual abuse
Musculoskeletal and soft tissue
    injuries
Acute ear infections
Digestive system and acute uri-
    nary conditions

Cardiovascular Risk Factors
Family history
Hypertension
Dyslipidemia
Obesity/diabetes mellitus
Lifestyle

Health/Risk Behaviors
Injury prevention
Safety belts and helmets
Occupational hazards
Recreational hazards
Firearms
Hearing
Breast self-examination
Skin exposure to ultraviolet rays
Suicide: depressive symptoms
Tobacco, alcohol, other drugs

Immunizations

Periodic
Tetanus-diphtheria booster (Every
    10 years)

*High Risk Groups**
Measles, mumps, rubella (MMR)
    vaccine
Hepatitis B vaccine
Influenza vaccine
Pneumococcal vaccine

Continued

Box 9-1 RECOMMENDED PREVENTIVE GUIDELINES FOR WOMEN'S HEALTH CARE

AGES 19-39 YEARS

Leading Causes of Death
Motor vehicle accidents
Cardiovascular disease
Homicide
Acquired immunodeficiency
  syndrome (AIDS)
Cerebrovascular disease

Screening

History
Reason for visit
Health status: medical surgical,
  family
Dietary/nutritional assessment
Physical activity
Tobacco, alcohol, other drugs
Abuse/neglect
Sexual practices

Physical Examination
Height
Weight
Blood pressure
Oral cavity
Neck: adenopathy, thyroid
Breasts, axillae
Abdomen
Pelvic and rectovaginal examina-
  tion
Skin*

Laboratory Tests
Periodic
Pap test (physician and patient discretion after 3 consecutive normal tests if low risk)
Mammography (every 1-2 years
  until age 50, yearly beginning at
  50)
Cholesterol, high-density lipoprotein cholesterol (every 5 years)
Fecal occult blood test
Sigmoidoscopy (every 3-5 years
  after age 50)

*High-Risk Groups**
Hemoglobin
Bacteriuria testing

Cancer

Leading Causes of Morbidity
Nose, throat, and upper
  respiratory conditions
Musculoskeletal and soft tissue
  injuries (including back
  and upper and lower extremity)

AGES 40-64 YEARS

Mammography
Fasting glucose test
Sexually transmissible disease
  testing
Human immunodeficiency virus
  (HIV) testing
Tuberculosis skin test
Lipid profile
Thyroid-stimulating hormone test
Colonoscopy

Evaluation and Counseling

Sexuality
High-risk behaviors
Contraceptive options
Genetic counseling
Prevention of unwanted pregnancy
Sexually transmissible disease
Partner selection
Barrier protection
Sexual functioning

Fitness
Hygiene (including dental)
Dietary/nutritional assessment
Exercise: discussion of program

Psychosocial Evaluation
Family relationships
Domestic violence
Job/work satisfaction
Retirement planning
Lifestyle/stress
Sleep disorders

Cardiovascular Risk Factors
Family history
Hypertension
Dyslipidemia
Obesity/diabetes mellitus
Lifestyle

Viral, bacterial, and parasitic
  infections
Acute urinary problems
Sexually transmissible diseases

Health/Risk Behaviors
Hormone replacement therapy
Injury prevention
Safety belts and helmets
Occupational hazards
Recreational hazards
Sports involvement
Firearms
Hearing
Breast self-examination
Skin exposure to ultraviolet rays
Suicide: depression symptoms
Tobacco, alcohol, other drugs

Immunizations

Periodic
Tetanus-diphtheria booster (every
  10 years)
Influenza vaccine (annually
  beginning at age 55)

*High-Risk Groups**
Measles, mumps, rubella (MMR)
  vaccine
Hepatitis B vaccine
Influenza vaccine
Pneumococcal vaccine

Leading Causes of Morbidity
Nose, throat, and upper respirato-
  ry conditions
Osteoporosis
Arthritis
Hypertension
Orthopedic deformities, including
  back and upper and lower
  extremities
Hearing and vision
  impairment

Leading Cause of Death
Heart disease

*See Table 9–2, *High-Risk Factors.*

unnecessary follow-up interventions with their own risks, and costs (U.S. Preventive Services Task Force, 1996).

To justify the time, discomfort, and expense of screening, the following criteria are useful for evaluating effectiveness (Frame & Carlson, 1975):

1. The condition must affect the quality and quantity of life greatly.
2. Acceptable methods of treatment must be available to patients.
3. The condition must have an asymptomatic phase during which detection and treatment significantly reduce morbidity and mortality.
4. Treatment in the asymptomatic phase must yield a therapeutic result superior to that obtained by delaying treatment until symptoms appears.
5. Tests that are acceptable to the woman must be available at reasonable cost to detect the condition in the asymptomatic period.
6. The incidence of the condition must be sufficient to justify the cost of the screening.

The nurse practitioner also should be aware that performing tests without closely tracking results and providing follow-up testing is not effective. Developing a system of tracking to ensure follow-up of patients is critical. Laboratories that analyze screening tests must adhere to national standards for accuracy in testing and reporting of results. Testing done on site must be in compliance with quality control standards.

IMPLEMENTATION OF PREVENTIVE CARE

Every health care provider needs to incorporate recommended guidelines into the daily delivery of care. The guidelines focus the nurse practitioner's efforts to achieve the goals of the recommendations based on age and risk, and they serve as a tool for the health care team members to communicate the accomplishments of each health care visit. A flowsheet developed from the guidelines enables the nurse practitioner to track and deliver preventive services promptly. The flowsheet is placed in the woman's chart and encompasses all the recommended screening tests, immunizations and prophylaxis, and counseling services. The feasibility of the guidelines is important, and care should concentrate on what can be provided reasonably.

Effectiveness is a major consideration in setting priorities for interventions. The difficulty in setting priorities for different age groups comes from the risk and the variation in effectiveness of some preventive services. These variables make recommending a uniform periodic health examination for all persons impossible.

In establishing preventive care guidelines, the nurse practitioner incorporates a needs assessment of the risk factor profile for the population served. A local state health department often can provide relevant health data on specific populations.

Monitoring and evaluating preventive care is an integral part of primary care. Software has been developed based on preventive care modules to track preventive care and has the ability to generate reminders for the health care provider and patient. Many larger organizations have databases to generate profiles on the patient population they serve and to measure specific outcomes. Periodic or ongoing objective feedback on actual compliance with the guidelines may be helpful to evaluate effectiveness and identify specific strategies to improve outcomes.

The nurse practitioner is a coparticipant in the health care of a woman throughout the life span. The nurse can identify and communicate specific health care recommendations, but the woman actively participates in making her own decisions, reporting progress and health-related problems. The responsibility shifts to the woman. The nurse practitioner must understand and recognize that barriers to achieving the goals may exist for some women because of the context of their lives. Understanding the woman's experience of health is important in setting forth realistic goals. The environment for delivering care should ensure privacy for the woman. Focusing on personal health behavior such as sexual behavior, tobacco use, diet, exercise, and injury prevention are more likely to reduce the risks of future illness and injury than any other types of preventive intervention.

Surveys have shown that too many women are not getting the care they need. One in every three women has not had the recommended mammogram or Pap smear. Seventy percent of women do not take in enough calcium to prevent osteoporosis (Frigoletto, "Primary Care," 1996). Nurse practitioners must take every opportunity to deliver preventive services, especially to persons with limited access to care. Those individuals at highest risk for many preventable diseases and disabilities—such as cervical cancer, tuberculosis, human immunodeficiency viral infection, and poor nutrition—are the same individuals least likely to receive adequate preventive services (U.S. Preventive Services Task Force, 1996).

Screening

Preventive services are divided into three categories: screening tests, counseling interventions, and immunizations and chemoprophylaxis. Only screening tests are discussed in this chapter. Specific recommendations for counseling, immunizations, and screening tests are identified based on age and risk factors in Box 9-1.

The assessment begins with the nurse practitioner eliciting a comprehensive health history (see Chapter 8) before conducting the physical examination and appropriate diagnostic tests. The history provides a useful way of screening for a number of common health problems or risk factors in a quick, inexpensive manner. The nurse practitioner tailors the frequency and content of the examination to the individual's health risks and identifies areas of routine questioning for each age group (see Box 9-1). The notion of a periodic complete physical examination may not yield results as great as once thought; however, parts of the physical examination have been studied in terms of their sensitivity and usefulness in detecting preclinical diseases. This chapter reviews the portions of the physical examination that are deemed effective.

Areas of Examination

Blood Pressure

Sphygmomanometry, the measurement of blood pressure, remains the most appropriate and inexpensive method of assessing for hypertension. ACOG recommends that blood pressure be measured as part of the periodic evaluation visit, which should occur yearly or as appropriate. Blood pressure screening is more significant for the woman more than 40 years old. Approximately 50 million Americans have elevated blood pressure warranting monitoring or drug therapy. Several large, randomized clinical studies have demonstrated that lowering blood pressure in hypertensive adults, even in cases of mild hypertension, is beneficial and that death from several common diseases can be reduced through detection and treatment of high blood pressure (U.S. Preventive Services Task Force, 1996).

Although sphygmomanometry is highly accurate when performed correctly, false positives or negatives can occur. Errors may be caused by the nurse, the instrument, or the patient. Sphygmomanometry is performed according to recommended technique (Joint National Committee, 1999). Diagnosis of hypertension is not based on a single measurement but requires confirmation during at least two subsequent visits over several weeks (unless systolic blood pressure is 210 mm Hg or higher and diastolic is 120 mm Hg or higher). The initial evaluation of hypertension consists of a complete history and physical examination, laboratory tests, and an electrocardiogram.

Oral Cavity

The oral exam has two purposes: identifying any types of lesions and evaluating for dental disease. The term *oral cancer* includes a diverse group of tumors arising from the oral cavity such as cancers of the lip, tongue, pharynx, and oral cavity. Oral cancer is responsible for 20% of all cancer deaths in the United States. The incidence is twice as high in men as in women, with the highest incidence in African-American males. In the United States, 90% of oral cancer cases are attributed to the use of tobacco and, to a lesser extent, alcohol. ACOG recommends that for women 40 years of age and older the oral cavity be part of the routine health examination and that dental hygiene be included in counseling in the yearly visit or as appropriate. Evidence to recommend for or against screening asymptomatic patients for oral cancer is limited, as is evidence on the frequency of false-positive results once a lesion is found. All patients should be advised to discontinue the use of all forms of tobacco and to limit consumption of alcohol (U.S. Preventive Services Task Force, 1996).

Dental and oral health problems are common. By age 17, 84% of American children have decay in their permanent teeth, and up to one third of all children have gingivitis. Adults continue to be at risk for dental decay. In most situations dental problems are preventable, and the dental and oral health status of adults is determined largely by the quality of preventive and treatment services received during childhood. The U.S. Preventive Services Task Force (1996) recommends that all persons be encouraged to visit a dental care provider regularly, with the optimal frequency determined by the person's dentist. The health care provider, when examining the mouth, examines the patient for obvious signs of oral disease such as dental cavities, inflamed or cyanotic gingival tissue, malalignment or crowding of teeth, and mismatching of upper and lower dentures.

The oral cavity examination includes inspection and palpation of the lips, gingival and buccal mucosa, palate, floor of the mouth, tongue (especially the lateral margins), and pharynx. If a patient is wearing dentures, the dentures are inspected in the mouth for fit and are removed during examination of the oral cavity. The nurse practitioner uses a bright light for visualization and performs the examination systematically from anterior to posterior, inspecting all aspects of the oral cavity.

Thyroid

Hyperthyroidism and hypothyroidism account for considerable morbidity in the United States. Thyroid dysfunction affects 1% to 4% of the adult population and is more common in women, persons who have Down syndrome, older adults, and individuals with a family history of thyroid dysfunction. Those persons who have upper body irradiation are at a higher risk for thyroid nodules and thyroid cancer. ACOG recommends that the thyroid-stimulating hormone (TSH) limits should be obtained every 3 to 5 years from all women aged 65 years and older and from younger women with autoimmune conditions or family histories of thyroid disease. The U.S. Preventive Services Task Force (1996) does not recommend routine screening for thyroid disease with the thyroid function test for asymptomatic adolescents or adults because insufficient evidence exists for such a recommendation.

Nurse practitioners should be alert for subtle symptoms and signs of thyroid dysfunction when examining women. Symptoms of thyroid dysfunction involve the nervous, cardiovascular, and gastrointestinal systems. For hyperthyroidism, physical findings include a resting tachycardia, fine tremor, and possibly slightly enlarged and tender thyroid. Signs and symptoms of hypothyroidism may be lethargy, weight gain, depressed mood, and hair loss (Greenspan & Strewler, 1997). The preferred test is measurement of TSH using a sensitive immunometric or similar assay as the initial screen and obtaining a free thyroxine (FT_4) or free thyroxine index level (FT_4I) only if the TSH level is abnormal. Medications and clinical conditions can affect the interpretation of the thyroid screening tests. Evidence of subclinical hypothyroidism may be related to unfavorable lipid profiles. The nurse practitioner should assess thyroid values within the context of the woman's hormonal status.

ACOG recommends thyroid palpation as part of the periodic health examination because thyroid disease is encountered regularly. Screening begins in women over the age of 18. The thyroid examination includes inspection and palpation with the woman in a seated position with her neck slightly flexed. The nurse practitioner observes the neck as the woman takes a sip of water: a thyroid mass may move up and down with swallowing. The nurse practitioner palpates the woman's neck while standing behind the woman, using the fingertips of the left hand to push the trachea slightly to the right and the fingers of the right hand to retract the sternocleidomastoid muscle. While the woman takes a sip of water, the nurse practitioner palpates the medial and lateral margins of the thyroid with the fingertips of right hand. The procedure is reversed for the left side. On physical examination the palpable bulbous portion of each lobe of the normal thyroid gland measures about 2 cm vertically and 1 cm horizontally above the isthmus. Any mass or tenderness may suggest a malignancy, but this finding is rare. Most single thyroid nodules prove to be benign adenomas. Autonomously functioning nodules are virtually always benign but produce increased amounts of thyroid hormone (Miklius & Daniels, 1995).

Breasts

Breast cancer is the most common type of cancer among women in the United States and the second leading cause of cancer death after lung cancer. A woman's average risk is one chance in eight of developing breast cancer over her lifetime, with mortality increasing with age. Major risk factors for breast cancer are age over 50 and a family history (first-degree relative) of breast cancer. The history includes identification of risk factors and determination of any recent direct trauma, duration of any lesion or biopsies, presence of fever, and presence and nature of any nipple discharge. ACOG recommends that women more than 18 years old have yearly clinical breast examinations during the periodic evaluation or as appropriate. The American Cancer Society recommends that women have a breast examination every 3 years from age 20 to 39 years and yearly after age 40.

Breast examination involves bilateral inspection and palpation of the breast and areola and the auxiliary and supraclavicular areas while the woman is in the upright and supine positions. The nurse practitioner palpates all areas of each breast systematically with deep and shallow palpations. The nurse practitioner looks for and notes any of the following:

- Fixation of the skin to underlying structures as the woman leans forward
- Dimpling of the skin when the woman presses downward on her hips
- Disparity in the size or contour of the breast
- Previous surgical scars
- Any palpable masses
- Nipple discharge
- Nipple retraction symmetry and position
- Edema
- Other distortions of the skin surface
- Inflammation
- Excoriation of the nipple

Any palpable breast lump, even with a normal mammogram, requires careful evaluation, including possible biopsy.

The three screening tests usually considered for early detection of breast cancer are clinical breast examination, x-ray mammography, and breast self-examination. (O'Malley & Fletcher, 1987). Estimates of the sensitivity and specificity of these maneuvers depend on number of variables, including the size of the lesion, the characteristics of breast being examined, the age of the woman, the extent of follow-up to identify false negatives, the skill and experience of the examiner or radiographic interpreter, and the quality of the mammogram (U.S. Preventive Services Task Force, 1996).

Mammography may be used as a screening device or an adjunct in diagnosis of a palpable mass. Mammography is the only screening method to detect subclinical or occult breast cancer. Screening for breast cancer every 1 to 2 years with mammography alone or mammography and annual breast examination is recommended for women ages 50 to 69. Although all organizations agree that women age 50 or older should be screened, the recommended age for starting screening mammography has been a source of much controversy. The American Cancer Society recommends that women begin annual mammography at age 40. The American College of Obstetricians and Gynecologists, American Medical Association, and National Cancer Institute recommend a screening mammogram every 1 to 2 years for women 40 to 49 years of age (*Put Prevention into Practice,* 1998).

Pelvic Organs

Several but not all major authorities consider routine pelvic examination to be a necessary component of the physical examination. The American Cancer Society recommends that the pelvic examination be performed every 1 to 3 years for women age 18 to 39 years and annually for women more than 40 years of age. ACOG recommends that women who are sexually active or 18 years of age and older should have annual pelvic examinations as part of the routine examination. Gynecological problems before age 18 may necessitate a pelvic examination. In those situations, issues of confidentiality are discussed with the adolescent and/or parent.

Cervix

The pelvic examination also involves screening for cervical, uterine, and other gynecological cancers and colon cancer. In addition, a Pap smear is conducted to detect neoplastic cells in cervical and vaginal secretions.

Cervical cancer causes approximately 4600 deaths yearly in the United States, and approximately 12,800 new cases occur per year according to the Cancer Information Service of the National Cancer Institute (Greenlee, Murray, & Bolden, 2000). The incidence of invasive cervical cancer has decreased an estimated 70%, due in large part to organized early detection programs. The greatest risk factor for developing cervical cancer is never or seldom having a Pap smear, particularly among groups of elderly African-American women and middle-aged women of lower socioeconomic status. Other risk factors for cervical cancer include first intercourse at an early age, having multiple sexual partners, smoking, and passive smoking (U.S. Preventive Services Task Force, 1996). Many of these factors place the woman at risk for altered cellular immunity.

Routine screening for cervical cancer is recommended with Pap smears for all women who are or have been sexually active and who have a cervix. The American Cancer Society, ACOG, and National Cancer Institute recommend that all women begin having a Pap smear at the onset of sexual activity or at 18 years of age, whichever occurs first. After a woman has had three or more consecutive satisfactory normal annual examinations, the Pap smear may be performed less frequently at the discretion of the woman and health care provider. This recommendation has been directed at women who are in a low-risk category. The U.S. Preventive Services Task Force recommends that Pap smears be performed appropriately at an interval of 1 to 3 years based on the presence of risk factors: early onset of sexual intercourse, history of multiple sexual partners, and low socioeconomic status. Pap smears may be discontinued at age 65, but only if the provider can document previous Pap screening in which smears have been consistently normal.

Women with a prior hysterectomy for a benign condition, adequate histological evidence that the cervix has been removed, and no previous abnormal Pap smears require no further screening for cervical cancer. Women who have had vaginal or cervical neoplasia at hysterectomy and those with prior endometrial cancer are at higher risk for developing vaginal neoplasia and need to continue to have vaginal smears. Infection with human immundeficiency virus and certain types of human papilloma virus also increases the risk of cervical cancer (American Cancer Society, 1993).

Depending on the technique used, Pap smears have a sensitivity of 50% to 90% and a specificity of 90% to 99% in detecting cervical cancer but are only moderately effective in detecting endometrial cancer. A large proportion of false-negative Pap smears are thought to be caused by poor technique (as many as half of all false negatives) and inadequate laboratory interpretation (Koss, 1993). Many authorities recommend that laboratories use the Bethesda system developed by the National Cancer Institute, which attempts to standardize classification categories and provides for reporting on aspects of the sample (Kruman & Solomon, 1994). Because the lead time for developing precancerous changes to invasive carcinoma takes 8 to 9 years, almost all precancerous or early stage malignancies initially missed can be detected by repeat testing (*Put Prevention into Practice*, 1998).

Once a woman has an abnormal Pap smear and the adequate follow-up has occurred, the next step is to delineate further the extent of the problem with a colposcopy. Sometimes abnormal cells can be found in the endocervix and a biopsy of the tissue is taken for pathology interpretation (Northrup, 1998).

Ovaries

One of every 70 women will develop ovarian cancer. In 1997 approximately 26,800 women in the United States were diagnosed with ovarian cancer and 14,600 American women died. Ovarian cancer is the leading cause of death from gynecological pelvic malignancies (American College of Obstetricians and Gynecologists, 1996; *Put Prevention into Practice*, 1998). A woman's risk of ovarian cancer is increased by nulliparity; older age at the time of first pregnancy or live birth; fewer pregnancies; and a personal history of breast, endometrial, or colorectal cancer. Ovarian cancer often shows no signs or symptoms until late in development and is often considerable in size by the time of detection.

The pelvic examination is of unknown sensitivity and specificity in detecting ovarian cancer. Although health care providers occasionally can detect ovarian cancer, small, early stage tumors often are not detected by palpation because of the deep anatomical location of the ovary (U.S. Preventive Services Task Force, 1996). The pelvic examination also may produce false positives when benign adnexal masses are found. In the premenopausal woman, most pelvic masses are not ovarian carcinoma. A pelvic mass discovered in a postmenopausal woman is much more likely to be ovarian cancer (Kellerman, 1997). The Pap smear occasionally may reveal malignant ovarian cells and is considered to be a valid screening test for ovarian carcinoma. An abnormal finding warrants referral to the appropriate medical specialty.

Routine screening for ovarian cancer by ultrasound, the measurement of serum tumor markers, or pelvic examination is not recommended. Insufficient evidence exists to recommend for or against screening of asymptomatic women at increased risk for developing ovarian cancer. No direct evidence from prospective studies has shown that women with early stage ovarian cancer detected through screening have lower mortality from ovarian cancer than do women with more advanced disease (U.S. Preventive Services Task Force, 1996).

Endometrium

Routine screening for endometrial cancer does not have any proven benefit. Women generally are advised to report all abnormal uterine bleeding, and those with such findings should be evaluated by endometrial sampling or other diagnostic testing. Endometrial carcinoma, or cancer of the uterus, is the fourth most common cancer in women and the most common genital cancer in women age 45 and older (American College of Obstetricians and Gynecologists, 1996). The Pap smear, used for screening for cervical cancer, is too insensitive for detection of endometrial cancer to be used as a screening technique. However, the Pap smear occasionally identifies endometrial abnormalities. Fortunately, most endometrial cancer is found early, at stage I, when the survival rate is approximately 90%. ACOG recommends performing annual pelvic examinations. Risk factors associated with endometrial cancer have been linked to the taking of unopposed estrogen, higher estrogen replacement therapy, tamoxifen therapy, and genetic mutations associated with hereditary nonpolyposis colon cancer. Risk may persist up to 5 years after taking a high dose of estrogen. Other risk factors include increasing age, postmenopausal state, and obesity (Burke et al., 1997; Von Gruenigen & Karlen, 1995). Bimanual examination also may detect some cases of endometrial cancer, although the efficiency and effectiveness of such detection has not been well studied.

The woman should empty her bladder before the pelvic examination. Bimanual examination of the internal organs is uncomfortable if the bladder is full, and palpation of the pelvic organs is difficult. The nurse practitioner should advise the woman not to douche or use vaginal medications or other inserts 2 to 3 days before the examination. The woman generally lies in a lithotomy position. The examination of the genitalia has essentially two phases: inspection and palpation. The nurse practitioner begins the internal examination by inserting a finger into the vaginal vault to palpate the cervix and sidewalls of the vagina for induration, masses, and tenderness. The nurse practitioner should select and warm the speculum before inserting it. The speculum allows the nurse practitioner to inspect the cervix and vagina. The Pap smear is done during this phase of the examination. The next part of the examination, the bimanual, is the palpation of the pelvic organs between the nurse practitioner's hands to assess the location, size, and mobility of the internal genitalia and for any tenderness. The nurse practitioner inserts the tip of a gloved finger into the vaginal opening and presses downward, waiting for the muscle to relax. The other hand is placed on the woman's abdomen and used to press the abdominal and pelvic contents. The finger is partially withdrawn from the vagina and inserted into the rectum to palpate the rectovaginal septum.

Rectum

Colorectal cancer in women is the third most common malignancy and the second most common cause of cancer death, accounting for about 140,000 new cases and about 55,000 deaths each year (Parker, Tong, Bolden, & Wing, 1997). The individual risk for women is 6%, only slightly less than the 7% in men. The risk of colon cancer increases after age 40 years, and 90% of cases are in individuals age 50 or older. Increased incidence is noted with familiar syndromes, ulcerative colitis, first-degree family history of adenoma or colorectal cancer, and a personal history of adenomas or of ovarian, endometrial, or breast cancer. Less than 10% of colorectal cancer can be palpated by digital rectal examination.

About 75% of all colorectal cancer occurs in persons with no predisposing factors for the disease (Colorectal Cancer Screening, 1996). ACOG recommends that rectal examination and fecal occult blood testing (FOBT) be included in the routine examination of women 50 years of age and older as part of the pelvic examination. Depending on a woman's age, whether the FOBT sample is rehydrated, and whether an initial screening or a rescreening is being performed, FOBT yields positive results in 1% to 16% of cases, according to the American College of Physicians data analysis. In reevaluation of women with positive FOBT, colorectal cancer is found in 2% to 17%. These results suggest that women who have positive results on FOBT should have a full colonoscopy (American College of Physicians, 1997). Another recommendation by the College is that screening for FOBT not be done in persons who are likely to have misleading results, such as those with active hemorrhoidal bleeding or symptoms that already suggest colorectal cancer.

The nurse practitioner does the rectal examination after the vaginal examination, inspecting the anal orifice, palpating the anal sphincter, and evaluating muscle tone. The rectal-vaginal examination has additional efficiency in assessing the posterior fornix for pelvic masses. A lubricated, gloved index finger is inserted into the anal opening to palpate all sides of the rectum for polyps.

Screening for colorectal cancer is recommended for all persons age 50 or older. Effective methods include FOBT, sigmoidoscopy, and colonoscopy. Hemoccult testing involves testing for a positive reaction on a card impregnated with guaiac. Most experts advocate obtaining a hemoccult test at the time of the annual rectal examination on three test cards that the woman sends back to the office. The nurse practitioner instructs the woman to avoid salicylates or antiinflammatory agents and the eating of large amounts of red meats, which may produce a false positive. Insufficient evidence is available to determine which of these screening methods is preferable or which combination produces greater benefits. Sigmoidoscopy screening is recommended every 3 to 5 years and is a procedure performed by a trained examiner that enables visualization of the lower part of the colon and rectum. If findings are abnormal, a colonoscopy is warranted.

Screening with colonoscopy is for those individuals at a higher risk for colorectal cancer. The indications and timing of screening vary somewhat among various organizations. Most organizations recommend colonoscopy starting at age 40 for those with asymtomatic first-degree family members with colorectal cancer. The American Cancer Society and the American Society of Colon and Rectal Surgeons recommend that persons with one or more first-degree relatives who receive a diagnosis of colorectal cancer at 55 years of age or younger undergo screening colonoscopy every 3 to 5 years beginning at age 35 to 40 years (Fuchs et al., 1994). If complete colonoscopy reveals no clinically important colorectal neoplasm, further colorectal cancer screening may be deferred for 5 or more years. If colonoscopy detects a high-risk lesion, colonoscopic surveillance is warranted after the lesion is removed (American College of Physicians, 1997). Screening as early as age 18 is recommended for those who have had ulcerative colitis for 10 years or more or who have a history of colon cancer, adenomatous polyps, or familial polyposis syndrome (U.S. Preventive Services Task Force, 1996).

Genitalia (Sexually Transmitted Diseases)

Almost 12 million cases of sexually transmitted diseases (STDs) occur annually in the United States. Sexually transmitted diseases are common and may have harmful effects. Chlamydia, gonorrhea, and syphilis are treated easily when diagnosed early but have serious sequelae if left untreated. See Chapter 15 for evaluation and treatment. Human immunodeficiency virus (HIV) infection is a serious public health problem. Although HIV has no cure, early diagnosis and treatment can delay the onset of acquired immunodeficiency syndrome (AIDS) and can help delay onset of symptoms and avoid transmission of the virus to others.

Regardless of the woman's age all women are screened for STDs. The risk factors for STDs are assessed during the gathering of the health history (see Box 9-1). Women who are poor or medically underserved and racial and ethic minorities contract a disproportionate number of STDs and the disabilities associated with them. Groups at the highest risk for STDs include sexually active women under 25, women who have multiple sexual partners, those with a history of sexually transmitted diseases, prostitutes and their sex partners, users of illicit drugs, and inmates of detention centers (*Put Prevention into Practice*, 1998).

Women often may not be aware of the disease or may be asymtomatic. The nurse practitioner should advise all adolescents and women about risk factors for STDs and counsel about effective measures to reduce the risk of infection. Screening along with diagnosis, counseling, and treatment are essential components in STD and HIV prevention.

ACOG recommends screening for all age groups, especially with a focus on high-risk groups. The nurse practitioner should offer testing for individuals at risk according to recommendations on screening for syphilis, gonorrhea, hepatitis B virus, HIV, and chlamydia infection. ACOG also recommends that HIV and STD counseling be included for all women as a part of their routine preventive services, whether pregnant or not.

Prenatal care involves preventing, screening, and testing for sexually transmitted diseases. The nurse practitioner informs pregnant women at risk about the potential risk to the fetus of HIV and other STDs (chlamydia, gonorrhea, syphilis, hepatitis B, and herpes) and the significance of screening for HIV and STDs during pregnancy. The standard of care is to offer HIV testing to all women who seek prenatal care (Acheson, 1997; U.S. Preventive Services Task Force, 1996).

The causative agent of syphilis cannot be cultured; screening relies on serology. A serological test for reagin (RPR, VDRL) is a sensitive screening test but is not specific. Occasionally, uninfected individuals may have reactive tests. Because nontreponemal serodiagnostic tests may be falsely positive, all reactive results in asymptomatic patients are confirmed with a more specific treponemal test such as fluorescent treponemal antibody absorption. Routine serological screening is recommended for all pregnant women because syphilis infects the fetus transplacentally. Screening also is recommended for persons at risk for known exposure to syphilis; those with positive or suspected infection should be screened for other STDs as well (Freund, 1995; U.S. Preventive Services Task Force, 1966).

HIV screening requires serological studies for the presence of antibodies. Enzyme immunoassay is the most widely used screening test for HIV-1 infection. When a positive result occurs, the results are validated by a confirmatory test, usually by Western blot tests. HIV screening always is performed with individualized counseling before and after the screening.

Skin

Skin cancer is the most common type of cancer in the United States and accounts for about 2% of all cancer deaths (American Cancer Society, 1999). The incidence of skin cancer is increasing faster than that of any other cancer in the United States with the exception of lung cancer in women (Morton, 1996). More than 1 million new cases of skin cancer are diagnosed each year. Three main types of skin cancer are basal cell carcinoma, the most prevalent; squamous cell carcinoma; and malignant melanoma. More than 95% of all basal cell and squamous cell carcinomas, referred to as nonmelanomatous skin cancer, are highly treatable and rarely metastasize. Melanoma, the deadliest form of skin cancer, affects women ages 25 to 29 years and poses a higher risk for development of additional skin cancer. Skin cancers are detected easily and often are cured by excisional biopsy. Local tissue destruction may cause disfigurement or functional impairment if these tumors are not detected early (Committee on Guidelines of Care, 1992; Karagas, Greenberg, Mott, Baron, & Ernster, 1998). Improved survival from melanoma is related directly to detection at an early stage of disease.

The American College of Obstetricians and Gynecologists and the U.S. Preventive Services Task Force recommend that skin examinations be performed on individuals with a family history or personal history of skin cancer, increased occupational or recreational exposure to sunlight, or clinical evidence of precursor lesions. The American Cancer Society recommends that skin examinations being given every 3 years for those 20 to 39 years old and yearly after age 40. Insufficient evidence exists to recommend for or against routine screening for skin cancer by primary care providers or counseling patients to perform periodic self-examinations (U.S. Preventive Services Task Force, 1996). The primary focus is educating patients about appropriate precautions with exposure to sunlight.

The principal screening test for skin cancer is clinical examination of the skin. Individuals with fair hair and light skin are known to be at increased risk of melanoma. A history of chronic sun exposure including painful or blistering sunburns in youth, freekles, atypical moles, certain congenital moles, or a family or personal history of skin cancer increase a woman's susceptibility. Melanoma is known to have a familial component, and evidence now indicates that genetic factors play an important role. Subsets of the population have been identified, with some groups having a predicted lifetime risk of melanoma of 80% to 100% (Slade, Marghoob, & Salopek, 1995).

In the early stages, melanoma is easy to detect and treat. Once advanced, however, melanoma spreads rapidly. In women, melanoma most commonly appears on the legs, back, arms, and face (Frigoletto, "Message," 1996). Detection of a suspicious lesion constitutes a positive screening test, which then should be confirmed by skin biopsy. Health care providers should remain alert for skin lesions with malignant features: asymmetry, border irregularity, color variability, diameter >6 mm, or rapidly changing lesions. Factors affecting the yield for skin cancer are the proportion of the body surface examined and the frequency of the examination.

The nurse practitioner should perform the following in a skin examination:

- Examine the skin of the head, upper torso, and upper extremities while the woman is seated
- Part the hair and inspect the scalp
- Examine and inspect the skin of the face and neck, taking special note of the eyelids, forehead, ears, nose, and lips
- Examine the upper extremities, shoulders, and back completely
- Inspect the skin on the chest and abdomen while the woman is supine

The nurse practitioner may examine the remaining skin of the back, legs, and genital and perianal areas with the woman lying on the side, ensuring that all skin areas have been examined.

Height and Weight

Most authorities, including U.S. Preventive Services Task Force, recommend periodic height and weight measurements. The American Heart Association recommends a body weight measurement every 5 years. Obesity is defined as having a body fat content of 20% or more above the desirable body weight.

Approximately 32 million American adults, 24% of men and 27% of women, are overweight. Mortality rates are increased even for individuals with weights only 10% above desirable weight. Some groups use body mass index as a measurement of weight and height, and the index is highly correlated with body fat. The height-weight calculation helps to determine whether a person is at a healthy weight or has too much body fat. Studies have shown that an increase in body mass index is associated with an increased risk of comorbid conditions. These conditions include but are not limited to coronary heart disease, certain forms of cancer, stroke, hypertension, hypercholesterolemia, and non–insulin-dependent diabetes mellitus. Obesity is associated with congestive heart failure, gallbladder disease, gout, sleep apnea, other pulmonary disease, and ostreoarthritis (U.S. Preventive Services Task Force, 1996). Extreme obesity shortens life.

Weight loss through changes in diet, increased physical activity, and other intervention can decrease the risk of most forms of morbidity associated with obesity. Weight loss must be sustained to be beneficial (*Put Prevention into Practice*, 1998).

In addition to obesity, the nurse practitioner should assess for other eating disorders. Many American women report that they are dieting or that they manipulate food intake to lose weight. Eating disorders such as bulimia and anorexia nervosa exist on a continuum from mild disorder to extreme dysfunction. Assessment is often difficult because of secrecy or a woman's lack of concern about the problem. Prevalence rates of 2% to 10% exist in many primary care populations. Symptoms characteristically begin when the woman is between 17 and 25 years old. Women commonly first present with symptoms in their 30s and 40s. Two questions assist in eliciting information from patients: "Do you ever eat in secret?" and "Are you satisfied with your eating patterns?" (Andolsek, 1997).

The nurse practitioner can obtain the woman's height more accurately with the woman in barefeet or in socks or stockings only. The nurse practitioner should take care to ensure that the woman is standing erect. Standiometers that are fixed to the wall yield more consistent results over time. Height-measuring rods attached to a scale become less precise in measurement over time.

Periodic calibration of equipment for height and weight is recommended. A balance beam or electronic scale (not spring-type scale) is recommended. Weight is measured most accurately with the woman wearing minimal or no clothing.

Cholesterol

Most of the prospective observational studies have reported a positive association between total cholesterol levels and coronary heart disease (CHD) in women. However, data from studies have been based predominately on men and relatively few women. Epidemiological studies have shown that cholesterol lipoprotein subfractions play an important role in CHD. Low-density lipoprotein (LDL) cholesterol is directly associated with CHD and high-density lipoprotein (HDL) cholesterol is inversely associated with CHD incidence. The findings from these studies suggest that lowering LDL and raising HDL cholesterol would benefit women and men. These studies show that a total cholesterol greater than 260 mg/dL increases a woman's risk of mortality by four times. A decreased level of HDL cholesterol is a particularly strong predictor of increased risk of CHD in women. The majority of lipid abnormalities are not associated with specific symptoms or signs. However, portions of the history and physical examination can be helpful in identifying high-risk patients and those with specific lipid abnormalities. A diet history can detect excess lipid intake and can provide insight into simple but effective changes to reduce dietary lipid intake.

ACOG recommends that adults 19 years or older have their cholesterol level measured every 5 years until 64 years of age and then every 3 to 5 years thereafter. The U.S. Preventive Services Task Force recommends periodic measurement of total serum cholesterol for women ages 45 to 65 years. Periodic screening is important when cholesterol levels are increasing, that is, for perimenopausal women and women who have gained weight. Women who are ill, pregnant, or nursing should not be screened because their cholesterol level may not be representative of usual levels. Patients with type 2 diabetes mellitus or poorly controlled type 1 diabetes have hypertriglyceridemia.

Cholesterol tests are performed on venous blood samples. The woman need not vary her usual eating habits before screening for total cholesterol or HDL cholesterol. Women undergoing lipoprotein analysis should fast (water and black coffee are acceptable) for 12 hours before testing. For those women with a total cholesterol greater than 200 mg/dL and HDL less than 35 mg/dL, a full lipid profile should be analyzed to determine the relative contribution of LDL, HDL, and very low-density lipoprotein. If the woman has a cholesterol level greater than 200 mg/dL and known cardiovascular disease or more than two risk factors listed following for atherosclerosis, a full lipid profile is warranted.

- Age ≥45 for men; ≥55 for women (or premature menopause without estrogen therapy)
- Family history of premature CHD
- Smoking
- Hypertension
- HDL cholesterol ≤35 mg/dL
- Diabetes

A total cholesterol level greater than 240 mg/dL is sufficient to warrant a complete lipid profile (Summary of Second Report of NCEP Expect Panel, 1993).

Urinalysis

Screening for asymptomatic bacteriuria by urine culture is recommended for all pregnant women. Insufficient evidence exists to recommend for or against routine screening for asymptomatic bacteriuria in diabetic or ambulatory elderly women, but recommendations against such screening may be made on other clinical judgments. Routine screening for asymptomatic bacteriuria in other persons is not recommended (U.S. Preventive Services Task Force, 1996). Screening for proteinuria has little value because most causes are benign or untreatable. Screening for diabetes with urinalysis is inaccurate and better accomplished with plasma glucose measurements. Most authorities recommend urinalysis only for certain conditions in specific high-risk populations (*Put Prevention into Practice*, 1998).

The most common tests for detecting bacteria in asymptomatic persons are dipstick urinalysis and direct microscopy. The dipstick test is rapid and inexpensive and requires little technical expertise. Urine screening tests generally are performed on a clean-catch specimen. ACOG recommends a urinalysis, including microscopic examination and infection screen, at the first prenatal visit, with the need for additional laboratory evaluations including urine culture determined by findings obtained from the history and physical examination.

Urine screening is available to detect occult hematuria, which can indicate urinary tract malignancies. Malignancies increase significantly after age 40 and are twice as frequent in men as in women. However, other etiological reasons for hematuria exist, such as exercise, menstrual period, and renal cysts. The sensitivity of dipstick tests for hematuria is good (91% to 100%), but specificity can be as low as 65%. Urine collected early in the morning, at least 6 hours after previous voiding and after 8 hours of fasting, is most likely to reveal abnormalities (*Put Prevention into Practice*, 1998).

Glucose Tolerance Test

Approximately 16 million persons in the United States have diabetes, and approximately 90% of these have non–insulin-dependent (type 2) diabetes mellitus. Presently not enough evidence exists for or against screening in asymptomatic adults and for gestational diabetes. Except for pregnant women, few patients in clinical practice undergo full screening for diabetes. Most cases are uncovered through investigation when the woman has symptoms or if blood work has been done for another purpose. Some clinicians presently screen individuals at high risk for diabetes, such as obese men and women over the age of 50, patients with a strong family history of diabetes, and members of certain ethnic groups. Type 2 diabetes mellitus is more common among African-American, Hispanic, and Native-American persons. In individuals without risk factors, screening for asymptomatic disease is much less likely to be beneficial. The glucose tolerance test is often helpful in diagnosing diabetes (*Put Prevention into Practice*, 1998).

ACOG recommends that fasting plasma glucose levels be determined periodically in patients who are at high risk, such as those with a family history of diabetes, high-risk ethnicity, history of gestational diabetes, and macrosoma. The American Diabetes Association (2001) recommends screening every 3 years for all adults ages 45 and older. Testing at a younger age for high-risk patients includes those persons with previously impaired glucose tolerance, hypertension, hypercholesterolemia or hyperlipidemia, or a history of gestational diabetes mellitus or who as infants weighed more than 9 lb at birth.

The time of specimen collection is important because blood glucose concentration rises rapidly after eating and then falls. Blood specimens are usually taken 10 to 12 hours after the last meal or 2 hours postprandial. The American Diabetes Association (2001) recommends that further testing be done on women with fasting plasma glucose results of 115 mg/dL or more. If a fasting sample is not available, random blood sampling may be used in screening. A random glucose test result in excess of 200 mg/dL is considered elevated and warrants further follow-up (U.S. Preventive Services Task Force, 1996).

Pregnancy can induce an insulin-resistant state that may result in gestational diabetes mellitus. Screening usually takes place at 24 to 28 weeks of gestation. Earlier screening may occur in high-risk patients who have history of gestational diabetes or delivery of an infant weighing more than 9 lb. The screening test consists of the woman drinking a 50-g oral glucose load followed by a 1-hour plasma glucose determination. If the value is not within the normal parameters, then the woman is referred for a 3-hour formal glucose tolerance test (Walters, Estridge, & Reynolds, 1995).

REPRODUCTIVE DIAGNOSTIC TESTS

Pregnancy Test

Immunological tests for confirming pregnancy are designed to detect human chorionic gonadotropin (hCG), which is a hormone produced by the placenta and present in the serum and urine of a pregnant woman shortly after fertilization.

Most pregnancy tests use antigen-antibody methods to detect hCG. A commercially prepared antibody to hCG (anti-hCG) is used to detect hCG (the antigen) in the patient specimen. The most common methods of detecting hCG are pregnancy test kits based on modified enzyme immunoassay techniques or agglutination inhibition techniques.

Depending on the sensitivity of the pregnancy test, the test can be performed before a period is missed. Over-the-counter home pregnancy tests can detect pregnancy as soon as 1 day after a menstrual period has been missed. Serum tests (radioimmunoassay and radioreceptorassay) using radiolabeled hCG as a marker can detect pregnancy 7 days after conception. Unless the woman is at high risk for conditions such as an ectopic pregnancy or has a medical condition, quantitative serum tests usually are not ordered.

False positives or negatives can occur. Manufacturers' instructions must be followed regarding storage, procedure, and expiration dates. Positive and negatives controls should be run with specimens to ensure reliability. False positives can be caused by certain drugs or medications: marijuana, methadone, tranquilizers, antidepressants, and even large doses of aspirin. Occasionally some rare cancers, trophoblastic diseases, ovarian cysts, and thyroid disorders can cause false positives. Pregnancy tests remain positive for about 10 days after a miscarriage or abortion. False negatives can occur if the urine is too dilute or has been at room temperature. Occasionally an ectopic pregnancy also leads to a false negative in a urine pregnancy test (Wallach, 1996; Walters, Estridge, & Reynolds, 1995).

Many women believe that confirming a pregnancy shortly after a skipped period is desirable. Most of the vital fetal development takes place in the first 3 months. Knowing that a woman is pregnant may influence her behavior and the outcome of the pregnancy. Women thinking of terminating the pregnancy can benefit additionally from early results because outcomes for termination are safer earlier.

Ultrasonography

Ultrasound is a diagnostic procedure in which high-frequency sound waves are bounced off certain internal structures of the body. The reflections of these sound waves are recorded to form a picture.

Routine screening of all pregnancies with ultrasound examinations at 18 weeks of gestation leads to earlier detection of multiple gestation, more accurate dating, and detection of possible fetal malfunction. A third-trimester scan can be used to screen for intrauterine growth retardation and fetal malpresentation as well as previously undetected multiple gestation and malfunctions. ACOG recommends that ultrasound examinations be performed for specific medical indications and not for routine use (American College of Obstetricians and Gynecologists, 1996).

Ultrasonography is used widely for pregnant women. In the United States, according to 1992 natality data, 58% of mothers who had live births receive ultrasonography. Insufficient evidence exists to recommend for or against routine ultrasound examinations in the second trimester in low-risk pregnancies, and routine third-semester ultrasound examinations are not recommended (U.S. Preventive Services Task Force, 1996).

In addition to assessing development during pregnancy, ultrasound measures the flow of blood and assists in diagnosing ovarian cysts, uterine fibroids, and pelvic pain. Ultrasound is used to diagnose various cancers and to examine a wide variety of organs, including the breast, thyroid gland, pancreas, and kidneys. Masses as large as 8 to 10 cm are missed by experienced examiners. High-resolution ultrasound can be invaluable for guiding fine needle aspiration, making delineating palpable breast lumps and diagnosing nonpalpable breast masses easier (Northrup, 1998; Wysocki & Davis, 1999). Transvaginal ultrasonography in particular is used to diagnose early pregnancy and pelvic masses (Hendricks, Von Escchen, & Grady, 1995). Ultrasound may be helpful in evaluating a woman who is obese or unable to cooperate during a physical examination.

Endometrial Biopsy

An endometrial biopsy involves removing and evaluating endometrial tissue. The biopsy is accomplished by aspirating or scraping tissue from the uterine lining using an instrument inserted from the cervix into the uterus. The tissue is aspirated by suction. The biopsy is performed within the clinical setting. The woman may experience cramping at the time of tissue removal.

Biopsy is done in selected circumstances, especially to evaluate the cause of abnormal vaginal bleeding. Abnormal findings may be the result of endometrial cancer, hyperplasia, endometrial polyp, or some forms of infertility. Women using combined estrogen-progestin regimens are expected to have uterine bleeding, but, if the bleeding is determined to be pathological, endometrial biopsy may be performed. Appropriate interpretation of endometrial biopsy is important for managing postmenopausal bleeding. Women who have endometrial cancer or adenomatous hyperplasia are referred to a gynecologist or gynecologist-oncologist. Cystic hyperplasia or proliferative endometrium requires an increase in the dosage of progestin, and a biopsy is performed 4 to 6 months later (Lemcke, Marshall, & Pattison, 1995).

A biopsy can be done to evaluate for infertility. If a basal body temperature chart and progesterone test suggest a problem with ovulation, the next step is performing a biopsy. The presence of a thickened endometrium as menstruation approaches indicates that ovulation has occurred. A biopsy may be used to evaluate a luteal-phase defect.

Hormonal Evaluation

Understanding the menstrual cycle is important in determining and evaluating problems resulting in menstrual disturbances, such as amenorrhea or ovulatory dysfunction. Amenorrhea can result from many causes. Women with irregular or absent menses may have ovulatory dysfunction. Many of these problems resolve spontaneously, but further evaluation and referral is warranted if these problems persist.

When the menstrual flow is affected, pregnancy, premature menopause, medication use, thyroid dysfunction, and a prolactin-producing pituitary tumor must be excluded from the diagnosis. Laboratory evaluation is warranted to rule out possible causes. The level of follicle-stimulating hormone (FSH) is determined to evaluate for premature menopause. Normal serum TSH and prolactin levels preclude thyroid disease and hyperprolactinemia (Greenspan & Strewler, 1997).

Documentation of ovulation can be obtained through tracking the basal body temperature. In addition, evaluation of luteinizing hormone (LH) is important in determining ovulation. Ovulation may be documented by obtaining commercially available urine LH tests. The midcycle surge of pituitary LH is the impetus for ovulation and is detectable in the urine. Serum LH testing is also available. Any abnormal findings warrant further evaluation and follow-up.

During perimenopause and menopause the pituitary gland and the ovaries undergo a gradual change during which the incidence of ovulation decreases and FSH and LH levels gradually increase. FSH and LH are not reliable diagnostic indications of menopause. Blood estrogen levels should be determined.

Osteoporosis Examination

Prevention of osteoporosis in women ages 45 to 65 has become increasingly important. Fractures are responsible for a large proportion of morbidity in the elderly. Loss of mobility and a sense of well-being because of chronic pain or acute injury may lead to loss of function in other systems and a loss of independence. The woman may voluntarily limit her activity because of a fear of falling, again altering quality of life (Sakornbut, 1997).

Insufficient evidence exists at this time to recommend for or against routine screening for osteoporosis with bone densitometry in postmenopausal women. Recommendations against routine screening may be made on clinical judgment. Postmenopausal women should be advised of the importance of smoking cessation, regular exercise, and adequate calcium intake. Weight bearing is important to maintenance of healthy bone mass. Although fracture or kyphosis is usually the first sign of osteoporosis, the health care provider is responsible for knowing which patients have early osteoporosis or who are at risk so as to achieve early intervention.

Bone densitometry has been used as a means of predicting risk of osteoporosis. Techniques include radiographic absorptiometry of the hand; dual energy photon absorptiometry of the spine, hip, or total body; and dual energy roentgenographic absorptiometry of the spine, hip, or total body. Dual energy roentgenographic absorptiometry is precise, has a short procedure time (5 to 10 minutes), and uses a low radiation dose. The cost and inconvenience of screening may be justified if screening reduces the burden of osteoporosis.

ACOG does not recommend routine screening for osteoporosis, which is consistent with the recommendations of the Canadian Task Force and American College of Physicians. However, the latter organizations and the World Health Organization recommend bone densitometry studies as a means of directing nonhormonal therapy for osteoporosis. All women should be counseled on diet and exercise as part of routine preventative visits. Women 65 and older should be counseled on fall prevention.

SUMMARY

Disagreement among various experts about screening recommendations makes decisions about screening asymtomatic women difficult for health care providers to make. Other variables that the health care provider should consider are associated risks, costs, time involved, and the possibility of false positives.

To implement preventive health care effectively, the women's health care nurse should be aware of and sensitive to the context in which a woman lives. As a co-participant in the delivery of care, the woman determines her own health care needs based on information she receives and her choices. The nurse's role is to be knowledgeable about the existing recommendations set forth and to provide the woman with information about the screening tests. The women's health care nurse may then assist the woman in obtaining the necessary services.

The woman and the nurse face a multitude of influences concerning decisions on health and disease. Women may vary in their perceptions of health, depending on their cultural beliefs, sexual orientation, and social and economic status. Women may use alternative forms of healing because of traditional cultural beliefs or perhaps because of exposure to alternative health care. In addition, economics influences what services are available and the frequency with which a woman might access these services. Although the influence of sociocultural experiences on individual responses is valuable, it is important that one not make assumptions that might influence the relationship between the nurse and the recommendations chosen.

REFERENCES

Acheson, L. (1997). Caring for the pregnant woman and planning for the delivery. In J. Rosenfeld (Ed.), *Women's health in primary care: Special considerations for nurse practitioners and physician assistants.* Baltimore: Williams & Willkins.

American Cancer Society. (1993). *Cancer facts and figures.* Atlanta, GA: Author.

American Cancer Society. (1999). *Cancer facts and figures.* Atlanta, GA: Author.

American College of Obstetricians and Gynecologists. (1996). *Guidelines for women's health care.* Washington, DC: Author.

American College of Physicians. (1997). Suggested techniques for fecal occult blood testing and interpretation in colorectal cancer screening. *Annals of Internal Medicine, 126,* 808–810.

American Diabetes Association. (2001). Clinical practice recommendations, 2001. *Diabetes Care, 24,* 521–579.

Andolsek, K. (1997). Eating disorders. In J. Rosenfeld (Ed.), *Women's health in primary care: Special considerations for nurse practioners and physician assistants* (pp. 205–225). Baltimore: Williams & Wilkins.

Burke, W., Petersen, G., Lynch, P., Botkin, J., Daly, M., Garber, J., et al. (1997). Recommendations for follow-up care of individuals with an inherited predisposition to cancer: I. Hereditary for nonpolyposis colon cancer. *Journal of the American Medical Association, 277*(11), 915–919.

Colorectal Cancer Screening. (1996). *Summary, evidence report no. 1.* Rockville, MD: Agency for Health Care Policy and Research.

Committee on Guidelines of Care. (1992). Guidelines of care for basal cell carcinoma. *Journal of the American Academy of Dermatology, 26,* 117–120.

Expert Panel on Women's Health. (1997). Women's health and women's health care: Recommendations of the 1996 AAN Expert Panel on Women's Health. *Nursing Outlook, 45*(1), 7–15.

Frame, P. S., & Carlson, S. J. (1975). A critical review of periodic health screening using specific screening criteria. *Journal of Family Practice, 2,* 29–36.

Freund, K. M. (1995). Screening in primary care for women in preventive medicine. In P. Carr, K. M. Freund, & S. Somani (Eds.), *The medical care of women* (pp. 1–13). Philadelphia: W. B. Saunders.

Frigolletto, F. (1996, June 3). A message about skin protection. *ACOG Women's Health Column,* 1–2.

Frigoletto, F. (1996, July 1). Primary care for women. *ACOG Women's Health Column,* 1–2.

Fuchs, C., Giovannucci, E., Colditz, G., Hunter, D., Speizer, F., & Willett, W. (1994). A prospective study of family history and the risk of colorectal cancer. *New England Journal of Medicine, 331*(25), 1669–1674.

Greenlee, R. T., Murray, T., & Bolden, S. (2000). Cancer statistics, 2000. *CA: A Cancer Journal for Clinicians, 50*(1), 7–33.

Greenspan, F., & Strewler, G. (Eds.). (1997). *Basic and clinical endocrinology* (5th ed.). Stamford, CT: Appleton and Lange.

Hendricks, S., Von Esschen, M., & Grady, M. (1995). Preconception counseling and cases of common medical disorders in pregnancy. In D. Lemcke, J. Pattison, L. Marshall, & D. Crowley, (Eds.), *Primary care of women* (pp. 518–530). Norwalk, CT: Appleton and Lange.

Heudebert, G. (1993). Prevention in primary care. In Berg, D. (Ed.), *Handbook of primary care medicine.* Philadelphia: J. B. Lippincott.

Joint National Committee on Detection, Evaluation, and Treatment of High Blood Pressure. (1999). The sixth report of the Joint National Committee on Detection, Evaluation, and Treatment of High Blood Pressure. *Archives of Internal Medicine, 1*(4), 342–345.

Karagas, M. R., Greenberg, E. R., Mott, L. A., Baron, J. A., & Ernster, V. L. (1998). Occurrence of other cancer among patients with prior basal cell and squamous cell skin cancer. *Cancer Epidemiology, Biomarkers, and Prevention, 7*(2), 157–161.

Kellerman, R. (1997). Ovarian cancer. In J. Rosenfeld (Ed.), *Women's health in primary care* (pp. 479–489). Baltimore: Williams & Wilkins.

Koss, L. G. (1993). Cervical (Pap) smear. *New Directions, Cancer, 71*(Suppl. 1), 1406–1412.

Kruman, R. J., & Solomon, D. (1994). *The Bethesda system for reporting cervical/vaginal cytologic diagnosis: Definitions, criteria, and explanatory notes for terminology and specimen adequacy.* New York: Springer-Verlag.

Lemcke, D., Marshall, L., & Pattison, J. (1995). Menopause and hormone replacement therapy. In D. Lemcke, J. Pattison, L. Marshall, & D. Crowley (Eds.), *Primary care of women.* Norwalk, CT: Appleton and Lange.

Madlow-Kay, D. (1997). Preventive health care. In J. Rosenfeld (Ed.), *Women's health in primary care* (pp. 75–92). Baltimore: Williams & Wilkins.

Miklius, A., & Daniels, G. (1995). Management of thyroid nodules. In P. Carr, K. M. Freund, & S. Somani (Eds.), *The medical care of women* (pp. 217–225). Philadelphia: W. B. Saunders.

Morton, B. A. (1996). Vaccine therapy for malignant melanoma, *CA: A Cancer Journal for Clinicians, 46*(4), 225–244.

National Cholestereol Education Program (NCEP) Expert Panel (1993). Summary of the second report of NCEP Expert Panel on detection, evaluation and treatment of high blood cholesterol in adults. *Journal of the American Medical Association, 269*(23), 3015–3023.

Northrup, C. (1998). *Women's bodies, women's wisdom.* New York: Bantam Books.

O'Malley, M., & Fletcher, S. (1987). Screening for breast cancer with breast self-examination. *Journal of the American Medical Association, 257,* 2197–2203.

Office of Public Health and Science, Office of Disease Prevention and Health Promotion. (1998). *Put prevention into practice: Clinician's handbook of preventive services.* Washington, DC: U.S. Department of Health and Human Services.

Parker, S. L., Tong, T., Bolden, S., & Wing, P. A. (1997). Cancer statistics. *CA: A Cancer Journal for Clinicians, 47,* 5–27.

Sakornbut, E. (1997). Preventive health care. In J. Rosenfeld (Ed.), *Women's health in primary care* (pp. 739–761). Baltimore: Williams and Wilkins.

Slade, J., Marghoob, A., & Salopek, T. (1995). A typical mole syndrome: risk factor for cutaneous malignant melanoma and implications for management. *Journal of the American Academy Dermatology, 32,* 479–493.

U.S. Preventive Services Task Force. (1996). *Guide to clinical preventive services* (pp. 763–769). Baltimore: William and Wilkins.

Von Gruenigen, V. E., & Karlen, J. R. (1995). Carcinoma of the endometrium. *American Family Physician, 1,* 1531–1536.

Wallach, J. (1996). *Interpretation of diagnostic tests* (6th ed.). Boston: Little, Brown.

Walters, N., Estridge, B., & Reynolds, A. (1995). Basic medical laboratory techniques. Albany, NY: Delmar.

Wysocki, S., & Davis, A. (1999). *Clinical challenges in women's health: A handbook for nurse practitioners.* Jamesburg, NJ: NP Communications.

RESOURCES

Lab Tests Online: *http://www.labtestsonline.org*

McClatchey. (2002). *Clinical laboratory medicine text and self-assessment review.* Philadelphia: Lippincott Williams & Wilkins.

National Guideline Clearinghouse, Agency for Healthcare Research & Quality: *www.ahcpr.gov*

Chapter 10

Physical Assessment

Margaret Burns

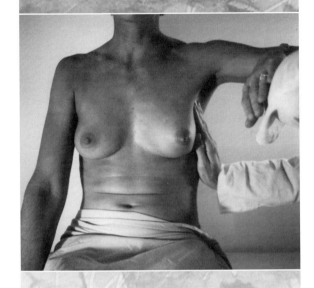

One of the essential qualities of the clinician is interest in humanity, for the secret of the care of the patient is in caring for the patient.

Dr. Francis Peabody

INTRODUCTION

The physical examination serves as a screening device for detecting abnormalities that are unknown to the woman and for identifying signs that may suggest illness or deformity. The examination is done along with the health history, risk assessment, screening, and targeted interventions. Findings serve to affirm any potential concern that might have been revealed through the health history. Some portions of the physical examination may be useful for screening or for determining further diagnostic procedures. The examination may prompt further discussion between the health care provider and the woman to uncover additional concerns. Based on the information obtained, the health care provider may include a more comprehensive examination of specific body systems. The physical examination usually is conducted from head to toe but can be adapted to meet the needs of the woman examined. This chapter focuses on those body systems most often examined for the primary care of women, based on recommendations of the American College of Obstetricians and Gynecologists (1996). The areas examined include the skin, head, face, mouth, neck, cardiopulmonary system, breasts, abdomen, and pelvic area. The cardiopulmonary system is included in this chapter because such an examination is indicated before a woman begins hormone therapy. A more comprehensive examination of other systems is warranted if the health history so indicates. Positive findings may indicate further diagnostic studies are needed. Normal variations for women during the life cycle are discussed.

ASSESSMENT OF BODY SYSTEMS

Skin

Skin assessment is integrated into the complete examination. The health care provider performs skin examination not as a separate step but along with other aspects of the physical examination. The health care provider inspects the outer skin surface before concentrating on the underlying structures. Careful inspection usually provides the most significant data. Palpation enables the nurse to assess the temperature and integrity of the skin and to note elevated lesions. The skin holds information related to the circulation and nutritional status of the body, signs of systemic disease, and topical data on the integument itself. Separate body areas that have skin folds, such as large breasts and an obese abdomen and groin, warrant close inspection. These areas are dark and warm and provide perfect conditions for irritation or infection. Inspection of the feet and toenails is warranted, for they are often forgotten.

The health care provider begins the physical assessment of the skin by observing the woman's general overall appearance from a distance of 3 to 6 feet, noting complexion, general color, color variations, and general appearance. Baseline knowledge is important in assessing color or pigment changes. The best lightning for a skin examination is sunlight, but strong, direct interior lighting (at least 60 W) is acceptable, perferably from an incandescent bulb, not a fluorescent one.

The health care provider needs to ask the woman about her skin color. Lighter-pigmented women usually appear ivory to pink, with possible olive or yellow overtones. Exposed areas are usually darker than nonexposed areas. Darker-pigmented women appear tan to dark brown. The lips may have a bluish hue in women of Mediterranean descent. African-American women may have a blue or reddish hue to lips and mucous membranes. Hyperpigmentation freckles on the face and arms are common in light-skinned women. The health care provider assesses the skin and pays particular attention to any lesions, which are described according to characteristics, exudate, pattern of arrangement, location, and distribution. Some skin disorders are recognizable by distribution over the body and by the primary lesions.

Normal Range of Findings

Adolescent. The increased activity of the sebaceous glands leads to oiliness and acne. Acne is the most common skin problem of adolescence. Acne may appear in children as early as 7 or 8 years old; the lesions increase in number and severity and peak at 14 to 16 years of age in girls. Many women have acne late into their teens and early 20s.

Aging Female. As a woman becomes older, she may develop common variations of hyperpigmentation. Lesions, often referred to as age spots but incorrectly called liver spots, are small, flat, brown macules. These lesions tend to cluster on the forearms and hands after years of prolonged sun exposure and are not malignant and do not require any treatment.

Keratosis results in lesions that are raised, thickened areas of pigmentation that appear crusty, scaly, and warty. Most appear on the trunk of the body but also may be found on the hands and feet and on unexposed and sun-exposed areas. These lesions do not become cancerous.

Head and Face

The health care provider begins the examination by inspecting the woman's face and head for size, shape, symmetry, and any tics or other abnormal movements. Inspection includes noting the head position. The normal size of the head varies considerably among individuals. In the adult the head size accounts for approximately 12% of overall body size. A horizontal jerking or bobbing motion may be seen in association with a tumor or with aortic insufficiency. The woman who constantly positions her head at an angle may be experiencing hearing or vision difficulties. A head held at an angle may result from the shortening of the sternocleidomastoid muscle (torticollis).

When palpating the skull, the health care provider assesses for tenderness, masses, depressions, and lesions. Using a rotary motion, the health care provider palpates the skull systematically starting from the frontal (forehead) region to the occipital (lower back of the head) region, being sure to include the temporal (temple) and parietal (upper back of the head above the occiput) regions.

Brief inspection of the scalp is adequate to identify underlying tenderness and to assess the character of the hair. A thorough inspection and palpation is suggested if the woman has a history of trauma and symptoms such as pain and persistent aching of the scalp. The scalp should not be dry or flaky. The health care provider should examine areas behind the ears at the hairline and at the crown of the head and should note any pattern of hair loss.

The health care provider inspects the facial features (eyelids, eyebrows, palpebral fissures, nasolabial folds, and mouth) for shape and symmetry and notes the woman's facial expression and contours. The health care provider observes for asymmetry, involuntary movements, edema, and masses. Numerous conditions can distort the shape of the face, including edema, thyroid disorders, adrenal dysfunction, chronic illness, dehydration, and malnutrition.

The health care provider then inspects the facial muscles as she instructs the woman to use the muscle groups innervated by the cranial nerves V and VII (trigeminal and facial), having the woman smile, frown, close both eyes, wrinkle her forehead, puff out her cheeks, and raise her eyebrows (facial cranial nerve) while the temporal and mastoid muscles are palpated for strength as the woman clenches her teeth and moves her jaw laterally (trigeminal cranial nerve). A paralyzed, weakened side of the face remains immobile, while the innervated side of the face wrinkles. The lips rise only on the intact side. The health care provider should suspect facial nerve paralysis when all of the face is affected and facial nerve weakness when weakness is confined to the lower face. Abnormal findings warrant the health care provider to perform a more comprehensive neurological and mental status examination.

When examining for facial hair, the nurse takes the woman's age and ethnic origin into account and notes any changes in the shape of the face or unusual features, such as edema, puffiness, coarsened features, prominent eyes, hirsutism, lack of expression, excessive perspiration, pallor, or pigmentation variation. Further follow-up is warranted with such findings because certain disorders cause characteristic changes in facial appearance.

Of the four pairs of sinuses, only the frontal and maxillary sinuses can be examined externally; the sphenoid and ethmoid sinuses are assessed by intranasal inspection. The health care provider palpates for sinus tenderness by pressing up in the frontal sinuses, above the midline of the eyebrow but avoids exerting pressure on the eyes. The health care provider next presses up in the maxillary sinuses at the soft tissue under the zygomatic bone and palpates the sinuses bilaterally for any tenderness, warmth, or swelling. For additional information, the health care provider may percuss the sinuses by tapping them lightly.

Mouth

The health care provider begins the oral examination by placing a glove on the dominant hand because the mouth requires internal inspection and palpation. If the woman is wearing dentures, they must be removed before the examination.

A systematic assessment of the mouth and oropharynx begins with the inspection of the external boundaries of the mouth, cheeks, and lips. The health care provider asks the woman to open her mouth slightly to inspect the lips more fully. Normally the lips are symmetrical and are more highly pigmented than the surrounding facial skin. The health care provider observes the lips for color and moisture and notes any lumps, ulcers, cracking, or scaling. The most common lesions are associated with chapped lips and cold sores (herpes).

The health care provider inspects the woman's mouth with a good light and a tongue blade. The health care provider needs to move the lips outward and upward or downward, one at a time to inspect the inner mucosa beyond the deep pigmentation of the external lips, including the buccal mucosa, gums, and teeth.

The mucous membrane is pinkish red, smooth, and moist. The Stensen duct may appear as a whitish-yellow protrusion located opposite the first upper molar. The health care provider should inspect the oral mucosa for color, ulcers, white patches, and nodules, which may need further evaluation by a dental practitioner. Frequently, a white, waxy line or scarring that is whitish or pinkish appears to protrude above the buccal surface and is visible on the buccal membrane where the upper and lower teeth meet. This line is known as the line of alba and is normal.

Leukoplakia, a condition of patchy white lesions on the mucosal membranes of the mouth, is found more commonly in smokers and heavy users of alcohol. Typically, it has a white leathery appearance. If the health care provider finds such lesions, the woman should be referred to a general dentist to rule out oral cancer.

The health care provider should inspect and palpate the gums, which should be slightly stippled (orange peel) pink with a clearly defined tight margin at each tooth. The gum surface should be free of lesions, inflammation, and bleeding. Using gloves, the health care provider palpates the gums for any lesions, induration, thickening, or masses and observes carefully for any extreme enlargement and bulging (hypertrophy) or retraction (atrophy). Easily bleeding, swollen gums that have enlarged crevices are associated with gingivitis or periodontal disease.

The health care provider should inspect and count the natural teeth. Adults normally have eight teeth on each side of the upper and lower jaws. While inspecting, the health care provider notes the location of any missing teeth and identifies any excess debris on the teeth (plaque). Loose teeth can result from an inflammatory process or trauma. The color of the teeth is generally ivory but variations exist. Yellow teeth can result from tobacco or caffeine use.

The tongue is normally pink, moist, intact, and free of lesions. The tongue often has a thin, white coating that is considered normal. The white coating should not be confused with thrush, which is thicker and cannot be displaced by gently scraping with a tongue blade. The numerous papillae (small, nipple-shaped elevations) of the tongue create the characteristic rough texture. Certain papillae toward the back of the tongue are larger than the others. The geographic tongue, a normal variation, has superficial denuded circles or irregular areas exposing the tips of papillae.

Palpation of the entire tongue and the floor of the mouth is important because tumors may not be seen initially. The health care provider should ask the woman to extend her tongue naturally and then the provider gently compresses the tongue little by little from front to back using the gloved hand.

The health care provider should request the woman to touch the tip of her tongue to the palate area directly behind the upper incisors so that the sublingual area may be inspected for lesions, masses, or discoloration and varicosities. The undersurface of the tongue should be completely smooth. The health care provider should wrap the tongue with a piece of gauze and gently pull the tongue laterally to inspect the sides of the tongue.

The health care provider then asks the woman to tilt her head slightly to inspect the palate and uvula. Using a penlight, the health care provider inspects the hard palate, which is usually white or pale pink, and then the soft palate. The palate is usually moist, intact, and free of any lesions. The uvula, a midline continuation of the soft palate, varies in length and thickness. The uvula should be free of lesions and hang down from the soft palate in front of the posterior pharynx. The health care provider should request the woman to say "Ah." The uvula should remain in the midline during phonation. Deviation could indicate tenth (vagus) cranial nerve damage.

Lastly, the health care provider inspects the tonsils, which lie deep in the oropharynx. The tonsils are normally pink and blend into the coloring of the pharynx. If the tonsils have not been removed, they appear as small, irregular surface growths with multiple small crypts (recesses). Both tonsils should be free of inflammation, lesions, and exudate. The health care provider should stimulate the gag reflex by placing a tongue blade on the back of the tongue. A normal response indicates that the ninth (glossopharygeal) and tenth (vagus) cranial nerves are intact.

Neck

The physical examination of the neck includes the examination of the thyroid gland and lymph nodes of the neck. The health care provider begins the examination with an overall inspection of the neck for the size and the position of the trachea and thyroid. The thyroid gland straddles the trachea in the middle of the neck and has two lobes, both conical, each curving posteriorly between the trachea and the sternocleidomastoid muscle. The lobes are connected in the middle by a thin isthmus lying over the second and third tracheal rings.

The techniques used to examine the thyroid gland include inspection, palpation, and auscultation. The health care provider assesses the thyroid for enlargement, tenderness, nodules, and bruits. The normal thyroid gland is not visible or palpable (or only slightly so). Examining the thyroid may be easier on a neck that is long and slender. If the woman's neck is short, or if the woman has had surgery, the examination may be more difficult.

The health care provider asks the woman to be seated with her neck slightly flexed to enhance the relaxation of the sternocleidomastoid muscle. The health care provider then observes the lower section of the neck. Using a standing lamp to shine light tangentially across the neck, the health care provider looks for any swelling. The health care provider asks the woman to swallow because an enlarged thyroid gland may be visible in the neck during swallowing.

Following inspection, the health care provider palpates the neck for an enlarged thyroid. With the woman sitting straight with her neck slightly forward and to the right, the health care provider stands behind the woman and uses the fingertips of the left hand to push the trachea slightly to the right and the fingers of the right hand to retract the sternocleidomastoid muscle. While the woman takes a sip of water, the health care provider palpates the medial and lateral margins of the thyroid. The process is repeated on the left side of the neck. The thyroid gland is fixed to the trachea and rises during swallowing. This feature distinguishes the thyroid from other structures in the neck. The health care provider palpates the thyroid to evaluate for size, shape, consistency, symmetry, tenderness, and any nodules. The thyroid feels soft but elastic. If the health care provider suspects an enlarged thyroid, she auscultates over the lateral lobes of the thyroid gland, using the bell of the stethoscope to detect a bruit. Increased blood flow to the thyroid gland produces vibrations that may be heard as a soft rushing sound. The health care provider next examines the lymph nodes. Examination of the thyroid includes a determination of lymphadenopathy.

Normal Range of Findings

Adolescent. The thyroid of a young child may be palpable. The thyroid glands of adolescents and adults are similar. The health care provider should use the techniques described for adults to note the size, shape, position, mobility, and any tenderness of the thyroid.

Pregnant Female. The thyroid gland enlarges slightly during pregnancy and may become palpable because of hyperplasia of the tissue and increased vascularity. A thyroid bruit may be noted.

Aging Female. The thyroid becomes more fibrotic with aging and may feel more nodular or irregular with palpation. Any single nodule may be a cyst or a benign tumor but warrants further investigation. One nodule raises the suspicion of a malignancy.

Lymph Nodes of the Neck

The health care provider begins the lymph node evaluation by inspecting the skin for lesions and by palpating for masses along the chains of lymph nodes. The nodes are assessed usually by examining both sides at once (by palpating using a gentle circular motion with the pads of the fingers) for enlargement, tenderness, and mobility.

The nodes generally are not palpable, but, if they are palpable, they should feel movable, discrete, soft, and not tender. Knowledge of the lymphatic system is important because whenever a node is enlarged or tender, the health care provider should look for a source such as an infection in the area where the node drains. If a lymph node is palpable, the health care provider should assess the location, size, consistency, mobility, and tenderness of the node. A node can be rolled up and down or side to side. Neither a muscle nor an artery can be moved this way.

The head and neck have a rich supply of lymph nodes. The lymph nodes are as follows (Figure 10-1):

■ **Preauricular**: In front of the ear
■ **Posterior auricular (mastoid)**: Superficial to the mastoid process
■ **Occipital**: At the base of the skull
■ **Jugulodigastric (tonsillar)**: At the angle of the mandible
■ **Submandibular (submaxillary)**: Halfway between the angle and tip of the mandible
■ **Submental**: In the midline a few centimeters behind the tip of the mandible
■ **Superficial cervical**: Overlying the sternocleidomastoid muscle
■ **Deep cervical**: Deep under the sternocleidomastoid muscle and often inaccessible for examination
■ **Posterior cervical**: Along the edge of the trapezius muscle
■ **Supraclavicular**: Deep in the angle formed by the clavicle at the sternocleidomastoid muscle

Breasts

The breast examination involves bilateral inspection and palpation of the breasts and areolae and the auxiliary and supraclavicular areas. Examination of the breast is performed in the upright and supine positions. The woman may express embarrassment or fear about having her breasts examined. Embarrassment may stem from a sense of modesty or dissatisfaction with her breast development. Fear may be related to what the

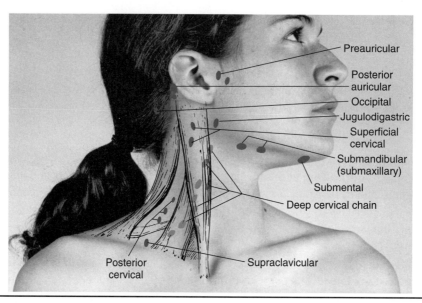

Figure 10-1 Lymph nodes of the head and neck. (From Jarvis, C. [1996]. *Physical examination and health assessment* [2nd ed., p. 273]. Philadelphia: W. B. Saunders.)

health care provider may discover on the examination. The health care provider should ensure privacy during the examination. Explaining the breast examination before the examination itself may relieve the woman's discomfort and allow her to anticipate the components of the examination. Before the breast examination, the health care provider will have been able to assess the woman's level of knowledge and practice regarding breast self-examination in the health history. Education usually is conducted simultaneously with the examination.

Inspection

The breasts are examined better visually under good lighting, with the woman sitting or standing with her hands on her hips. Generally the woman is seated, disrobed to the waist. Inspection of the breast focuses on symmetry and contour; position of the nipples; skin changes such as puckering, dimpling, or scaling of the skin; scars; nipple discharge; nipple retraction; and appearance of a mass. The breast should be relatively symmetrical, although variations are normal. The breast is round and smooth, and the surface contour should appear even and uninterrupted. The color of the breast, except for the nipple and areola, is uniform with the woman's skin in other covered parts of the body. Vascular patterns are diffuse and symmetrical. Hypervascular patterns may be noted on pregnant, obese, and very fair-skinned individuals. Focal or unilateral patterns are abnormal and may be produced by dilated superficial veins from increased blood flow to a malignancy.

The areolae and nipples are inspected for size and shape. The areola can range from light pink to dark brown, depending on the woman's skin color and hormonal influences. In pregnancy the areolae enlarge and darken. The areola and nipple are generally equal in size, round or oval, with a smooth surface. Montgomery tubercles (sebaceous glands that produce a waxy secretion) may be placed irregularly around the areolae. If the breasts are symmetrical, nipples usually point in the same direction, normally outward. The nipples should appear soft and smooth and should have no crusting. Inversion of one or both nipples, if present from puberty, is normal. Inversion may pose difficulty for nursing an infant but is not clinically significant.

To detect dimpling that may be otherwise invisible, the health care provider asks the woman to lift her arms slowly over her head. Tension in the breast through contraction of the pectoral muscle assists in eliciting dimpling if a mass is present. Both breasts should move symmetrically. With the woman's arms lowered and palms pressed together at waist level, the health care provider again should look for signs of retraction. If breasts are larger or pendulous, a third position may be useful. The health care provider asks the woman to stand and lean forward; the breasts should move forward symmetrically. The health care provider should find no evidence of fixation of the breasts to the chest wall.

Normal Range of Findings

Adolescent. At puberty, growth of the periductal tissue, enlargement of lobules, and deposition of fat cause breast growth. The areola and nipple become more pigmented at this time. Completely developed breasts are conical, and some superficial veins are present. When examining an adolescent girl, the health care provider should assess breast development according to Tanner's sex maturity rating (see Chapters 7 and 11). Adolescent girls often are concerned about their breast development. Explaining the sequence of breast development and where the girl might be in relation to the developmental sequence may be helpful.

Breasts of the nonpregnant woman change with fluctuations in hormones during the monthly menstrual cycle. In the 3 to 4 days before onset of menses, the breast may feel tight, heavy, and sore. The breast volume will be the smallest on days 4 to 7 of the menstrual cycle.

Pregnant female. Numerous changes occur in the breasts during pregnancy. The changes start during the second month and are an early sign of pregnancy. The hormonal changes stimulate the expansion of the duct system and supporting fatty tissue. Breast size may increase 2 to 3 times prepregnancy size. Striae caused by rapidly increasing skin tension on the breast may become more visible. The areolae become darker and their diameter increases. Montgomery tubercles become more prominent, often as sebaceous glands hypertrophy. The venous pattern is more prominent during pregnancy and becomes visible as a blue network beneath the skin surface. After about 4 months, colostrum may be expressed from the nipples. Colostrum initially is clear to yellowish but becomes cloudy later in pregnancy.

Aging female. Before menopause a moderate decrease in glandular tissue and some decomposition of alveolar and lobular tissue occurs. This process continues after menopause, and glandular tissue is replaced by connective tissue. The decrease in glandular tissue results in a decrease in breast size. Simultaneously the breast loses elasticity and tends to hang more loosely from the chest wall. The breast looks more flattened. The nipples become smaller and flatter and lose some erectile ability.

Palpation

Palpation of the breast begins with the axillary, subclavicular, and supraclavicular lymph nodes and usually is performed after the neck is examined. To conduct this portion of the examination effectively, the woman remains seated. While the health care provider supports and lifts the woman's left arm with her left arm, the health care provider cups the fingers of her right hand and places them high into the woman's axilla. The health care provider encourages the woman to relax her arm because contracted muscles may obscure slightly enlarged nodes. The health care provider moves down firmly to palpate in four directions: along the chest wall, along the anterior border of the axilla, along the posterior border of the axilla, and along the inner aspect of the upper arm. Of the axillary nodes, these are most often palpable. One or more soft, small (<1 cm), nontender nodes frequently are felt. Following the same sequence, the health care provider then examines the right axilla, using the left hand again, supporting and lifting with the right arm.

The health care provider palpates the supraclavicular nodes while the woman is sitting and relaxed with neck flexed slightly forward. The woman's head should be turned slightly toward the side. The supraclavicular nodes may be felt in the angle formed by the clavicle and sternocleidomastoid muscle.

The primary purpose of the palpation of the breasts is to discover masses. The palpation should be performed systematically. Two commonly used patterns of palpation are (1) to start with the nipple and move out from the center to the periphery of the breast, similar to spokes on a wheel, or (2) to move out from the nipple and around the breast in a spiral or concentric circle pattern. The exact sequence selected for palpation is not critical, but developing a systematic approach that always begins and ends at a fixed point is extremely beneficial for the health care provider. The health care provider should take care to palpate the tail of Spence, which extends from the upper outer quadrant to the axilla. A higher portion of malignancies occurs in the upper quadrant of the breast. The health care provider should perform a light palpation and then repeat the examination with deeper, heavier palpation (Figure 10-2).

The health care provider should palpate all the breast tissue with the woman in the upright and supine positions. The woman should sit with her arms hanging freely at the sides for examination in the upright position first. The health care provider palpates the breast using a bimanual technique with the finger pads. One hand supports the inferior aspect of the breast, while the other hand palpates the breast. Next, the health care provider examines each breast with the woman in a supine position with the arm on the side to be examined raised over the head. The health care provider's fingers,

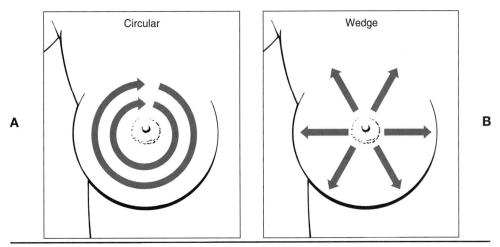

Figure 10-2 Methods for palpating the breast. **A,** Palpation in concentric circles. **B,** Palpation out from the center in wedge sections. (From Seidel, H. M., Ball, J. W., Dains, J. E., & Benedict, G. W. [1999]. *Mosby's guide to physical examination* [4th ed., p. 500]. St. Louis: Mosby.)

while examining the breast, should remain on the breast throughout. The fingers move from one point to another. For large breasts the health care provider again may want to immobilize the inferior surface of the breast with one hand. If a breast mass is felt, the health care provider should characterize the mass by its location, size, shape, consistency, tenderness, mobility, borders, and retraction. The location is indicated by using a clock orientation or by using quadrants, and the distance from the nipple in centimeters is documented. The size of the mass is identified by length and width in centimeters. Consistency is evaluated as soft, hard, or rubbery.

The health care provider carefully palpates the areolar areas to determine the presence of underlying masses and should check for nipple discharge by gently squeezing the nipple. Discharge may be easier to elicit in the upright position. If the nipple discharge is not associated with normal changes in pregnancy or postpartum, the health care provider should collect a specimen of the discharge. When discharge is present on the nipple, the health care provider can bring a slide in contact with the nipple and rub it across the nipple, allowing the discharge to collect on the slide.

If the woman reports that she has discovered a breast lump, the health care provider should examine the unaffected breast first. The baseline consistency of the unaffected breast serves as a comparison to the affected breast. Referral for further diagnostic tests generally is warranted.

The last part of the breast examination is to have the woman demonstrate breast self-examination. Critique of the technique can be performed as well as answering any specific questions that the woman may have. The American College of Obstetricians and Gynecologists recommends that women examine their breasts monthly.

Chest and Lungs

The health care provider generally examines the chest and lungs in the traditional sequence of inspection, palpation, percussion, and auscultation. The examination is performed by comparing the findings from one side with the other as the woman sits upright, generally disrobed to the waist. The woman can use a gown or drape to cover her breasts when the posterior and lateral portions of the chest are examined. When the woman cannot sit up without aid, assistance may be required so that the examination of the posterior side of the chest is performed in the upright position. The examination should be performed in a warm, well-lighted, quiet room. Additional lighting is essential to aid in closer inspection of specific areas. A stethoscope is necessary to assess the chest and lungs.

Inspection

Inspection is for measuring and assessing the pattern of respiration and for assessing the skin and overall configuration, symmetry, and integrity of the thorax. Inspection begins with observing the woman's chest for color, shape or contour, breathing patterns, and muscle development. The color should be even and consistent with the color of the woman's face, with an allowance for sun-exposed areas on the chest and back. The health care provider inspects the skin, nails, and lips and notes any cyanosis or pallor. These areas may provide clues to a respiratory or cardiac disorder. The health care provider should note any lesions and inquire about any changes in appearance and should inspect the chest wall for any scars possibly attributable to surgery. The health care provider notes the shape and symmetry of the chest from inspecting the back and front portions of the chest. The shape or contour should have a downward appearance that equals about a 45-degree slope relative to the spine. The scapulae are placed symmetrically in the hemithorax. Inspecting the woman's anterior chest for deviations in size or shape is important. Normally, the anteroposterior diameter is less than the lateral diameter. If the contour of the chest changes, as in chronic lung disease, the contour of the chest can be described as barrel chest with noted increase in the anterior-posterior diameter. With a barrel chest, the ribs are more horizontal, the spine is somewhat kyphotic, and the sternal angle is more prominent.

Other changes in the chest wall contour may result from structural problems in the spine, rib cage, or sternum. Two common chest changes are pectus excavatum (funnel chest), an indentation of the lower sternum above the xiphoid process, and pectus carinatum (pigeon chest), a prominent sternal protrusion.

The health care provider should note any abnormal retractions of the interspaces during inspiration. Retraction of interspaces may indicate some obstruction of free air inflow. Retraction is more apparent in the lower interspaces. Bulging of interspaces on expiration occurs when air outflow is obstructed or may result from tumor, aneurysm, or cardiac enlargement.

The health care provider should assess the woman's respiration for rate, rhythm, depth, and effort. The rate is generally between 12 and 20 respirations per minute. The health care provider should assess the duration of any periods lacking spontaneous respiration and note any abnormal respiratory problems such as tachypnea (persistent, rapid, shallow breathing) or bradypnea (abnormally decreased respiration). Expansion of the chest should be bilaterally symmetrical, and the woman should be able to breathe easily. The health care provider should check the woman for use of accessory muscles by looking for supraclavicular retraction and for contraction of the sternocleidomastoid muscle. Normally, none of these signs is present. The health care provider should listen to the woman's breathing, noting any additional sounds during the respiratory cycle.

Palpation

Palpation of the thoracic muscles and skeleton further assesses for other structural abnormalities, such as pulsations, bulging, and tender areas and assesses tactile fremitus and respiratory expansion. The thorax should be bilaterally symmetrical with some elasticity of the rib cage. The sternum and xiphoid should be relatively inflexible, but the thoracic spine should be rigid.

Palpation first begins with evaluating the position of the trachea. The health care provider assesses the trachea by palpating for lateral deviation while standing in front of the woman. The health care provider places an index finger in the suprasternal notch and moves the finger laterally left and right in the spaces bordered by the upper edges of each clavicle and in the spaces above to the inner borders of the sternocleidomastoid muscles. The spaces are symmetrical, and the trachea should be in the midline above the suprasternal notch. Palpation may show that the trachea is not at the midline. The position of the trachea could have resulted from a collapse of lung tissue, thyroid enlargement, or fluid accumulation in the air spaces of the lungs. A tumor, a collapsed lung, or nodal enlargement may shift the trachea to one side.

Moving down from the trachea, the health care provider palpates systematically from the lateral shoulder region to the infraclavicular region to the sternum and down its lateral margins toward the rest of the thoracic cage including the axillary region. During the examination, the health care provider palpates from the area of one hemisphere to the corresponding area of the other until all major locations have been examined. The health care provider uses the palmar surface of the hand or the base of the fingers to palpate sequentially the large muscle masses, intercostal spaces, and costochondral junctions near the sternum. On palpation, the muscles should feel firm and smooth. The health care provider palpates the suprasternal nodule to determine the presence and intensity of aortic arch pulsation in tracheal position.

Simultaneously palpating for tenderness, the health care provider assesses the quality of the tactile fremitus. Fremitus is the palpable vibration transmitted through the bronchopulmonary tree to the chest wall by phonation. The health care provider should ask the woman to repeat the words *ninety-nine* or *one, two, three* while the chest walls are palpated systematically. Palpation occurs with the palmar surfaces of the fingers or the ulnar aspects of a closed fist. The health care provider can use two hands to assess both sides of the chest or use one hand moving alternately to compare one side of the chest to the other. The health care provider should palpate each area systematically.

The health care provider should identify and locate any areas of increased, decreased, or absent fremitus. Fremitus varies among persons, but symmetry is most important. The vibration should be consistent in the corresponding area. Fremitus is typically stronger in the interscapular area than in other portions of the lungs and stronger on the right side than left side because the right side is closer to the bronchial bifurcation. Fremitus disappears below the diaphragm. The health care provider should avoid palpating over the scapula because the bone lessens sound transmission.

Increased tactile fremitus is caused when a solid mass or the presence of fluids within the lungs occurs and may be the result of lung consolidation or a tumor. Fremitus is increased in conditions that decrease the distance between the lungs and the palpating fingers. Decreased or absent tactile fremitus occurs when the distance between the palpating hand increases or interference with sound transmission occurs. Decreased fremitus occurs with diminished production or transmission of sounds. Conditions such as excess air in the lungs, pleural effusion, pleural thickening, pneumothorax, bronchial obstruction, or emphysema decrease the fremitus.

The health care provider confirms symmetrical chest expansion by placing warm hands on the anterolateral chest walls with thumbs extending along the costal margins, pointing to the xiphoid process. The health care provider places the thumbs posteriorly at the level of the tenth rib, with the palms on the posterolateral chest, so that the thumbs are 3 to 5 cm apart before inspiration. The health care provider can feel and observe the amount and symmetry of the thoracic expansion during quiet and deep respiration and next should ask the woman to take a deep breath, to feel the symmetry of respiration as the thumbs are separated an additional 3 to 5 cm during deep inspiration. A loss of symmetry in movement of the thumbs may denote a problem on one or both sides.

Percussion

Percussion is the tapping of an object to produce a sound and a palpable vibration. Percussion helps to identify the boundaries of the lungs to determine the relative amount of air, liquid, or solid material in them. Percussion penetrates only 5 to 7 cm into the chest. The health care provider conducts the examination by comparing all areas, using one side as a control for the other. While the woman remains in an upright position, the health care provider percusses the anterior thorax by placing the hands over the lung apices in the supraclavicular areas, proceeding downward and moving from side to side at 3-to 5-cm intervals. The health care provider then requests the woman to raise her arms over her head. While the woman is in this position, the health care provider percusses the lateral thorax starting at the axilla and moving down the side to the rib cage, percussing between the ribs. The health care provider percusses the posterior thorax by progressing in a zigzag fashion from the supracapular to the interscapular to the infrascapular region. The health care provider should avoid the scapular because muscle and bone produce a flat tone. Resonance, the predominate sound in healthy lung tissue, is a hollow, loud, low pitch with longer duration.

Tympany, a hollow sound, results from percussion over the stomach. Percussion sounds that are abnormal over lung tissue are hyperresonance of emphysematous lung tissue or dullness from consolidation of fluid or a solid mass, which may occur with pneumonia or atelectasis.

Auscultation

Auscultation of the lungs is an important technique for assessing air flow throughout the tracheobronchial tree. The health care provider auscultates the anterior, lateral, and posterior thorax to detect normal and abnormal breath sounds. With the woman sitting, the health care provider asks her to breathe through her mouth more deeply and more slowly than usual. The health care provider warms the diaphragm of the stethoscope before placing it over the thoracic landmarks and performs auscultation systematically by listening over the apices and the posterior, lateral, and anterior chest. Using the pattern suggested for percussion, the health care provider moves from one side to the other and compares symmetrical areas of the lungs. If a sound is abnormal, the health care provider should auscultate adjacent areas to describe the extent of the abnormality more fully. Assessment requires one full breath at each placement of the stethoscope. The health care provider should observe the woman for signs of hyperventilation and alter the process if the woman becomes light-headed.

Normal breathing sounds include bronchial, bronchovesicular, and vesicular sounds. Bronchial sounds, heard over the trachea, are high-pitched and harsh, with expiration being longer than inspiration. Bronchovesicular sounds, heard over the main bronchus, are medium-pitched and continuous, with inspiration and expiration being the same length. Vesicular breathing sounds are low pitched and are heard best over the base of the lungs during inspiration, which is longer than expiration (Table 10-1).

The health care provider should note any adventitious sounds, which normally are not heard and are superimposed on the usual breathing sounds. The common terms used to describe the adventitious sounds are crackles (rales), rhonchi, wheezes, and friction rubs.

A *crackle* is an abnormal respiratory sound often heard during inspiration and characterized by discrete sounds. Crackles may be fine, high pitched, and relatively short in duration. Crackles are *fine* when they occur by air passing through moisture in small passages and alveoli and are *coarse* when they occur by air passing through moisture in the bronchioli, bronchi, and trachea. If crackles are apparent, the health care provider should note their loudness, pitch, and duration and describe the number (timing in the respiratory cycle and location) of the crackles.

Sibilant wheezes are continuous sounds that are high pitched and musical and are heard during inspiration or expiration. These sounds are caused by a high-velocity air flow through the narrow airways of the bronchioles. *Sonorous wheezes (rhonchi)* are deeper and more pronounced during expiration. Wheezes originate in the larger bronchi, are low pitched, and may be altered by coughing. Crackling does not dissipate with coughing. If wheezes are apparent, the health care provider should note their timing and location.

Table 10-1 | **CHARACTERISTICS OF BREATHING SOUNDS**

AREA OF THE LUNG	DURATION OF SOUND	INTENSITY OF EXPIRATORY SOUND	PITCH OF EXPIRATORY SOUND	LOCATIONS WHERE SOUND IS HEARD NORMALLY
Vesicular	Inspiratory sounds last longer than expiratory ones	Soft	Relatively low	Over most of both lungs
Bronchovesicular	Inspiratory and expiratory sounds are about equal	Intermediate	Intermediate	Often in the first and second interspaces anteriorly and between the scapulae
Bronchial	Expiratory sounds last longer than inspiratory ones	Loud	Relatively high	Over the manubrium, if heard at all
Tracheal	Inspiratory and expiratory sounds are about equal	Very loud	Relatively high	Over the trachea in the neck

Modified from Bates, B., Bickley, L. S., & Hoekelman, R. A. (1995). *A guide to physical examination and history taking* (6th ed.). Philadelphia: J. B. Lippincott.

Friction rub occurs outside the respiratory tree and has a loud, dry, grating, low-pitched sound that can be heard during inspiration and expiration. A friction rub heard over the lungs may be caused by inflamed pleura rubbing against the chest wall or an inflamed pericardium; heard over the pericardium, the sound may suggest pericarditis; and heard over the lung, the sound may suggest pleurisy. The respiratory friction rub disappears when the breath is held, the pericardial rub does not.

In determining abnormal bronchovesicular or breathing sounds, the health care provider can assess for the abnormality through transmitted voice sounds. The health care provider asks the woman to say *ninety-nine*. Usually the sounds transmitted through the chest are muffled and indistinct. Increased transmission of voice sounds indicates that the lung has consolidation.

Normal Range of Findings

Pregnant female. By the third trimester, the thoracic cage is more prominent because of the increased costal angle. The lower rib cage of the pregnant woman appears to flare out. As the uterus enlarges, the woman's breathing patterns become more thoracic. Respiration rate and depth may increase during the second and third trimesters.

Aging female. The anteroposterior chest increases in size in relation to the lateral diameter, causing the thoracic structure to become rounder in appearance. Changes also occur in the thoracic and lumbar spines. Chest expansion might be decreased somewhat, but expansion is symmetrical. Calcification of the rib articulation may cause the woman to use her accessory muscles.

The older woman may fatigue easily, especially during auscultation when deep mouth breathing occurs. The health care provider should exercise caution to prevent the woman from becoming dizzy.

CARDIOVASCULAR EXAMINATION

Examination of the cardiovascular system includes observing and palpating the pulses. The health care provider compares each pulse with the contralateral pulse; compares the pulses of the upper extremities with those of the lower; and examines pulsation in the radial and carotid arteries, the jugular vein, and the heart. Techniques for assessing the heart include inspection, palpation, and auscultation. The cardiovascular examination usually starts with the measurement of the heart rate and blood pressure. Generally the health care provider takes both measurements along with the other vital signs at the beginning of the physical examination. Routine screening for peripheral arterial disease in asymptomatic persons is not recommended. The health care provider should evaluate a woman at increased risk who has clinical evidence of vascular disease.

A quiet location is important for a thorough examination of the cardiovascular system because heart sounds are quiet and low in pitch and are difficult to hear when extraneous noises are present. A comfortable room temperature is important to prevent the woman from shivering, which interferes with discerning heart sounds. Lighting is important for detecting visible pulsation. For most of the cardiac examination, the woman is supine, with the upper body raised by elevating the head of the examination table. The woman also sits in the forward position and lies on her left side during the examination. The health care provider stands to the right of the woman during the examination to facilitate hand placement and auscultation of the pericardium.

Generally the health care provider conducts the cardiovascular assessment in the following order:

■ Pulses and blood pressure
■ Neck vessels
■ Pericardium

Pulses

The health care provider may easily evaluate all major arterial pulses during the routine physical examination. Palpation of arterial pulses can indicate heart rate, rhythm, pulse contour (wave form), amplitude or quality, symmetry of bilateral pulses, and sometimes obstruction of blood flow. The normal rate varies with age and other factors but usually the range is 60 to 90 beats per minute in adults. The pulses should feel regular in rhythm and equal in strength bilaterally. Pulses with normal amplitude are easily palpable and are obliterated only with strong finger pressure. The contour of the pulse wave is pliable, and healthy arteries have a smooth rounded or domed shape. Evaluation of the radial pulse is a routine part of the physical examination. While assessing the woman's vital signs, the health care provider palpates the radial pulse to assess the heart rate.

After palpation of the radial artery, the health care provider assesses the other major pulse points to determine blood flow. Pulses are best palpated over arteries that are close to the surface of the body and are over bones. The pulses generally assessed are those of the carotid, brachial, radial, femoral, popliteal, dorsalis pedis, and posterior tibial arteries. The health care provider assesses peripheral vascular pulses while assessing the sufficiency of the peripheral vascular perfusion, which usually is integrated with the examination of the other body parts. If a pulse is difficult to find, the health care provider should try varying the pressure and feeling carefully throughout the area. The health care provider also evaluates the pulse for symmetry. The skin of an extremity may appear unusually white or pale and feel cool to the touch when the blood supply to the extremity is blocked by some arterial obstruction. Other abnormal changes in the skin and nails may be present.

Neck Vessels

The vascular structures of the neck accessible to examination are the carotid arteries and the jugular veins. Examination of these vessels provides information about the vessels themselves and yields important information on heart activity. The health care provider uses the techniques of inspection, palpation, and auscultation to examine the carotid arteries and of inspection to examine the jugular veins.

Carotid Arteries

The health care provider inspects the neck for the amplitude of the carotid pulsation, which may be visible just medial to the sternocleidomastoid muscles. The fingertips palpate the carotid pulse just below and medial to the angle of the jaw in the lower third of the neck, pressing posteriorly to feel the pulse. The health care provider palpates one carotid artery at a time to avoid excessive carotid massage, which can precipitate a potentially dangerous slowing of the heart rate or drop in blood pressure. Carotid massage may be particularly dangerous in the older woman who may already have compromised cardiovascular function. If the health care provider has difficulty feeling the pulse, she can ask the woman to move her head toward the side being examined to relax the sternocleidomastoid muscle. The health care provider feels the contour and amplitude of the pulse. The contour should include a smooth up stroke and down stroke. The findings should be the same bilaterally.

For middle-aged or older persons or those who show symptoms or signs of cardiovascular disease, the health care provider should auscultate each carotid artery for the presence of a bruit. A bruit requires further evaluation. A bruit produces a blowing sound heard over an artery that indicates increased arterial flow or arterial stenosis. The sound of a bruit is usually low pitched and difficult to hear. Using the bell of the stethoscope, the health care provider asks the woman to hold her breath briefly. Carotid artery bruits are best heard at the lateral end of the clavicle and the posterior margin of the sternocleidomastoid muscle.

Jugular Veins

After evaluating the carotid pulses, the health care provider inspects the jugular venous pulse. The woman lies supine at a 30- to 45-degree angle or wherever visualization of pulsation is best. The external jugular veins are not any more prominent than 1 to 2 cm above the level of the manubrium. The health care provider uses tangential lighting to delineate the pulses, and, because the wave forms are subtle, directs the light at an angle across the neck where the jugular veins are located. Turning the woman's head slightly away from the side being inspected yields better visualization of the vessels.

Although the external jugular vein is easier to visualize, the internal jugular vein, especially on the right side, attaches more directly to the superior vena cava and is more reliable for assessment. The health care provider should identify the external jugular vein on each side of the neck and then find the pulsation of the internal jugular vein, which is in the suprasternal notch area or around the attachments of the sternocleidomastoid muscles on the sternum and the clavicle. The pulsations are visible through the surrounding soft tissue in this area. The health care provider must distinguish the internal jugular vein pulsation from that of the carotid artery.

The highest point of pulsation in the internal jugular vein is determined by using a centimeter ruler and measuring the vertical distance between the manubriosternal joint (angle of Louis) and comparing it with the highest level of jugular vein pulsation on both sides. The health care provider places a straight edge intersecting the ruler at a right angle to assist in an accurate measurement and reads the level of intersection on the vertical ruler. Normal jugular venous pulsation is 2 cm or less above the sternal angle. Venous pressure measured greater than 3 or possibly 4 cm above the sternal angle is considered elevated. Abnormal distention may be caused by increasing pressure in the right side of the heart.

If the health care provider cannot find the pulsations in the internal jugular veins, the external jugular veins provide a reference point. The health care provider observes the external jugular veins to determine the point that pulsation appears to collapse, making observations on each side of the neck and documenting the vertical distance of these points from the sternal angle (Table 10-2).

Auscultation

Auscultation over an artery for a bruit is indicated when the health care provider is following the radiation of a murmur or is assessing for signs of obstruction. Murmurs are usually low pitched and difficult to hear. The health care provider uses the bell of the stethoscope and asks the woman to hold her breath for several seconds. Auscultation for a bruit is assessed at the carotid, jugular, temporal, abdominal, aortic, renal, and femoral arteries.

Pericardium

In assessing the pericardium, the health care provider systematically begins with inspection, palpation, percussion, and auscultation. First, the health care provider inspects the pericardium with the woman supine with a light source tangential to the woman to visualize any flicker of movement. Visible pulsation and any evidence of heaves or lifts of the chest can give clues to the size and symmetry of the heart. Lifts and heaves may be present with left ventricular hypertrophy. One may or may not see the

Table 10-2	CHARACTERISTICS OF CARDIOVASCULAR PALPATION OF THE NECK
INTERNAL JUGULAR PULSATIONS	**CAROTID PULSATIONS**
Rarely palpable	Palpable
Soft, rapid, undulating quality, usually with two elevations and two troughs per heart beat	A more vigorous thrust with a single outward component
Pulsations eliminated by light pressure on the vein(s) just above the sternal end of the clavicle	Pulsations not eliminated by pressure on the vein(s) just above the sternal end of the clavicle
Level of the pulsations changes with position, dropping as the patient becomes more upright	Level of pulsations does not change with position
Level of pulsations usually descends with inspiration	Level of pulsations is not affected by inspiration

Modified from Bates, B., Bickley, L. S., & Hoekelman, R. A. (1995). *A guide to physical examination and history taking* (6th ed.). Philadelphia: J. B. Lippincott.

apical impulse, which can be obscured easily by obesity, large breasts, and great muscularity. The apical pulse is generally visible in thin adults and children. The pulsation is created as the left ventricle rotates against the chest wall during systole. A visible apical pulse is located at the fourth or fifth intercostal space at or inside the midclavicular line. The apical pulse is generally synchronous with the carotid impulse and the first heart sound (S1).

Palpation

The health care provider should have warm hands while placing the woman in the supine position. The health care provider feels the pericardium gently using the proximal half of the hand and palpates the entire pericardium systematically starting at the apex, moving toward the left sternal border and then to the base of the heart, and searching for any other pulsation. The characteristics of the apical impulse helps the health care provider determine the size of the left ventricle. The health care provider notes the heart rate and rhythm, feels for the apical pulse, and identifies its location by the intercostal space and the distance from the midsternal line. The impulse is gentle and brief, not lasting as long as systole. The health care provider also palpates for any abnormal heaves, retractions, or thrills.

Percussion

Percussion is of limited value in defining the borders of the heart or determining its size. Usually one begins percussion at the anterior axillary line, moving along the intercostal spaces toward the sternal borders. Normally the left border of cardiac dullness is at the midclavicular line in the fifth interspace and slopes toward the sternum as one progresses upward so that by the second interspace the border of dullness coincides with the left sternal border. The right border of dullness matches the sternal border.

Auscultation

Because all heart sounds are low in frequency, the health care provider needs to perform auscultation in a quiet room. Auscultation generally is performed in five cardiac areas, using the diaphragm first and then the bell of the stethoscope. The five designated auscultatory areas are the following (Figure 10-3):

1. Aortic valve area at the second right intercostal space
2. Pulmonic valve area at the second left intercostal space
3. Second pulmonic area at the third left intercostal space
4. Tricuspid valve area at the left lower sternal border
5. Mitral valve area at the apex of the heart at the fifth intercostal space at the left midi-clavicular area

The examination focuses on these five locations, but the health care provider should not limit the auscultation to only these five locations because the sounds produced by the valves may be heard throughout the pericardium. The health care provider should auscultate in any areas where an abnormality is observed. Generally the examiner moves the stethoscope along and at each pause listens selectively for each component of the cardiac cycle.

In evaluating heart sounds, the health care provider should listen for a few cycles to assess the overall rate and rhythm of the sounds. The key to a successful cardiac examination is identification, characterization, and interpretation of the heart sounds.

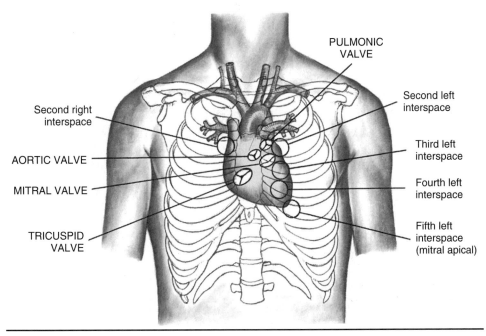

Figure **10-3** Areas for auscultation of the heart. (From Seidel, H. M., Ball, J. W., Dains, J. E., & Benedict, G. W. [1995]. *Mosby's guide to physical examination* [3rd ed., p. 393]. St. Louis: Mosby.)

The main sounds are vibrations caused by closure of valves and by the turbulence of blood flow (Seidel, Ball, Dains, & Benedict, 2003).

During auscultation, the health care provider should characterize the heart sounds by their frequency, intensity, duration, and timing in the cardiac cycle. The health care provider instructs the woman to breathe normally but hold the breath during expiration and listens for the first heart sound while palpating the carotid pulse. S1 should be synchronous with the carotid pulse. The health care provider should note the intensity and any variation or any splitting of S1. An experienced health care provider may be able to discriminate the sound of each valve closing. The first heart sound is louder in the mitral and tricuspid areas and softens in the aortic and pulmonic areas.

The health care provider compares the loudness of the heart sound at each location to differentiate systole from diastole. The health care provider concentrates on S1, the beginning of systole for any additional sounds, and next on diastole, which is longer than systole. S1 immediately follows diastole. The second heart sound occurs at the beginning of diastole. S2 is produced with the aortic and pulmonic valves. This sound is louder in the aortic and pulmonic areas.

The health care provider then focuses on S2, again listening for intensity, splitting, the effects of respiration, and any variation. S2 may have a split sound because the aortic and pulmonic valves do not close at exactly the same time. A normal S2 occurs during inspiration but disappears with expiration.

During auscultation, the health care provider usually examines the woman in the upright, supine, and left lateral positions. The upright forward leaning position is best for hearing high-pitched sounds related to semilunar valve problems such as aortic and pulmonic valve murmurs. While the woman is supine, the health care provider usually stands to the right. If heart sounds seem faint or undetectable, the health care provider can reposition the woman. After the woman is supine, she should roll to the left side. This position is best for hearing low-pitched sounds related to atrioventricular valve problems, such as mitral valve murmurs and extra heart sounds. The health care provider listens at the second left and second right intercostal spaces at the sternal border to detect a high-pitched diastolic murmur of aortic or pulmonic valve insufficiency.

Normal Range of Findings

Functional murmurs are encountered in mature adults, but not with the frequency that they are seen in children and young pregnant women. In many normal healthy children and young adults, auscultation may reveal a split S2. Splitting occurs during inspiration when right ventricular ejection takes slightly longer than left ventricular ejection and causes a slight delay in the pulmonic valve closing. The inspiratory delay is long enough to discriminate the two components of S2.

Physiological S3 is common in children and occurs in early diastole. S3 is characterized as dull and is best heard at the apex. In all cases, distinguishing an innocent murmur from a pathological one is important. Signs of asthma, cardiac rhythm irregularities, and gallops are all important evidence of disease. Cardiac murmurs warrant further follow-up.

Pregnant Female. The resting pulse rate of a pregnant woman usually increases 10 to 15 beats per minute and blood pressure decreases. The systolic and diastolic blood pressure decreases to normal or below normal in the first half of pregnancy. The blood pressure generally rises in the second half of pregnancy, and one cannot be sure whether the cause is preeclampsia or the natural rebound of chronic hypertension. Blood pressure readings elevated from those recorded before pregnancy should cause the health care provider to suspect pregnancy-induced hypertension. Functional murmurs may appear in the pregnant woman because of the increased blood volume and workload. More audible splitting of S1, S2, and S3 may be heard readily after 20 weeks of gestation. A grade II systolic murmur is audible in 90% of women over the pulmonic area soon after delivery. The murmur intensifies during inspiration or expiration.

The enlarged uterus of the pregnant woman causes the heart to shift to the left. The apical impulse is audible more upward and more lateral by 1 to 1.5 cm. During palpation of the pulses, the health care provider should note edema and varicosities, especially in the legs.

Aging Female. With age the heart rate slows and the normal blood pressure may increase. The heart rate may be slower because of increased vagal tone or more rapid, ranging from 40 to more than 100 beats per minute. Occasional ectopic beats are fairly common and may or may not be significant. The systolic and diastolic pressure increase. The increase in systolic pressure rise is greater because of the increased rigidity of the vascular tree.

During inspection of the sternoclavicular area, the health care provider may observe pulsations caused by calcification and dilation of the aorta. The superficial vessels of the forehead, neck, and extremities may feel prominent and ropelike during palpation. The health care provider uses caution in palpating and auscultating the carotid artery and avoids increased pressure to the artery.

With aging, the thorax often increases in the anteroposterior diameter, making palpating the point of maximum intensity (PMI) more difficult. Additional heart sounds warrant further follow-up.

ABDOMINAL EXAMINATION

When examining the abdomen, the health care provider keeps in mind that the placement of the organs and structures is important to assessing this system. The abdomen is a large, oval cavity extending from the diaphragm to the brim of the pelvis. The lower edge of the thorax partially protects the liver, spleen, kidneys, adrenal glands, and pancreas. The health care provider performs the examination of the abdomen with the woman lying comfortably on her back with her head supported by a pillow, the genitalia and breasts covered, and the arms at the woman's side because raising the arms may stretch the abdominal muscles, making the abdomen harder to examine. Ordinarily the woman's knees are not drawn up unless the woman is uncomfortable with the lower extremities flat. The woman may assume this position if she is nervous. The health care provider's goal is to work with relaxed abdominal muscles to allow an adequate examination. To avoid abdominal tensing, the stethoscope and hands should be warm. The woman should empty her bladder before the examination.

The four basic steps of the abdominal examination, in sequence, are inspection, auscultation, percussion, and palpation. The health care provider generally works from the right side of the woman, except for inspection, when all possible angles are observed. For convenience in description, the abdominal wall is divided into four quadrants by a vertical and horizontal line bisecting the umbilicus.

Inspection

Abdominal assessment begins by inspecting the woman's entire abdomen, noting overall contour and skin integrity, appearance of the umbilicus, and any visible pulsation. The health care provider generally inspects the abdomen from a seated position on the right of the woman. This position allows a tangential view that enhances shadows and contouring. Inspection includes skin color, which may be slightly lighter than exposed areas, and fine white or silver striae, which may be visible and result from pregnancy or an increase in weight. The health care provider should note contour discolorations, including rashes.

The umbilicus should be located centrally and normally may be flat, rounded, or concave. The abdomen should be evenly rounded or symmetrical without visible peristalsis. Normal peristalsis is not visible. The health care provider should be aware that variation in contour depends on body type and should note any localized distention or irregular contours for further assessment. A protuberance of the abdomen may be symmetrical or asymmetrical. An asymmetrical protuberance is usually a localized bulging or swelling of the abdominal area caused by an enlarged organ, an abdominal tumor or cyst, or hernia. Having the woman raise her head and shoulders while remaining supine allows detection of any umbilical or incisional hernias.

Auscultation

Auscultation assesses bowel sounds and vascular sounds. The health care provider performs auscultation in a systematic manner, using the four quadrants of the abdomen as a guide. Bowel sounds are high pitched and therefore are appreciated best with the diaphragm of the stethoscope. The mixing and moving forward of the liquid and air in the intestines produce brief bursts of gurgling in all four quadrants, normally anywhere from 2 to 3 times per minute up to 10 to 15 times per minute. Bowel sounds are reported as being active, hyperactive, or hypoactive. The health care provider should auscultate with the bell of the stethoscope over the aorta, renal arteries, iliac arteries, and femoral arteries for bruits.

Percussion

Abdominal percussion helps determine the size and location of abdominal organs and detects excessive accumulation of fluid and air in the abdomen. Percussion is used independently or concurrently with palpation for evaluation of specific organs and can affirm palpation findings. Percussion elicits several kinds of sounds. Tympany is a low-pitched sound of long duration arising from percussion of a gas-filled organ and is the predominate sound caused by the air-filled stomach or intestines. After general percussion of the abdomen, the health care provider percusses the liver, spleen, and stomach in depth. The health care provider begins percussion of the liver at the right midclavicular line over an area of lung resonance, percusses down the interspaces, proceeds to an area of dullness, and marks the spot where the sound changes. The health care provider usually can percuss the upper border of the liver between the fifth and seventh interspaces and the lower edge of the liver about 7 cm from the upper border at the costal margin.

The health care provider marks and measures the areas outlining the liver to estimate the vertical span of the liver. The usual span is approximately 7 cm. A span greater than this may indicate liver enlargement. Liver size can vary depending on the person's size and sex. The measure is only a gross estimate because errors can occur when the dullness results from pleural effusion, lung consolidation, or gas in the upper quadrant, leading to underestimation of size. The health care provider can assess the descent of the liver by asking the woman to take a deep breath and hold the breath while the health care provider percusses upward on the abdomen at the midclavicular line. The areas of lower border dullness move downward 2 to 3 cm. Percussing the liver edge is a helpful guide in planning how to place the hands for palpation of this area.

The health care provider percusses the spleen from the ninth to eleventh intercostal space just behind the left midaxillary line, beginning at the areas of lung resonance. The health care provider percusses the lower intercostal space in the left axillary line before and after the woman takes a breath. The sound identified should be tympany. With splenic enlargement, tympany changes to dullness because inspiration brings the spleen forward and downward. The gastric air bubble is in the area of the left lower anterior rib cage and left epigastric region. Tympany produced by the gastric bubble is lower in pitch than the tympany of the intestines.

Palpation

The health care provider performs palpation to judge the size, location, and consistency of certain organs and to screen for an abnormal mass or tenderness. The examination begins with light palpation. The recommended technique for palpation is to start with the lowest portion of the abdomen and to bounce the fingertips upward at 2-or 3-inch intervals roughly along the midinguinal line to the costal margin. Very light palpation with the fingertips rarely produces tenderness, even in an inflamed abdomen. The health care provider should always start in the lower-most quadrant of the abdomen and progress slowly to the costal margins. The health care provider performs light palpation by pressing the abdominal wall with the pads of the fingers lightly but firmly enough to indent the wall. After exploring the entire abdomen adequately by light palpation, the health care provider performs deep palpation using the same criteria.

To overcome the resistance of a large or obese abdomen, the health care provider often uses a bimanual technique, placing one hand on top of the other. The top hand does the pushing while the bottom hand is relaxed to the sense of palpation.

Assessment for Peritoneal Irritation

If a woman identifies an area of abdominal pain in her medical history, that area should be palpated last. Premature palpation of a painful area may produce a spasm, causing rigidity of the abdominal wall. While palpating around the abdomen, the health care provider should discriminate between voluntary and involuntary rigidity. Voluntary guarding can occur when the woman is cold, tense, or ticklish. Attempting to work with the woman in relaxing the abdominal muscles is beneficial to the examination. Persistent rigidity is more indicative of involuntary rigidity and may indicate peritonitis. To evaluate hypersensitivity the health care provider gently lifts a fold of skin away from the underlying muscle or stimulates the skin with a pin or other object and has the woman describe the feeling. In the event of hypersensitivity, the woman will perceive pain or exaggerate the response to the sensation of this maneuver.

The health care provider assesses for rebound tenderness when the woman reports any abdominal pain or when palpation elicits tenderness. The health care provider should choose a site away from the painful area, hold her hand in at a 90-degree angle to the abdomen, and press firmly and deeply into the abdomen and then suddenly and quickly let go. The health care provider asks the woman if the pain is worse with deep palpation or with the rapid release of pressure. Pain that is more intense with the release indicates rebound pain. The tenderness is often significant in peritonitis.

Throughout the palpation portion of the examination, the health care provider asks the woman if any of the maneuvers are painful. Often more information is gathered by observing the woman's reaction to palpation.

On identifying a mass, the health care provider should do the following:

- Distinguish the mass from a normally palpable structure or an enlarged organ
- Use both hands to determine the size of the mass
- Describe the mass in terms of the location, size, shape, consistency, tenderness, mobility, pulsation, and movement with respiration
- Place, if possible, the fingertips of both hands on either side of the mass to determine if pulsation is present

The health care provider can sense pulsation in the fingertips as a pulsatile flow expanding a structure such as the aorta.

Liver

The health care provider places her left hand behind the woman at the eleventh and twelfth ribs, supporting this area and the adjacent soft tissues below. The woman rests on the health care provider's hand while the health care provider presses her left hand forward, elevating the liver toward the abdominal wall. The health care provider places her right hand on the woman's abdomen lateral to the rectus muscle. The health care provider's fingers point toward the woman's head and extend so that the tips of the fingers are on the right midclavicular line below the level of liver dullness. Gently the health care provider presses the fingers in and up and instructs the woman to take a few breaths and then take a deep breath. The health care provider will feel the liver edge as the diaphragm pushes the liver down to meet the fingertips. The liver will feel like a firm, regular ridge with a smooth surface. Often the liver is not palpable.

An alternate technique for palpating the liver is for the health care provider to stand up at the woman's shoulders to her right and facing the woman's feet. The health care provider hooks her fingers over the right costal margin below the level of liver dullness and asks the woman to take a deep breath. The health care provider will feel the liver edge across the fingertips.

If the abdomen is distended or the abdominal muscles are tense, the usual technique for discovering the lower liver edge may not be productive. Although not highly reliable, another method uses auscultation by which the health care provider can distinguish the difference in sound over a solid or hollow organ. The scratch test assesses the size of the liver. The health care provider places the stethoscope over the liver and with the opposite hand scratches lightly over the abdominal area with short transverse strokes. The sound is magnified over the liver.

Spleen

The spleen is normally soft and nonpalpable in the woman and is located behind the left side at the eleventh and twelfth ribs. The health care provider, while still on the woman's right, reaches across with the left hand and places it beneath the woman over the left costovertebral angle. With fingers extended, the health care provider places the palmar surface of the right hand on the woman's abdomen below the left costal margin and with the fingertips presses inward toward the spleen, while requesting that the woman take a deep breath. The health care provider attempts to feel the edge of the spleen as it moves downward toward the fingertips. The health care provider should use caution in palpating the spleen to avoid rupture. With the woman lying on her right side with her legs somewhat flexed at her hips and knees, the health care provider repeats the palpation of the spleen. In this position the spleen moves forward and downward into a palpable location.

Kidneys

To assess each kidney for tenderness, the health care provider first examines them with the woman sitting. Assessment of the kidneys usually occurs with the back examination or at the end of the posterior lung examination. The examination of the kidneys includes inspection and fist percussion of the back for renal problems. The flanks are symmetrical, and any fullness or asymmetry may result from renal disorders. Discoloration of this area is not considered normal.

Fist percussion in each costovertebral angle evaluates kidney tenderness. The health care provider places the palm of her hand over the right costovertebral angle and strikes her hand with the ulnar surface of the fist of the other hand. The maneuver is repeated over the left costovertebral angle. Direct percussion with the fist also can be used directly over the costovertebral angle. No pain or tenderness should occur during this maneuver.

The remaining aspect of the kidney examination is performed on the woman in the supine position. To capture the left kidney, the health care provider stands at the woman's right side, reaches across with the left hand and places it over the left flank, and places the right hand at the woman's left costal margin. As the woman takes a deep breath, the health care provider then elevates the left flank with the left hand and palpates deeply with the right hand. The health care provider attempts to feel the lower pole of the kidney with the fingertips when the woman inhales. A normal left kidney is rarely palpable.

When palpating the right kidney, the health care provider places the left hand under the woman's right flank and the right hand at the costal margin. The right kidney is more easily palpable because of its anatomical location. If the kidney is palpable, it should be smooth, firm, and not tender.

Gallbladder

The normal gallbladder cannot be felt. However, a distended gallbladder can be palpated below the liver margin at the lateral border of the rectus muscle. An enlarged gallbladder indicates cholecystitis, whereas a large but nontender gallbladder suggests obstruction of the common bile duct. In a woman with inflammation of the gallbladder, pain will occur. The Murphy sign elicited through a bimanual technique further supports the diagnosis. The health care provider holds her fingers under the liver border. As the descending liver pushes the inflamed gallbladder onto the examining hand, the woman will experience sharp pain and will abruptly stop midway through inspiration. Pain also may occur in women with hepatitis.

Pancreas

The pancreas cannot be palpated in the well woman because of its small size and location in the retroperitoneal position. A pancreatic mass may be described as a vague sensation of fullness in the epigastrium.

Urinary Bladder

Generally the urinary bladder is not palpable unless the bladder is distended. The woman should empty her bladder before the examination. A distended bladder is smooth and round. Percussion may be performed to define the outline of the distended bladder.

Aorta

With the woman supine, the health care provider palpates deeply slightly to the left of the midline to feel for aortic pulsation. If pulsation is prominent, the health care provider tries to determine the direction of pulsation. A prominent lateral pulsation suggests an aortic aneurysm. The pulse should be in an anterior direction. With fingers extended, the health care provider places the palmar surface of the hands on the midline and presses the fingers inward on each side of the aorta. In thinner women, the health care provider may use the thumb and fingers to palpate the aortic pulsation. In women over 50, the health care provider should try to assess the width of the aorta by pressing deeply with one hand on each side of the aorta. In this age group, a normal aorta is not more than 3 cm wide, excluding the thickness of the abdominal wall. The average size is approximately 2.5 cm.

Normal Range of Findings

Pregnant Female. As the uterus enlarges, the muscles of the abdominal wall stretch and ultimately lose some tone. When assessing a pregnant woman, the health care provider needs to be knowledgeable of the variations associated with pregnancy. Striae gravidarum vary from one pregnant woman to another and appear as the skin stretches to accommodate the growing uterus. Striae are caused by separation of the underlying connective tissue and are pink or purple; they generally fade after delivery and become white. A line of pigmentation at the midline (linea nigra) often develops. During the third trimester, the rectus abdominis muscles may separate at the midline. The umbilicus may flatten or protrude.

The enlarged uterus displaces upward and posteriorly, thereby repositioning the appendix upward and laterally, high and to the right of the McBurney point. Peristalsis slows during pregnancy, so bowel sounds may be diminished. The gallbladder may become distended, accompanied by decreased emptying time and change in tone. Auscultation of the fetal heart can be heard with Doppler as early as the tenth week of gestation. The contour of the pregnant abdomen may be asymmetrical, and fetal movement may be observed.

Aging Female. Positioning of an elderly female for an abdominal assessment depends on the woman's physical condition and comfort. Abdominal assessment is usually the same, except that muscle tone becomes more relaxed with aging, allowing for easier palpation. The liver size decreases after age 50. Hepatic blood flow decreases because of the decline in cardiac output associated with aging.

PELVIC EXAMINATION

Preparation

The examination of the genitalia may be perceived by the woman as being different from the rest of the examination. Finding out previous experience with pelvic examinations helps the health care provider to understand the woman's feelings, concerns, or fears. Taking time initially is important to make the woman as relaxed as possible. Answering her questions and explaining the purpose of the examination ahead of time has been found to be helpful. A nonjudgmental approach decreases the woman's anxiety and embarrassment. The health care provider should establish rapport with the woman, listen actively, avoid interruptions, and maintain eye contact before and during the examination. Some women, because of cultural differences, may not reciprocate eye contact.

Determining the woman's level of knowledge of the physical examination and the anatomy of genitalia guides the health care provider to determine the extent of preparation and explanation required. Showing and explaining the equipment to be used may tend to allay fear. Plastic specula make a loud click when locked or released, and forewarning helps to avoid surprises. Interaction and feedback about the examination and any discomfort is important so that the health care provider can change technique or stop the examination to assist the woman in further relaxation. The health care provider may need to readjust the speculum or try a different size if the woman is uncomfortable. Questioning a woman extensively during the pelvic examination may increase the woman's anxiety.

The health care provider should place equipment nearby and within easy reach and should gather all the equipment before placing the woman in the lithotomy position.

Equipment

The health care provider should have a strong light source with a vaginal speculum of appropriate size.

Equipment includes the following:
1. Gloves
2. Speculum
   - The Graves' speculum is useful for most adult women and is available in varying lengths and widths.
   - The Pederson speculum has narrow blades and is useful for a virginal or a post-menopausal woman with a narrow vaginal orifice or is comfortable for a woman who has said she has had previous discomfort.
3. Drapes
4. Water-soluble lubricant
5. Goose-neck lamp
6. Large cotton-tipped applicators

Materials for cytological sampling include the following:
1. Sterile cytobrush or cotton-tipped applicator to obtain endocervical specimen for the Papanicolaou (Pap) smear
2. Wooden or plastic cervical spatula to obtain cell samples for Pap smear
3. Glass slide with frosted end for specimen of cervical and vaginal areas
4. Cytology spray fixative
5. Specimen container for *Gonorrhea* and *Chlamydia* culture (slide or tube)
6. Normal saline to prepare discharges for presence of specific organisms (slide or tube)
7. Potassium hydroxide (KOH) to prepare discharge on slides to assess for presence of *Candida*
8. Cover slips for normal saline and KOH; glass slides

Positioning the examining lamp is important for the inspection of the external and internal genitalia. A speculum with an attached light source is the best method for visualization. The health care provider should follow universal precautions throughout the examination and with the equipment. Washing hands before and after the examination and wearing gloves throughout the examination and afterward is mandatory. Some clinicians prefer to double glove. Wearing eye protection is encouraged.

The room temperature should be comfortable and privacy ensured. The health care provider should inform the woman if an assistant will be present during the examination. The recommendation for the health care provider is to have a chaperone present during this portion of the examination. The health care provider can ask the woman if she would prefer that someone to be in the room to provide support for her. The health care provider's hands and all materials touching the woman should be warmed.

The woman should empty her bladder before the examination. Bimanual examination of the internal organs is uncomfortable if the bladder is full, and palpating the pelvic organs is difficult. The health care provider should advise the woman not to douche, use vaginal medications or other inserts or tampons, or have intercourse 2 to 3 days before the examination.

The health care provider places the legs of children a frog-leg position and places adult women in the lithotomy position on an examination table with stirrups. The health care provider asks women to move their buttocks to the edge of the table and assists them with placing their legs in the stirrups. The health care provider places her hand at the edge of the table and instructs the woman to move down the examination table until the woman touches the health care provider's hand. Some women are more comfortable with leaving their shoes or socks on. The woman's arms are placed at her sides or across her abdomen. Having the woman's arms over her head may tighten the abdomen muscles. A pillow should support her head. During the inspection and palpation of the external genitalia, the health care provider sits on a stool facing the woman's genitalia. During the bimanual and rectovaginal examination, the woman remains in the lithotomy position, but the health care provider stands between the woman legs.

A drape can cover the woman's stomach, knees, and symphysis, exposing only the external genitalia. Depressing the drape between the knees allows the health care provider to watch the woman's facial expressions throughout the examination. Many women prefer to be in a more upright position versus laying flat on the examination table. Asking the woman for her preference is important. Many health care providers keep a hand mirror available for the woman to visualize aspects of the examination. A car mirror, which can be purchased at a local auto shop, is particularly helpful because of the size and length, and it is less cumbersome to the health care provider during the examination.

Being as gentle as possible in performing the examination is important because many women view the pelvic examination as an intrusive procedure. The health care provider may need to wait until the woman is ready. Touching the outer thigh and moving down to the genitalia is a strategy that many clinicians use in beginning the inspection of the genitalia. The health care provider palpates the horizontal chain of nodes inferior to the inquinal ligament and the vertical chain along the upper thigh. Nodes in this area that are smaller than 1 cm in diameter may be normal if they are soft, discrete, and moveable.

External Genitalia

The examination of the genitalia has essentially two phases: inspection and palpation. During palpation, and at certain times during the inspection, the health care provider touches the woman's genitalia with one hand. The health care provider usually chooses the dominant hand. Sometimes using a cotton-tipped applicator to move the skin downward during the assessment is helpful. The health care provider starts by inspecting all the skin for lesions and parasites. Using a gloved finger, the health care provider spreads the hair and labia to inspect all skin surfaces. The skin should be smooth and clear, with the hair distribution in the usual female pattern of an inverted triangle. The health care provider should note the character and distribution of the hair.

Following inspection of the hair pattern, the nurse informs the woman by touching the leg and through verbalization that inspection of the genitalia will continue. The health care provider inspects the external genitals slowly and systematically, separating the labia majora by using the thumbs of both hands or the thumb and the second and third digits of one hand. The health care provider inspects the labia minora, clitoris, urethal meatus, paraurethal or Skene glands, hymen, vaginal orifice, and Bartholin glands.

The labia majora and minora may be considered as a whole or as individual surfaces. The labia normally are symmetrical, full in appearance during adulthood, and atrophic in postmenopause. The tissue should be soft and not tender. After a vaginal birth, the labia may appear slightly shriveled and gaping. The mucous membranes may appear dry or moist but are normally dark pink. The skin of the vulvar area is slightly darker than the skin of the rest of the body. Abnormal findings include abnormal exudate, asymmetrical tender masses, focal hyperpigmentation, depigmentation, erythema, excoriation, ulceration, and leukoplakia (focal, whitish thickening of the epithelium). The health care provider should evaluate any mass for consistency, mobility, shape, size, tenderness, and texture and should evaluate abnormal exudate for color, odor, viscosity, and amount.

The health care provider inspects the clitoris for size and length and examines the adjacent areas for lesions. The clitoris is enlarged in masculinizing conditions. The prepuce covering the clitoris should be easily retractable by palpation. The health care provider observes for any inflammation, lesions, atrophy, or adhesions. Moving downward, the urethral opening appears slitlike or as an irregular opening. The urethral meatus usually is located midline but may be close to or slightly within the vaginal introitus. The health care provider assesses the vestibule and identifies the Skene glands (paraurethal) lateral to the urethal meatus. These glands are not usually visible.

Inspecting the vaginal introitus, the health care provider focuses on the Bartholin gland ducts located at the 5 and 7 o'clock positions. The health care provider notes any tenderness, swelling, erythema, lesions, tissue thickening, and palpable abnormalities and uses a cotton-tipped applicator swab to move labial and hymeneal tissues during the inspection.

The health care provider palpates the urethra by placing a finger on the anterior surface of the vaginal opening and gently applying pressure while bringing the finger toward the vaginal orifice. The health care provider inspects for erythema, polyps, and discharge and milks the paraurethal ducts by exerting upward pressure moving the finger outward. Discharge from the urethra on inspection or with compression is abnormal. The health care provider rotates the hand without removing the finger and palpates the lateral tissue between the index finger and thumb. The health care provider should palpate each Bartholin gland separately, paying particular attention to the posterolateral portion of the labia majora where the Bartholin glands are located. Discharge, erythema, and prominence of glandular ducts are abnormal. The health care provider should culture any discharge.

Assessing Muscle Tone

The health care provider asks the woman to squeeze the vaginal opening around her finger and explains that she is assessing muscle tone. The health care provider should anticipate that muscle tone in a nulliparous woman will be tighter than in a multiparous woman. Next, the health care provider separates the vaginal orifice with the middle and index fingers and asks the woman to strain or bear down to elicit bulging or urinary incontinence. Lastly, the health care provider inspects and palpates the perineum. Normally, the perineum should feel thick and smooth in the nulliparous woman and thin and more rigid in a multiparous woman. The area should not be tender to touch. The health care provider assesses for inflammation, fistulas, lesions, or growths. A well-formed and healed episiotomy scar, midline or mediolateral, may be evident in a multiparous woman who has had vaginal births. The rectum has coarse skin and an increased pigmentation.

Internal Examination

The health care provider begins the internal examination by inserting a finger into the vagina to locate the position of the cervix. Locating the cervix manually assists the health care provider in positioning the speculum more accurately in the vagina and determining the appropriate size of the speculum. Lubricating the finger with warm water assists in the comfort of the woman, but the health care provider should not consider using other lubricates if specimens are to be taken. Lubricants are bacteriostatic and can distort the cytological specimen.

Insertion of Speculum

The health care provider informs the woman by touching her and inserts two fingers of the hand, most preferable the dominate hand, just inside the vaginal opening and gently applies pressure downward. The health care provider requests that the woman take a few deep breaths to relax her muscles to ease the insertion of the speculum. The health care provider selects and warms the speculum. At the time of insertion both the blade tips of the speculum are aligned and the bases are closed fully and secured. With the other hand, the health care provider slowly guides the closed speculum past the fingers at a somewhat oblique angle and directed at 45-degree angle downward. This technique avoids pressure on the urethra. The health care provider should be careful not to pull on the pubic hair or pinch the labia with the speculum.

The health care provider removes the fingers from the introitus and rotates the speculum to a horizontal angle, inserting the speculum the length of the vaginal canal. The health care provider opens the blades of the speculum by squeezing the handles together and adjusting the blades to cup the cervix, bringing the cervix into full view, and maintains the open position of the speculum by tightening the thumb screw.

Inspection of the Cervix

The health care provider inspects the cervix for color, position, size, surface characteristics, any secretions, masses, bleeding and discharges, and size and shape of the os. The cervix is normally an evenly distributed pink color. A bluish color may denote an increase in vascularity and is a sign of pregnancy. The cervix is paler in color after menopause or is associated with anemia. Symmetrical, circumscribed erythema surrounding the os may indicate a normal condition of exposed columnar epithelium called *ectropion.* No lesion should be present except for occasional Naboth cysts. The cysts are yellowish, 1-cm nodules that may appear as multiple modules but are firm and not tender. The direction of the cervix corresponds with the position of the cervix. A cervix pointing anteriorly indicates a retroverted uterus; one pointing posteriorly indicates an anteverted uterus.

The position of the cervix is generally in the midline but may point in anteriorly or posteriorly. Deviations may indicate mass, adhesions, pregnancy, or normal variation. The size of the cervix is 2.5 cm, protruding into the vagina by 1 to 3 cm. This finding is more likely to be seen during a speculum examination than felt during palpation. The cervix is normally firm but resilient and can be moved from 1 to 2 cm in any direction without discomfort. Abnormal findings include an asymmetrical shape or enlargement not attributable to a vaginal delivery, induration, limited mobility, protrusion into the vaginal vault by more than 3 cm, tenderness, and any abnormal mass.

If secretions are copious, the health care provider should swab the area with a thick-tipped swab. This method sponges away secretions, and the health care provider will have a clearer view of the cervix.

Vaginal Smears and Cultures

Often during examination with the speculum the health care provider obtains vaginal specimens for smears and cultures. The vagina normally contains bacteria such as *Lactobacillus, Staphylococcus, Escherichia coli,* and some *Candida.* The vagina has numerous intrinsic mechanisms that control the overgrowth of pathogens and maintain a healthy balance. Smears are done according to the risk of the woman and, if the woman is symptomatic, to detect a causative agent.

The health care provider obtains the Pap smear before other specimens so that no disruption or removal of cells occurs followed by the gonococcal and other smears, if indicated. The Pap smear screens for cervical cancer. Specimens are not obtained during the woman's menses or if a heavy discharge is present. The woman should not have douched; used vaginal creams, foams, or tampons; or had intercourse for 2 days before collecting the specimen (Huff, 2000). The frosted ends of the slides of the specimen are labeled with the woman's name and the location of the specimen. The date of specimen, date of birth, last menstrual period (LMP), hormone use, or if pregnant, prior abnormal Pap smear or cervical treatment, recent history of cancer therapy, history of immunosuppression are included as clinical information on the specimen requisition for the cytology laboratory.

With the cervical smear method, the health care provider collects a sample from the ectocervix with the bifid end of the spatula. The health care provider inserts the longer projection of the spatula or the groove into the cervical os, rotates the spatula 360 degrees keeping it against the entire cervix, and withdraws the spatula and spreads the specimen from one side of the spatula on the glass slide. The health care provider should use a single-stroke method to thin out the specimen on the slide, not a back-and-forth technique.

Next, the health care provider introduces the endocervical brush into the cervical os until the bristles closest to the handle are exposed and rotates the brush in one direction 180 degrees, one quarter to one half of a turn to minimize the bleeding. The woman may feel a slight pinch. The health care provider moves the brush and rotates the brush gently onto the glass or places the material in a preservative vial as instructed by the laboratory for its layer technique. The health care provider rotates the brush in the direction opposite to that in which the specimen was taken.

The health care provider then moistens cotton swabs first with saline to saturate the fibers so as not to trap cells and uses the ThinPrep method. After swabbing the cervical os, the health care provider thinly spreads the specimen across the slide. Rapid fixation of the cells is critical and is to be done within a few seconds to minimize air drying. The health care provider may place the slide in an ethanol solution or use spray fixative, spraying from a distance of 9 to 12 inches to cover the slide (Huff, 2000). For a woman who has undergone a hysterectomy with the removal of the cervix, the health care provider can collect the Pap smear from the vagina and vaginal pool.

The ThinPrep Pap smear is a fluid-based method used for collecting and preparing cervicovaginal samples. The collection device(s) are rinsed in Cytyc's ThinPrep PreservCyt medium and a thin-layer slide is prepared using the ThinPrep 2000, automated processor (Massarani-Wafai, Bakos, Wojcik, & Selvaggi, 2000). The health care provider obtains the specimen in the manner described. If the spatula or brush is used, each should be placed in the liquid preservative as soon as possible. Once placed in the liquid tube, the nurse practitioner rotates the device in the solution 10 times while pushing against the PreservCyt vial wall, with the goal of removing as many cells from the device and into the solution (Huff, 2000).

Gonorrhea Culture Specimen

Immediately after the Pap smear the health care provider obtains the *Gonorrhea* culture. The health care provider inserts a sterile cotton applicator into the cervical os, rotates it 360 degrees, and leaves it in place 10 to 30 seconds to allow for absorption of secretions and organisms. The health care provider then withdraws the swab and spreads the specimen in a large Z pattern over the culture medium (Thayer Martin), rotating the swab at the same time, or places it into a culture tube, depending on laboratory procedure. The health care provider labels the tube or plate and follows the routine for transporting and warming the specimen. The sample for the culture must be taken from the endocervical canal, not from the vagina. If indicated, an anal or oropharyngeal culture may be obtained after the vaginal speculum has been removed. The health care provider inserts a fresh, sterile cotton swab about 2.5 cm into the rectum and rotates it 360 degrees, holds it in place for 10 to 30 seconds, and withdraws the swab and prepares the specimen as described for the vaginal culture.

Chlamydia Enzyme Immunoassay Specimen

The health care provider collects the *Chlamydia* specimen after the gonococcal specimen, if both are indicated. The health care provider inserts the appropriate swab (provided with or specified by kit) into the cervical os, rotates the swab for 10 to 30 seconds to allow for absorption of an adequate sample, removes the swab and places it into the appropriate tube containing the specimen reagent, labels the specimen according to the recommendations for transport. The health care provider fills out the appropriate requisition to accompany the specimen.

Saline Mount and Potassium Hydroxide Procedures

To screen for other sexually transmitted diseases, or if one notes any other abnormal vaginal discharge, the health care provider can obtain a saline mount or "wet prep" and a KOH preparation.

To prepare the wet mount, the following vaginal microscopy procedure is recommended (Secor, 1997):

1. Use a double slide holder and two frosted-tip glass slides.
2. Place 2 to 3 drops of saline on front slide.
3. Place 2 to 3 drops of 10% to 20% KOH on back slide.
4. Take a sample from the posterior fornix using a wooden or plastic spatula.
5. Test pH using 1-inch strip of phenaphthazine (Nitrazine) by Squibb.
6. Stir sample into saline 3 to 4 times until light opaque color (dilute).
7. Stir sample into KOH 10 to 20 times until creamy white (concentrated).
8. Immediately check the whiff test from the spatula.
9. Apply cover slips gently just before viewing the smear.
10. Identify and quantitate number of lactobacilli for 2 to 3 minutes.

The health care provider will be evaluating the saline slide for findings indicative of bacterial vaginosis. Bacterial vaginosis has a pH of 4.5 to 5.5 and is associated with a loss of hydrogen peroxide–producing lactobacilli, a massive overgrowth of pathogens, clue cells within epithelia cells, and positive whiff or amine loss. Trichomoniasis is associated with the presence of a parasitic protozoan *Trichomonas* and with a loss of lactobacilli, predominantly replaced by diphtheroids, streptococci, staphylococci, and anaerobes.

The health care provider will use the KOH specimen to diagnose infection with *Candida albicans*. The KOH destroys structures such as epithelial cells and white blood cells; any fungi present appear as tangled masses resembling hair or threads.

Withdrawal of the Speculum

Inspection of the vagina occurs during insertion, while the speculum is open, and again during its removal. The health care provider loosens the thumbscrew but continues to hold the speculum blades open. Slowly the health care provider withdraws the speculum, rotating it to inspect the vaginal mucosa fully and noting the color and any inflammation, discharge, ulcers, or masses.

As with cervical discharge, vaginal discharge is normally odorless, nonirritating, thin or mucoid, and clear or cloudy. The presence of some whitish, creamy discharge (leukorrhea) is normal. The health care provider should inspect the speculum for odor and discard in the proper container, placing metal speculums in soaking solution and dicarding plastic speculums in universal red-marked plastic bags.

Palpation of the Internal Genitalia: Bimanual Vaginal Examination

The bimanual examination involves palpation of the pelvic organs between the health care provider's two hands. The health care provider palpates the internal genitalia to assess location, size, mobility, and any tenderness or mass. The woman remains in the lithotomy position, but the health care provider moves from a sitting to a standing position between the woman's legs.

The health care provider informs the woman of the internal digital examination, changes gloves or removes the outer glove, and lubricates the index and middle fingers. The health care provider then spreads the labia with the thumb and index finger of the opposite hand, inserts the tips of the gloved fingers into the vaginal opening and presses downward, again waiting for the muscle to relax, and gradually inserts the full length of the fingers. The health care provider palpates the vaginal walls with the index and middle fingers. The most sensitive aspect of the health care provider's fingers is the palmar position of the fingertips.

The health care provider places the other hand on the woman's abdomen and presses the abdominal and pelvic contents forward. Using the fingers, the health care provider locates the cervix, feels the cervix by moving fingers around and then feels the fornices. Normally the cervix is 7 to 9 cm from the vaginal orifice. If the vaginal orifice comes well up to the upper end or third joint of the finger, the cervix is in normal position. The health care provider feels the cervix for size, contour, consistency, surface, mobility, and location. The cervix should be in the midline, pointing anteriorly or posteriorly. The normal cervix feels similar to hard connective tissue. Pregnancy softens the cervix beginning at the lower end and gradually involves the entire cervix. Moving the cervix several centimeters in either direction should not elicit pain. Pelvic pain may denote an inflammatory process. Diminished mobility may result from scarring or malignant infiltration and inflammatory exudate in the pelvis or uterine tumor. Laceration or overstretching of pelvic floor supports increases mobility. The os is patent and may admit a fingertip of 0.5 cm. Deviation from normal may indicate stenosis of the os. The fornices surrounding the cervix are pliable and smooth. Any hardened, nodular, or irregular surface is considered abnormal.

With the fingers in the anterior fornix, the health care provider assesses the uterus, palpating the size, shape, surface characteristics, consistency, mobility, and tenderness of the uterus and fundus and determining the position or the location of the fundus of the uterus. When the cervix is pointing along the vaginal axis and the fundus lies in the same plane as the vagina, the uterus is said to be in *midposition*. The fundus may not be palpable, depending on the amount of adipose tissue and degree of abdominal muscle relaxation. When the cervix is aimed anteriorly and the fundus is noted posterior to the vaginal plane and is not palpable, the uterus is said to be *retroverted*. When the cervix is aimed posteriorly and the fundus is rotated anteriorly to the vaginal plane, the uterus is said to be *anteverted*. The uterus can take two positions when the fundus is at an angle to the cervix. When the cervix points along the axis of the vaginal canal and the fundus is not palpable, the uterus is said to be *retroflexed*. When the cervix points along the axis of the vaginal canal and the fundus is bent forward and is palpable at the pubis, the uterus is said to be *anteflexed*.

After palpating the fundus, the health care provider spreads the fingers within the vagina and presses into and upward within all the fornices to palpate the lateral uterine wall. The uterus is pear shaped and 5 to 8 cm long. The uterus in a multiparous woman will be larger. No tenderness or masses should be noted on palpation. The health care provider then gently bounces the uterus between intravaginally and abdominally placed hands for mobility and tenderness. The uterus is a freely movable organ, and no tenderness should be elicited. The health care provider should avoid frequent shifting of the position of the abdominal fingers, which may result in increased resistance of the abdominal muscles, and should be cautious not to depress the abdominal wall too close to the pubis.

After palpating the uterus, the health care provider examines separately the left and right adnexal areas and ovaries, placing the fingers of the abdominal hand on the right lower quadrant, the index and middle fingers (intravaginal) in the right lateral fornix, pressing the external and abdominal hand in and down over the corresponding suprapubic area, and trying to push the adnexal structure toward the intravaginal fingers. The effect of this configuration is to cup the adnexal tissues between the hands moving in an inferior and lateral direction. At the same time, the external hand is pressed downward and both hands sweep toward the pubis. The hand on the abdomen acts as resistance and the intravaginal hand palpates the organs between the hands. The entire process is performed in a single motion and then repeated on the opposite side.

The ovaries, if palpable, should feel smooth, firm, ovoid, and no longer than 4 to 6 cm. Adnexal tissue is normally mobile. Tenderness, enlargement, and nodularity are not normal. Any mass the health care provider cannot identify positively as a normal adnexal structure should be considered abnormal pending further investigation.

Normal Range of Findings

Infant and Adolescent

At birth the female external genitalia are engorged because of the high amounts of maternal estrogen. Within several weeks the external genitalia recede and remain small until puberty. Slight growth of the internal and external genitalia parallels the increase in body size.

At puberty the adolescent female begins to undergo changes related to endocrine function. Estrogen stimulates the growth of cells in the reproductive tract and the development of secondary sex characteristics. During puberty, the reproductive organs increase in size and weight and become capable of functioning.

The secondary sexual characteristics increase, with the clitoris becoming more erectile and the labia minora more vascular. The labia majora and mons pubia become more prominent, and pubic hair develops. At the same time breast development occurs. Sexual changes usually proceed according to a predictable pattern. The first signs of puberty begin between ages 8½ and 13 years and take about 3 years to complete. The sequence of sexual changes in females is as follows:

■ Broadening of the bony pelvis
■ Breast development
■ Development of the uterus, vagina, labia, and clitoris
■ Pubic hair development
■ Maximum height spurt
■ Menarche

Tanner's table on breast and pubic development (see Chapter 11) is helpful in teaching girls to anticipate the sequence of sexual development. The average age of menarche is 12 years 6 months to 12 years 10 months with the normal age between 9 years 11 months and 15 years 6 months. Just before menarche, vaginal secretions increase. Normal kinds of discharge may need to be differentiated from those of an infectious nature. The onset of menstruation occurs at an earlier age in the Southern hemisphere. Other factors affecting the onset of menstruation are heredity, health, nutritional status, and weight. African-American females tend to begin puberty at an earlier age than white females.

Referral is warranted if pubertal development occurs before 7 years of age or after 13 years of age, pubertal changes fail to progress, or if menarche is absent after 17 years of age in one whose sexual development has been otherwise normal.

Pregnant Female

Shortly after the first missed menstrual period, the pregnant female begins to undergo changes resulting from an increase in uterine blood flow and lymph, causing pelvic congestion and edema. The uterus, cervix, and isthmus soften, and the cervix looks bluish (Chadwick sign). The vaginal changes are similar to the cervical changes and result in a bluish color. Cervical and vaginal secretions increase and have an acidic pH because of an increase in lactic acid production by the vaginal epithelium. A thick, tenacious mucus forms in the space of the cervical canal (mucous plug).

The high levels of estrogen and progesterone are necessary to support pregnancy and are responsible for the increase in size of the uterus. The uterus increases in capacity by 500 to 1000 times its nonpregnant state, excluding the fetus and placenta. The early growth of the uterus encroaches on the space occupied by the bladder. After 10 to 12 weeks of gestation, the uterus is too large to remain in the pelvis. At 20 weeks of gestation the uterus becomes larger and ovoid and moves out of the pelvis into the abdominal cavity. The uterus displaces the intestines superiorly and laterally.

Aging Female

Concurrent with endocrine changes, ovarian function diminishes in women in their 40s, and menstruation ceases on the average between age 45 and 52. Menopause is the cessation of menses for 1 year. During this time circulating estrogen levels decline, causing dramatic physical changes. The labia and clitoris become smaller, and pubic hair turns gray and becomes sparser. The mons pubis looks smaller because the fat pads atrophy. Other hormone levels also change. Adrenal androgen and ovarian testerone levels decrease greatly after menopause, which may cause a decrease in libido, muscle mass, and strength.

Changes occur not only externally but also internally. The vaginal opening decreases in size and gradually constricts. Vaginal atrophy occurs after menopause, resulting in a pale pink mucosa, and the vaginal pH becomes more alkaline. The vagina narrows, shortens in length, and loses its rugation. Decreased vaginal secretions leave the vagina dry and at risk for irritation. The cervical tissue begins to atrophy and in postmenopausal women, the cervix becomes flush with the vaginal wall. The uterus becomes smaller, and the endometrium thins. The ovaries decrease in size 1 to 2 cm and are not palpable after menopause. Ovulation usually ceases 1 to 2 years before menopause.

Rectal Examination

Following palpation of the internal genitalia, the examiner inspects the anal orifice and palpates the anal sphincter and the rectum. The health care provider changes gloves between the intravaginal examination and the rectovaginal examination to prevent migration of vaginal flora to the rectum. With one finger in the vagina the health care provider presses the middle finger against the anus and asks the woman to bear down. As the woman does, the health care provider slips the top of the finger into the rectum just past the sphincter, palpates the anorectal junction and just above it and, after asking the woman to tighten and relax the anal sphincter, notes the tone of the anal sphincter. The health care provider then inserts the finger fully into the rectum. If a retroverted or retroflexed uterus was found during palpation of the internal genitalia, the health care provider attempts to palpate the fundus through the anterior wall of the rectum and also palpates each rectal wall for abnormal masses.

The health care provider palpates the areas of the rectovaginal septum and cul-de-sac, which should be a firm, smooth, pliable structure.

Completion of the Examination

The health care provider assists the woman into a sitting position and offers her a sanitary pad or tissues to wipe herself. The health care provider shares with the woman briefly the findings but has the woman dress before discussing in more complete details the findings of the examination and recommendations for her health plan.

A more comprehensive examination of other systems is warranted if indications are uncovered within the health history or revealed at the time the examination is being conducted. After practicing and acquiring proficiency in the physical examination, the health care provider develops a systematic pattern for performing an integrated physical examination. Conducting the examination systematically and efficiently saves time, and the health care provider is less likely to omit a procedure or not evaluate a body part. The health care provider considers elements of efficiency but is sensitive to cues from the woman while conducting the examination. The health care provider's goal is to ensure the woman's comfort and privacy during the examination.

After the examination is performed, the health care provider integrates the findings from the history and physical examination. The health care provider formulates general recommendations about the plan of care but does not proceed until after discussing the findings with the woman, for both decide the plan of care. Learning what the priority is from the woman's perspective is important in determining and planning the care. Often the health care provider may have to negotiate with the woman or her family because values and priorities may differ when determining the plan of care.

SUMMARY

This chapter presented information on the use of a physical examination as a screening device for detecting abnormalities that are unknown to the woman and for identifying signs that may suggest illness or deformity. Physical examination is done along with the health history, risk assessment, screening and targeted interventions to obtain a complete database on a woman's physical health status. This information is critical to caring for the whole woman; therefore nurse practitioners must have excellent skills in physical examination.

REFERENCES

American College of Obstetricians and Gynecologists. (1996). *Guidelines for women's health care*, Washington, DC: American College of Obstetricians and Gynecologists.

Huff, B. C. (2000). Screening for cervical cancer. It's time to check your Pap technique. *AWHONN Lifelines*, 53–55.

Massarani-Wafai, R., Bakos, R., Wojcik, E. M., & Selvaggi, S. M. (2000). Evaluation of cellular residue in the ThinPrep PreservCyt vial. *Diagnostic Cytopathology, 23(*3), 208–212.

Secor, R. M. (1997, May). Wet mount flowsheet and instructions. *Clinical Excellence for Nurse Practitioners, 1(*3), 1–6.

Seidel, H., Ball, J., Dains, J., & Benedict, G. W. (2003). *Mosby's guide to physical examination* (5th ed.). St. Louis: Mosby.

BIBLIOGRAPHY

American Nurses' Association (1993). *Clinician's handbook of preventive services* (2nd ed.). Waldorf, MD: U. S. Department of Health and Human Services.

Barkauskas, V., Stoltenberg-Allen, K., Baumann, L., & Darling-Fisher, C. (1994). *Health and physical assessment.* St. Louis: Mosby.

Bates, B., Bickley, I., & Hoekelman, R. (1999). *A guide to physical examination and history taking* (7th ed.). Philadelphia: J. B. Lippincott.

Fuller, J., & Schaller-Ayers, J. (1999). *Health assessment: A nursing approach* (3rd ed.). Philadelphia: J. B. Lippincott.

Jarvis, C., (2000) *Physical examination and health assessment* (3rd ed.). Philadelphia: W. B. Saunders.

Reeder, S., Martin, L., & Koniak-Griffin, D. (1997). *Maternity nursing: Family, newborn, and women's health care* (18th ed.). Philadelphia: Lippincott-Raven Publishers.

Seidel, H., Ball, J., Dains, J., & Benedict, G. W. (1999). *Mosby's guide to physical examination* (4th ed.). St. Louis: Mosby.

Silverman, M., Hurst, J., & Willis (Eds.). (1996). *Clinical skills for adult primary care.* Philadelphia: Lippincott-Raven Publishers.

RESOURCES

Virtual Hospital: *www.vh.org/*
Martindale's Health Science Guide—2002: *www.sci.lib.vci.edu/HSG/HSGuide.html*
Physical Exam Study Guides, University of Florida: *www.medinfov.ufl.edu/year one/bes/clist/index.html*
National Center for Education in Maternal and Child Health: *www.ncemds.georgetown.edu*

Chapter 11

Nutrition

Susan Miller

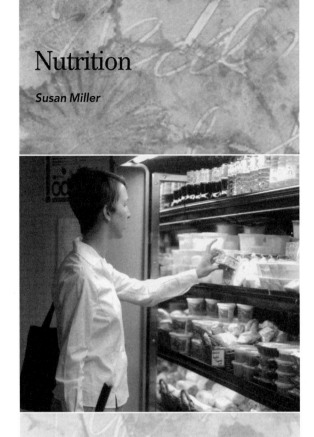

We are indeed much more than what we eat, but what we eat can nevertheless help us to be much more than what we are.

Adelle Davis

INTRODUCTION

Nutrition is central to a woman's health and must be an integral part of the health agenda. Many experts agree that health problems that affect women—such as osteoporosis, heart disease, and female cancers—have strong links to nutrition. Nutrition may hold the key to the prevention and treatment of these devastating chronic diseases. Bernadine Healy (1995) notes that nutrition is probably the single biggest factor in the health and well-being of a woman at any stage of her life. Women need nutritional knowledge not only to prevent disease but also to empower themselves to achieve optimum health and well-being.

This chapter provides information on the critical nutrient needs for adolescent, menopausal, and older women. Basic guidelines are presented to assist the nursing professional with assessing individual nutritional needs. Adolescent nutrition focuses on nutrients essential for optimal growth and future disease prevention. Nutritional profiles for the pregnant teen and adolescent athlete, as well as the phenomena of eating disorders, are covered. Nutrition for the middle years presents nutritional trends among women and the connection between nutrition and chronic disease. Nutritional requirements for pregnancy, lactation, and premenstrual syndrome are examined. Finally, the last section explores changes in the postmenopausal woman and how these changes relate to nutritional health.

NUTRITION DURING ADOLESCENCE

Adolescence is the 10-year period (ages 10 to 21) when the process of physically developing from a child to an adult occurs. Rate of growth during adolescence is matched only by that of the first year of life. The rapid growth in height, weight, and body composition and sexual maturation all require increased energy and nutrients. Proper nutrition is crucial during this time to achieve optimal growth and height attainment and to prevent chronic disease in adulthood. Adolescence is a time to build adequate nutrient stores to support future pregnancies and is also a time of great variation among individuals. All teenagers do not hit physiological and sexual development at the same time. Therefore evaluating nutritional needs based on physical maturity rather than on chronological age is important (Tanner, 1987). Tanner's sexual maturity ratings are helpful for this.

GROWTH AND DEVELOPMENT

Pubertal Events

Tanner (1962) classified pubertal events into a range of stages noted in Table 11-1.

Each of these stages can be used to evaluate an individual's place in the sexual maturation process. Tanner's stages are better predictors of nutrient needs than is chronological age. For instance, after stage 4 when menarche usually has occurred, growth has slowed down dramatically and nutrient needs are not as high. Because menarche occurs at different ages among girls, what may be an appropriate nutrient recommendation for one will not be for another. Height, weight, achievement of menarche, and changes in body composition are associated with these stages of pubertal growth.

Table 11-1	STAGES OF PUBERTY	
STAGES OF PUBERTY	**GROWTH AND DEVELOPMENT**
Stage 1 (Prepubertal) Age range 8-11	No outward signs of development. Ovaries are enlarging and hormone production is beginning.
Stage 2 Age range 8-14, average 11-12	The first visible signs of puberty appear, including the beginning of breast growth, "breast buds," and pubic hair.
Stage 3 Age range 9-15, average 12-13	Pubic hair increases, darkens, and coarsens. Breasts and genitalia enlarge.
Stage 4 Age range 10-16, average 13-14	Pubic hair growth takes on the triangular shape of adulthood. Underarm hair is likely to appear in this stage as is menarche.
Stage 5 Age range 12-19, average 15	Adult characteristics of breasts, pubic hair, and genitalia have been attained. Menstrual periods are well established, and ovulation occurs monthly.

From Tanner, J. M. (1962). *Growth at adolescence* (2nd ed.). Oxford: Blackwell Scientific.

Height

Approximately 15% to 20% of the final adult height is achieved during adolescence. Peak height velocity, or the period of greatest gain in height, usually occurs during Tanner stages 2 and 3 (Story & Alton, 1996). Nutrient needs are highest during peak height velocity. Menarche usually occurs 1 year after peak height velocity.

Weight and Body Composition Changes

During peak weight velocity, weight gain for females reaches approximately 50% of the ideal adult weight (Gong & Spear, 1988). Although boys gain proportionately more lean muscle mass during peak weight velocity, the influence of estrogen and progesterone causes girls to deposit more fat than muscle tissue. The normal range for body fat when adolescents reach adulthood is 23% for women as opposed to 12% for men (Rees, 1992).

Other body composition changes that add to an increase in weight include skeletal growth. Forty-five percent of total bone growth occurs during adolescence (Gong & Heald, 1994). Changes in height, weight, and body composition lead to an increased demand for energy and nutrients.

Nutrient Requirements

Nutrient needs during adolescence are higher than at any other time in life (Story, 1992). Unfortunately, data concerning specific nutrient needs for adolescence are limited and are based on chronological age rather than on physical maturation. Because of the wide variability in growth rate among teenagers, increasing or decreasing certain nutrients according to the level of growth the individual has attained may be necessary.

Recent national surveys have documented nutrient intake in sample populations of teenagers. One of the largest and most extensive nutrient intake studies conducted in the United States is the Third National Health and Nutrition Examination Survey, 1988-1991. This study found that among adolescent girls, mean nutrient intake for protein and for several major vitamins such as vitamin A and vitamin C was adequate. Mineral intake, however, was found to be low. Minerals are especially crucial during the adolescent growth phase. Calcium is needed for skeletal growth, iron is needed for increased hemoglobin levels and new muscle tissue, and zinc is essential for new skeletal and muscle tissue and plays a vital role in sexual maturation (Gong & Heald, 1994). Because of documented low intake, the minerals calcium, iron, zinc and the vitamin folate will be discussed.

New Reference Values

The Food and Nutrition Board of the Institute of Medicine, National Academy of Sciences, in cooperation with Health Canada, began in the 1990s an extensive review of nutrient requirements and their evidenced association with health outcomes. The results have led to a redefining of the Recommended Daily Allowances (RDAs) in a set of at least four nutrient-based reference values refashioned as the Dietary Reference Intakes (DRIs). The DRIs are quantitative estimates of nutrient intakes to be used for planning and assessing diets for healthy persons. DRIs differ from the former Recommended Daily Allowances in the following ways:

1. In addition to preventing deficiency, if specific data on safety and efficacy exist, the reduction in the risk of chronic disease also is included in the formulation of the recommendation.
2. Upper levels of intake have been established if data regarding adverse effects from too much of the nutrient exist.
3. Components of food that may not meet the traditional concept of a nutrient but may have health benefits also are being reviewed, and, if enough data exist, a reference intake will be established.

The four new reference values are as follows (Food and Nutrition Board, 2000):

1. **Recommended Dietary Allowance:** The average daily dietary intake that is sufficient to meet the nutrient requirement of nearly all (97% to 98%) healthy individuals in a particular life stage and gender group.
2. **Adequate Intake (AI):** A recommended intake value based on observed or experimentally determined approximations or estimates of nutrient intake by a group (or groups) of healthy persons that are assumed to be adequate. AIs are used when an RDA cannot be determined.
3. **Tolerable Upper Intake Level:** The highest level of daily nutrient intake that is likely to pose no risk of adverse health effects for almost all individuals in the general population. As intake increases above the tolerable upper intake level, the potential risk of adverse effects increases.
4. **Estimated Average Requirement:** A daily nutrient intake value estimated to meet the requirement of half of the healthy individuals in a life stage and gender group.

Calories

Energy needs vary among individuals and throughout adolescence. Because increments in height represent the greatest predictor of anabolic needs, using calories per unit of height may be the best determiner of energy needs. For females ages 11 to 14, 14.0 kcal/cm height is recommended, and for females 15 to 18, 13.5 kcal/cm height (Food and Nutrition Board, 1989). Exercise and activity levels also must be taken into consideration.

Adequate calorie levels are essential for the female teenager to achieve optimum growth and nutrition. Pugliese, Lifshitz, Fort, Grad, and Marks-Katz (1983) found delayed puberty and growth failure because of malnutrition among girls aged 9 to 17 who were on a self-imposed restriction of calories. Murphy, Rose, Hudes, and Viteri (1992) noted an association between low energy intake and poor diet quality.

Calcium

Because 99% of calcium is found in skeletal bone, this mineral is critical during adolescence. Forty-five percent of the adult skeletal mass is accumulated during adolescence (Gong & Heald, 1994). Studies have indicated that the risk of osteoporosis is associated with how much skeletal mass the woman accumulates by the time she reaches peak bone density between 25 and 30 years of age (Cerrato, 1992). Therefore reaching teenagers early in life with the message of calcium consumption may be one of the keys to prevention.

Because current research is not adequate to establish an RDA or an Estimated Average Requirement for calcium, an AI has been set. For individuals age 9 to 18 years, the AI for calcium is 1300 mg/day (Food and Nutrition Board, 1997). Box 11-1 lists good sources of calcium.

Individuals who have lactose intolerance, a condition in which milk is not digested adequately because of a lack of the intestinal enzyme lactase, can consume low-lactose milk products available in major grocery stores. For adolescents, obtaining calcium from food is more desirable than using supplements because calcium rich foods are also rich in protein, vitamins, and minerals. Teenage females may believe that milk products are fattening and should be avoided. Education and counseling on low-fat milk products would help to alleviate this fear.

Iron

Iron is imperative for the synthesis of new tissue and increase in red blood cells associated with growth. Blood loss because of menses also increases the need for iron. National surveys such as the Nationwide Food Consumption Survey found that iron intake among adolescent girls met only two thirds of the RDA (Wright, Guthrie, Wang, & Bernardo, 1991). The RDA of iron for adolescent girls 14 to 18 years of age is 15 mg/day (Food and Nutrition Board, 2001). Adolescent girls who are restricting calories for dieting purposes also may be restricting foods high in iron, such as red meat. Low dietary iron intake may diminish iron stores and ultimately lead to anemia.

Symptoms of iron-deficient anemia include the following:

▪ Fatigue
▪ Headache
▪ Reduced attention span
▪ Reduced physical performance

Assessing for anemia usually is done by determining blood hematocrit and hemoglobin levels. Because these tests can be influenced by factors such as dehydration, serum ferritin levels are a more accurate predictor of iron-deficient anemia (Harris, 1995). Managing anemia involves dietary changes (Box 11-2).

Box 11-1 SOURCES OF CALCIUM

▪ Milk (1 cup = 300 mg)
▪ Calcium-enriched orange juice (1 cup = 300 mg)
▪ Yogurt (1 cup = 415 mg)
▪ Turnip greens (½ cup = 125 mg)
▪ Broccoli (½ cup = 89 mg)
▪ Almonds (1 ounce = 80 mg)

Box 11-2 DIETARY SOURCES FOR MANAGING ANEMIA

Best sources (heme iron)
Lean red meat
Fish
Poultry

Good sources (non-heme iron)
Grains enriched with iron (i.e., iron-fortified cereal)
Dried fruits
Beans
Tofu
Spinach

Substances that inhibit the absorption of iron should not be consumed at the same time. These include calcium sources, polyphenols (substances found in tea and coffee), bran, and antacids. Combining a good source of vitamin C like orange juice along with dietary sources of iron enhances absorption.

Treatment for anemia usually includes iron supplements. Ferrous sulfate is the most efficient and economical form of iron therapy. If anemia does not improve within 6 to 8 weeks, a physician or nurse practitioner should reevaluate the adolescent (Harris, 1995).

Folate

Folate is necessary for deoxyribonucleic acid and ribonucleic acid synthesis and amino acid metabolism, and so folate is critical for the growing female adolescent. Perhaps the most significant reason for adequate folate intake is the potential for teen pregnancy. In 1992 the U.S. Public Health Service recommended that women of childbearing years between the ages of 15 and 44 increase consumption of folic acid to reduce neural tube defects such as spina bifida and anencephaly (Centers for Disease Control, 1992). Werler, Shapiro, and Mitchell (1993) found that first occurrences of neural tube defects were reduced by approximately 60% with 0.4 mg folic acid supplementation before pregnancy and during the early stages because neural tube defects occur early in pregnancy. In 1996 the Food and Drug Administration mandated that all enriched grain products be fortified with folic acid (Food and Drug Administration, 1996). This fortification, however, is not adequate to meet the new recommendation of 400 µg. Folic acid from foods and from supplements must be included to reach this level. The Tolerable Upper Intake Level for adults is set at 1000 µg/day of folate from fortified food or as a supplement exclusive of food folate (Food and Nutrition Board, 1998; Box 11-3).

Zinc

Zinc is also an important component for protein synthesis, growth, and sexual maturation. Zinc deficiency can lead to growth retardation and delayed

---

Box 11-3 SOURCES OF FOLATE

Asparagus
Beans
Broccoli
Liver
Orange juice
Spinach

---

sexual maturation (Sandstead, 1994). The RDA for zinc has been set at 11 mg/day for ages 14 to 18 years (Food and Nutrition Board, 2001).

Good sources of zinc include the following:
■ Lean meat and poultry
■ Low-fat dairy products
■ Legumes
■ Whole grains

EATING BEHAVIOR

Current Dietary Patterns

Adolescence is a time when dietary choices and patterns are altered drastically. Teens experience greater independence and more peer influence, eat more meals away from home, and have greater accessibility to fast food. All of these factors influence dietary choices at a time when good nutrition is critical. Studies have pointed to childhood dietary patterns as affecting disease patterns in later life. Cancer, heart disease, osteoporosis, and diabetes may have origins in adolescence (World Health Organization, 1997). Therefore including nutrient rich foods believed to promote optimum health, proper weight, and disease prevention is crucial during this time.

In a study of 3350 students, researchers found that more than half ate 5 times during the day and 98% ate at least 3 times a day (Devaney, Gordon, & Burghardt, 1995). This finding suggests that for many adolescents snacking is an integral part of their food consumption. Snacking has been discouraged in the past because of earlier findings that snacks contributed calories but few nutrients (Thomas & Call, 1973). Bigler-Doughten and Jenkins (1987) found that although snacks were generally low in calcium, iron, vitamin A, and vitamin C, they were providing one fourth to one third of the energy intake of the population in study. For female adolescents in their peak growth velocity, extra calories are essential and snacking helps provide for this need. Consequently, snacking should not be discouraged but should instead be directed toward healthier selections that contribute nutrient density to the diet.

Changing social structures, teenagers with busier lives and schedules, and attempts to control weight lead to more missed meals. According to the National Adolescent Student Health Survey (American School Health Association, 1988) the evening meal was consumed most regularly, with lunch second and with 18% of participants indicating they never eat breakfast.

Recommended Dietary Patterns

Healthful eating means choosing foods that contain the appropriate amounts of essential nutrients and calories needed to prevent deficiencies and excesses. The caloric intake for a day should consist of 50% to 60% carbohydrates, 15% to 20% protein, and 15% to 25% fat. For most female teens, simply providing information on the amounts of nutrients they need will have little meaning. The Food Guide Pyramid (1996), developed by the U.S. Department of Agriculture and the U.S. Department of Health and Human Services, provides a visual way to translate the RDAs into what and how much to eat (Figure 11-1).

The grain group, which makes up the base of the pyramid, should also make up most of the intake of calories for a day. Breads and cereals provide fuel for the body in the form of carbohydrates, and in their more natural state are good sources of fiber.

Fruits and vegetables form the next layer, with a recommended intake of 5 to 9 servings per day. Fruits and vegetables are rich sources of vitamins and minerals as well as carbohydrates and fiber. According to the American Cancer Society, encouraging the habit of eating fruits and vegetables beginning at an early age potentially can improve the health of Americans by reducing the risk of cancer and other chronic diseases (Subar et al., 1991).

Milk and meat products form a small layer, and although they do provide essential nutrients such as protein, calcium, riboflavin, and vitamin B_{12}, they do not need to be consumed in large quantities. Low-fat milk and meat sources should be encouraged.

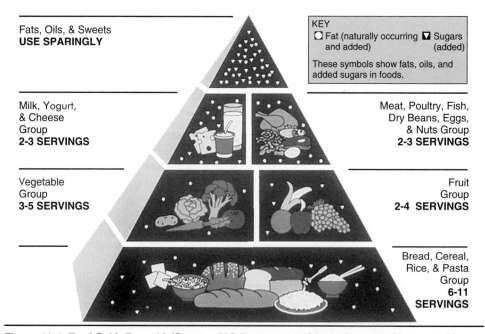

Figure 11-1 Food Guide Pyramid. (Courtesy U.S. Department of Agriculture, Washington, DC.)

The top of the pyramid contains fats and oils that should be used in small quantities. Fat provides more than twice the number of calories (9 kcal/g) than do carbohydrates (4 kcal/g) or protein (4 kcal/g). Many fast-food choices fit in this category and therefore should be limited. With a healthful diet, however, no reason exists to eliminate these foods altogether because they tend to provide much enjoyment for teens. Education and counseling should focus on how to make them a limited part of a healthful lifestyle.

Eating Disorders

Adolescence, when changing body image and the search for self-identity are at their peak, can be a prime time for the appearance of eating disorders. Teenagers are similar to toddlers: Both are exploring the world, view the world in terms of themselves, and are striving to gain independence from mom and dad and other authority figures. Eating patterns and choices reflect these psychological and emotional changes. Teens skip meals because of busy lifestyles and weight concerns. They are starting to purchase and prepare more food on their own. They also have ready access to convenience and fast foods. Some abnormal eating patterns are to be expected. Eating disorders are manifestations of deeper psychological problems within the individual (McDuffie & Kirkley, 1996).

Eating disorders such as anorexia, bulimia, and obesity are characterized by gross deviations in eating patterns (Palmer, 1990). Eating disorders can be examined along a continuum of behavior with obesity at one end and anorexia at the other (Rees, 1992). Along the spectrum are varying weights and varying levels of eating disorder. Many adolescents may not fall at the ends of the spectrum, classifying them as eating disordered, but their eating behavior may still be abnormal enough to need intervention. Recognizing this aspect is important for the health professional. Wherever the individual falls on the spectrum, female adolescents with eating disorders are using food for purposes other than nourishment.

Prevalence and Risk

An estimate of the prevalence of eating disorders is approximately 1.2 million adolescents and young adult females in the United States (Palmer, 1990). Eating disorders are found among all socioeconomic levels and all races. African-American and American-Indian females, however, are more likely to be satisfied with their bodies and less likely to engage in unhealthy weight control practices (Story, French, Resnick, & Blum, 1995).

Story and others (1991) found that chronic dieters were more likely than other students to report using unhealthy weight-loss techniques. Unhealthy weight-loss methods include vomiting; use of laxatives, diuretics, and diet pills; and excessive caloric restriction and exercise routines.

Anorexia Nervosa

Anorexia is typified by self-imposed starvation and distorted images of body weight and shape. Anorexia, which in its most literal sense means lack of appetite, is actually a misnomer. Individuals with anorexia do not lack appetite; they instead exhibit an extreme amount of control over their intake of food. Anorexia is seen mostly in young females and rarely is seen in males. Approximately one half of cases are seen before the age of 20 and three fourths of cases before the age of 25 (Lucas & Huse, 1994). The cause of anorexia is complex and may involve biological, familial, sociocultural, and psychological origins.

The American Psychiatric Association (1994) has set forth four diagnostic criteria, each of which must be present for the diagnosis for anorexia:

- Refusal to maintain normal height-for-age body weight. Weight loss reaches less than 85% of the expected weight
- Vehement fear of gaining weight and becoming fat, even though underweight
- Disturbed body image: feels fat and denies the seriousness of current low body weight
- Absence of three consecutive menstrual cycles

Intervention and treatment for the anorexia is crucial; without them many die. Estimated mortality from anorexia ranges between 1% and 15% from suicide and medical complications such as electrolyte disturbance, acute kidney failure, and cardiac complications (Palmer, 1990). The goal of treatment needs to focus on regaining weight to optimal levels while treating psychological symptoms. Treatment needs to be a multifaceted joint effort of aggressive medical management, psychotherapy, behavioral management, and nutritional counseling.

Bulimia Nervosa

The bulimic individual is usually of normal weight and attempts to maintain that weight while gorging and bingeing on food. Normal weight is maintained through purging or vomiting and using laxatives to induce diarrhea. Bulimic behavior (purging after bingeing) occasionally may be used by adolescents as a means of weight control (Polivy & Herman, 1987) without meeting criteria for bulimia diagnosis. The American Psychiatric Association (1994) has set the diagnostic criteria for bulimia:

- Recurrent episodes of binge eating, which is characterized as eating an abnormal amount of food with a sense of lack of control over eating during the episode
- Recurrent use of improper weight control behavior such as self-induced vomiting, laxatives, diuretics, enemas, fasting, or excessive exercise
- Bingeing and purging behavior occurs at least twice a week for 3 months
- Overconcern with body weight and shape
- The disturbance does not occur solely during incidents of anorexia nervosa

The cause of bulimia nervosa has been researched extensively and debated. Several factors may contribute to the development or maintenance of the bingeing/purging syndrome. Dansky, Brewerton, Kilpatrick, and O'Neil (1997) found higher rates of bulimia nervosa in women who had been victims of sexual or aggravated assault. Other studies have reported that patients with bulimia have reduced serotonin activity, which may play a role in the pathophysiology of bulimia (Weltzin, Fernstrom, & Kaye, 1994). Serotonin is one of several neuromodulators of feeding. Serotonin-active antidepressant medications have been shown to decrease binge eating and may be a useful in a comprehensive treatment plan for bulimia.

Persistent vomiting behavior can lead to irritation of the throat, damage to the teeth, and swollen salivary glands from constant exposure to the acidic vomitus. Life-threatening situations can include electrolyte imbalance and kidney damage. Treatment focuses on terminating the binge behavior and normalizing eating behavior. As in anorexia, treatment for bulimia needs to be multifaceted, including psychotherapy and nutritional therapy.

Obesity

At the other end of the spectrum lies the overweight female adolescent. Data from four national surveys have indicated significant increases in adolescent obesity (Gortmaker, Dietz, Sobol, & Wehler, 1987). Obesity in children and adolescents has increased from approximately 15% in 1976 to 1980 to 24% in 1988 to 1994 (Crane, Hubbard, & Lewis, 1999). Obesity is defined as above the 95th percentile weight for height or triceps skinfold greater than or equal to the 85th percentile. Gortmaker, Must, Perrin, Sobol, & Dietz (1993) found that being overweight in adolescence increased the risk of being overweight in adulthood and also increased the risk of morbidity for several conditions such as heart disease, atherosclerosis, and colorectal cancer. Women who were overweight as adolescents were more likely to have a compromised functional capacity from conditions such as arthritis.

A variety of psychological, genetic, environmental, and physiological factors may be contributing to the obese condition. Recently, with the discovery of the obese gene in mice, the argument for a genetic component to obesity has been strengthened (Zhang, et al., 1994). Studies on the body mass index (BMI) of twins reared apart also have concluded that strong genetic influences may determine body weight (Stunkard, Harris, Pedersen, & McClearn, 1990).

Other influences of adolescent obesity include the following:

■ Abundance of high-fat fast foods, convenience foods, and school lunch program foods (American Dietetic Association, 1996)
■ Increased television viewing (Gortmaker, Dietz, Sobol, & Wehler, 1987)
■ General decline in physical activity (Schlicker, Borra, & Regan, 1994)

Whatever the causes of obesity, obese female adolescents suffer from psychological repercussions. Young women who are overweight are less likely to be married, complete fewer years of education, and have lower household incomes and higher rates of poverty (Gortmaker, Must, Perrin, Sobol, & Dietz, 1993).

Satter (1996) recommends that assumptions and paradigms about adolescent fatness be altered. The current assumption is that fatness is always unhealthy and should be treated. The new emerging view is that fatness may be a normal genetic condition for some. Fatness should not be defined on a growth grid or chart but should instead be evaluated based on what is excessive for the individual. The adolescent's task is to grow at a stable level, even if growth is at the higher end of the growth chart. Parental and health professional responsibilities include helping teens maintain homeostasis within their genetic makeups. Encouraging healthful eating and activity lets teens develop the weight that is right for them. Providing an atmosphere of trust rather than control and manipulation over their eating is crucial.

SPECIAL NUTRITIONAL PROFILES

Adolescent Athlete

Athletics for adolescents can play a big part in building self-esteem, building team values, and providing positive physical activity for their growing and developing bodies. Proper nutrition and information about hydration and ergogenic aids assist in helping female adolescents reach their full growth and athletic potential without hazardous consequences.

A diet adequate in calories is essential for teen athletes. Calories must be adequate to cover the needs for increased physical activity and increased growth and development. An increase of 1500 to 3000 calories beyond baseline needs is recommended (Loosli & Benson, 1990). A diet based on the Food Guide Pyramid will meet the demands.

Perhaps one of the biggest concerns for the female adolescent athlete is adequate hydration. Vigorous exercise may delay the thirst mechanism, making replacing fluids essential, with a plan for periodic consumption (American Dietetic Association, 1993). General guidelines for fluid consumption include the following:

- Drink 2 cups fluid 2 hours before exertion.
- Drink 2 cups 15 to 20 minutes before a game or competition.
- Drink 4 ounces to 6 ounces every 15 minutes throughout the event.

Plain, cool water is best for most activities lasting 1 hour or less. Individuals participating in events lasting longer than 1 hour or those done in extreme temperature and humidity may benefit from consumption of a sports beverage (Clark, 1995).

Ergogenic aids are substances believed by some to increase the ability of the body to perform athletically. Female teen athletes looking for the competitive edge may be lured into using these products. Examples include amino acids, bee pollen, protein powders, chromium picolinate, and creatine. None has been proved scientifically to work (Eichner, 1997). Many have not been around long enough (e.g., chromium picolinate) to prove long-term safety. The use of ergogenic aids by female adolescent athletes should be discouraged.

Special attention should be given to screening female adolescent athletes for eating disorders, the prevalence of which among female athletes may be as high as 15% to 62% (Wichmann & Martin, 1993). Predominance of eating disorders is especially high in those sports that require the body to be displayed, such as gymnastics, figure skating, ballet, and diving. Screening is especially important in light of the recent recognition of the "female athlete triad" (Smith, 1996). Coined by the American College of Sports Medicine, the term describes disordered eating, amenorrhea, and osteoporosis, and the disorder affects girls in many sports. Irreversible bone loss and possible death may result.

Pregnant Adolescent

Between 1998 and 1999 the teenage birth rate was 49.6 births per 1000 women ages 15 to 19 (U.S. Department of Health and Human Services, 2000). Even though this rate is down 20% from the most recent high in 1991, many of these babies were born premature, had low birth weight, and required intensive care or died at birth (American Dietetic Association, 1994). Pregnancy during adolescence is a critical time for intervention by parents and health professionals to ensure a healthful pregnancy outcome.

One of the strongest predictors of a healthful outcome is the birth weight of the infant, which in turn depends on how much weight the mother gains and her initial height-weight relationship when the pregnancy began. Appropriate weight gain recommendations for pregnant adolescents are based on pregnancy body mass index (BMI) and are discussed further in the section on pregnancy. Despite adequate weight gain, pregnant teens may still give birth to low-birth-weight babies for reasons such as the following:

■ Competition for nutrients between the growing adolescent and the growing fetus (Scholl, Hediger, Schall, Khoo, & Fischer, 1994)
■ Erratic nutritional behavior of adolescents
■ Smoking and drug and alcohol abuse

Caloric needs for pregnant teens can be determined by the RDA per centimeter of height. For 11-to 14-year-olds, 15.9 kcal/cm height is recommended; for 15-to 18-year-olds, 15.3 kcal/cm height is recommended (Food and Nutrition Board, 1989).

Evidence suggests that pregnant teens may improve dietary practices during pregnancy (Skinner & Carruth, 1991). However, supplementation and dietary sources need to be recommended for iron, calcium, vitamins B_6 and C, and folate (American Dietetic Association, 1994). Pregnant adolescents who face economic challenges as well should be referred to supplemental food programs such as Women, Infants, and Children. The program provides not only nourishing food but also appropriate education for the pregnant teen.

NUTRITION THROUGH THE REPRODUCTIVE YEARS

Women in their middle years face changes from all directions. Many are pregnant or are considering starting a family. Many are in the midst of working and a career and are trying to balance family life. Economics, time constraints, knowledge, and dietary choices are factors that affect a woman's pursuit of optimal health.

Economics

The number of women who are raising families by themselves has increased. In 1970, single mothers headed 12% of all families with children under the age of 18. By 1992 this percentage had increased to 26% (Lino & Guthrie, 1994). Women who are single heads of household have a much higher poverty rate than families with a male head of household. In 1992, 52% of all poor families had a female head of household (Bureau of the Census, 1991). Female single heads of household were more likely to receive government assistance with food and to shop more infrequently and were significantly less likely to consume fruits, vegetables, and milk products (Lino & Guthrie, 1994).

Time Constraints: Eating Away from Home

More and more women are working outside of the home, leaving less time for food preparation. Between 1977 and 1985 the percentage of women ages 19 to 50 who ate away from home on a given day increased from 45% to 57% (Haines, Hungerford, Popkin, & Guilkey, 1992). Information from the Continuing Survey of Food Intakes by Individuals revealed that women who ate predominantly away from home consumed more fat, in particular, saturated fat, and cholesterol. Calcium, fiber, folacin, and vitamin C were also consumed less than by women who ate predominantly at home (Wilkinson-Enns, & Guenther, 1988).

Knowledge and Dietary Choices

The composition of the diet of U.S. women has changed over the past decade. Women have more diversity in their diet as well as a higher number of low-fat foods (Popkin, Haines, & Reidy, 1989). Even with a plethora of diet and health messages being presented to women, improvements can be made. Popkin and others (1989) found an increase in women consuming higher-fat foods such as certain cheeses, desserts, and salty snacks. Alaimo and others (1994) found sodium intake higher than recommended and fiber intake lower than recommended. Clearly women need access to information that is translated easily into wise food choices.

Special Nutritional Considerations

Women have particular nutritional needs because of their physiological makeup. Proper nutrient intake is essential for healthful outcomes in pregnancy and lactation and during the menstrual cycle.

Pregnancy

Affect of maternal nutritional status. Pregnancy is a time of nutritional demand unmatched by any other time in a woman's life. The belief that the baby was the perfect parasite and would simply take whatever nutrition it needed from the mother has been refuted by the now recognized connections between birth problems and nutrition.

Observations from the now historical Dutch famine that influenced maternal nutritional status on birth outcome provided insight into timing and duration of malnutrition on the health of the infant. Susser and Stein (1994) summarized the effects of the famine that occurred for a 6-month period during the winter from 1944 to 1945. The famine was a deliberate result of the Nazi occupation. The researchers concluded that poor nutrition in the later trimesters resulted in poor fetal growth and that poor nutrition in the early trimesters affected development of the embryo and the rate of birth defects.

Caloric needs. An increase in calories is essential to the physiological needs of the pregnant woman. The Food and Nutrition Board (1989) of the National Research Council recommends an increase of 300 kcal/day to cover the needs of the pregnant woman's physical changes and the growing fetus. This increase in calories may not be enough for women who begin pregnancy underweight or in poor nutritional health. The Food and Nutrition Board caloric recommendations also may not be appropriate for women who begin pregnancy very overweight. Caloric needs should be adjusted to achieve optimum weight gain.

Weight gain. The amount of weight gained during pregnancy varies among individuas and affects the birth weight of the infant (Abrams & Selvin, 1995). Weight-gain guidelines determine appropriate weight gain using BMI (Olson, 1994). The Institutes of Medicine recommend the following weight gain levels:

■ Low BMI (<19.8), 12.5 to 18 kg
■ Normal BMI (19.8 to 26.0), 11.5 to 16 kg
■ High BMI (26.0 to 29.0), 7 to 11.5 kg

Protein. Additional protein is needed during pregnancy for the mother and the fetus. Maternal protein is needed for the support of increased blood volume, uterus, and breasts. The Food and Nutrition Board (1989) of the National Research Council suggests approximately 60 g of protein a day. To calculate individual allowances, the daily need would be 1.3 g protein/kg of pregnant body weight.

Avoiding dubious substances. Pregnancy is a time when many health professionals caution women about using questionable substances. Most studies conclude that caffeine use of less than 300 mg/day before birth has no effect on the health of the fetus. Levels above 300 mg/day may affect the birth weight of the infant (Hinds, West, Knight, & Harland, 1996). Limited data is available on the effects of using heavy artificial sweetener during pregnancy. Pregnant women should be advised to use caution and common sense when including saccharin and aspartame in their diet.

Alcohol consumed during pregnancy has been shown to have a variety of harmful effects on the fetus. Heavy alcohol exposure produces growth retardation and physical and mental abnormalities commonly called *fetal alcohol syndrome* (Larrson, Bohlin, & Tunell, 1985). Even mothers who only drink socially can produce infants who are at greater risk for growth or behavior changes (Blume, 1985). Abstinence from alcohol is the only reasonable and safest course during pregnancy.

Lactation

Breastfeeding is the natural sequel to pregnancy. Approximately 500 extra calories are needed to sustain breast-feeding (Food and Nutrition Board, 1989). Moderate to severe caloric restriction, especially in the early weeks of lactation, compromises the woman's ability to produce breast milk.

Breast milk provides a nutritionally superior food for the infant that is always safe and fresh and contains immunological properties that help protect the baby against illness. Breast milk is less likely to be allergenic to the baby than milk formula substitutes. Women who breast-feed benefit from lactation amenorrhea, close bonding with their infants, and possible protection against premenopausal breast cancer (Newcomb et al., 1994). The American Dietetic Association ("Promotion of Breast-feeding," 1997) recommends sustained, exclusive breast-feeding for 4 to 6 months and optimally breast-feeding with weaning for at least 12 months.

Even with the obvious advantages to breast-feeding, convincing some women to breast-feed their infants is still difficult. Many barriers exist to establishing increased breast-feeding rates among women in the United States. Deterrents include physicians who are trained inadequately in lactation support, short postpartum hospital stays that limit exposure to breast-feeding support and education, and unsupportive employers (American Dietetic Association, "Promotion of Breast-feeding," 1997; Hills-Bonczyk et al., 1994).

More importantly, breast-feeding within U.S. society is simply not accepted as a cultural norm. In the opinion of many, breast-feeding in public is not a favorable sight. Breast-feeding mothers need to be free of closet nursing and the strong social unacceptability of breast-feeding (Hills-Bonczyk et al., 1994). Also, with decreasing rates of breast-feeding, an entire generation of women has little or no breast-feeding experience to pass on to subsequent potential breast-feeders. Lactation consultants are becoming more common in helping women find support and information on breast-feeding (Diamond, 1997).

Premenstrual Syndrome

Premenstrual syndrome (PMS) refers to a group of symptoms that occur during the luteal or premenstrual phase and disappear soon after the onset of menstruation. PMS appears to be related to hormonal changes in the menstrual cycle, and symptoms include depressed mood, anxiety, appetite changes, and insomnia.

Dietary recommendations and supplements have been suggested as ways of alleviating PMS symptoms (Box 11-4).

These recommendations are made on the theory that PMS may result from nutritional deficiencies or excesses. Mira, Stewart, and Abraham (1988) found no evidence for a nutritional (deficiency of magnesium, zinc, retinol, vitamin E, or vitamin B_6) cause of PMS, however.

Box 11-4 DIETARY CHANGES AFFECTING PREMENSTRUAL SYNDROME

Eliminate	*Increase*
Refined sugar	Fish
Salt	Poultry
Red meat	Whole grains
Animal fat	Legumes
Alcohol	Green leafy vegetables
Caffeine	Soy products
Dairy products	
Tobacco	

Other nutritional supplements such as calcium and vitamin E have not been shown in well-designed clinical studies to improve PMS symptoms (Tangney, 1996).

Moving Toward a Healthful Lifestyle

Recommended Daily Allowance vs. Dietary Guidelines

In the first half of the twentieth century, research focused on nutrient deficiencies and the nutrient levels needed to prevent them. The RDAs of nutrients were the result. Because of these efforts, nutrient deficiency diseases decreased as the major causes of mortality. Today chronic diseases such as heart disease and cancer are the major causes of death. Research now focuses on how diet plays a role in the cause and prevention of chronic diseases. From this effort the Dietary Guidelines for Americans (2000, fifth edition) has become one of the useful guides to promoting better health and reducing chronic disease risk.

The Dietary Guidelines present 10 guidelines under an umbrella of three basic messages referred to as the "ABCs for Good Health":

- **A**im for fitness
- **B**uild a health base
- **C**hoose sensibly

Dietary Guidelines for Americans

The Dietary Guidelines are translated easily into everyday food choices by using the Food Pyramid Guide.

NUTRITION AND THE POSTMENOPAUSAL YEARS (45 TO 60)

Menopause is the medical term for the end of a woman's menstrual periods. As a natural part of the aging process, the ovaries gradually decrease the production of estrogen hormones, leading to the cessation of menstruation. Menopause usually occurs between the ages of 45 and 60. Because estrogen has a protective effect against diseases such as heart disease and osteoporosis, the postmenopausal years are a time when many women begin to take their health seriously as the threat of chronic disease becomes more real.

Diet and Chronic Disease

Although causality of dietary factors and disease is hard to prove, epidemiological, clinical, and laboratory evidence indicates that diet influences the risk of several major chronic diseases (Committee of Diet and Health, 1989). Evidence is strong for a dietary connection with atherosclerotic cardiovascular diseases and hypertension and highly suggestive for some cancers (e.g., esophageal, stomach, large bowel, breast, and lung).

Obesity

Obesity appears to be the precursor to many chronic diseases such as type II diabetes, hypertension, coronary heart disease, gallbladder disease, osteoarthritis, and endometrial cancer (Committee of Diet and Health, 1989). In 1990, diet and activity patterns were the second highest contributors (behind tobacco) to mortality in the United States (McGinnis & Foege, 1993). The prevalence of overweight and obese adults in the United States is now estimated to be 61% (Centers for Disease Control and Prevention, 1999).

Overweight and obesity have different definitions. *Overweight* refers to an excess of body weight (including water and tissues), whereas *obesity* refers to an excess of body fat. The body mass index (BMI) is currently an easily obtained measurement used to define body fatness. BMI is determined by dividing weight (in kilograms) by height (in meters) squared. Healthy levels of body fat have been associated with BMIs of 19 to 25. BMIs of 25.0 to 29.9 indicate overweight, whereas BMIs greater than or equal to 30.0 among adults 20 years and older indicate obesity.

Some chronic diseases are predictable by the distribution of fat on the body. Increased abdominal fat carries a higher risk for high blood pressure, diabetes, early onset of diabetes, early onset of heart disease, and certain types of cancers than do comparable fat deposits on hips and thighs. A waist-to-hip ratio compares the amount of fat deposits around the waist with the amount of fat deposits on the hips. A waist-to-hip ratio greater than 0.8 in women may indicate increased health risks (American Dietetic Association, "Weight Management," 1997).

Traditional avenues of weight loss have not been successful. No current treatment programs appear capable of producing permanent weight loss (Goodrick, Poston, & Foreyt, 1996). Individuals who have lost weight tend to regain as much as two thirds of it within a year and almost all of it within 5 years (Bruce & Wilfley, 1996).

The American Dietetic Association recommends adopting a weight management modality that includes healthful eating of low-fat foods, whole grains, fruits, and vegetables; eating behavior based on internal regulation (hunger and satiety); and exercise consisting of 30 minutes of enjoyable activity every day (American Dietetic Association, 1997). Successful programs focus on correcting low self-esteem, which can accompany repeated weight loss attempts, and on physical health rather than weight loss.

Pharmacological treatment of obesity is sometimes recommended for those individuals with a BMI over 30 or a BMI of 27 with comorbidities. Finding effective and safe weight-loss drugs, however, has been difficult. The serotonin-based anorexiants dexfenfluramine hydrochloride and fenfluramine hydrochloride were withdrawn from the market last year because of their association with cardiac valvulopathy (Food and Drug Administration Press Release, 1997). Another medication that has shown some success has been a serotonin-norepinephrine reuptake inhibitor marketed under the name Meridia. The newest candidate on the weight loss market is a gastrointestinal lipase inhibitor that prevents absorption from the gut of about 30% of dietary fat. Long-term success and safety have yet to be determined on these drugs. Furthermore, if any weight-loss medications are not used within a comprehensive program that includes changes in diet and physical activity, weight is regained after withdrawal from the medication.

Diabetes

The number of individuals with diabetes has been increasing steadily over the past decade. At present, 10.5 million persons have been diagnosed with diabetes and 5.5 million persons are estimated to have the disease but are undiagnosed (King, Aubert, & Herman, 1997). Diabetes is the seventh leading cause of death in the United States, usually from diabetes-associated cardiovascular disease. Diabetes in women is associated with a three- to fourfold increase in coronary heart disease compared with nondiabetic females (American Diabetes Association, 1996).

Diabetes is classified as one of four types. Type 1 diabetes accounts for 5% to 10% of all diagnosed cases and usually occurs in children and adolescents. Type 1 diabetes manifests itself when the pancreas stops making insulin, and insulin administration is needed to live. Type 2 diabetes accounts for 90% to 95% of all diagnosed cases and usually occurs in adults more than 30 years of age and presents itself when the pancreas continues to make insulin but the body tissues are not able to use it effectively. Previously, type 1 diabetes was referred to as juvenile or insulin-dependent diabetes and type 2 diabetes as adult-onset or non-insulin-dependent diabetes. Gestational diabetes develops in 2% to 5% of all pregnant women but disappears after the pregnancy. Other specific types of diabetes result from specific genetic syndromes, surgery, drugs, malnutrition, infections, and other illnesses. These types of diabetes account for 1% to 2% of all diagnosed cases.

Complications of diabetes may consist of heart disease, stroke, high blood pressure, blindness, kidney disease, nervous system disease, amputations, and dental disease. State-of-the-art nutrition therapy for all types of diabetes involves manipulating nutrient intake and food consumption patterns to optimize pre- and postprandial blood glucose levels, lipid levels, and blood pressure. For type 1 diabetes, the American Diabetes Association (2000) recommends that individuals using insulin eat at consistent times throughout the day, synchronized with the time-action of the insulin preparation used. For type 2 diabetes, individuals should select dietary choices and patterns that maintain glucose, lipid, and blood pressure goals. Approximately 90% of those with type 2 diabetes are overweight; therefore, food selections also must promote weight loss. Individuals with diabetes can use the Dietary Guidelines for Americans, Food Guide Pyramid, and the Diabetes Food Guide Pyramid to make healthful food choices.

Because of the risk for cardiovascular disease, additional information must be given to individuals with diabetes concerning the selection of dietary fats. The American Diabetic Association advises that 80% to 90% of calories should be distributed between dietary fat and carbohydrates with less than 10% of calories coming from saturated fat and less than 10% of calories coming from polyunsaturated fats. The remaining 60% to 70% of calories should be distributed between monounsaturated fats and carbohydrates. For some, eating a high percentage of carbohydrates on a daily basis may exacerbate triglyceride levels. If an individual experiences increased levels of low-density lipoproteins (LDL) and triglycerides, a moderate increase in monounsaturated fat may be appropriate. Monitoring blood lipid levels and body weight is important, however, when making any dietary fat modifications.

Exercise has been shown not only to enhance weight loss in those with diabetes but also to improve the ability of muscle to use glucose at the cellular level (Clark, 1992). One must take care, however, to time eating and exercise to avoid a hypoglycemic reaction.

Female Cancers

For women in their middle years (45 to 65 years), cancer remains a major threat. Since 1990, cancer has taken nearly 5 million lives. Cancer is the second leading cause of death in the United States, exceeded only by heart disease (National Center for Health Statistics, 2000). Female cancer sites and their possible link to dietary choices and patterns will be considered.

Cancer has many causes. One theory is that female cancers result from several insults on a specific tissue site throughout a lifetime. Significant events may happen in childhood or even in infancy to affect the genesis of the disease (Freudenheim et al., 1994). For female cancers the insult may involve steroidal hormones, particularly estrogen, which in turn are affected by reproductive events and dietary factors. Cancer and steriodal hormones appear to be interrelated. For instance, an early age onset of menarche may be associated with an increased risk of breast cancer. Diet may play a part in adolescent girls starting menarche at an earlier age (Sanchez, Kissinger, & Phillips, 1981). Diet during pregnancy and the postpartum period may influence the nutritional status of the cervical tissue, ultimately affecting the initiation of cervical cancer (Freudenheim & Potischman, 1996).

Diet also may influence hormone levels apart from reproductive events. Alcohol raises estrogen levels, which may contribute to the disease process. Shu and others (1993) discovered that a diet high in animal protein and animal fat might play an important role in the cause of endometrial cancer. In their study population, Asian women who live in Western countries and have adopted a Western diet that includes more animal products have a higher incidence of endometrial cancer. The researchers theorize that animal fat and protein may alter endogenous hormone levels. Possibly the carcinogens present in animal products also could contribute to the development of cancer.

Research concerning fat intake and breast cancer risk has shown puzzling results. A strong positive correlation exists between the per capita availability of fat and the incidence of breast cancer. However, epidemiological studies (case-control and cohort) offer conflicting results regarding the causal relationship between fat intake and breast cancer (Hankin, 1993). Still, in the minds of many researchers, the decision to negate fat as a cancer risk factor is not yet appropriate.

Rather than a high-fat diet, increased body weight (which may result from a high-fat diet) may instead be the associated risk factor. Ballard-Barbash, Schatzkin, Taylor, and Kahle (1990) discovered in their sample of U.S. women that an increase of 8 kg/m^2 in body mass was identified with a 250% increase in breast cancer risk. Adiposity is thought to result in increases in bioavailable estrogen.

Dietary recommendations to reduce cancer risk focus on reducing dietary fat and animal foods and replacing them with foods from plant sources such as beans, high-fiber grains, fruits, and vegetables. Rohan, Howe, Friedenreich, Jain, and Miller (1993) found that women with high intakes of dietary fiber had a reduced risk of breast cancer. Fiber may reduce risk by binding with estrogen in the gut, making the estrogen unavailable to the body. Fruits and vegetables contain not only fiber but also nutrients that may protect against cancer. Freudenheim and others (1996) discovered that premenopausal women with a high intake of vegetables had a decreased risk of breast cancer. Carotenoids, vitamins C and A, and many other unknown food components in fruits and vegetables may be responsible for this protection. When supplements of vitamins C and E and folic acid were taken, no association of breast cancer risk was found. The researchers theorize that components found together in vegetables may have a synergistic effect on breast cancer risk. Fruits and vegetables rich in carotenoids typically are dark green, dark yellow, dark orange. The American Cancer Society recommends consuming five or more servings of fruits and vegetables each day. More than 140 million Americans are not eating the recommended daily amount (Subar et al., 1991).

Cardiovascular Disease

Cardiovascular disease (CVD), defined as diseases of the blood vessels, is the leading cause of death in women. In 1998, CVD claimed the lives of 503,927 women. When CVD is diagnosed in women, the prognosis is poorer than for men because women are more likely to die from a heart attack.

For men, annual rates of first major cardiovascular events rise from 7 per 1000 men at ages 35 to 44 to 68 per 1000 at ages 85 to 94. Women do not reach comparable rates until 10 years later in life (American Heart Association, 2000). The presence of estrogen has long been recognized as a protective factor against heart disease, which is why the incidence of heart disease for women increases after menopause and later in life than for men.

The evidence is clear that a Western diet high in fat and animal foods plays a major role in promoting heart disease. Research has provided solid evidence that cholesterol, saturated fat, and possible trans-fatty acids increase the risk of CVD (Gaziano & Manson, 1996). The National Cholesterol Education Program (2001) has issued clinical practice guidelines on the detection, management, and treatment of high blood cholesterol in adults, also known as the Adult Treatment Panel III.

Adult Treatment Panel III guidelines take a more aggressive approach to identifying those at risk for cardiovascular disease and in need of cholesterol-lowering treatment than previously published guidelines in 1988 and 1993. Although the guidelines address altering the major blood lipids associated with cardiovascular disease, they primarily target lowering LDL cholesterol. In all adults age 20 years or older, a fasting lipoprotein blood profile (total cholesterol, LDL cholesterol, high-density lipoprotein cholesterol, and triglycerides) should be obtained. Blood lipid levels are classified as optimum if total cholesterol is less than 200 mg/dL, high-density lipoprotein cholesterol is greater than 60 mg/dL (less than 40 mg/dL is considered a risk factor), LDL cholesterol is less than 100 mg/dL, and triglycerides are less than 150 mg/dL.

Adult Treatment Panel III recommends a multifaceted lifestyle approach to reduce the risk of cardiovascular disease designated as therapeutic lifestyle changes. Dietary recommendations are found in Box 11-5.

Other dietary options for lowering LDL cholesterol include using foods that contain plant stanols and sterols or that are rich in soluble fiber. Plant stanols and sterols have been added to certain margarines and salad dressings; foods high in soluble fiber include cereal grains, beans, peas, legumes, and many fruits and vegetables. A portion of the population may require LDL cholesterol–lowering medication in addition to therapeutic lifestyle changes to reach the designated goal for LDL cholesterol.

Osteoporosis

Of the 20 to 25 million Americans who suffer from osteoporosis, 80% are women (Heaney, 1996). Osteoporosis is a condition in which skeletal bone mass decreases and becomes fragile, resulting in bone fractures, and occurs specifically in women who are at the onset of menopause. Women can lose one third of their spinal bone mass in the first 6 years after menopause. One of the most common bone fracture sites for osteoporosis, the hip, incurs a 16% mortality rate and extensive loss in independence. About half of all hip-fracture survivors lose the ability to live independently. Women who are underweight and of Northern European ancestry are at greatest risk for osteoporosis. Although a strong genetic component exists, achieving maximum bone health is thought to minimize the effects of osteoporosis.

Bone health has three aspects: nutrition, hormones, and lifestyle. Lifelong dietary patterns may affect skeletal health. Calcium is the principal building matrix for bones, and not getting enough results in porous, fragile skeletal bone. By the age of 35, bones are as strong as they will ever be. Bone mass is maintained until menopause, when estrogen levels decrease. Estrogen receptors in bone cells and in organ systems help regulate bone remodeling and calcium homeostasis (Notelovitz, 1997). Decreased estrogen levels have a major impact on the turnover of bone and render a women more susceptible to greater bone porosity. Optimal calcium intake throughout a woman's life

---

Box 11-5 DIETARY RECOMMENDATIONS TO REDUCE RISK OF CARDIOVASCULAR DISEASE

- Reduce intakes of saturated fats (<7% of total calories)
- Polyunsaturated fats, up to 10% of total calories
- Monounsaturated fats, up to 20% of total calories
- Total fat, 25%-35% of total calories
- Carbohydrates, 50%-60% of total calories
- Fiber, 20-30 g/day
- Protein, 15% total calories
- Cholesterol, <200 mg/day
- Total calories: Balance energy intake and expenditure to maintain desirable body weight and prevent weight gain.

is needed to maximize peak bone mass, maintain adult bone, and minimize bone loss after menopause.

The new recommendations for calcium are 1000 mg/day for adults 19 to 50 years old and 1200 mg/day for adults more than 51 years of age. Because research was not adequate to determine an Estimated Average Requirement or an RDA, the new calcium recommendations are listed as Adequate Intakes. An upper limit was established at 2500 mg/day (Food and Nutrition Board, 1997).

Calcium is obtained easily by consuming milk and dairy foods (described in the calcium section). Low-fat sources are available and should be encouraged. Nondairy sources such as leafy greens (collards, kale, and broccoli) and calcium-fortified orange juice are also good sources of calcium.

For those who have trouble digesting milk or getting enough calcium-rich foods in their diet, supplements may be appropriate. Calcium carbonate is the most frequently used as a supplement because it is the cheapest and most efficient form. One should take care to avoid calcium supplements that contain oyster shell, dolomite, or fossil-shell calcium carbonate because they may be contaminated with aluminum and lead (Whiting, 1994). Trying to get at least half of one's calcium needs from food and the other half from supplements is best. Calcium supplementation is most efficient when doses are no greater than 500 mg and are taken with a meal.

Additional suggestions for getting the most from the calcium consumed include avoiding combining calcium-rich foods or supplements with the following:

- High-fiber foods
- Oxalic acid (found in spinach and rhubarb)
- Caffeine

Foods made from soybeans such as tofu, soy milk, soy flour, and soyburgers also may help reduce the risk of osteporosis as well as of cancer and heart disease. Soybeans contain phytosterols, saponins, and isoflavones, which act to help retain bone mass, inhibit cancer development, and reduce the risk of atherosclerosis. Researchers have found that an average intake of 47 g soy protein per day significantly decreased serum concentrations of total blood cholesterol, LDL cholesterol, and triglycerides (Anderson, Johnstone, & Cook-Newell, 1995).

Soybeans also contain a number of anticarcinogens. Although the epidemiological data are inconsistent, most of the data reviewed by Messina, Persky, Setchell, and Barnes (1994) pointed toward the consumption of nonfermented soy products as protective against or not associated with cancer risk: "While a definitive statement that soy reduces cancer risk cannot be made at this time, there is sufficient evidence of a protective effect to warrant continued investigation."

NUTRITION AND THE OLDER WOMAN

The elderly population has grown exceedingly large. The U.S. Census Bureau projects that this population of adults will grow even larger by the middle of this century. In 1994, one in eight Americans were elderly, but by 2030 this statistic will change to one in five (Hobbs, 1997). Between 1900 and the present, life expectancy for women increased from 48 to 78 years (U.S. Senate Special Committee on Aging, 1988).

Although women are living longer, they are not necessarily living better. Women experience more disability and morbidity than do older men (*Report of the National Institutes of Health*, 1992). For instance, among noninstitutionalized persons over the age of 75, 33% of women needed help with one or more activities of daily living as opposed to 23% of men. Eighty-five percent of all nursing home residents are women (Hobbs, 1997). Factors such as institutionalization and co-morbidity can contribute to poor nutritional health. Some studies (Abbasi & Rudman, 1994; Lowik et al., 1992) have found lower nutritional status among institutionalized elderly women as opposed to those living independently. The inability to receive good nutrition eventually leads to subclinical malnutrition and with it the inability to adequately defend against sickness and disease or heal from traumatic injuries.

Energy Requirements

Physical changes that occur because of aging or menopause can affect nutritional needs. Aging is associated with changes in body composition, mainly the reduction in skeletal muscle mass and consequently of energy needs. Fat-free mass is the main determinant of energy expenditure and declines approximately 15% between the third and eighth decades of life (Evans, 1995). Fat-free mass reduction leads to a reduced metabolic rate and lowered energy requirements, as do chronic conditions or disabilities that prevent or hinder physical activity in elderly women.

Protein

The current RDA for protein, 0.8 g/kg/day, is based on younger subjects and may not be appropriate for older women. More importantly, inadequate protein intake may contribute to the decline of muscle mass and a reduction in muscle strength, which is a major cause of disability among the elderly (Evans, 1997). Campbell, Crim, Dallal, Young, and Evans (1994) suggest a higher intake of 1.0 g to 1.25 g/kg/day of high-quality protein to maintain nitrogen equilibrium and reduce loss of muscle tissue.

Vitamins and Minerals

Physiological and functional changes during aging result in changes in vitamin and mineral needs. Intakes of vitamin B_6, folate, and vitamin B_{12} have been increased in the current DRIs because of their relationship with blood homocysteine levels. Elevated plasma homocysteine levels are considered an independent risk factor for cardiovascular disease. Research has shown an inverse association with vitamin B_6 and folate and the risk of myocardial infarction (Verhoef et al., 1996). The current level for vitamin B_6 is 1.5 mg and for folate, 400 µg. Greater intakes of vitamins B_6 and B_{12} (2.4 µg) and of folate have been shown to prevent some decline in cognitive function associated with aging (American Dietetic Association, 2000). Rich dietary sources of vitamin B_6 are chicken, fish, pork, and eggs. Folate is found in leafy green vegetables and fruits. Additional studies have suggested that higher intakes and plasma levels of vitamin C may protect against early mortality from heart disease in the elderly population (Sahyoun, Jacques, & Russel, 1996).

As estrogen levels decrease in the postmenopausal woman, the protective effect of the hormone against osteoporosis declines. AIs for calcium (as mentioned earlier) may need to be increased to protect against bone mineral loss. Daily supplementation of soy protein found in soybean foods may help reduce the incidence of osteoporosis and also may reduce the frequency of hot flashes in postmenopausal women that are associated with declining estrogen levels.

Achieving Quality Not Just Quantity

How to achieve the best quality of life as opposed to simply living longer is foremost on the minds of many researchers. Evans (1997) suggests that regular exercise may be the key component to helping the elderly maintain functional status and independence. Reaching optimum function is also essential to fight off disease and disability and improve quality of life. Food intake for the elderly woman has not only nutritional significance but also social and emotional significance. Many factors affect food choices (Box 11-6). The most significant strides will be made toward improving quality of life when nutrition, exercise, and mental health are viewed as interrelated and an integral part of an elderly woman's health.

SUMMARY

Good nutrition for women is important throughout their lives. Although all women need the same nutrients, they need them in varying amounts at the different stages of development. Research is critical in determining these amounts and in examining the nutrition-related disease processes in women. Only recently have researchers acknowledged that a woman's hormonal environment changes the way a disease process works and responds to therapy. Surprisingly, women have been excluded from many of the major health studies, for example, the Multiple Risk Factor Intervention Trial (Kjelsberg, Cutler, & Dolecek, 1997).

The Women's Health Trial is one (and probably the largest) response to the political backlash of women's exclusion. The trial is the largest women's study ever attempted,

---

Box 11-6 FACTORS AFFECTING FOOD CHOICES FOR THE ELDERLY WOMAN

Psychological	Dental status
Social activity	Chronic disease
Loneliness	
Mental awareness	***Socioeconomic***
	Age
Physiological	Income
Appetite	Availability of transportation

involving more than 40 centers nationwide with 162,000 American women, ages 50 to 79 who will be followed for an average of 9 years. Over 15 years, researchers will attempt to test the impact of low-fat diets, estrogen, calcium, and vitamin D on the incidence of breast cancer, osteoporosis-induced hip fractures, and CVD (U.S. Department of Health and Human Services, 1999).

The nursing professional is many times the first health professional an individual encounters in a medical setting. Nurses are critical to the recognition and assessment of nutritional problems and are the vital link for referral to the nutrition health professional.

REFERENCES

Abbasi, A. A., & Rudman, D. (1994). Undernutrition in nursing home: Prevalence, consequences, causes and prevention. *Nutrition Reviews, 52*(4), 113–122.

Abrams, B., & Selvin, S. (1995). Maternal weight gain pattern and birth weight. *Obstetrics & Gynecology, 86*(2), 163–169.

Alaimo, K., McDowell, M. A., Briefel, R. R., Bischof, A. M., Caughman, C. R., Loria, C. M., et al. (1994). *Dietary intake of vitamins, minerals and fiber of persons ages 2 months and over in the United States: Third National Health and Nutrition Examination Survey, Phase I, 1988–91* (advance data from vital and health statistics, No. 258). Hyattsville, MD: National Center for Health Statistics.

American Diabetes Association. (1996). *Diabetes 1996: Vital statistics.* Alexandria, VA: Author.

American Diabetes Association. (2000). Nutritional recommendations and principles for individuals with diabetes mellitus. *Diabetes Care, 23,* S43–S46.

American Dietetic Association. (1993). Nutrition for physical fitness and athletic performance for adults. *Journal of the American Dietetic Association, 93*(6), 691–696.

American Dietetic Association. (1994). Nutrition care for pregnant adolescents. *Journal of the American Dietetic Association, 94*(4), 449–450.

American Dietetic Association. (1996). Child and adolescent food and nutrition programs. *Journal of the American Dietetic Association, 96*(9), 913–917.

American Dietetic Association. (1997). Promotion of breast-feeding. *Journal of the American Dietetic Association, 97*(6), 662–666.

American Dietetic Association. (1997). Weight management. *Journal of the American Dietetic Association, 97*(1), 71–74.

American Dietetic Association. (2000). Nutrition, aging and the continuum of care. *Journal of the American Dietetic Association. 100,* 580.

American Heart Association. (2000). *Heart and stroke statistical update.* Retrieved July 16, 2001, from *http://www.americanheart.org/statistics/cvd.html.*

American Psychiatric Association. (1994). *Diagnostic and statistical manual of mental disorders* (4th ed.). Washington, DC: APA.

American School Health Association, Association for the Advancement of Health Education, & Society for Public Health Education. (1988). *The National Adolescent Student Health Survey: A report on the health of America's youth.* Oakland, CA: Third Party Publication.

Anderson, J. W., Johnstone, B., & Cook-Newell, M. (1995). Meta-analysis of the effects of soy protein intake on serum lipids. *New England Journal of Medicine, 333*(5), 276–282.

Ballard-Barbash, R., Schatzkin, A., Taylor, P. R., & Kahle, L. L. (1990). Association of change in body mass with breast cancer. *Cancer Research, 50,* 2152–2155.

Bigler-Doughten, S., & Jenkins, R. M. (1987). Adolescent snacks: Nutrient density and nutritional contribution to total intake. *Journal of the American Dietetic Association, 87,* 1678–1684.

Blume, S. B. (1985). Is social drinking during pregnancy harmless? There is reason to think not. *Advances in Alcohol & Substance Abuse, 5*(1–2), 209–219.

Bruce, B., & Wilfley, D. (1996). Binge eating among the overweight population: A serious and prevalent problem. *Journal of the American Dietetic Association, 96,* 58–61.

Bureau of the Census, U. S. Department of Commerce. (1991). *Poverty in the United States: 1991.* Washington, DC: Government Printing Office.

Campbell, W. W., Crim, M. C., Dallal, G. E., Young, V. R. & Evans, W. J. (1994). Increased protein requirements in elderly people: New data and retrospective reassessments. *American Journal of Clinical Nutrition, 60*(4), 501–509.

Centers for Disease Control. (1992). Recommendations for the use of folic acid to reduce the number of cases of spina bifida and other neural tube defects. *Morbidity and Mortality Weekly Report, 41*, (No. RR–14).

Centers for Disease Control, National Center for Health Statistics—Health E Stats. (1999). *Prevalence of overweight and obesity among adults: United States, 1999.* Retrieved July 16, 2001, from *http://www.cdc.gov/nchs/products/pubs/pubd/hestats/obese/obsr99.htm.*

Cerrato, P. L. (1992). Teens can shape their postmenopausal years. *RN. 55*(8), 65–67.

Clark, N. (1992). Eating right with type II diabetes. *Physician and Sportsmedicine, 20*(9), 17–18.

Clark, N. (1995). Water the ultimate nutrient. *Physician and Sportsmedicine, 23*(5), 21–22.

Committee of Diet and Health, Food and Nutrition Board, Commission of Life Sciences, National Research Council. (1989). *Diet and health: Implications for reducing chronic disease risk.* Washington, DC: National Academy Press.

Crane, N. T., Hubbard, V. S., & Lewis, C. J. (1999). American diets and year 2000 goals. In E. Frazão (Ed.), *America's eating habits: Changes and consequences.* (Agriculture Information Bulletin No. 750). Washington, DC: Food and Rural Economics Division, Economic Research Service, U. S. Department of Agriculture.

Dansky, B. S., Brewerton, T. D., Kilpatrick, D. G., & O'Neil, P. M. (1997). The National Women's Study: Relationship of victimization and posttraumatic stress disorder to bulimia nervosa. *International Journal of Eating Disorders, 21*(3), 213–228.

Devaney, B. L., Gordon, A. R., & Burghardt, J. A. (1995). Dietary intakes of students. *American Journal of Clinical Nutrition, 61*(Suppl.), 205S–212S.

Diamond, L. (1997). Lactation consulting: Is it for you? *Journal of the American Dietetic Association, 97*(6), 591–592.

Eichner, E. R. (1997). Ergogenic aids: What athletes are using—and why. *Physician and Sportsmedicine, 25*(4), 70–80.

Evans, W. J. (1995). What is sarcopenia? *Journal of Gerontology* [Series A, *Biological Sciences & Medical Sciences*; Special Issue], *50*, 5–8.

Evans, W. J. (1997). Nutrition, exercise, and healthy aging. *Journal of the American Dietetic Association, 97*(6), 632–638.

Food and Drug Administration. (1996). Food standards: Amendment of standards of identity for enriched grain products to require addition of folic acid. *Federal Register, 61*, 8781–8797.

Food and Nutrition Board. (1989). *Recommended dietary allowances* (10th ed.). Washington, DC: National Academy Press.

Food and Nutrition Board, Institute of Medicine. (1997). *Dietary reference intakes for calcium, phosphorus, magnesium, vitamin D, and fluoride.* Washington, DC: National Academy Press.

Food and Nutrition Board, Institute of Medicine. (1998). *Dietary reference intakes for thiamin, riboflavin, niacin, vitamin B$_6$, folate, vitamin B$_{12}$, pantothenic acid, biotin, and choline.* Washington, DC: National Academy Press.

Food and Nutrition Board, Institute of Medicine. (2000). *Dietary reference intakes: Use in dietary assessment.* Washington, DC: National Academy Press.

Food and Nutrition Board, Institute of Medicine. (2001). *Dietary reference intakes for vitamin A, vitamin K, arsenic, boron, chromium, copper, iodine, iron, molybdenum, nickel, silicon, vanadium, and zinc.* Washington, DC: National Academy Press.

Food Guide Pyramid. (1996). Washington, DC: U. S. Department of Agriculture and U. S. Department of Health and Human Services.

Freudenheim, J. L., Marshall, J. R., Graham, S., Laughlin, R., Vena, J. E., Bandera, E., et al. (1994). Exposure to breastmilk in infancy and the risk of breast cancer. *Epidemiology, 5*(3), 324–331.

Freudenheim, J. L., Marshall, J. R., Vena, J. E., Laughlin, R., Brasure, J. R., Swanson, M. K., et al. (1996). Premenopausal breast cancer risk and intake of vegetables, fruits, and related nutrients. *Journal of the National Cancer Institute, 88*(6), 340–348.

Freudenheim, J. L., & Potischmen, N. (1996). Cancer. In D. A. Krummel & P. M. Kris-Etherton (Eds.), *Nutrition in women's health* (pp. 463–496). Gaithersburg, MD: Aspen.

Gaziano, J. M. & Manson, J. E. (1996). Diet and heart disease: The role of fat, alcohol, and antioxidants. *Cardiology Clinics, 14*(1), 69–83.

Gong, E. J., & Heald, F. P. (1994). Diet, nutrition, and adolescence. In M. E. Shils, J. A. Olsen, & M. Shike (Eds.), *Modern nutrition in health and disease* (8th ed.). Philadelphia: Lea & Febiger.

Gong, E. J., & Spear, B. A. (1988). Adolescent growth and development: Implications for nutritional needs. *Journal of Nutrition Education, 20*(6), 273–278.

Goodrick, G. K., Poston, W. S. C., & Foreyt, J. P. (1996). Methods for voluntary weight loss and control: Update. *Nutrition, 12*, 1–4.

Gortmaker, S. L., Dietz, W. H., Jr., Sobol, A. M., & Wehler, C. A. (1987). Increasing pediatric obesity in the United States. *American Journal of Diseases of Children, 141*(5), 535–540.

Gortmaker, S. L., Must, A., Perrin, J. M., Sobol, A. M., & Dietz, W. H. (1993). Social and economic consequences of overweight in adolescence and young adulthood. *New England Journal of Medicine, 329*(14), 1008–1012.

Haines, P. M., Hungerford, D. W., Popkin, B. M., & Guilkey, D. K. (1992). Eating patterns and energy and nutrient intakes of U. S. women. *Journal of the American Dietetic Association, 92*(6), 698–707.

Hankin, J. H. (1993). Role of nutrition in women's health: Diet and breast cancer. *Journal of the American Dietetic Association, 93*(9), 994–999.

Harris, S. (1995). Helping active women avoid anemia. *Physician and Sportsmedicine, 23*(5), 35–47.

Healy, B. (1995). *A new prescription for women's health.* New York: Viking.

Heaney, R. P. (1996). Osteoporosis. In D. A. Krummel & P. M. Kris-Etherton (Eds.), *Nutrition in women's health* (pp. 418–439). Gaithersburg, MD: Aspen.

Hills-Bonczyk, S. G., Tromiozak, R. R., Avery, M. D., Potter, S., Savik, K., & Duckett, L. J. (1994). Women's experiences with breastfeeding longer than 12 months. *Birth, 21*(4), 206–212.

Hinds, T. S., West, W. L., Knight, E. M., & Harland, B. F. (1996). The effect of caffeine on pregnancy outcome variables. *Nutrition Reviews, 54*(7), 203–207.

Hobbs, F. B. (1997). *U. S. Census Bureau: The official statistics—The elderly population.* http://www.census.gov/population/www/pop-profile/olderpop.html.

King, H., Aubert, R., & Herman, H., (1997). Global burden of diabetes, 1995–2025: Prevalence, numerical estimates and projections. *Diabetes Care, 21*, 1414–1431.

Kjelsberg, M. O., Cutler, J. A., & Dolecek, T. A. (1997). Brief description of the Multiple Risk Factor Intervention Trial. *American Journal of Clinical Nutrition, 65*(Suppl.), 191S–195S.

Larrson, G., Bohlin, A. B., & Tunell, R. (1985). Prospective study of children exposed to variable amounts of alcohol in utero. *Archieves of Disease in Childhood, 60*(4), 16–21.

Lino, M., & Guthrie, J. (1994). The food situation of families maintained by single mothers: expenditures, shopping behavior, and diet quality. *Family Economics Review, 7*(1), 9–20.

Loosli, A. R., & Benson, J. (1990). Nutritional intake in adolescent athletes. *Pediatric Clinics of North America, 37*(5), 1143–1152.

Lowik, M. R. H., Van den Berg, H., Schrivjer, J., Odink, J., Wedel, M., & Van Houten, P. (1992). Marginal nutritional status among institutionalized elderly women as compared to those living more independently (Dutch Nutrition Surveillance System). *Journal of the American College of Nutrition, 11*(6), 673–681.

Lucas, A. R., & Huse, D. M. (1994). Behavioral disorders affecting food intake: Anorexia nervosa and bulimia nervosa. In M. E. Shils, J. A. Olsen, & M. Shike (Eds.), *Modern nutrition in health and disease* (8th ed.). Philadelphia: Lea & Febiger.

McDuffie, J. R., & Kirkley, B. G. (1996). Eating disorders. In D. A. Krummel. & P. M. Kris-Etherton (Eds.), *Nutrition in women's health* (pp. 58–97). Gaithersburg, MD: Aspen.

McGinnis, J. M., & Foege, W. H. (1993). Actual causes of death in the United States. *Journal of the American Medical Association, 270*(18), 2207–2212.

Messina, M., Persky, V., Setchell, K., & Barnes, S. (1994). Soy intake and cancer risk: A review of the in vitro and in vivo data. *Nutrition and Cancer, 21*(2), 113–131.

Mira, M., Stewart, P. M., & Abraham, S. F. (1988). Vitamin and trace element status in premenstrual syndrome. *American Journal of Clinical Nutrition, 47*, 636–641.

Murphy, S. P., Rose, D., Hudes, M., & Viteri, F. E. (1992). Demographic and economic factors associated with dietary quality for adults in the 1987-88 Nationwide Food Consumption Survey. *Journal of the American Dietetic Association, 92*(11), 1352–1357.

National Center for Health Statistics. (1999). *Vital statistics of the United States, 1997.* Vol. 10. *Mortality,* Part A. Washington, DC: Public Health Services.

National Center for Health Statistics. (2000). *Vital statistics of the United States, 1998.* Vol 11. *Mortality,* Part A. Washington, DC: Public Health Services.

National Cholesterol Education Program. (2001). *Third report of the Expert Panel on Detection, Evaluation, and Treatment of High Blood Cholesterol in Adults* (NIH Publication No. 01-3670). Bethesda, MD: National, Heart, Lung, and Blood Institute. National Institutes of Health.

Newcomb, P. A., Storer, B. E., Longnecker, M. P., Mittendorf, R., Greenberg, E. R., Clapp, R., et al. (1994). Lactation and a reduced risk of premenopausal breast cancer. *New England Journal of Medicine, 330*, 81–87.

Notelovitz, M. (1997). Estrogen therapy and osteoporosis: Principles and practice. *American Journal of Medical Science, 313*(1), 2–12.

Olson, C. M. (1994). Promoting positive nutritional practices during pregnancy and lactation. *American Journal of Clinical Nutrition, 59*(Suppl.), 525S–531S.

Palmer, T. A. (1990). Anorexia nervosa, bulimia nervosa: Causal theories and treatment. *Nurse Practitioner, 15*(4), 12–18.

Polivy, J., & Herman, C. P. (1987). Diagnosis and treatment of normal eating. *Journal of Consulting Clinical Psychology, 55*, 635.

Popkin, B. M., Haines, P. S., & Reidy, K. C. (1989). Food consumption trends of U.S. women: Patterns and determinants between 1977 and 1985. *American Society for Clinical Nutrition, 49*, 1307–1319.

Pugliese, M. T., Lifshitz, F., Grad, G., Fort, P., & Marks-Katz, M. (1983). Fear of obesity: A cause of short stature and delayed puberty. *New England Journal of Medicine, 309*(9), 513–518.

Rees, J. M. (1992). Nutrition in adolescence. In S. R. Williams & B. S. Worthington-Roberts (Eds.), *Nutrition throughout the life cycle* (2nd ed.). St. Louis: Mosby.

Report of the National Institutes of Health: Opportunities for research on women's health summary report. (1992). (NIH Publication No. 92-3457A). Washington, DC: U.S. Department of Health and Human Services.

Rohan, T. E., Howe, G. R., Friedenreich, C. M., Jain, M., & Miller, A. B. (1993). Dietary fiber, vitamins A, C, and E, and risk of breast cancer: A cohort study. *Cancer Causes & Control, 4*(1), 29–37.

Sahyoun, N. R., Jacques, P. F., & Russell, R. M. (1996). Carotenoids, vitamins C and E, and mortality in an elderly population. *American Journal of Epidemiology, 144*(5), 501–511.

Sanchez, A., Kissinger, D. G., & Phillips, R. I. (1981). A hypothesis on the etiological role of diet on age of menarche. *Medical Hypotheses, 7*(11), 1339–1345.

Sandstead, H. H. (1994). Understanding zinc: Recent observations and interpretations. *Journal of Laboratory & Clinical Medicine, 124*(3), 322–327.

Satter, E. (1996). Internal regulation and the evolution of normal growth as the basis for prevention of obesity in children. *Journal of the American Dietetic Association, 96*(9), 860–864.

Schlicker, S. A., Borra, S. T., & Regan, C. (1994). The weight and fitness status of United States children. *Nutrition Reviews, 52*(1), 11–17.

Scholl, T. O., Hediger, M. L., Schall, J. I., Khoo, C-S., & Fischer, R. L. (1994). Maternal growth during pregnancy and the competition for nutrients. *American Society for Clinical Nutrition, 60*, 183–188.

Shu, X. O., Zheng, W., Potischman, N., Brinton, L. A., Hatch, M. C., Gao, Y. T., et al. (1993). A population-based case-control study of dietary factors and endometrial cancer in Shanghai, People's Republic of China. *American Journal of Epidemiology, 137*(2), 155–165.

Skinner, J. D., & Carruth, B. R. (1991). Dietary quality of pregnant and nonpregnant adolescents. *Journal of the American Dietetic Association, 91*(6), 718–720.

Smith, A. D. (1996). The female athlete triad: Causes, diagnosis, and treatment. *Physician and Sportsmedicine, 24*(7), 67–86.

Story, M. (1992). Nutritional requirements during adolescence. In E. R. McAnarney, R. E. Kreipe, D. P. Orr, & G. D. Comerci (Eds.), *Textbook of adolescent medicine* (pp. 75–84). Philadelphia: W. B. Saunders.

Story, M., & Alton, A. (1996). Becoming a woman: Nutrition in adolescence. In D. A. Krummel, & P. M. Kris-Etherton (Eds.), *Nutrition in women's health.* Gaithersburg, MD: Aspen.

Story, M., French, S. A., Resnick, M. D., & Blum, R. W. (1995). Ethnic/racial and socioeconomic differences in dieting behaviors and body image perceptions in adolescents. *International Journal of Eating Disorders, 18*(2), 173–179.

Story, M., Rosenwinkel, K., Hirnes, J. H., Resnick, M., Harris, L. J., & Blum, R. V. (1991). Demographic and risk factors associated with chronic dieting in adolescents. *American Journal of Diseases of Children, 145*(9), 994–998.

Stunkard, A. J., Harris, J. R., Pedersen, N. L., & McClearn, G. E. (1990). The body-mass index of twins who have been reared apart. *New England Journal of Medicine, 322*(21), 1483–1487.

Subar, A. F., Heimendinger, J., Patterson, B. H., Krebs-Smith, S. M., Pivonka, E., & Kessler, R. (1991). *5 a day for better health: 1991 5 a day baseline study of America's fruit and vegetable consumption,* Bethesda, MD: National Institutes of Health.

Susser, M., & Stein, Z. (1994). Timing in prenatal nutrition: A reprise of the Dutch famine study. *Nutrition Reviews, 52*(3), 84–94.

Tangney, C. C. (1996). Diet, the menstrual cycle, and sex steroid hormones. In D. A. Krummel & P. M. Kris-Etherton (Eds.), *Nutrition in women's health* (pp. 141–173). Gaithersburg, MD: Aspen.

Tanner, J. M. (1962). *Growth at adolescence* (2nd ed.). Oxford: Blackwell Scientific.

Tanner, J. M. (1987). Issues and advances in adolescent growth and development. *Journal of Adolescent Health Care, 8*, 470–478.

Thomas, J. A., & Call, D. L. (1973). Eating between meals: A nutrition problem among teenagers? *Nutrition Reviews, 31*(5), 137–139.

U.S. Department of Health and Human Services. (1999). *Facts about the women's health initiative.* (NIH Publication No. 99-4074). Washington, DC: Government Printing Office.

U.S. Department of Health and Human Services. (2000). *New CDC report shows teen birth rates continue to drop.* Retrieved July 15, 2001, from *http://www.hhs.gov/news.*

U.S. Senate Special Committee on Aging. (1988). *Aging America: Trends and projections* (1987–88 ed.). Washington, DC: Government Printing Office.

Verhoef, P., Stampfer, M. J., Buring, J. E., Gaziano, J. M., Allen, R. H., Stabler, S. P., et al. (1996). Homocysteine metabolism and risk of myocardial infarction: Relation with vitamins B_6, B_{12}, and folate. *American Journal of Epidemiology, 143*(9), 845–859.

Weltzin, T. E., Fernstrom, M. H., & Kaye, W. H. (1994). Serotonin and bulimia nervosa. *Nutrition Reviews, 52*(12), 399–408.

Werler, M. M., Shapiro, S., & Mitchell, A. A. (1993). Periconceptional folic acid exposure and risk of occurrent neural tube defects. *Journal of the American Medical Association, 269*(10), 1257–1261.

Whiting, S. J. (1994). Safety of some calcium supplements questioned. *Nutrition Reviews, 52*(3), 95–97.

Wichmann, S., & Martin, D. R. (1993). Eating disorders in athletes: Weighing the risks. *Physician and Sportsmedicine, 21*(5), 126–135.

Wilkinson-Enns, C., & Guenther, P. M. (1988). Women's food and nutrient intakes away from home. *Family Economics Review, 1*, 9–12.

World Health Organization. (1997). *World Health Report 1997: Executive summary—Conquering suffering, enriching humanity.* Geneva, Switzerland: Author.

Wright, H. S., Guthrie, H. A., Wang, M. Q., & Bernardo, V. (1991). The 1987–88 Nationwide Food Consumption Survey: An update on the nutrient intake of respondents. *Nutrition Today, 26*, 21–27.

Zhang, Y., Proenca, R., Maffei, M., Barone, M., Leopold, L., & Friedman, J. M. (1994). Positional cloning of the mouse obese gene and its human homologue. *Nature, 372*(6505), 425–432.

RESOURCES

FDA: *www.fda.gov*

American Dietetic Association: *www.eatright.org*

American Society for Nutritional Sciences (ASNS): *www.faseb.org/asns*

National Center for Education in Maternal and Child Health (NCEMCH): *www.ncemch.georgetown.edu*

United States Department of Agriculture (USDA): *www.usda.gov*

Food and Nutrition Information Center (FNIC): *www.nal.usda.gov/fnic*

American Diabetes Association: *www.diabetes.org*

American Heart Association: *www.americanheart.org*

U.S. Department of Health and Human Services. (2000): *Healthy people 2010:* *www.health.gov/healthypeople.*

U.S. Department of Agriculture. (2000): *Nutrition and your health: Dietary guidelines for Americans* (5th ed.; Home and Garden Bulletin No. 232). Washington, DC: Government Printing Office.

Chapter 12

Exercise and Fitness for Women

Erin Miller

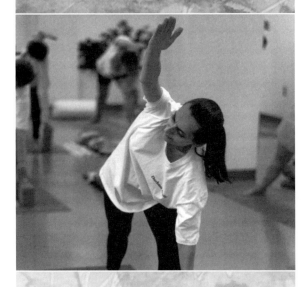

An idealist believes the short run doesn't count. A cynic believes the long run doesn't matter. A realist believes that what is done or left undone in the short run determines the long run.

Sydney J. Harris

INTRODUCTION

According to the International Health, Racquet, & Sportsclub Association (IHRSA), America is the fattest nation on the face of the earth. And in the last 20 years, America has become the fattest nation in civilized history. What does this mean? To begin with, it means that 97 million Americans—55% of American adults—have been classified by the National Institute on Health as carrying so much extra poundage that their weight constitutes a serious threat to their health (McCarthy, Moore, & Howland, 1999). It means that 58 million American adults have now been classified as "clinically obese." As such, they are much more vulnerable to almost every conceivable health problem. Obesity is now killing over 300,000 Americans every year, a crisis of epidemic proportions (McCarthy et al., 1999).

Stress is also becoming a deadly disease in American society. Thirty-eight percent of Americans now state that they "always feel rushed." Some 60% feel that stress is negatively affecting their health, and 78% say that they need to reduce the amount of stress in their lives (McCarthy et al., 1999). Not surprisingly, Americans lead the world in per capita consumption of stress-related medications.

Every day, millions of older Americans become progressively disabled. With each passing year, they lose more and more of their ability to perform such basic functions as walking or getting in and out of a car or chair. Their risk of complete disability, both mental and physical, increases each and every day.

America's health care system is filled with contradictions. For example, millions of Americans are subject to such chronic illnesses as hypertension, arthritis, diabetes, osteoporosis, heart disease, depression, anxiety, and sleep disorders. And yet for all of these conditions, there is an acknowledged, proven, cost-effective therapy—exercise. Sadly, most of the women (and men) who suffer from these conditions lack the confidence, competence, and support needed to use this therapy.

America also spends more on medical care than any other nation in the world. In 1998, Americans spent more than a trillion dollars on health care—almost 15% of the nation's gross national product (GNP) (McCarthy et al., 1999). Whether measured in per capita spending (almost $4000 per person per year) or percentage of GNP, the United States spends 30% to 70% more on medical care than any other industrialized nation in the world (McCarthy et al., 1999). Yet, despite this outlay, America ranks nowhere near the top in the longevity of its citizens, public satisfaction with the nation's health care system, or any basic measure of healthy living.

In many ways, America's health care system is the envy of the Western world. Many of its leading hospitals and leading physicians are justly regarded as world leaders in every branch of medicine. America leads the world in medical research and medical technology. Yet today America's health care system spends 98% to 99% of its resources on diagnosis and treatment—on taking care of people after they become ill—rather than on preventing illness in the first place. Even today, America's primary care physicians receive virtually no training in prevention, health promotion, and health education. Nor are they taught how to motivate patients to take better care of themselves. These physicians, who comprise the front line of American medicine, receive no reward or recognition for helping their patients to live healthier lives.

Dr. C. Everrett Koop, the former U.S. Surgeon General, puts the implication of this failure in the starkest possible terms: "Under America's present health care system you had better take charge of your own health because no one else is going to do it for you."

THE FORCES OF INACTIVITY

America has an educational system that produces more inventors, entrepreneurs, Nobel Prize winners, scientific and literary leaders, and technological breakthroughs than any other country in the world. But it is also an educational system that, year after year, in state after state, has progressively abandoned its commitment to providing daily physical exercise for its girls (and boys) aged 6 to 18. As a result, America's children are now following their parents' example and are becoming the fattest young people on the face of the globe. Today, roughly one in five American children is clinically obese (McCarthy et al., 1999). This percentage increases every decade.

America is the greatest food-producing country in the history of civilization. Its food production and food marketing industries, the most technologically advanced in the world, spend billions of dollars every year relentlessly encouraging Americans to eat more, drink more, and snack every chance they get. This industry invents scores of new foods, new snacks, and new drinks every year. America's restaurants compete to see which can offer the greatest number of helpings, the biggest portions, and the most extensive menus.

America has the largest and most aggressive television industry in the world. Its programming is incessantly marketed in every conceivable medium. Millions of Americans now have between two and five television sets in their homes. Experts predict that Americans will soon choose from as many as 500 television channels, each one luring viewers to settle in, become more sedentary, and lose themselves in lethargy. Americans are the most enthusiastic television viewers in the world. Today, America's children spend 10 times more hours watching television than they spend in all forms of outdoor activity (McCarthy et al., 1999).

America has become the greatest automobile culture in world history. Americans are more dependent on automobiles than any other people on the face of the globe. Millions of American families now have two or three cars to make sure that no one ever has to walk, bike, or make any physical effort beyond turning the ignition key of their car when they want to get somewhere. The entire culture of suburban living is predicated on nonstop car travel. Once daily walking was a normal part of everyday urban or rural life. Now most walking occurs to and from a car.

America invented, and continues to lead, the modern computer industry. With each passing year, more and more Americans spend more and more of their work lives staring into a computer screen. The computer is an enormously positive and productive force in the business and educational life of our society. But it is one more force conspiring to make every American less active with each passing year.

These are the grim array of forces that are facing women of today. Almost every force in society—automobiles, computers, entertainment, food production and consumption—urges Americans to become sedentary and fat. And so here lies the great challenge: To prepare ourselves to resist immense cultural forces which, left to their own devices, threaten to drag the country down into a collective lifestyle consisting of two primary activities: sitting and eating.

PLAN OF ACTION: TO WAGE A WAR AGAINST SEDENTARY LIVING—A 5-STEP PROGRAM

Step I: Get Moving!—The Quantity of Cardiovascular Exercise

The third edition of the American College of Sports Medicine's (ACSM) *Guidelines for Exercise Testing and Prescription* (1998) and the 1990 *ACSM Position Stand on the Quality and Quantity of Exercise* are well accepted as primary sources of recommendations for exercise training programs to develop and maintain physical fitness. The scientific basis for these exercise recommendations is well developed and reviewed extensively in the *ACSM Position Stand*. It has been estimated that approximately 250,000 deaths per year can be attributed to sedentary living habits and that only 22% of adults are sufficiently active to derive the health benefits associated with participation in regular physical activity (ACSM, 1998).

Based on the high prevalence of sedentary living habits and the numerous studies showing reductions in chronic disease associated with increased leisure time, physical activity, and/or cardiorespiratory fitness, the Centers for Disease Control and Prevention (CDC) and the ACSM developed new physical activity recommendations for adults that are intended to complement the exercise prescription guidelines of the ACSM. The essence of the new recommendations is captured in the following excerpt from the report (Phillips, 1999):

Every U.S. adult should accumulate 30 minutes or more of moderate intensity physical activity on most, preferably all, days of the week. This recommendation emphasizes the benefits of moderate intensity and of physical activity that can be accumulated in relatively short bouts. Adults who engage in moderate-intensity [exercise]—i.e., enough to expend approximately 200 calories per day—can expect many of the health benefits described herein.

A discussion of these recommendations must begin by reviewing the operational definitions for several important terms found within the statements. First, the term *physical activity* refers to "any bodily movement produced by skeletal muscles that results in energy expenditure" (ACSM, 1998). *Exercise* is considered a subclass of physical activity and is defined as "planned, structured, and repetitive bodily movement done to improve or maintain one or more components of physical fitness" (ACSM, 1998).

Step II: Get in the Zone—The Quality of Cardiovascular Exercise

Many may ask, "What is moderate-intensity exercise?" The definition of moderate-intensity is a little vague, but, generally, moderate equates to a 3 to 6 metabolic equivalent (MET) intensity range when walking 3 to 4 mph (ACSM, 1998). Light activities are described as requiring less than 3 METs. Heavy or vigorous activities are those requiring more than 6 METs. Clinicians often use METs to describe exercise intensity. A single MET is equivalent to the amount of energy expended during 1 minute of rest (ACSM, 1998). Therefore exercise at a metabolic rate that is five times the resting VO_2 rate is equivalent to 5 METs. In a strict sense, the absolute energy expenditure during exercise at a 5-MET intensity would depend on body size (i.e., a large individual would likely have a large resting VO_2 when compared to a smaller individual). For simplicity, individual differences in resting energy expenditures are often overlooked, and 1 MET is considered equivalent to a VO_2 of 3.5 ml/kg/min (ACSM, 1998). Hence 1 MET represents an energy expenditure of approximately 1.2 kcal/min for a 70-kg person (ACSM, 1998).

A simpler approach to monitoring intensity is to use the *Rate Of Perceived Exertion Scale*. Because it is most often impractical to effectively monitor METs, and formulas used to calculate heart rates are frequently inaccurate because of genetic variability, the Rate of Perceived Exertion Scale can be a much more accurate way to evaluate intensity level.

Using a simplified 1 to 10 scale, with 1 representing no effort (e.g., sitting) and 10 representing exhaustion, those wishing to get a moderate-intensity workout according to the ACSM guidelines will want to exercise so they feel as if their effort is between about 4 and 6. Levels 1 to 3 represent the *Easy Zone*. This is the pace used during warm-up, cool-down, and recovery breaks. You can maintain this pace a long, long time with very little or light effort. Levels 4 to 6 represent the *Endurance Zone*, a moderate, comfortable aerobic pace. You can "endure" this pace for at least 15 to 20 minutes and as long as 60 minutes. You can still talk, but you are not breathless. It is still completely aerobic. Levels 7 to 8 represent the *Endurance Edge*. This level is comfortably hard (athletes would refer to this as thereshold). You can maintain or "endure" this pace for 5 to 8 minutes. You can still talk, but you will need to pause for breaths between phrases. Breathing is harder. It is still primarily aerobic, but a slightly higher percentage of anaerobic metabolism is being used than in the Endurance Zone. Levels 9 to 10 represent the *Elite Zone*. This zone is very intense. It might not feel difficult until you slow down and sense your heart beating hard (i.e., as when you perform the 50-yard dash at 100% effort). You can maintain this pace for only a short time (perhaps a maximum of 2 to 3 minutes). You prefer not to talk, but if you do, you can only comfortably say a few words.

Especially as exercisers are getting to know their own physical limits, cross checking both effort levels and heart rates can be helpful to determine what is best for them. That is particularly true because age-graded maximum heart rate calculations are only estimates, and a participant's heart rate might actually be lower or higher by 10 to 15 beats (Blahnik et al., 2001).

It is important to encourage participants to tune in to how easy or hard the workout feels, then to check their heart rates to see if it corresponds numerically with that perception. Eventually, they will be able to determine which heart rate ranges correspond to Easy, Endurance, Endurance Edge, and Elite zones, and they can fine-tune their workout efforts even more precisely (Greene & Winfred, 1996).

When you exercise at a high rate, your cells respond by using oxygen at a faster rate, and your body burns more calories. If you train your cells to work at this faster rate by exercising intensely on a daily or almost daily basis, then they will continue to burn calories at a higher rate even when you aren't exercising (Kybartas, 1997).

Step III: Strength Training Assessment (Box 12-1)

For many women past age 35, a loss of strength and a lack of vigor are painfully familiar. The main reason most people slow down when they get older is that they lose about a third of their muscle mass between ages 35 and 80 (Nelson, 1998). Aging plays a major role. However, inactivity is also major factor and can be addressed.

The first signs of inactivity are subtle: legs tire more quickly during a brisk walk; briefcases and grocery bags seem heavier. After a few decades, even such simple acts as standing up from a low sofa may become difficult.

Irwin Rosenberg, M.D., director of the Tufts Center on Aging coined a word for the transformation: *sarcopenia*, from the Greek *sarco* for "flesh" or "muscle," and *penia* for "loss" (Nelson, 1998). Unlike heart disease and cancer, sarcopenia does not actually kill. But more than any other single factor, muscle loss is responsible for the frailty and diminished vitality we associate with old age.

Box 12-1 STRENGTH TRAINING ASSESSMENT

- Have you lost strength over the past decade?
- Do you ever say, "I know I should exercise, but I just don't have the energy"?
- At the end of a normally busy day, do you feel tired and worn out?
- Do you notice fat where there used to be muscle?
- Do you feel older than you would like?
- Is it more difficult to maintain your weight, even though you are eating less?
- Are your favorite sports harder and less fun than they used to be?
- Do you look at your female relatives and worry that someday you will be just as limited physically as they are now?

Research has shown that sarcopenia can be prevented to a very great extent, and if the process has begun it can be reversed (Nelson, 1998).

If you've lost strength, you can regain it.

If your energy has sagged, you can raise it.

If you've lost muscle and gained fat, you can reverse it.

If you've become flabby, you can get trim.

If you feel older than you like, you can feel younger, stronger, and more vigorous—perhaps better than you've ever felt in your entire life.

Strength training will result in gains in strength and vitality as well as other healthful outcomes (Draper, 2001).

Strength Training Halts Bone Loss and Even Restores Bone

Each year after menopause, a woman typically loses 1% of her bone mass and even more during the first 5 premenopausal years (Nelson, 1998). Over time, she may develop osteoporosis, a condition in which bones become so porous they easily break. Strength training helps prevent osteoporosis. In a study done by Miriam E. Nelson of the School of Nutrition Science and Policy at Tufts University, the women who didn't exercise lost 2% of their bone density over the year of the study. The women who strength trained not only didn't lose bone, they gained 1% (Nelson, 1998).

Strength Training Improves Balance

The ability to maintain balance also declines with passing years. The change happens so slowly that it may not be noticed until women are in their seventies. Falling, the result of deteriorated balance, is a significant hazard in later life. In Nelson's study (1998), the women who didn't exercise showed an 8.5% decline in balance over the study period. In contrast, the women in the strength training group improved their balancing ability by 14%.

Strength Training Helps to Prevent Bone Fractures

Improvements in strength, bone density, and balance have special significance for women because they dramatically reduce the risk of fractures, a serious problem for older women. A woman of 70 has a 30% risk of breaking her hip if she lives another 20 years (Nelson, 1998).

Hormones, calcium supplements, and medications offer a degree of protection from bone loss. However, strength training not only builds bone, it also reduces the risk of fractures by improving strength and balance to help prevent falls. What's more, all those benefits come without side effects.

Strength Training Energizes

Nelson (1998) also found that the nonexercise group had become 25% less active by the end of the study, and the strength training group had become 27% more active. The stronger you are, the easier it is to move (Nelson, 1998).

As highlighted by the 1996 Surgeon General's Report, physical activity helps decrease disease and disability, improves mental health, and actually increases longevity. Nelson (1998) encourages sedentary women to begin strength training before they attempt cardiovascular activities. She feels that if their muscles are weak, aerobic exercise will be difficult. But after a month or two of strength training, they often find that an aerobic workout has become fun.

Strength Training Trims and Tightens

Although weight loss and body shaping were not goals of Nelson's study, participants were asked to maintain their weight over the year. Although their weight did not change, their appearance did. Instead of dropping pounds, the women who strength trained lost inches.

Strength Training Helps to Control Weight

Gaining muscle not only promotes aerobic activity, which burns calories, but also boosts metabolism. That's because muscle is active tissue and consumes calories; stored fat, on the other hand, is inert and uses very little energy. Unfortunately, dieters often lose muscle along with fat. In a small preliminary study, it was found that women who strength trained while following a weight reduction program maintained muscle as the pounds melted away (Nelson, 1998).

Strength Training Helps Your Heart

Heart disease is the number one killer of women. It is well documented that cardiovascular or aerobic exercise is essential for cardiac health, and now it is known that strength training helps also because it makes the body leaner. The better the muscle-to-fat ratio, the lower the risk of heart disease. Even individuals who already have cardiac problems can benefit from adding strength training exercises.

Patients studied in a cardiac rehabilitation center were divided into two groups; half got the usual care, including a walking program, the others also did strength training three times per week. After 12 weeks, the usual care group was slightly stronger, but those who strength trained showed dramatic increases. Moreover, their aerobic improvement was much greater, even though both groups had followed the same walking program (Nelson, 1998).

Strength Training Relieves Arthritis Symptoms

Women with arthritis not only can lift weights; it actually improves their symptoms (Nelson, 1998). A study was completed with individuals who suffered from moderate to severe rheumatoid arthritis. Although walking and other weight-bearing exercise was painful for them, they were able to strength train, which decreased their pain and improved their range of motion (Nelson, 1998). The program also restored strength and muscle, which is especially important for people with arthritis because often they use muscle-depleting drugs, such as corticosteroids (Nelson, 1998).

Strength Training Treats Depression

Aerobic exercise is an extremely healthy way to boost the spirits, and strength training has been found to have the same effect. A study was conducted to see if strength training could improve mood. All the participants were clinically depressed. Half were assigned to discussion groups; the others did strength training. Since everyone got a lot of supportive attention, they all showed improvement after 3 months (Nelson, 1998); however, the change was significantly greater for those who strength trained. It's unclear if they felt better because they were stronger, or if strength training produced helpful biochemical changes in their brains; most likely it was a combination of both (Nelson, 1998).

Bone Health Over the Life Cycle (Nelson, 1998)

From birth to 25:

Women add more bone than they lose, and bone mass is at its maximum at around age 25.

Age 25 to 35:

If women are healthy they maintain bone density, neither gaining nor losing.

Age 35 to menopause:

Women reach a turning point. For the first time in their lives, they have a natural tendency to lose bone, about half a percent each year. If women don't take measures to prevent it, they will undergo the transformation called osteopenia (*osteo* means "bone" and *penia* means "loss"). It is similar to sarcopenia (muscle loss).

The first 5 years after menopause:

During this short period, unless women do something about it, they will lose 1% to 2% or even more of their bone mass every year. This is the most critical time for preventive measures.

Age 55 to 70:

Bone loss slows down, but women will still lose an average of about 1% per year.

Age 70 and older:

The average rate of loss slows further, to less than half a percent per year. Refer to Chapter 17 for a thorough discussion of osteoporosis. In summary, women lose both bone and muscle mass as a result of the aging process.

Recognizing the need for a well-rounded training program to develop and maintain muscular as well as cardiovascular fitness, the ASCM recommends resistance training at moderate to high intensity sufficient to develop and maintain muscle mass. One set of 8 to 12 repetitions consisting of 8 to 10 exercises with major muscle groups at least 2 days per week is the recommended minimum (ACSM, 1998).

Step IV: Nutrition and Exercise

No exercise program is complete without attention to nutrition. Although nutrition is covered in Chapter 11, here are a few basic guidelines.

Good nutrition, like good training, is simple—learn the basics and practice them consistently.

- Avoid saturated fats, excessive salt, and simple sugars. This eliminates 99% of fast foods, munchies, and soft drinks.
- Eat a basic breakfast of complex carbohydrates, protein, and fat to establish a consistent metabolism for the day and provide fuel and muscle-sustaining ingredients. Protein builds and maintains muscle, and carbohydrates and fat supply fuel for energy. Women need a wholesome meal in the morning or their bodies will draw on their muscle stores as a source of energy, which can result in muscle deficit (Draper, 2001).
- Eat every 2 1/2 to 3 hours throughout the day, each meal consisting of protein, fat, and carbohydrate. Avoid skipping meals!
- Women need a higher intake of protein over carbohydrate to build a leaner body. One way to calculate the minimum number of grams of protein necessary to maintain one's current lean body mass is to multiply bodyweight $\times$ 0.6-0.8.
- Avoid between-meal snacking. Snacks should not become a substitute for a complete meal.
- Simple carbohydrates (e.g., sugar, honey, soft drinks, candy, and cake) provide a quick energy pickup but the energy level drops just as quickly. Excessive sugar may result in variability in insulin metabolism, leading to fatigue, poor performance, and fat storage.
- Eat before and after a workout. Eat a small, easily digested meal about an hour before exercise. With protein and carbohydrate in their system, women will be able to exercise longer and with more enthusiasm. Similarly, women need to eat a meal within 45 minutes to an hour after exercise, particularly if they have been doing intense strength training, to provide the muscle-building materials (protein and carbohydrates) to repair depleted tissue and begin the process of building new muscle.
- The most important body ingredient is plain water. The quality of body tissues, their performance, and their resistance to fatigue are absolutely dependent on the quality and quantity of the water consumed. Women should consume 8 to 10 12-ounce glasses of water per day (approximately one half gallon).
- Sleep, rest, and relaxation are of prime importance. It is during periods of sound sleep that the body recuperates and builds muscle tissue.
- Women need to be educated about the concept of weight. It is the ratio of lean body mass (bones, internal organs, and muscle) to fat that counts. Women should be instructed to weigh themselves only once a week, on the same day. Weight will fluctuate from day to day largely on the basis of the amount of water that's in their system.

A healthy diet and exercise complement each other. They work synergistically to promote a healthy lifestyle. Exercise increases metabolism and burns more calories. When women are fit, their bodies utilize nutrients more effectively.

Step V: The Five Stages of Change

There are five stages of change that women pass through as they adopt an exercise regimen: precontemplation, contemplation, preparation, action, and maintenance. In the precontemplation stage, women don't know anything about the value of exercise and need information about its health benefits. Women in the contemplation stage want to begin an exercise program, but need information on how to get started. The preparation stage is when women have already decided to start an exercise program and need assistance with the concrete steps specifically related to the program they selected. Women in the action stage are in the first 6 months of the exercise program, and they need assistance to measure their progress and stay motivated. The maintenance stage is when exercise has become a routine part of their lives. Women during this stage often feel an incredible sense of empowerment and spiritual well-being. They've accomplished something important for themselves.

Women struggle to start and maintain an exercise program for themselves. It often requires significant planning and commitment. Box 12-2 contains suggestions for planning an exercise program and Box 12-3 has guidelines for maintaining an exercise program. Table 12-1 is a summary of exercise recommendations across the lifespan.

Box 12-2 SUGGESTIONS FOR BEGINNING AN EXERCISE PROGRAM

- Write down all the reasons why you want or need to exercise.
- Make a list of the equipment you will need.
- Get out the phone book and write down places to shop. Plan a time to buy the equipment and put it on your calendar.
- Check your schedule. Decide what days of the week and what times you want to exercise. Write the appointments on your calendar.
- If you want to exercise with a friend, decide when you are going to call and write it on your calendar.
- Make any necessary arrangements to clear your workout times. For instance, if you need to discuss child care with your husband, give yourself a deadline for doing it.
- Finally, keep all of your appointments.

Box 12-3 SUGGESTIONS FOR MAINTAINING AN EXERCISE PROGRAM

- *Keep Fitness Logs*—Studies have shown that if you record your progress in a fitness program, you are much more likely to be successful.
- *Enjoy Your Workouts*—Many women take pleasure from the pure sensation of lifting weights. Keep it fresh. Always look for new ways to enjoy yourself while exercising.
- *Work Out with a Friend or Form a Group*—Having an exercise partner is the next best thing to having a personal trainer. It gives you the structure of a regular schedule and a commitment to someone else.

Table **12-1**	**SUMMARY EXERCISE RECOMMENDATIONS FOR WOMEN ACROSS THE LIFESPAN**		
LIFE STAGE	**DEFINITION**	**EXERCISE RECOMMENDATIONS**	**TYPE OF EXERCISE**
Adolescence	6 years following puberty	3 or more sessions per week of activities that last 20 minutes or more at moderate to vigorous levels of exertion 2-3 days a week of light resistance strength training, high repetitions per set (no less than 6-8 reps per set) Avoid heavy weight training, power lifting, or bodybuilding at this age	Walking Jogging Stair climbing Basketball Racquet sports Cycling Strength (resistance) training Flexibility training
Adulthood Early Middle Late	 20-29 years 30-44 years 45-64 years	30 minutes or more of moderate-intensity physical activity on most, preferably all, days of the week (enough to expend approximately 200 calories per day)	Walking Jogging Cycling Weight training Racquet sports Stair climbing Dance Swimming Strenuous housework Cross-country skiing
Pregnancy	Refer to Chapter 16	Refer to Chapter 16	Refer to Chapter 16
Senescence Elderly Older Elderly Very Old	 65-74 years 75-84 years 85 years and older	Emphasis on increased frequency vs. duration (5-7 days per week) 20-40 minutes per session, may need to shorten duration (10-15 minutes) repeated 2-3 times a day Low to moderate intensity levels	Minimal or non-weightbearing, low-impact activities, such as cycling, swimming, chair, and floor exercises Walking Stretching Strengthening (moderate resistance)

Im (2001) in her review of research on physical activity in women found that three major problematic themes emerged from the analysis: (1) no consideration of women's own experiences, (2) implicit androgenic and ethnocentric assumptions, and (3) no meaningful interaction for the women. All of these themes need to be avoided in designing exercise programs for women.

In order for women to be successful in long-term exercise and fitness programs, the programs must be designed to be personalized for each women, taking into consideration her own personal experiences, her needs for interaction and feedback, and her perception of fitness from her own feminine and cultural context.

SUMMARY

American women have become increasingly sedentary, which has resulted in high rates of obesity and the negative health outcomes associated with it. As women age, muscle mass and bone mass decrease, which increases their risk for falls, fractures, and the negative health outcomes associated with them. Exercise and fitness can prevent and reverse these problems. This chapter described a five-step plan for women across the lifespan to develop an exercise fitness program that will improve their health and ultimately may save their lives.

REFERENCES

American College of Sports Medicine. (1998). *ACSM's resource manual for guidelines for exercise testing and prescription* (3rd ed.). Baltimore: Williams & Wilkins.

Blahnik, J., Kolovou, T., McHugh, L., Glick, R., Mylreq, M., Sheron, A., et al. (2001). *Precision cycling instructor training manual.* Irvine, CA: Star Trac.

Draper, D. (2001). *Brother iron, sister steel.* Aptos, CA: On Target Publishing.

Greene, B., & Winfrey, O. (1996). *Make the connection.* New York: Hyperion.

Harris, S. J., & Bakshian, A. (1995). *American speaker's 100 best quotes for 1996.* Washington, DC: Georgetown Publishing House.

Im, E. (2001). Nursing research on physical activity: a feminist critique. *International Journal of Nursing Studies, 38*(2), 185–194.

Kybartas, R. (1997). *Fitness is religion.* New York: Simon & Schuster.

McCarthy, J., Moone, D., & Howland, B. (1999). *50 million members by 2010.* San Francisco: The Publication Group.

Nelson, N. E. (1998). *Strong women stay young,* New York: Bantam Books.

Phillips, B. (1999). *Body for life.* New York: HarperCollins Publishers.

RESOURCES

Associations

American College Of Sports Medicine
P.O. Box
Indianapolis, IN 46206-1440
(317) 637-9200

American Heart Association
7272 Greenville Ave.
Dallas, TX 75231-4599
(800) AHA-USA1

American Hiking Association
1015 31st Street NW
Washington, DC 20007
(703) 385-3242

Bicycle Federation of America
1818 R Street NW
Washington, DC 20009
(202) 332-6986

Institute For Aerobics Research
12330 Preston Road
Dallas, TX 75230
(800) 527-0362

The Melpomene Institute for Women's Health Research
1010 University Avenue
St. Paul, MN 55104
(612) 642-1952

National Association for Sport and Physical
  Education
1900 Association Drive
Reston, VA 22091
(703) 476-3410

National Handicapped Sports
451 Hungerford Drive, Suite 100
Rockville, MD 20850
(301) 217-0960

National Women's Health Resource Center
5514 10th Street NW
Washington, DC 20004
(202) 628-7814

President's Council on Physical Fitness and
  Sports
Department of Health and Human Services
450 5th Street NW
Washington, DC 20001
(202) 272-3421

Information on the Internet

American College of Sports Medicine
www.1ww.com/acsmcrc
(800) 486-5643

AFPA—American Fitness Professionals and
  Associates
www.afpafitness.com
(800) 494-7782

American Council On Exercise
www.acefitness.org
(858) 535-8227

Aquatic Fitness Professionals
www.aquacert.org
(303) 621-2931

C.H.E.K. Institute
www.chekinstitute.com
(800) 552-8789

Creative Health Products
www.chponline.com
(800) 287-5901

International Council on Active Aging
(866) 335-9777
www.icaa.cc

Women's Exercise Research Center
www.gwu.edu/~exci/werc.html

Women's Sport and Fitness
www.women.com/body/wsf/canemail.html

Chapter 13

Immunization

Karen C. Smith

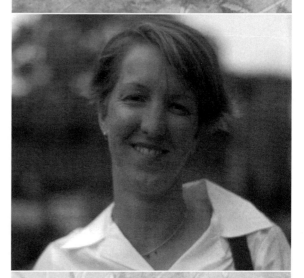

Sustained laughter stimulates an increased release of endorphins -the body's own natural morphine. We feel better when we laugh because endorphins actually diminish physical and psychological pain. Endorphins also stimulate the body's immune system to increase its disease-fighting ability.

Adapted from Norman Cousins

INTRODUCTION

Women are exposed to vaccine-preventable diseases throughout their lifetimes. Comprehensive women's health care involves the use of immunization within health prevention programs. Immunizations traditionally receive a lot of well-deserved attention during childhood years but may not be used consistently in adults. There is now enhanced interest in adult vaccines because of increasing evidence documenting their efficacy and because new products are available for use. Recommendations for some of the standard immunizations continue to evolve. New and appropriate emphasis is being given to the role of preventive health in managed care as well as in traditional provider settings. Furthermore, immunization rates are now being followed as quality assurance indicators in the outpatient setting.

Substantial opportunities exist to improve compliance with current immunization recommendations. Unfortunately, the rates for both giving and documenting adult immunizations on an appropriate schedule are poorer than expected. Lewis (1988) published results from surveys done to assess utilization of routine immunizations in adults. The compliance rate for adult diphtheria-tetanus (Td) boosters was under 24% (Lewis, 1988). The Centers for Disease Control and Prevention (CDC) reported influenza vaccination rates in those age 65 or older were estimated to be 33% in 1989, rising to 63% plus in 1997 (Centers for Disease Control and Prevention, 2000d). Use of influenza vaccines in targeted individuals *under* age 65 remained below 30% in 1993 and 1997 (Centers for Disease Control and Prevention, 1996c; Centers for Disease Control and Prevention, 2000d). Immunization rates in health care workers (targeted to receive vaccine to reduce the likelihood of exposing high-risk persons in the health care setting) remained low at 34% in 1997. Pneumococcal immunization rates increased only from 15% to 28% between the years 1989 and 1993 in those over age 65 (Centers for Disease Control and Prevention, 1995c).

Nursing roles increasingly include surveying women's prior immunization records, counseling patients about their current and future immunization needs, and adequately documenting vaccines given (Kottke, Brekke, & Solberg, 1993). The need for documentation goes beyond keeping a simple record. That the information be stored in a retrievable, highly visible portion of the medical chart (such as a lifetime immunization record page) for future reference is imperative. Adolescents and adults may benefit from clearly defined periodic health examinations to update immunizations and to coordinate other preventive care (McGinnis & Griffith, 1996). A visit when the patient is an adolescent may serve to update the Td booster and provide varicella, MMR (measles, mumps, and rubella), and hepatitis B vaccinations, if indicated, and to address some of the psychosocial changes at that phase of life (Centers for Disease Control and Prevention, 1996a). Likewise, a screening visit at age 50 provides an opportunity to update a Td booster, if needed, to initiate annual influenza vaccinations, and to assess the need for early pneumococcal immunization (indicated in about one third of women at that age because of chronic medical problems). Colon cancer screening tests commonly are initiated at that age, and a reassessment of cardiovascular risk factors is also appropriate. At age 65, initiation or update of the pneumococcal vaccine may be combined with a geriatrics needs evaluation and Td booster if due (Centers for Disease Control and Prevention, 1995a; Task Force on Adult Immunization, 1994a). The criteria used to identify vaccine recipients and vaccine schedules and doses are listed in Boxes 13-1 and 13-2.

DIPHTHERIA AND TETANUS

Tetanus continues to occur in the United States, and, in 1989 and 1990, 117 cases were reported to the CDC. In 24% of cases the outcome was fatal. Adequate tetanus immunization prevents disease, and universal immunization is recommended. Special target groups include individuals not likely to have received primary immunization and the elderly because immunity may wane with age. The cost of hospitalization care for a single episode of tetanus may approximate the cost of administering 50,000 doses of Td vaccine (Centers for Disease Control and Prevention, 1994b).

Use of the diphtheria vaccine conjugated with tetanus in adult and pediatric preparations has effectively eliminated respiratory diphtheria from the United States (Task Force on Adult Immunization, 1994b). Fewer than five cases a year are reported now. Diphtheria is on the rise in some Third World nations, including parts of the former Soviet Union. The New Independent States of the former Soviet Union reported

Box 13-1 DOSES AND ROUTES OF ADMINISTRATION FOR VACCINES

Td: For primary immunizations, two initial doses of 0.5 mL are given intramuscularly (IM), 4 to 8 weeks apart, and a booster is given 6 to 12 months after the second vaccine.

Influenza: The dose is 0.5 mL, given IM.

Pneumococcal vaccine: The dose is 0.5 mL, given IM or subcutaneously.

Hepatitis B:

■ *Adults*

The vaccine dose (of any of the three preparations) is 1.0 mL and should be administered into the deltoid muscle. The two vaccines (10 μg of Recombivax HB [Merck, Sharp, and Dohme] or 20 μg of Engerix-B [SmithKline Beecham]) are given in three doses, with the first two administered 4 weeks apart and the last received at 6 months. New Jersey USA Engerix-B also may be given in a rapid series of three doses on initiation and at 1 and 2 months with excellent short-term immunity, but a fourth dose then is indicated at 12 months. For postexposure protection, 0.06 mL/kg (up to 5 mL) of hepatitis B immune globulin is given with the first dose of vaccine.

■ *Adolescents*

Recombivax (11 to 15 years) is given as two 1.0-mL (10 μg) doses IM, 4 to 6 months apart, or as three 0.5-mL (5 μg) doses IM on initiation and at 1 and 2 months. Engerix-B (11 to 19 years) is given as 0.5 mL (10 μg) on initiation and at 1 and 6 months, or the adult dose 1.0 mL (20 μg) if given in the rapid series four-dose sequence (see the description for adults).

Hepatitis A: The dose is 1.0 mL IM. If a booster dose is desired for long-term immunity, a single booster is given 6 months after the injection.

Varicella: In adults, this vaccine is given in two doses (0.5 mL subcutaneously), 1 to 2 months apart.

MMR: The dose of the combination vaccine is 0.5 mL, given subcutaneously.

Box 13-2 TARGET POPULATIONS FOR INFLUENZA VACCINE

■ Adults over age 50

■ Residents of nursing homes and any other long-term care facilities (including adult day-care centers) where persons with chronic medical conditions reside

■ Individuals requiring hospitalization or medical treatment for chronic metabolic conditions, including diabetes mellitus, chronic renal disease, hemoglobinopathies, or immunosuppression such as that induced by human immunodeficiency virus infection, malignancy, or medication (e.g., chemotherapy or prednisone)

■ Individuals with chronic cardiovascular compromise or chronic pulmonary disorders, including asthma

■ Individuals who may transmit influenza to persons at high risk of disease or complications, including health care workers, employees of chronic-care facilities, household members, or caregivers of persons at high risk

■ Pregnant women in their second or third trimester during flu season or women who are in their first postpartum months during flu season

■ Adolescents (up to 18 years) who take chronic or intermittent aspirin therapy for chronic diseases to avoid Reye syndrome

■ General population: Any person who desires the vaccine to prevent illness or time off work may be immunized, unless contraindicated

Source: Centers for Disease Control and Prevention. (2000d). Prevention and control of influenza. *Morbidity and Mortality Weekly Report, 49* (RR-3), 1–38.

more than 50,000 cases in 1995 (Centers for Disease Control and Prevention, 1995b). Travelers should be certain their immunization status is up to date. In adults the Td adsorbed vaccine is used. Thereafter, Td boosters are given every 10 years. Providing a final, single Td booster at age 50 or 65 may be adequate, if a primary series including a booster in late adolescence or early adulthood has been completed. For protection against tetanus after wounds or burns, a Td vaccine should be administered if a vaccination cannot be documented within the prior 10 years. If the wound is deep and dirty, a booster should be provided if none can be documented within the previous 5 years. If prior vaccination is remote or incomplete, a Td vaccine should be given with tetanus immune globulin for passive immunization. If the wounded individual has never received tetanus immunization, tetanus immune globulin should be given and a Td vaccine series should be initiated concurrently (Task Force on Adult Immunization, 1994b; U.S. Preventive Services Task Force, 1994). Table 13-1 gives a lifespan immunization summary for women.

A history of neurological or immediate hypersensitivity reaction is a contraindication to subsequent vaccination. Although complications are not reported, women probably should not receive the vaccine in the first trimester of pregnancy unless it is necessary

Table 13-1 LIFESPAN IMMUNIZATION SUMMARY FOR WOMEN

VACCINATION	ADOLESCENCE	CHILDBEARING YEARS	AGE 50	AGE 65
Td	Booster every 10 years (see text)	Booster every 10 years (see text)	Booster every 10 years (see text)	Booster every 10 years (see text)
MMR	Update if needed	Update if needed	Not applicable	Not applicable
Varicella	Evaluate for likely immunity and need for vaccine	Evaluate for likely immunity and need for vaccine	Not applicable	Not applicable
Influenza	Immunize high-risk adolescents yearly (see text)	Immunize high-risk females yearly (see text)	Annual vaccine	Annual vaccine
Pneumococcal	Immunize high-risk adolescents (see text)	Immunize high-risk females (see text)	Immunize high-risk females (see text)	Single vaccine or booster
Hepatitis B	Universal immunization	Immunize high-risk adults (see text)	Immunize high-risk adults (see text)	Immunize high-risk adults (see text)
Hepatitis A	Immunize high-risk adolescents (see text)	Immunize high-risk adults (see text)	Immunize high-risk adults (see text)	Immunize high-risk adults (see text)

for wound prophylaxis. History of a severe local (Arthus-type) reaction is not an absolute contraindication, but such individuals should not receive boosters before 10 years have elapsed. Tetanus vaccine alone is available, if preferred, for wound prophylaxis (Task Force on Adult Immunization, 1994b).

INFLUENZA

Epidemic influenza occurs nearly annually in the winter and is responsible for 20,000 deaths per year in the United States. Pneumonia and influenza together rank high as a cause of death in the United States, the sixth leading cause in 1993 (Centers for Disease Control and Prevention, 1995d). An overall increase in the number of pneumonia and influenza deaths between 1979 and 1992 occurred because of an increase in the population more than 65 years of age in that interval. Eighty percent to 90% of excess deaths caused by pneumonia and influenza affect persons older than age 65. Approximately 10,000 to 50,000 excess deaths attributable to influenza alone occur during flu epidemic years. The calculations of Medicare showed the annual cost of influenza-related care during epidemic years to be *$750 million to $1 billion* (Centers for Disease Control and Prevention, 1994a). Efficacy of the vaccine for reducing hospitalization was demonstrated in the Medicare Influenza Vaccine Demonstration Project (Centers for Disease Control and Prevention, 1993). Efficacy of the vaccine against infuenza for healthy working adults was shown to provide health-related and economic benefits (Nichol et al., 1995). Immunization protection from disease is 50% to 60% in the elderly (perhaps as low as 30% to 40% in frail elderly). Immunization is 80% effective in preventing *death* from influenza. In 1991 the U.S. Public Health Service set a goal of a 60% immunization rate by the year 2000 for influenza and pneumococcal vaccine for those in high-risk categories, including individuals older than 65 (Centers for Disease Control and Prevention, 1995e; Centers for Disease Control and Prevention, 1997b).

Newly formulated vaccines are available each year in late September or early October. The vaccine consists of one B strain and two A strains of influenza. The A strains represent the two most prevalent antigen types, H1N1 and H3N2. *H* and *N* refer to the surface antigens *hemagglutinin* and *neuraminidase*. The viral strains are grown in eggs, and the actual vaccines are composed of inactivated virus or virus subparticles. The vaccine is protective within 2 weeks after administration. The recommended vaccination period is generally early October to mid-November (Centers for Disease Control and Prevention, 1996c; Task Force on Adult Immunization, 1994b; U.S. Preventive Services Task Force, 1994). The CDC now advocates scheduling any large organized vaccine campaigns for late October through November of each season. Relying on earlier dates may not be feasible because of unpredictable supplies of effective vaccine early in the year.

As of the 2000 to 2001 influenza season, the CDC lowered the age recommended for universal immunization from 65 to 50. The rationale was based on several observations. First, surveys indicated that immunization rates rose when specific age groups were targeted. This had not been true when only disease groups (such as diabetes or asthma) were targeted as high-risk conditions for vaccine administration. In fact, immunization rates of individuals ages 50 to 64 with specific medical indications for receiving influenza vaccine remained flat at 40% to 41% in the late 1990s. Second, at least 30% of persons over age 50 already had a medical indication for vaccination. Third, data indicate that immunizing large groups of persons against influenza reduces work absenteeism and the number of individuals who may expose an at-risk population to influenza.

Contraindications to vaccine use are straightforward. Individuals known to have an anaphylactic reaction to chicken feathers, eggs, or other vaccine components should not receive influenza vaccination (desensitization may be considered in rare instances). The vaccine should not be given to those with serious febrile illness. Minor infections, however, even with low-grade fevers, are not an indication to withhold the vaccine. Side effects are uncommon and include fever, malaise, or myalgia (constitutional symptoms) occurring 6 to 12 hours after injection and lasting 1 to 2 days. Other complications of the vaccine include soreness at the site, for up to 48 hours, and rare immediate hypersensitivity. Guillain-Barré syndrome no longer is associated statistically with influenza vaccines; the rate of occurrence is felt to be 1 in 100,000 and possibly only coincidentally (Centers for Disease Control and Prevention, 2000d; Task Force on Adult Immunization, 1994b; U.S. Preventive Services Task Force, 1994).

PNEUMOCOCCAL VACCINE

Streptococcus pneumoniae is the most commonly isolated pathogen in community-acquired pneumonias (CAPs). CAPs cost the United States $10 billion a year. Ninety percent of that cost is for inpatient care. Four billion dollars of the CAPs expense may be attributed directly to identified episodes of streptococcal pneumonia infections. This organism is a likely pathogen in many more cases of CAPs where the causative agent is not isolated (Chenoweth, Saint, Martinez, Lynch, & Fendrick, 2000). The number of annual pneumococcal infections is high: 500,000 cases of pneumonia, 50,000 cases of bacteremia, and 3000 cases of meningitis. Pneumococcal infections cause approximately 40,000 deaths annually (Centers for Disease Control and Prevention, 1997a; Task Force on Adult Immunization, 1994b). Vaccine efficacy has been difficult to demonstrate in smaller studies, but case control analyses have shown 56% to 80% protection against infection. The 23-valent vaccine protects against the pneumococcal serotypes that cause nearly 90% of the infections in the United States. Data suggest that those with severe immunodeficiencies are less likely than healthy adults or patients with chronic medical conditions to develop immunity after a single dose of vaccine. Newer recommendations to repeat boosters in certain individuals may partially offset the lower protection rate in the immunocompromised (Centers for Disease Control and Prevention, 1997a).

The current vaccine contains purified capsular materials of 23 serotypes of *S. pneumoniae.* That the standard adult vaccine is *not* interchangeable with a new 7-valent pneumococcal protein conjugate vaccine now offered to infants and young children is important to emphasize. Table 13-1 and Box 13-3 give indications for use and dosing information for the pneumococcal vaccine. Guideline changes as of 1997 add indications for a booster dose in certain recipients of this vaccine. Adolescent and adult women with severe immunosuppression (Box 13-3) should receive *one* booster at least 5 years after the first dose (Centers for Disease Control and Prevention, 1997a). Adults aged 65 or older who had an initial pneumococcal vaccine before age 65 should receive *one* booster after 5 years have elapsed.

No real contraindications to using the pneumococcal vaccine exist. Some minor local reactions have occurred at injection sites, and Arthus-type reactions have occurred with second immunizations, especially if given within 6 years of the first. Anaphylactic reactions occur in previously unimmunized individuals in five out of a million recipients. The rate is no higher in previously vaccinated persons when the second dose is given at least 5 years after the first (Centers for Disease Control and Prevention, 1997a; Task Force on Adult Immunization, 1994b).

HEPATITIS B

The CDC estimates a 5% lifetime risk of contracting hepatitis B in the United States (Centers for Disease Control and Prevention, 1995f; Task Force on Adult Immunization, 1994b). The overall hepatitis B vaccine efficacy is 85% to 90%. Universal immunization at an early age is now the national goal for eliminating most of the 200,000 to 300,000 cases that occur each year. An estimated 15,000 hospitalizations for acute infection and several hundred deaths from acute fulminant hepatitis occur each year; 5% to 10% of infected adults become chronic carriers. Chronic active hepatitis may occur in up to 25% of the carriers, leading to increased risk of premature death from cirrhosis or liver cancer. One million to 1.25 million carriers are now present in the United States and serve as the major reservoir for transmitting infection to others, mostly via intravenous or sexual routes (Centers for Disease Control and Prevention, 1995f; Task Force on Adult Immunization, 1994b; U.S. Preventive Services Task Force, 1994).

Box 13-3 TARGET POPULATIONS FOR PNEUMOCOCCAL VACCINE

- Adults over age 65
- Younger adults with chronic cardiac or pulmonary disease
- Adults of any age with the following or other significant immunosuppressive diseases: sickle cell anemia, lymphoma or other hematological malignancies, asplenia, diabetes mellitus, alcoholism, chronic liver disease (especially cirrhosis), chronic renal disease (specifically nephrotic syndrome or dialysis-dependent), and human immunodeficiency virus infection
- Residents of chronic-care facilities at high risk of infection or complications

Source: Centers for Disease Control and Prevention. (1997a). Prevention of pneumococcal disease: Recommendation of the ACIP. *Morbidity and Mortality Weekly Report, 46*(RR-8), 1–24.

The current vaccines are genetically engineered recombinant preparations. Vaccine efficacy after three doses approximates 95% in healthy adults under age 30. The vaccine is somewhat less effective in adults over age 30, obese individuals, smokers, and those with human immunodeficiency virus infections. Passive immunization (after suspected exposure to virus) is only reliably accomplished by hepatitis B immune globulin (HBIG). By contrast, serum immune globulin (gamma globulin) has less than one hundredth of the anti–hepatitis B surface antibody titer that is in HBIG and is not considered effective. In adults a three-dose vaccine schedule is recommended. The Advisory Committee on Immunization Practices approved an alternate immunization schedule for adolescents in the 11- to 15-year age range as of February 2000. Studies demonstrated that the new two-dose schedule provided equal efficacy to the standard three-dose course with the Recombivax HB formulation. One should note that each dose of the two-injection regimen contains twice the volume and antigen compared with the original three-injection regimen. With either vaccination schedule, reinitiating the series is not necessary if boosters are provided later than the recommended dates. If an adolescent has begun the three-dose series, she should complete that series rather than switch to two doses (Centers for Disease Control and Prevention, 2000c). Table 13-1 and Box 13-4 provide more information. If long-term immunity is important because of occupational or social factors, testing for hepatitis B surface antibody should be performed 6 months after the final dose of vaccine. If follow-up titers are negative, up to three additional boosters may be provided at 1- to 2-month intervals, with assessment of immunity done after each dose. Some of the nonresponders may have subclinical immunity; however, providing HBIG to such persons after any exposure is wise. No definite contraindications are known, and no reports of serious side effects from the vaccine or HBIG have been made. The minor adverse effects noted after hepatitis B vaccine mostly are limited to site soreness or malaise (rare). Occasionally a minor rash develops after HBIG injection (Task Force on Adult Immunization, 1994b).

Box 13-4 TARGET POPULATIONS FOR HEPATITIS B VACCINE

1. Adolescents (age 12 or older) who did not receive earlier immunization
2. Adults
   a. Women at risk from occupational exposure, including dental and health care workers and women at risk of body-fluid exposure (e.g., police officers)
   b. Lifestyle-exposure risk groups, including intravenous drug users, homosexual males, heterosexuals with a pattern of many partners (defined as two or more within the preceding 6 months) or those who acquire a sexually transmitted disease
   c. Environmental risk groups, including household members of individuals with hepatitis B (acute or carrier state), clients and staff of facilities caring for developmentally disabled persons, prison staff and inmates, and travelers to high-risk areas if exposure is considered possible
   d. Women receiving blood-product transfusions frequently or undergoing hemodialysis

Source: Centers for Disease Control and Prevention. (1995f). Update: Recommendations to prevent hepatitis B virus transmission–United States. *Morbidity and Mortality Weekly Report, 44*, 574–575.

HEPATITIS A

Hepatitis A is an RNA virus transmitted by the fecal-oral route, in contrast to hepatitis B and C, which are transmitted by sexual or parental exposure to infected products, including blood. Morbidity and mortality caused by hepatitis A are substantial. From 75,000 to 125,000 cases are reported each year in the United States, with 100 deaths and a cost of $200 million (Gardner et al., 1996). Risk of hepatitis A is certainly greater to travelers to foreign countries where hepatitis A is endemic. Vaccination provides long-term protection and is appropriate for prophylaxis when visits to these areas are frequent. Passive immunization for travelers who need only short-term protection for a rare trip may be achieved less expensively with serum immune globulin. Current availability of serum immune globulin varies, however, and hepatitis A vaccination of all travelers going to areas at risk is normal.

Certain women in the United States may be at risk of acquiring or experiencing complications from hepatitis A. These women should be offered the two-injection series of hepatitis A vaccine. Prior infection with hepatitis A confers immunity. The antibody status may be evaluated, if desired, before offering the vaccine. In aggregate, 33% of U.S. citizens have immunity to hepatitis A, and this may be determined by drawing a total or gamma globulin (not immunoglobulin M) antibody level to hepatitis A. The age-specific prevalence of immunity in adults is 18% in those ages 20 to 29, 49% in those ages 40 to 49, and 75% in those over age 75 (Centers for Disease Control and Prevention, 1996d). Table 13-1 and Box 13-5 provide more details.

A single injection of vaccine produces 80% to 90% immunity within 15 days and 96% immunity after 30 days. If a booster dose is given 6 to 12 months after the initial dose, seroconversion rates are virtually 100% (Centers for Disease Control and Prevention, 1996d; Innis et al., 1994). Side effects are minimal. This vaccine should be avoided if a person has a known allergy to alum or, in the case of the Havrix preparation, to 2-phenoxyethanol or if a person has a history of hypersensitivity to the first dose, in the setting of a concurrent severe acute illness, or in pregnancy (no data regarding safety exists) (Centers for Disease Control and Prevention, 1996d; Innis et al., 1994).

Box 13-5 TARGET POPULATIONS FOR HEPATITIS A VACCINE

- Certain travelers (see the text) and individuals who live in endemic areas
- Adolescent or adult women who have chronic liver disease or have occupational risks of exposure (mostly laboratory workers who handle fecal specimens) and intravenous drug users

Source: Centers for Disease Control and Prevention. (1996d). Prevention of hepatitis A through active or passive immunization. *Morbidity and Mortality Weekly Report, 45*(RR-15), 1–30. Innis, B. L., Snitbhan, R., Kinasol, P., Laorakpongse, T., Poopatanakool, W., Kosik, C. A., et al. (1994). Protection against hepatitis A by an inactivated vaccine. *Journal of the American Medical Association, 271,* 1328–1334.

VARICELLA

Varicella vaccine has been available for widespread use since 1996. The niche for this vaccine is predominantly in pediatric and adolescent populations. Young adult women also should consider receiving this new vaccine if they are not immune. More than 90% of adult women already are immune to varicella-zoster virus. A clinical history of prior infection is adequate evidence of immunity in most cases where risk of exposure is small. More than 70% of adults who are unsure of their immunity status are seropositive for varicella-zoster virus on testing (Centers for Disease Control and Prevention, 1996e). The CDC concludes that testing for immunity in adult candidates for the vaccine before offering the immunization is cost-effective (Varicella Vaccine, 1995). Table 13-1 and Box 13-6 give specific recommendations.

Susceptible women are defined as those without a history of varicella infection or those who lack antibody titers demonstrating immunity. The vaccine may have a use in a postexposure setting, if given within 72 hours of exposure. The vaccine is a live attenuated virus and so must not be given to immunocompromised or pregnant women or to women likely to become pregnant within a month after administration. Side effects to the vaccine include fever within 6 weeks after injection or local symptoms such as tenderness, swelling, or erythema in 25% to 33% of women and local or diffuse rash in up to 8% of women. The evidence is not consistent that the vaccine can precipitate outbreaks of zoster. Seroconversion is 78% after one dose in adolescents and adults and 99% after two doses. Prolonged immunity without booster doses is unknown. A history of anaphylaxis to neomycin or gelatin (both of which are included in the vaccine preparation in minute amounts) is a contraindication to vaccine use. The varicella-zoster vaccine has not been studied in the setting of human immunodeficiency virus infection. Adolescents should avoid salicylates for 6 weeks after immunization because of a theoretical risk of acquiring Reye syndrome after the varicella vaccine (Centers for Disease Control and Prevention, 1996a; Varicella Vaccine, 1995).

MEASLES, MUMPS, AND RUBELLA

Measles, mumps, and rubella (German measles) continue to occur in adolescents and adults in the United States. In 1995 the CDC reported 128 cases of rubella (not

---

Box 13-6 TARGET POPULATION FOR VARICELLA VACCINE (IF SUSCEPTIBLE TO INFECTION)

Health care workers in the following settings:
- Women who are household contacts of immunocompromised individuals
- Women who work or spend prolonged periods of time in environments that are high risk for varicella transmission (e.g., day-care workers)
- Young women in relatively closed environments such as college campuses or military facilities
- Nonpregnant women of child-bearing potential
- International travelers

Source: Varicella vaccine. (1995). *Medical Letter on Drugs and Therapeutics, 37*(951), 55–57.

congenital rubella), 309 cases of measles, and 906 cases of mumps. As of 1999, however, a panel of experts convened by the CDC concluded that measles (rubeola) was no longer endemic in the United States. One hundred cases of measles occurred in 1999, and most were demonstrated or suspected to be from imported sources. Confirmed rubella cases in the United States in 1999 totaled 267. Many of these were imported as well. Twenty-four cases of congenital rubella syndrome were documented in 1999 in the United States (Centers for Disease Control and Prevention, 2000a).

A single MMR vaccine should be given to any nonpregnant woman who is known to be susceptible to measles (rubeola) or German measles (rubella) (Centers for Disease Control and Prevention, 1996a; Measles Revaccination, 1989; Task Force on Adult Immunization, 1994b; U.S. Preventive Services Task Force, 1994). Populations known to be at risk include those born after 1956 who did not receive at least one MMR vaccine on or after age 15 months and those without serological evidence of immunity. Prior infection provides adequate protection. Certain adults are advised to consider revaccination if they have received only one previous MMR. These individuals are college students or military enrollees, workers or residents of facilities where infection rates may be high (including health care workers), and international travelers. Antibody testing for rubella and rubeola titers is readily available and may be used to identify susceptible individuals if immunization records are incomplete. Individual vaccines for rubella or measles may be appropriate if testing shows a person has immunity to only one of the two viruses. The MMR vaccine and the individual rubella and rubeola vaccines contain attenuated live viruses and therefore have certain contraindications. They should not be used in immunocompromised persons, including those with leukemia or human immunodeficiency virus infection (Centers for Disease Control and Prevention, 1996b). The vaccines also should not be administered to women who are pregnant or who may become pregnant within 3 months of receiving the vaccine. Women with a history of anaphylactic reactions to ingestion of gelatin or to exposure to neomycin are not candidates for the MMR because of possible adverse reactions.

SPECIAL POPULATIONS

Adolescent Females

The immunization timetable for adolescents depends on successful completion of the childhood vaccination schedule and anticipation of current and future needs. Guidelines of the American Academy of Pediatrics and the Advisory Committee on Immunization Practices state that by age 11 or 12, the childhood regimen of vaccines should be completed. Specific areas of concern include ensuring that a second MMR has been received, assessing for risk of varicella infection and the need for vaccination, and offering or completing hepatitis B immunization. The diphtheria-pertussis-tetanus series will have been completed by around age 6. Adolescents between ages 11 to 16 need to begin Td boosters. The possibility of pregnancy needs to be considered in all adolescent girls before administering live-virus vaccines. The doses of vaccines are the same for this population as for adults. An adolescent's chronic illness may make her eligible for some typically adult immunizations such as influenza or pneumococcal vaccines (Centers for Disease Control and Prevention, 1996a).

Pregnant Females

As stated previously, live viruses are contraindicated for pregnant women. Women receiving live-virus vaccines also require specific counseling to avoid pregnancy for at least 1 (for varicella vaccine) or 3 (for measles, mumps, and/or rubella vaccines) months (Centers for Disease Control and Prevention, 1996e; Gardner et al., 1996; Task Force on Adult Immunization, 1994b). Influenza vaccine is apparently safe throughout pregnancy but is not advocated during the first trimester for two reasons: One concern is that pregnancy loss is relatively high in the first trimester from multiple causes, and a recent vaccine might be implicated as a cause of miscarriage; another concern is that an increased risk associated with pregnancy and influenza infection has been demonstrated for the second and third trimesters (Centers for Disease Control and Prevention, unpublished data). Pregnant women who are identified as being *high risk* for pneumococcal or hepatitis B infection may receive either vaccine safely in pregnancy, but routine immunization with these agents usually is postponed until after delivery (Task Force on Adult Immunization, 1994b). No data exist regarding the use of hepatitis A vaccine in pregnancy (Gardner et al., 1996). The Td booster is appropriate to use in pregnant women for wound prophylaxis, but routine booster use generally is postponed until delivery. Lactation is not a contraindication for using of any of the vaccines described (Task Force on Adult Immunization, 1994b).

College Students

Awareness of outbreaks at colleges of meningococcal infection and the availability of a vaccine is increasing. Meningococcal infection is fortunately rare in the United States. Mortality, however, is 10%, and 9% to 11% of infections result in serious sequelae. Nationwide 2400 to 3000 cases occur annually at a population rate of 0.8 to 1.3 per 100,000. In the years 1994 through 1997 only four of 42 reported outbreaks occurred on college campuses. The rate of infection across the population is low enough that offering routine immunization for meningococcal infection does not appear cost-effective. The lower limit for cost-effectiveness for this vaccine is estimated to be 10 in 100,000. One subpopulation stands out as at risk: The rate of infection between 1997 and 1999 in college freshman who live in dorms was 4.6 per 100,000. This number is still below target range for cost-effectiveness but is substantially above normal population rates. The American College Health Association recommended in 1997 that college students living on campus be made aware of their increased risk of meningococcal infection and that they be offered the vaccine if they desired it. The vaccine is administered in one dose of 0.5 mL given subcutaneously. Protection is against four serotypes: A, C, Y, and W-135. Protection is less than 100% and doesn't include any coverage for type B, which was responsible for 24% of college-related infections. The injection is protective in 7 to 10 days. Side effects are minimal, mostly consisting of pain and redness at the site within the first 48 hours. Fevers occur in less than 5% of persons, and serious reactions (immediate hypersensitivity) occur in less than 0.1 in 100,000 recipients (Centers for Disease Control and Prevention, 2000b; Centers for Disease Control and Prevention, 2000e).

SUMMARY

Improvement of immunization rates in adult and adolescent women will reduce the frequency of some infectious diseases in our society. The opportunities of eradicating some infections such as smallpox (worldwide) and polio (in the Western Hemisphere, except for vaccine-associated infections) now are realized. Measles is no longer considered to be an endemic disease in the United States. More illnesses will be prevented or attenuated by the systemic use of the immunizations we have readily available. Our short-term challenge is achieving greater compliance rates and documentation of the vaccines mentioned in this chapter. Patient education on the value of immunizations continues to be a driving force in universal acceptance of preventive services, including immunizations. The nursing community has a major role in the promotion and use of these services.

REFERENCES

Centers for Disease Control and Prevention. (1993). Final results: Medicare Influenza Vaccine Demonstration—Selected states, 1988-1992. *Morbidity and Mortality Weekly Report, 42,* 601–604.

Centers for Disease Control and Prevention. (1994a). Implementation of the Medicare influenza vaccination benefit: United States, 1993. *Morbidity and Mortality Weekly Report, 43,* 771–773.

Centers for Disease Control and Prevention. (1994b). Tetanus: Kansas, 1993. *Morbidity and Mortality Weekly Report, 43,* 309–311.

Centers for Disease Control and Prevention. (1995a). Assessing adult vaccination status at age 50 years. *Morbidity and Mortality Weekly Report, 44*(29), 561–563.

Centers for Disease Control and Prevention. (1995b). Diphtheria epidemic: New Independent States of former Soviet Union, 1990-1994. *Morbidity and Mortality Weekly Report, 44,* 177–181.

Centers for Disease Control and Prevention. (1995c). Influenza and pneumococcal vaccination coverage levels among persons aged >65 years: United States, 1973-1993. *Morbidity and Mortality Weekly Report, 44,* 506–515.

Centers for Disease Control and Prevention. (1995d). Pneumonia and influenza death rates: United States, 1979-1994. *Morbidity and Mortality Weekly Report, 44,* 535–537.

Centers for Disease Control and Prevention. (1995e). Prevention and control of influenza. Part II. Antiviral agents: Recommendations of the ACIP. *Morbidity and Mortality Weekly Report, 43*(RR-15), 1–10.

Centers for Disease Control and Prevention. (1995f). Update: Recommendations to prevent hepatitis B virus transmission—United States. *Morbidity and Mortality Weekly Report, 44,* 574–575.

Centers for Disease Control and Prevention. (1996a). Immunization for adolescents. *Morbidity and Mortality Weekly Report, 45*(RR-13), 1–16.

Centers for Disease Control and Prevention. (1996b). Measles pneumonitis following MMR vaccination of a patient with HIV infection, 1993. *Morbidity and Mortality Weekly Report, 44,* 603–606.

Centers for Disease Control and Prevention. (1996c). Prevention and control of influenza. *Morbidity and Mortality Weekly Report, 45*(RR-5), 1–22.

Centers for Disease Control and Prevention. (1996d). Prevention of hepatitis A through active or passive immunization. *Morbidity and Mortality Weekly Report, 45*(RR-15), 1–30.

Centers for Disease Control and Prevention. (1996e). Prevention of varicella. *Morbidity and Mortality Weekly Report, 45*(RR-11), 1–25.

Centers for Disease Control and Prevention. (1997a). Prevention of pneumococcal disease: Recommendation of the ACIP. *Morbidity and Mortality Weekly Report, 46*(RR-8), 1–24.

Centers for Disease Control and Prevention. (1997b). Update: Influenza activity—United States, 1996-97 season. *Morbidity and Mortality Weekly Report, 46*, 76–78.

Centers for Disease Control and Prevention. (2000a). Measles, rubella, and congenital rubella syndrome. *Morbidity and Mortality Weekly Report, 49*(46), 1048–1050.

Centers for Disease Control and Prevention. (2000b). Meningococcal disease and college students. *Morbidity and Mortality Weekly Report, 49*(RR-7), 11–20.

Centers for Disease Control and Prevention. (2000c). Notice to readers: Alternate two-dose hepatitis B vaccination. *Morbidity and Mortality Weekly Report, 49*(12), 261.

Centers for Disease Control and Prevention. (2000d). Prevention and control of influenza. *Morbidity and Mortality Weekly Report, 49*(RR-3), 1–38.

Centers for Disease Control and Prevention. (2000e). Prevention and control of meningococcal disease. *Morbidity and Mortality Weekly Report, 49*(RR-7), 1–10.

Chenoweth, C. E., Saint, S., Martinez, F., Lynch, S. P. 3rd, & Fendrick, A. M. (2000). Antimicrobial resistance in *Streptococcus pneumoniae*: Implications for patients with community acquired pneumonia. *Mayo Clinic Proceedings, 75*(11), 1161–1168.

Gardner, P., Eickhoff, T., Poland, G. A., Gross, P., Griffin, M., La Force, F. M., et al. (1996). Adult immunizations. *Annals of Internal Medicine, 124*, 35–40.

Innis, B. L., Snitbhan, R., Kinasol, P., Laorakpungse, T., Poopatanakool, W., Kozik, C. A., et al. (1994). Protection against hepatitis A by an inactivated vaccine. *Journal of the American Medical Association, 271*(17), 1328–1334.

Kottke, T., Brekke, M. L., & Solberg, L. I. (1993). Making time for preventive services. *Mayo Clinic Proceedings, 68*, 785–791.

Lewis, C. E. (1988). Disease prevention health promotion practices of primary care physicians in the United States. *American Journal of Preventive Medicine, 4*(Suppl.), 9–16.

McGinnis, M., & Griffith, H. M. (1996). Put prevention into practice [Editorial]. *Archives of Internal Medicine, 156*, 130–132.

Measles revaccination. (1989). *Medical Letter on Drugs and Therapeutics, 31*(797), 69–70.

Nichol, K. L., Lind, A., Margolis, K. L., Murdoch, M., Mc Fadden, R., Hauge, M., et al. (1995). The effectiveness of vaccination against influenza in healthy, working adults. *New England Journal of Medicine, 333*, 889–893.

Task Force on Adult Immunization. (1994a). Adult immunization. *Annals of Internal Medicine, 21*, 540–544.

Task Force on Adult Immunization. (1994b). *Guide for adult immunization* (3rd ed.). Philadelphia: American College of Physicians.

U.S. Preventive Services Task Force. (1994). *Guide to clinical preventive services* (Vol. 2). Alexandria, VA: International Medical Publishing.

Varicella vaccine. (1995). *Medical Letter on Drugs and Therapeutics, 37*(951), 55–57.

RESOURCES

Centers for Disease Control and Prevention: *www.cdc.gov*

Engerix-B: *www.gsk.com* or *www.worldwidevaccines.com*

Morbidity and Mortality Weekly Report: *www.cdc.gov/mmwr/* (a weekly scientific publication containing data on health and safety topics)

U.S. Department of Labor: Occupational Safety and Health Administration: *www.osha.gov*

Vaccines, Recombivax HB: *www.merckvacines.com*

Chapter 14

Female Sexuality

Catherine Ingram Fogel

Techniques and methods are often discussed with only passing reference to what are the most vital things of all—the emotions our experiences arouse in us, our identity as people, our values, our relationships with others, and the social context in which all our private behavior occurs and which is reflected in our most private acts.

Sheila Kitzinger

INTRODUCTION

Women have the right to intimate and sexual lives and relationships that are voluntary, wanted, pleasurable, and noncoercive (Alexander, 1997). Sexual health promotion is an essential nursing function. Women often have expressed concerns regarding sexuality and sexual activity directly to nurses and in turn expect sexual information, counseling, or therapy. The goal of this chapter is to build a strong knowledge base from which nurses can address sexual concerns. This chapter focuses on the physiological and psychological processes inherent in sexual development, sexual desire, women's views of self and presentations to society, sexual response and factors that influence response, function, and dysfunction. Furthermore, a framework for practice is offered and management strategies for selected sexual health problems are provided.

SEXUALITY

Sexuality is an integrated, unique expression of self that includes physiological and psychological processes inherent in sexual development that encompasses a view of self as a female and presentation of self as a woman, sexual desire, sexual response, and sexual orientation (Fogel, 1998; Fogel & Lauver, 1990). Furthermore, sexuality is a basic part of a woman's life and an important aspect of her health throughout her life.

Few women are alive for whom sex has not been important at some time in their lives. Through her sexuality a woman expresses her identity and her need for emotional and physical closeness with others. Women express their sexuality differently at different times—alone, with one partner, or with many—and no two women express sexuality in exactly the same way. Expressed positively, sexuality can bring much pleasure, but sexuality also has the potential to cause great pain. Sexuality is not limited by age, attractiveness, partner availability or participation, or sexual orientation.

COMPONENTS OF SEXUALITY

The unique human quality that is sexuality has several dimensions, including sexual desire, sexual identity, and presentation of self. Sexuality includes more than heterosexual intercourse and involves a wide range of behaviors, including fantasy, self-stimulation, noncoital pleasuring, erotic stimuli other than touch, communication about needs and desires, and the ability to define what is wanted and pleasurable in a relationship (Alexander, 1997).

Sexual desire or libido is the innate urge for sexual activity, produced by the activation of a specific system in the brain and experienced as a specific sensation that motivates an individual to seek or respond to sexual experience (Kaplan, 1979). The amount of sexual desire experienced varies from woman to woman and differs across a woman's life. Sexual desire is learned by experiencing feelings of pleasure, enjoyment, dissatisfaction, or pain during sexual activity. Sexual desire develops from interest in sexual activity, preferred frequency of activity, and gender preference for a sexual partner (Fogel, 1998).

Sexual identity includes one's view of self as female, presentation of self as a woman, and sexual orientation. This identity is formed in early childhood and evolves throughout a woman's life as circumstances continue to shape identity. A woman's view of herself as female includes her gender identity (sense of self as a woman); her sense of having characteristics customarily defined as female, masculine, or both (sex role); and body image (a mental picture of one's body and its relationship to the environment) (Fogel, 1998; Fogel & Lauver, 1990). Although gender identity is influenced by biological or anatomical sex, an individual's gender identity is not necessarily consistent with her biological sex (Alexander & LaRosa, 1994).

Presentation of self as a woman (sex role behaviors) includes all those behaviors women use to indicate to society that they are women, such as dress, hairstyle, speech patterns, and walk. Sex role behaviors are a reflection of a woman's internalization of societal and cultural stereotypes and expectations of what a woman's behavior should be (Alexander & LaRosa, 1994). Sex role proscriptions and expectations shape sexual expression. Beliefs about women and men and assumptions regarding appropriate behaviors for both affect sexual behavior, communication patterns, and expectations of sexual relationships.

Sexual orientation refers to the preference an individual develops for a partner or for the gender of the person with whom one has an emotional and physical attraction and wishes to share sexual intimacy (Rynerson, 1990). Sexual preferences exist on a continuum ranging from complete orientation to the same sex, through bisexuality, to complete orientation to the other sex.

Sexual lifestyles provide the pattern and context for one's sexuality (Fogel & Lauver, 1990). Although many options exist for women today, not all are accepted equally by society:

- **Heterosexual marital monogamy.** This is the most frequently acknowledged pattern for women, and marriage with a monogamous partner is assumed to be most desirable by the majority in society.
- **Serial heterosexual monogamy.** This lifestyle consists of an established pattern of having one monogamous relationship followed by another.
- **Nonmonogamous heterosexual marriage.** Women who choose this lifestyle may participate in sexual activity with other individuals or couples while married to another.
- **Heterosexual coupling without marriage.** Women with this lifestyle have sexual relations with one or more male partners without marriage.
- **Single state.** Women with this sexual lifestyle may be unmarried, divorced, and widowed. This lifestyle often is assumed to be transitional by society.
- **Partnering with either a woman or a man (bisexual).** A woman's sexual and affectional preferences are directed toward individuals of either sex. Women may be married, have partners of both sexes simultaneously or serially, or have lesbian relationships as well as previous sexual relationships with men.
- **Partnering with a woman (lesbian).** A woman's sexual and affectional preferences are directed toward women. A woman may be coupled or single with one or many partners. The most common pattern is serial monogamy.
- **Celibacy.** This lifestyle involves the conscious choice to abstain from sexual activity. Women may view this choice positively as a means of giving oneself time and energy to devote total attention to other activities. Celibacy also may be involuntary when a woman is between relationships.

SEXUAL RESPONSE IN WOMEN

Sexual response involves capacity (or what a woman is capable of experiencing) and activity (or what she actually experiences). Emotion and physiology are interwoven in a woman's sexual response cycle. The two principal physiological responses to sexual stimulation are vasocongestion and muscle tension and are represented differently throughout the phases of the cycle. Furthermore, the phases of the sexual response have the potential to create a sense of enjoyment, satisfaction, and intimacy for a woman. The human sexual response cycle was first described by Masters and Johnson (Masters & Johnson, 1966) and focused on physiological responses to stimuli. Later authorities incorporated biological and psychological components (American Psychiatric Association, 1994; Kaplan, 1979). Although the physical sensations are common to all women, the sequence of physical and emotional sensations is experienced uniquely by each woman, and not every woman experiences each response. A woman may experience different affective and physical responses from cycle to cycle. Progressing through each of the phases is not necessary to achieve sexual fulfilment (Roberts, Fromm, & Bartlik, 1998). The sexual response is the same whether the stimulus is self-pleasuring or pleasuring from another woman, from a man, or from intercourse (Woods, 1995). The phases of sexual response are described subsequently and in Table 14-1. This more-inclusive model incorporating physiological and psychosocial factors includes the element of consent (Chalker, 1994).

Desire

The first phase of the sexual response cycle is characterized by desire for sexual activity (libido) and sexual fantasy and involves all of the thoughts, images, wishes, and imaging that are a part of sexual activity. Although no specific physiological changes are associated with this phase, the phase prepares a woman for sexual stimulation and excitement (American Psychiatric Association, 1994; Kaplan, 1979).

Excitement

The excitement phase consists of physiological changes of sexual arousal and is characterized by vaginal lubrication, external genitalia swelling, narrowing of lower third of the vagina, lengthening of upper two thirds of the vagina, and breast tumescence. The clitoris becomes engorged and highly sensitive. Some women may experience a sexual flush. Systemic responses during this phase include accelerated heart rate and respiration and increased blood pressure. This phase may be interrupted, prolonged, or ended by distracting stimuli (American Psychiatric Association, 1994; Masters & Johnson, 1966; Roberts, Fromm, & Bartlik, 1998).

Orgasm

Orgasm is the height of sexual pleasure and is experienced by a peaking of sexual pleasure followed by an involuntary release of sexual tension and rhythmic contractions of perineal muscles, uterus, and lower third of the vagina. In addition, heart rate, respiration, and blood pressure continue to be elevated. Orgasms commonly last between 3 and 60 seconds and may vary with each sexual experience and from woman to woman. Unlike men, women are capable of multiple and frequent orgasms during a single sexual encounter (Alexander, 1997; Chalker, 1994; Darling, Davidson, & Jennings, 1991). Orgasms experienced with sexual intercourse have been reported to be more satisfying and less intense than those experienced with masturbation (Darling et al., 1991; Davidson & Darling, 1989). Women generally place emphasis on the emotional and physical aspects of a relationship in addition to the orgasmic experience itself.

Resolution

With resolution women experience a sense of general relaxation and well-being. The phase is characterized by a bodily return to the preexcitement state. With adequate stimulation, women may again begin sexual response before complete resolution.

Table 14-1 SEXUAL RESPONSE CYCLE IN WOMEN

PHASE OF THE RESPONSE CYCLE	PHYSIOLOGICAL/PSYCHOLOGICAL CHANGES
Desire	Sexual fantasy and thoughts Sexual appetite, desire, and motivation Active awareness that sexual stimulation is wanted No physiological changes
Excitement (several minutes to several hours; intense excitement, 30 seconds to 3 minutes)	Subjective sense of anticipation and pleasure Tumescence and subsequent withdrawal of clitoris; labia redden and enlarge; vaginal lubrication; thickening of vaginal walls; expansion of inner two thirds of vagina; orgasmic platform of outer one third of vagina Uterus elevates in pelvis Anus tightens Sexual flush (mottling and reddening of skin) in up to 75% of women Nipple erection and enlargement of the breasts Increased heart rate, blood pressure, neuromuscular tension, perspiration, pupillary dilatation Uterine contractions just before orgasm
Orgasm (3 to 60 seconds)	Peak of sexual tension and pleasure; sense of release Vasocongestion and muscle tension peak and release Clitoris remains retracted; vagina and labia majora contract rhythmically (about every 3 to 4 seconds; 3 to 15 contractions) Strong uterine contractions from fundus toward lower uterine segment; minimal relaxation of external cervical os External urethral sphincter contracts External rectal sphincter may contract; continued anus tightening Well developed sexual flush Breasts remain enlarged Hyperventilation (up to 40 breaths/minute); tachycardia (up to 180 bpm); increased blood pressure (30 to 80 mm Hg systolic; 20 to 40 mm Hg diastolic)
Resolution (10 to 15 minutes; if no orgasm, up to 1 day)	Subjective sense of relaxation Vasocongestion subsides quickly and body returns to unaroused state Clitoris returns to normal position; orgasmic platform relaxes and shrinks; vagina shortens; labia return to normal Uterus decreases in size and descends; cervix drops into seminal pool Breast size decreases Sexual flush resolves Blood pressure, pulse, and respiration return to baseline Light perspiration (30% to 40% of women)

Sources: Lauver, D., & Welch, M. B. (1990). Sexual response cycle. In C. I. Fogel & D. Lauver (Eds.), *Sexual health promotion*. Philadelphia: W. B. Saunders. Roberts, L. W., Fromm, L. M. & Bartlik, B. D. (1998). Sexuality of women through the life phases. In L. A. Wallis & A. S. Kasper (Eds.), *Textbook of women's health*. Philadelphia: Lippincott-Raven. Zwelling, E. (1998). Sexuality during pregnancy. In F. H. Nichols & E. Zwelling (Eds.), *Maternal-newborn nursing theory and practice*. Philadelphia: W. B. Saunders.

FACTORS INFLUENCING SEXUALITY

A number of factors influence women's sexuality, including physiological development, sociocultural mores, health, and relationships.

Developmental Factors

Adolescence

Adolescence, ages 12 to 19 years, is a period of rapid physical change and potentially stressful psychosocial demands, including a time of awareness and change in sexual feelings. The development of adolescent sexuality focuses on five aspects (Masters, Johnson, & Kolodney, 1995; Zwelling, 1997):

■ Physical changes of puberty and their relationship to self-esteem and body image
■ Learning about normal bodily functions and sensual and sexual responses and needs
■ Developing one's sense of self as a woman (gender identity) and comfort with one's sexual orientation
■ Learning about sexual and romantic relationships
■ Developing a personal sexual value system

Sexuality often is defined through activities such as dating. During this time, adolescent females select companions, test ideas regarding themselves, and eventually experience sexual pleasure.

As adolescents develop a capacity for sexual intimacy, sexual curiosity and experimentation are common. Today adolescents are more sexually active than ever before and at an earlier age. In the United States, the mean age of first voluntary intercourse is 17.2 years for white females and 16.7 for African-American females (Seidman & Reider, 1994). Furthermore, 5% of white females and 12% of African-American females are sexually active before age 13 (Coker et al., 1994). Young women who begin sexual activity early have greater numbers of lifetime sexual partners (Seidman & Reider, 1994). Adolescents often face peer pressure to be sexually active; an additional motivation for sexual activity for girls may be a desire for sexual intimacy rather than a wish for the physical act of intercourse. Risks associated with early sexual activity are increased risk for contracting sexually transmitted infections, including human immunodeficiency virus, and unintended pregnancies.

Adulthood

In early adulthood, 20 to 40 years, women achieve maturity in a sexual role and in the relationship tasks started in adolescence, including developing intimacy with another individual and developing a long-term commitment to a sexual relationship. Important career and personal decisions are made and increasing responsibilities are assumed; balancing relationships, career, and children is often a concern. Women face choices regarding sexual lifestyles and often experience several before settling into one. During these years, a woman continues to develop her personal sexual value system and must learn to be tolerant of others' sexual values. At some point during a woman's 20s and 30s, she faces decisions about childbearing. Throughout these years, frequency of sexual activity decreases.

In midlife, 40 to 60 years, women's sexuality is as varied as are women (Doress-Worters & Ditzion, 1998; Sang, Warshow, & Smith, 1991; Taylor & Sumral, 1993). Some women report that sex is very good, possibly the best ever. Others report that sex is not the driving force it once was or that sex is less exciting and gratifying. Although decreased libido can affect a woman at any age, up to one third of postmenopausal women report a loss of sexual interest during menopause (Murray, 2000). The physiological changes associated with menopause, which occurs generally between age 40 and 60, can affect sexual desire, expression, and functioning. During the perimenopausal years, fluctuating levels of estrogen and related vasomotor instability can result in sleep disturbances associated with hot flashes; the resulting fatigue can affect sexual desire adversely. With menopause and decreasing estrogen levels, some women may notice decreased vaginal lubrication and increased vaginal dryness. For some women, lessened concern of becoming pregnant may increase sexual desire and lessen inhibitions. Additionally, postmenopausal women are not immune to the universal psychosocial stressors that have been shown to decrease libido in younger women (Butcher, 1999; Klock, 1999).

During older adulthood, after age 60, women continue to be sexual and enjoy sexual activities. Although sexual frequency may decline, sexual enjoyment sometimes increases with age and patterns of sexual behavior remain similar to those in midlife (Alexander & LaRosa, 1994; Steinke, 1988; Steinke, 1994). The need for excitement, pleasure, and intimacy does not fade with aging. A critical issue for older women's sexual expression and activity is availability of a partner. Another important factor is health because good health is associated positively with sexual interest and activity (Johnson, B. K., 1996). The prevailing cultural view of older women as asexual beings also can affect sexual expression and activity negatively and often becomes self-fulfilling prophecy. Furthermore, current cultural emphasis on youth, beauty, and thinness also contributes to the societal expectation of asexuality in older women.

The physiological changes associated with aging (i.e., decreased estrogen supply, decreased tissue elasticity, and thinning of vaginal tissues) can cause irritation or discomfort with penetration and contribute to lessened desire and activity. The vascular changes that occur in arousal and the intensity of muscular contractions with orgasm may diminish moderately after age 55 to 60 (Alexander, 1997). Loss of fatty tissue of labia and mons pubis may result in tenderness and easily damaged tissue or abrasions and also may decrease sexual libido and functioning. Orgasms may decrease in intensity and, in some women, become painful. Breast size also decreases and breasts may sag. Although these changes may alter a woman's sexual view of herself, they do not alter her ability to respond sexually.

Body changes may require that a woman and her partners alter how they engage in sexual activity. With aging, sexual practices may include the use of water-soluble lubricant, increased foreplay for arousal, different sexual positions, and planning intercourse for times when energy levels are highest.

Although sexual interest and activity may decrease somewhat with aging, many older women do maintain sexual relationships, if a partner is available. Older women with partners may find that opportunities for sexual expression within relationships increase as career and family pressure are reduced and that more time is available for sharing with a partner. Many older women become celibate for lack of a partner; however, their need for touch and closeness continues, and they must be encouraged to seek out opportunities for intimacy with another person.

Childbearing Influences

Women may experience changes in sexuality with each trimester of pregnancy. Levels of libido and frequency of sexual activity can vary with the trimester of pregnancy. During the first trimester, desire and functioning may be inhibited by nausea and vomiting, breast tenderness, fatigue, and anxiety about the pregnancy. In the second trimester, women often express heightened desire as they feel better, although some may be inhibited by increasing weight and bodily changes. Women may experience diminished sexual desire and activity during the third trimester associated with physical discomfort related to increasing size, especially near term.

The changes associated with pregnancy can contribute to changes in pregnant women's sexual response (Alteneder & Hartzell, 1997; Fogel & Lauver, 1990; Masters, Johnson, & Kolodney, 1995). In the first trimester, relief associated with becoming pregnant and the increased sensitivity of sexual organs because of the increased vascularity of the genital area can enhance sexual pleasure. Conversely, the discomforts of early pregnancy—food aversions, nausea and vomiting, breast tenderness, fatigue, and sleep disturbances—can decrease sexual desire and responsiveness. Generalized vasocongestion of the pelvic viscera and increased vaginal lubrication occurs by the end of the first trimester and persists throughout pregnancy, and vaginal lubrication develops more rapidly and extensively. Orgasm may be triggered more easily during pregnancy because of increased vascular flow to the genital tissues, particularly clitoral erectile tissues, and muscle tension; some women may experience their first orgasm during pregnancy. In the third trimester, women may experience continuous (tonic) uterine contractions with orgasm rather than the typical rhythmic contractions (Zwelling, 1997). The resolution phase may be longer because of increased pelvic vasocongestion that may not be relieved completely by orgasm.

Fears about the effect of intercourse on pregnancy maintenance and harming the fetus may decrease sexual interest or pleasure at any time during pregnancy. A woman's partner also may experience decreased interest in sexual activity as his view of a woman shifts from partner to mother. Both may experience reticence associated with the presence of a third person (the fetus) in their relationship.

Health care providers' taboos and restrictions on sexual activity during pregnancy were common in the past, and physicians and nurses often did not initiate discussion on the topic routinely unless a woman had specific questions or unless specific medical conditions contraindicated sexual intercourse. Historically, this attitude arose from the persistence of outdated information in textbooks and inconsistent research findings on the effects of sexual activity on pregnancy outcomes. However, more recently professional organizations have recognized that addressing sexuality is an essential component of holistic health care (Wilkerson & Shrock, 2000). Not addressing a woman's concerns about sexual expression during pregnancy can contribute to her lack of libido and inhibit sexual activity

Current recommendations are that sexual intercourse should be avoided during pregnancy when a woman has been diagnosed with a threatened or inevitable abortion, a history of habitual abortion or incompetent cervix before or without cerclage, or known placenta previa. Often women with a history of preterm labor or delivery are counseled against intercourse during pregnancy (Wilkerson & Shrock, 2000). However, recent research (Sayle, Savitz, Thorp, Hertz-Picciotto, & Wilson, 2001) has provided evidence against the hypothesis that sexual activity generally increases a woman's risk of preterm delivery between 29 and 36 weeks. Nurses should be alert to new research as it becomes available and counsel their patients appropriately.

During the postpartum, women report lessened sexual desire and decreased sexual activity for up to 6 months. Reasons for decreased desire and activity are physical discomfort, lessened physical strength, dissatisfaction with appearance, and fatigue (Ellis & Hewat, 1985; Fischman, Rankin, Socken, & Lenz, 1986). Early postpartum physical symptoms such as lochia, increased vaginal discharge, and episiotomy pain are not conducive to sexual desire or activity. Once the initial vaginal discharge has subsided, women may notice a marked vaginal dryness associated with decreased estrogen and progesterone. Although experienced by all postpartum women, vaginal dryness is most common in breast-feeding women. Women who experience vaginal dryness may require some form of lubrication to prevent dyspareunia. Finally, motherhood allows little privacy and little rest, both of which are necessary for sexual pleasure.

Sexuality is often a concern for many women and their partners during pregnancy and postpartum as they experience the changes associated with childbearing. At the same time, these changes offer an opportunity to obtain a sexuality assessment and provide education for a couple's changing needs (Alteneder & Hartzell, 1997).

Struggles with infertility and repeated attempts to conceive can affect sexual self-esteem, sexual expression, activity, and desire negatively. Women may find the concepts of woman and infertile to be mutually exclusive (Johnson, C. L., 1996). Fertility and virility seem to be inextricably linked in our society. A diagnosis of infertility may affect negatively a woman's sense of sexuality, her self-image, and even her marriage. For women who desire pregnancy, pressure and need to time intercourse may interfere with pleasure and communication as couples no longer have sex for pleasure but rather only for procreation. Years of attempting to conceive or bear a child makes spontaneous sex difficult to maintain. Sexuality is an important source of communication and growth in the development of a couple's relationship. When the desired end result of sexual activity is reproduction, sex can become mechanical or take on a demand type of value. Women may initiate sexual activity around the time of ovulation even if they are experiencing low or decreased desire. Feeling threatened or resentful of sex on demand, men may experience reactive impotence or an inability to perform sexually, especially around the time of ovulation. Hopelessness, isolation, and self-blame may accompany miscarriage, stillbirth, and infertility.

Sociocultural Influences

Women's sexuality exists within the context of cultural expectations, individual experiences, and biological potential. Family, culture, law, and religion shape women's attitudes and behavior regarding sex. Society and culture are inextricably interwoven with sexuality and influence it as much as do physiology and psychology. Social influences on sexuality begin first within the structure of the family. Through socialization of the individual, the family conveys its own, as well as societal, sexual attitudes and behaviors and can contribute to later sexual dysfunction. Restrictive family upbringing or a belief that expressions of intimacy or sexuality are shameful or taboo may contribute to a woman's inability to express herself sexually. Poor parent-child interactions can contribute indirectly to sexual problems through decreased self-esteem or ability to cope with intimacy (Sheaham, 1989), whereas unsatisfactory relationships with fathers may contribute to orgasmic difficulties (Bernhard, 1995). Messages such as "sex is something to endure" or "women who enjoy sex are no good" may inhibit sexual expression or enjoyment.

The larger structure of society and its culture also affect sexuality. Society defines what sexual behavior is and the norms for that behavior, guiding the behavior of the individuals. Current American cultural values present mixed messages to women: Be sexually responsive but within well-defined boundaries. Today, women are defined as dysfunctional if they are too promiscuous or if they are not sexual enough, for example, lack desire for an appropriate partner or do not become aroused or reach orgasm with that partner. A specific behavior may be defined as desirable by one cultural group and evil by another. Different views often exist regarding premarital, extramarital, and marital sex; appropriate sexual positions; accepted foreplay activities; and duration of coitus.

To the extent that sexual activity is a coerced activity, full sexual functioning is unlikely to occur. Coercion exists on a continuum from guilt induced by a partner's hurt feelings if refused to the extreme of rape. Male sexual coercion of females in our society is endemic. In almost all present societies, incest is prohibited. Incest contributes to sexual dysfunction, particularly when it involves threat or force, occurs at an older age when guilt is more apt to be present, is associated with strong negative feelings, or is repeated (Sheaham, 1989).

In part, women form their ideas of what is sexually appropriate and desirable from years of cultural scripting. These scripts are frequently different for men and women and can be the basis of many of the issues women experience in sexual relationships. The notions that men who are sexually aggressive are macho or studs and that sexually aggressive women are whores and easy are examples of such cultural beliefs. Current sex role stereotypes prescribe that men initiate sexual activity while women exercise control. Certainly, cultural practices that physically alter sexual response such as clitorectomy affect sexuality.

Sexual myths, common in every culture and society, are a source of sexual ignorance and misinformation and can be related to many sexual problems. Often they interfere with women reaching full sexual potential and establishing fulfilling sexual relationships. Many sexual myths exist today (Fogel, 1998; Smith, 1997), such as the following:

- Women should satisfy men; women's needs are secondary to men's. Furthermore, men are oversexed and women are undersexed; men initiate sex and women receive sex.
- Sexual pleasure is the responsibility of the partner. Related to this is the expectation that a partner should somehow be able to sense what a woman's needs are.
- Large amounts of sexual stimulation are needed to arouse a woman; a woman arouses more slowly than a man.
- Orgasms are different for men and women.
- Women who are raped asked for it; every woman wants to be raped; when a woman says no, she does not mean it.
- Little girls should not be told about sex because that will put ideas in their heads.
- Women are not interested in sex; they cannot have multiple orgasms.
- Women only want sex for procreative purposes.
- Women are so sexually aggressive that they can never be satisfied.
- Sex and intercourse are synonymous.
- A woman who initiates sex is immoral.
- A woman cannot enjoy sex unless she has an orgasm.
- Absolute norms exist for sexual expression.
- Masturbation is dirty.
- Women can only have an orgasm with intercourse.
- Men are more aroused by pornography and fantasy than women.
- Men and women have different sexual age peaks, or men wear out and women wear well.
- Having sex during menstruation is dangerous; sex during pregnancy can mark a child and should be avoided.
- Menopause or hysterectomy ends a woman's sexual life.
- Oral-genital sex indicates homosexual tendencies.

Some sexual myths are also specific to elderly women:

- Older women are not interested in or capable of sexual expression.
- Older women cannot make love even if they want to do so.
- Older women are fragile and might hurt themselves if they do attempt sexual relations.
- Older women are physically unattractive and sexually undesirable.
- Older women who do have sexual relations are shameful or dirty.

Religion also influences sexual attitudes, beliefs, and values and can exert a strong influence throughout a person's life. Religious proscriptions can contribute to sexual concerns or problems. For example, a view that sexual intercourse is acceptable only for procreation may raise concerns when a woman feels pleasurable sensations. Accepting or rejecting premarital sex, using contraception to prevent pregnancy, beliefs about monogamy for men and women, and condoning or rejecting homosexuality are examples of religious influences in a woman's life.

Laws usually are made in a society to regulate and control unacceptable sexual behavior. Often periods of societal change are necessary to alter sociocultural beliefs and change laws. One example of such a period was the 1960s and 1970s when women began to redefine their sexuality for themselves. New definitions that recognized that sexuality is created by individuals, not anatomically given and proscribed, began to be developed. During this time, women-centered definitions of sexuality that included sensuality, closeness, mutuality, and relationships emerged (Fogel, 1998).

Health-Related Influences

A number of health-related factors, including illness, surgery, disability, medications, and substance abuse, can influence sexuality and sexual performance.

Illness can affect sexuality in a number of ways, and a variety of medical conditions can cause sexual dysfunction in women (Box 14-1). Chronic illness with its associated fatigue, pain, and stress affects sexual desire and arousal more often than it affects orgasm. For example, treatment of gynecological cancer is associated with less frequent intercourse, sexual excitement, and arousal (Andersen, Anderson, & DeProsse, 1989; Schover, Fife, & Gershenson, 1989). Women with endometrial cancer have stressed the negative effect of symptoms such as vaginal bleeding on sexual expression; furthermore, the fatigue and lethargy associated with cancer treatment adversely influences sexual functioning (Lamb & Sheldon, 1994). Results of studies on the effect of a hysterectomy on sexuality vary considerably and no longer document negative effects only (Bernhard, 1992). Diabetic women report sexual difficulties, including orgasmic dysfunction, inadequate lubrication, performance anxiety that interferes with sexual functioning, and lower levels of sexual desire than nondiabetic women (LeMone, 1993; Watts, 1994; Young, Koch, & Bailey, 1989). Furthermore, alterations in glucose levels and monilial infections interfere with sexual activity.

In the United States, where breasts are sexual, a woman with breast cancer may have sexuality concerns; greater sexuality problems may be experienced by women who dislike their breasts, have a negative self-image, have been sexually abused, lack a support system, or are uncomfortable discussing personal or sexual concerns (Bernhard, 1995). In addition, sexually transmitted diseases can have a tremendous affect on a woman's sexuality. Drastic changes may occur in her sexual behavior, including choice of partner, use of condoms, and specific sexual practices.

Disability may affect sexuality in a number of ways. The disabled often are viewed as asexual by health providers and the public alike and thus are not encouraged to express their sexual feelings or to be sexually active. The attitude that a disability somehow neuters a woman interferes with her right to sexual feelings and sexual expression (Blackwell-Stratton, Breslin, Mayerson, & Bailey, 1988; Nosek et al., 1994; Sawin, 1998). Most disabled women are single (Bernhard, 1995). The length of time a woman has been disabled may affect her sexuality; the suggestion has been made that women whose disability occurred early in life are less likely to engage in various sexual activities that are those whose disability occurred later in life (DeHaan & Wallander, 1988). However, recent research on women with spinal cord injury found that women injured

Box 14-1 MEDICAL CONDITIONS THAT MAY INTERFERE WITH SEXUAL FUNCTIONING IN WOMEN

Neurological disorders (affects sex center in brain)
Arnold-Chiari malformation
Cardiovascular accident
Central nervous system tumors
Head trauma
Hypothalamic lesions
Temporal lobe epilepsy

Neurological disorders (spinal cord and peripheral nerves)
Amyotrophic lateral sclerosis
Herniated lumbar disk
Lumbar canal stenosis
Multiple sclerosis
Neoplastic spinal cord disease
Paraplegia and other spinal cord injuries
Peripheral neuropathies
Polio
Radical pelvic surgery
Surgical sympathectomy
Tabes dorsalis
Vitamin deficiencies

Cardiovascular and pulmonary disorders
Asthma
Cardiac disease
Coronary artery disease
Hypertension
Postcoronary syndrome
Poststroke syndrome

Endocrine disorders
Acromegaly
Addison disease
Cushing disease
Diabetes mellitus
Hypopituitarism
Pituitary tumor
Prolactin-secreting pituitary adenoma
Thyroid deficiency

Renal and urological disorders
Chronic interstitial cystitis
Chronic renal failure
Cystitis
Cystocele
Dialysis
Nephritis

Miscellaneous
Anemia
Arthritis
Degenerative diseases
Infections
Liver disease
Lower bowel disease
Malignancies
Malnutrition
Musculoskeletal disorders
Pelvic fracture
Radiation therapy

Sources: Kaplan, H. (1979). *Disorders of sexual desire and other new concepts and techniques in sex therapy.* New York: Brunner/Mazel. Kaplan, H. S. (1983). *The evaluation of sexual disorders: Psychological and medical aspects.* New York: Brunner/Mazel. Roberts, L. W., Fromm, L. M. & Bartlik, B. D. (1998). Sexuality of women through the life phases. In L. A. Wallis & A. S. Kasper (Eds.), *Textbook of women's health.* Philadelphia: Lippincott-Raven.

at an earlier age were more likely to have had sexual intercourse and to have resumed intercourse within 12 months of the injury than were older women (White, Rintala, Hart, & Fuhler, 1994). A critical issue for some women who are disabled is body image, because they may view their bodies as a problem and as a source of anxiety rather than pleasure. The reactions of others may suggest that a woman's body is unacceptable or unattractive (Nelson, 1995). The specific physical effects of a given disability on sexual activity differ with the disability. For example, women with spinal cord injuries may experience spasticity with orgasm, and those women with a complete spinal lesion will not experience clitoral or vaginal sensations or a traditional orgasm (Bernhard, 1989; Kettl et al., 1991; Sawin, 1998).

Many medications can alter sexual functioning and cause sexual dysfunctions, including anorgasmia and inadequate lubrication. The drugs that most commonly induce these affects are antidepressants, antihypertensives, antihistamines, neuroleptics, and antipsychotics (Bachmann, Coleman, Driscoll, & Renshaw, 1999). Table 14-2 provides a list of drugs that alter sexual function. Additionally, depending on the dosage and an individual's mental and physical state, some medications known to inhibit sexual function also may enhance it. Examples of such drugs include the benzodiazepine tranquilizers and chlorpheniramine (Roberts et al., 1998).

Substance use and abuse can have an adverse effect on sexual functioning and sexuality. Sexual dysfunctions can occur with substances such as alcohol, amphetamines, cocaine, opiods, sedatives, and tranquilizers. Chemical dependency in women is associated with issues such as incest and childhood sexual abuse, rape, and violent relationships as adults (Teets, 1990). Women who use illicit drugs have been labeled crack whores and described as compulsively exchanging sex for a drug. In reality, contrary to popular folklore that crack is an aphrodisiac, women who use crack cocaine report that the drug has an adverse effect on sexual desire and functioning (Henderson, Boyd, & Whitmarsh, 1995). Although crack use reduces sexual desire and physical ability to have sex and have an orgasm, crack use is associated with more frequent sex, trading sex for drugs and money, and having multiple partners.

Sexually transmitted diseases, including the human immunodeficiency virus, that are transmitted within the context of a dyadic, interpersonal relationship have the potential to affect a woman's sexuality and sexual functioning. A profound conditioning in our culture says that sex is love, sex is power, and sex makes you important (Kasl, 1989). Women who have been diagnosed with a sexually transmitted disease often experience depression, low self-esteem, guilt, lack of trust, and anger (Fogel, 1995). The adoption of safer sex practices necessitates altered sexual practices (Table 14-3). A fundamental characteristic of sexual risk-reduction practices is that individuals must give up behavior that is enjoyable, gratifying, highly reinforced, and often long-standing and replace that behavior with alternatives that are almost always less gratifying, more awkward or inconvenient, and harder to do than current behaviors (Kelly & Kalichman, 1995). Women may decide to be celibate to avoid risk, decrease the number of their partners or avoid certain partners, and change or avoid specific sexual activities that increase risk. The risk of sexual coercion may be greater for women in power-imbalanced relationships with men who resist using condoms. Sex roles and sexual double standards may hinder a woman's ability to ask for safer sex practices and contribute to a man's resistance to implement these practices.

Relationships and Partners

Relationship Issues

Women are more likely to associate sex with love and commitment, and a woman's subjective perception of sexual pleasure is influenced by her perception of her relationship with her partner. Women have reported that their most pleasurable sexual

Table **14-2**	**MEDICATIONS ADVERSELY AFFECTING SEXUAL FUNCTIONING**
CATEGORY AND GENERIC NAME	**TRADE NAME**
Anorectics	
Phentermine	Ionamin, Fastin
Fenfluramine	Pondimin
Phenylpropanolamine	Ephedra, Mormon Tea, Dexatrim, Ayds, and Acutrim
Diethylpropion	Tenuate
Mazindol	Sandrex
Anticancer Drugs	
Vinblastine	Methotrexate
5-Fluorouracil	Efudex
Tamoxifen	Nolvadex
Antihypertensives	
Reserpine	Serpasil
Methyldopa	Aldomet
Guanethidine	Ismelin
Beta-blockers	
Propranolol	Inderal
Atenolol	Tenormin
Metoprolol	Lopressor
Bisoprolol	Zebeta
Timolol	Timoptic
Betaxolol	Betoptic
Alpha$_1$-blockers	
Prazosin	Minipress
Doxazosin	Cardura
Alpha$_2$-blockers	
Clonidine	Catapres
Guanfacine	Tenex
Ace inhibitors	
Captopril	Capoten
Enalapril	Vasotec
Calcium channel blockers	
Amlodipine	Norvasc
Verapamil	Calan, Isoptin
Diltiazem	Cardizem
Antiulcer Medications	
Cimetidine	Tagamet
Famotidine	Pepcid
Nizatidine	Axid

Table 14-2	MEDICATIONS ADVERSELY AFFECTING SEXUAL FUNCTIONING—CONT'D

CATEGORY AND GENERIC NAME	TRADE NAME
Cold/Allergy Medications	
Chlorpheniramine	Chlor-Trimeton
Diphenhydramine	Benadryl
Pseudoephedrine	Sudafed
Antiolytics/Tranquilizers	
Benzodiazepines	
Antipsychotics/Neuroleptics	
Phenothiazines	
Chlorpromazine	Thorazine
Fluphenazine	Prolixin
Perphenazine	Trilafon
Thioridazine	Mellaril
Other	
Haloperidol	Haldol
Thiothixine	Navane
Resperidone	Risperdal
Psychotrophics	
Tricyclic antidepressants	
Clomipramine	Anafranil
Amitriptyline	Elavil
Doxepin	Sinequan
Imipramine	Tofranil
Nortriptyline	Aventyl
Desipramine	Nopramin
Monoamine oxidase inhibitors	
Isocarboxazid	Marplan
Phenelzine	Nardil
Tranylcypromine	Parnate
Serotonin uptake inhibitors	
Fluoxetine	Prozac
Paroxetine	Paxil
Sertraline	Zoloft
Fluvoxamine	Luvox
Venlafaxine	Effexor
Mood stablizers/anticonvulsants	
Lithium carbonate	
Valproate	Depakote
Carbamazepine	Tegretol
Phenytoin	Dilantin
Phenobarbitol	Dosette

Source: Roberts, L. W., Fromm, L. M., & Bartlik, B. D. (1998). Sexuality of women through the life phases. In L. A. Wallis & A. S. Kasper (Eds.), *Textbook of women's health*. Philadelphia: Lippincott-Raven.

feelings were in response to intercourse with a partner, though their most profound physical responses occurred through masturbation (Darling, Davidson, & Jennings, 1991).

Table 14-3   **SEXUAL RISK PRACTICES**

SAFEST	LOW RISK	POSSIBLY RISKY (POSSIBLE EXPOSURE)	HIGH RISK (UNSAFE)
Behavior	*Behavior*	*Behavior*	*Behavior*
Abstinence	Wet kissing	Cunnilingus	Unprotected anal intercourse
Self-masturbation	Vaginal intercourse with condom	Fellatio	Unprotected vaginal intercourse
Monogamous (both partners and no high-risk activities)	Anal intercourse with condom	Mutual masturbation with skin breaks	Fisting
Hugging, massage, and touching*	Fellatio interruptus	Vaginal intercourse after anal contact without new condom	Multiple sexual partners
Oral-anal contact	Urine contact with intact skin		Sharing sex toys and douche equipment
Dry kissing			
Mutual masturbation			
Drug abstinence			
Prevention	*Prevention*	*Prevention*	*Prevention*
Avoid high-risk behaviors	Avoid exposure to potentially infected body fluids	Dental dam or female condom with cunnilingus	Avoid exposure to potentially infected body fluids
	Consistently use condoms and spermicide	Use condom with fellatio	Use condoms and spermicide consistently
	Avoid anal intercourse	Use condoms and spermicide consistently	Avoid anal penetration
		Use latex gloves	If have anal penetration, use condom with intercourse and latex glove with hand penetration
			Avoid oral-anal contact
			Do not share sex toys, needles, or douching equipment; if sharing needles, clean with bleach before and after use

*Assumes no breaks in skin.
Adapted from Fogel, C. I. (1995). Sexually transmitted diseases. In Fogel, C. I., & Wood, N. F. (Eds.), *Women's health care.* Thousand Oaks, CA: Sage Publishers. Star, W. L. (1995). Sexually transmitted diseases. In W. L. Star, L. L. Lommel, & M. T. Shannon (Eds.), *Women's primary health care: Protocols for practice.* Washington, DC: American Nurses Publishing.

Relationship discord may precipitate sexual dysfunction, so much so that many sex therapists believe that sexual dysfunction is a symptom of underlying relationship dysfunction. Open communication of one's sexual preferences, feelings, and desires is essential for sexual satisfaction. One or both partners may experience difficulty after disclosure of sexual activity outside the relationship. Sexual communication difficulties can be exacerbated by distrust, feelings of betrayal, and fear of disease. Sexual dysfunction in one partner may precipitate dysfunction in the other partner; for example, erectile difficulty in the male often is accompanied by lack of vaginal lubrication, orgasmic difficulties, and impaired desire disorders in the female.

Loss of a Partner

Loss of one's partner can affect sexuality adversely. Many women define their identity through their relationships and thus loss of a partner can create loss of sense of self. Furthermore, the typical image of a widow is that of a grieving woman whose sexual life has ended. Factors that may be related to a woman's sexuality after loss of a partner are her extramarital sexual experiences, age, and sexual satisfaction in the marriage (Bernhard, 1995). Remarriage is correlated with age; the older a woman is when she loses a partner, the less likely she is to remarry.

SEXUAL DYSFUNCTION

Sexual Health

Before considering sexual dysfunction, one must define sexual health, which is difficult and for many is not considered until sexual activity is absent. Although experts do not agree on a definition of sexual health, the following definition developed by the World Health Organization provides a focus for nursing. Sexual health is the integration of somatic, emotional, intellectual, and social aspects of sexual beings in ways that are positively enriching and that enhance personality, communication, and love (World Health Organization, 1975). Essential elements of this definition include the capacity to enjoy and control sexual and reproductive behavior in accordance with a social and personal ethic; freedom from shame, fear, guilt, and misconceptions that inhibit sexual response and harm sexual relationships; and freedom from disease, illness, organic disorders, and deficiencies that interfere with sexual functioning. Essential to sexual health is an acceptance of one's gender identity, body image, sexual identity, and sexual orientation. Also important is the ability to communicate one's sexual feelings, need, and desires and to be comfortable with that. In short, sexual health may be considered the physical and emotional state of well-being that enables us to enjoy and act on our sexual feelings (Comfort, 1975).

Definitions of sexual health and sexual practices may contain value-laden terms susceptible to different interpretations. Cultural norms often dictate what is acceptable or normal behavior. Nurses must be aware of how they define normal and abnormal sexual practices before they can provide sexual health care. Distinguishing between aberrant and merely unconventional practices is not always easy. The following questions can be used when considering a particular behavior or practice (MacLauren, 1995):

■ What does the behavior mean to the woman?
■ Does the behavior enrich or impoverish the sexual life of the woman and those with whom she shares sexual relations?
■ Is the behavior tolerable to society?
■ Is the behavior between two consenting adults?

- Does the behavior cause physical or psychological harm to the woman or her partner?
- Does the behavior involve coercion?

Sexual dysfunction occurs when impaired, incomplete, or absent expressions of normally recurring human sexual desires and responses are associated with distress and discomfort. Thus sexual dysfunction may be defined as the persistent impairment of an individual's normal patterns of sexual interest and response and is inherently subjective (Roberts et al., 1998). Several factors characterize sexual dysfunction (Fogel, 1998):

- Dysfunction can occur in one or more of the phases of the sexual response cycle and is less common in the resolution phase.
- Dysfunction may occur during masturbation or during sexual activity with a partner.
- Dysfunction may occur throughout a woman's active sexual life (lifelong) or develop after a period of normal responsiveness (acquired).
- Dysfunction may occur once or repeatedly.
- Dysfunction may occur in all situations with all partners (general) or only in certain situations or with certain partners (situational).
- Dysfunction is most typically seen in individuals in their late 20s or early 30s.

The exact prevalence of sexual dysfunctions among women is not known because research is limited and findings conflicting. Furthermore, clinicians often hesitate to ask about sexual matters when providing health care, and women are often uncomfortable answering questions or reporting problems of a sexual nature. One estimate is that between 25% and 63% of women experience some degree of sexual difficulty at some time in their lives (Lauman, Paik, & Rosen, 1997). For example, transient, delayed, or absent sexual desire or excitement can occur with fatigue or illness, with preoccupation with the demands of career or financial concerns, or with drug or alcohol use. Furthermore, satisfaction with marriage does not ensure adequate sexual functioning or satisfaction (Heiman, 1995).

Causes of Dysfunction

Pathophysiological (organic) causes of sexual dysfunction are more common than those that are psychological or emotional. As previously discussed, illness and medications can impair a person's ability to respond sexually. However, traumatic sexual experiences such as incest, rape, and coercive sexual encounters may precipitate sexual difficulties. Other associated factors may be depression and life stresses. Conditions in one's environment, including poverty, fatigue, and overwork, that necessarily make sexual pleasure and interaction a low priority, can cause sexual dysfunction. Psychiatric illness can impair a woman's ability to enter into a mutually enjoyable sexual relationship. Anxieties, including performance anxiety and fear of partner rejection may also result in dysfunction (Kaplan, 1979). Poor communication between partners regarding sexual feelings, needs, and desires can precipitate or perpetuate an unsatisfactory sexual pattern or escalate problems by limiting knowledge of each other or restricting acceptable sexual behaviors.

Types of Dysfunction

Sexual dysfunction may arise from a disruption in any of the phases of the sexual response cycle, most commonly desire, excitement, and orgasm; in addition, sexual pain

---

Box 14-2 FEMALE SEXUAL DYSFUNCTIONS

Disorders of sexual desire
Hyposexual sexual desire: Persistent lack of desire for sexual activity
Sexual aversion disorder: Aversion to and avoidance of genital sexual activity; more severe form of sexual inhibition

Sexual arousal disorder
Inability to attain or maintain physiological sexual arousal

Inhibited female orgasm
Inability to experience orgasm following normal sexual excitement phase with sexual activity

Sexual pain disorders
Dyspareunia: Recurrent pain before, during, or after vaginal intercourse
Vaginismus: Involuntary vaginal muscle spasm accompanied by pain, interfering with or preventing coitus

---

Sources: Ayers, A. (1995). Sexual dysfunction. In W. L. Star, L. L. Lommel, & M. T. Shannon (Eds.), *Women's primary health care: Protocols for practice.* Washington, DC: American Nurses Publishing. Fogel, C. I. (1998). Women and sexuality. In E. Q. Youngkin & M. S. Davis (Eds.), *Women's health: A primary care clinical guide* (2nd ed.). Stamford, CT: Appleton & Lange. Heiman, J. R. (1995). Evaluating sexual dysfunction. In D. P. Lemke, J. Pattison, L. A. Marshall, & D. S. Cowley (Eds.), *Primary care of women.* Norwalk, CT: Appleton & Lange. Morrison, J. (1995). *DSM-IV made easy.* New York: Guilford Press. Roberts, L. W., Fromm, L. M. & Bartlik, B. D. (1998). Sexuality of women through the life phases. In L. A. Wallis & A. S. Kasper (Eds.), *Textbook of women's health.* Philadelphia: Lippincott-Raven.

disorders are considered to be sexual dysfunctions (Box 14-2). Sexual dysfunctions also are classified as lifelong or acquired and general or situational (Morrison, 1995).

Hypoactive sexual desire disorder is a prevalent sexual problem and one for which women most commonly seek assistance (Roberts et al., 1998). Sexual desire is influenced by many factors, including inherent sexual drive, self-esteem, previous sexual satisfaction, availability of a partner, and a good relationship with a partner in areas other than sex. Women with hypoactive sexual desire have little or no interest in sexual activities, do not become frustrated with lack of sexual activity, and rarely if ever initiate sexual stimulation alone or with a partner. Some women may respond to their partner's approaches and experience arousal and orgasm; others may not. Sexual activity occurs infrequently or only in compliance with a partner's wish for sexual activity (Ayers, 1995; Heiman, 1995). Although the cause is not known, depression, anxiety, and high levels of stress are associated with the disorder. Two common causes are relationship issues that create resentment and hostility and sexual trauma (abuse, assault, and incest).

Sexual aversion disorder is characterized by intense, persistent, or recurrent aversion to and avoidance of all or almost all genital contact with a sexual partner. Less common than hypoactive sexual desire disorder, this disorder may result from painful intercourse; sexual assault occurring in childhood or earlier in a woman's sexual life; feelings of anxiety, fear, or disgust; or relationship conflicts. Physical factors usually are not involved.

Sexual arousal disorder occurs in up to one third of all women (Morrison, 1995) and is characterized by an inability to attain or maintain adequate vaginal lubrication and swelling. Additionally, a woman may have little or no sense of sexual excitement, pleasure, or arousal. Biological factors may cause insufficient vaginal lubrication, including the hormonal changes associated with pregnancy, postpartum, lactation, and menopause; medications such as antihistamines and anticholinergics; or marijuana use before sexual activity (Ayers, 1995). Chronic vaginal infections such as monilial infection, bacterial vaginosis, or trichomoniasis also may be associated with inadequate lubrication.

Inhibited female orgasm, or the inability to experience an orgasm, is defined as a sexual disorder only when a woman reports receiving adequate sexual stimulation without orgasm. A significant minority of women report having difficulty achieving orgasm at some time in their lives. Women with this disorder do experience erotic feelings, vaginal lubrication, and genital stimulation. Primary (lifelong, general) orgasmic disorder rarely is caused by a physical condition; rather factors such as a restrictive home environment, negative cultural scripting, unrealistic performance expectations, inadequate knowledge of female anatomy or the sexual response cycle, and current relationship issues are involved. Physical causes of inhibited female orgasm include medications (see Table 14-2), illnesses such as diabetes or hypothyroidism (see Box 14-1), vaginal damage such as episiotomy scars, any physical cause of dyspareunia, or endometriosis (Morrison, 1995; Seagraves, 1988).

Dyspareunia is pain experienced in the labia, vagina, or pelvis during or after intercourse. Pain may be experienced before intercourse, with penetration, with thrusting, or after intercourse. Even after the actual pain is gone, the memory of the pain may continue and interfere with pleasure. The symptoms range from mild discomfort to sharp pain. The section on dypareunia covers this problem more fully.

Vaginismus involves the involuntary, spasmodic, sometimes painful contractions of the pubococcygeus and other muscles in the lower one third of the vagina and introitus (Heiman, 1995; Morrison, 1995). The degree of spasm ranges from partial (penetration is possible but painful) to complete (no penetration is possible). This disorder can occur at any point in the sexual response cycle when vaginal entry is attempted. Vaginismus may be associated with other sexual dysfunctions, including lack of desire, arousal, or orgasm. Although the incidence of this condition is not known, sex therapists believe the condition is more common than is documented because women do not seek help for it (Fogel, 1998). Often women do not seek help until they experience problems in their relationships or wish to become pregnant. Vaginismus may be caused by sexual trauma, phobias about sexual response or intercourse, conservative religious values, or hostile feelings toward one's partner. Although generally medical conditions are not a significant cause of vaginismus, infection or other sources of vaginal mucosal irritation can contribute to the problem. Once experienced, vaginismus can become repetitive in that a woman may anticipate further pain and a pain-fear-tension-pain syndrome develops that is self-maintaining.

Secondary/Other Sexual Dysfunctions

Most of the sexual dysfunctions discussed (with the possible exception of dyspareunia) have a psychological component or are caused solely by psychological factors or cannot be explained by a general medical or surgical condition. Some sexual problems do result from a medical condition such as when orgasm is inhibited by Cushing disease or hypoparathyroidism. Lack of sensation in the genital area from neurological disease or injury or scarring and adhesions from surgery can be a problem for some women. Alcohol, even in small amounts, can have a negative affect on sexual functioning, and psychoactive drugs such as cocaine can affect the sexual abilities of women.

SEXUAL ASSESSMENT

To provide satisfactory sexual health care, nurses must be comfortable with their own sexuality, aware of their own biases, and have a sincere desire to assist their clients. MacLauren (1995) recommends that health professionals become aware of their personal values and attitudes about sex and sexuality by asking themselves a series of questions such as "In my culture, communicating my sexual needs to my partner is considered [blank]" (see MacLauren, 1995, p. 109, for the complete list of questions). When providing sexual health care, nurses must not make assumptions regarding a woman's sexual attitudes, values, feelings, or behavior. Additionally, nurses need to know how various health problems, diseases, and their treatment affect sexual functioning and sexuality

Sexual health assessment includes a physiological, psychological, and sociocultural evaluation through obtaining a history, conducting a physical examination, and performing laboratory tests.

History

Sexual history is the most important aspect of the assessment process in relation to sexuality, yet nurses are often reluctant to ask about their patients' sexual histories or lifestyles (Warner, Rowe, & Whipple, 1999). Four factors that contribute to nurses not obtaining adequate information about a woman's sexuality are not seeing the woman's sexual history as relevant to her health problem, inadequate training, embarrassment, and fear of offending.

The nurse should take responsibility for introducing the topic of sexual health problems. As with any interview, establishing a positive tone before beginning is important. Rapport and trust need to be developed and sufficient time allowed for trust to build before soliciting information the woman may consider highly personal or intimate. The nurse should choose a location where the client can be comfortable and where privacy is assured; the client should be assured that there will be strict confidentiality. Collecting all the information at one time is not necessary; a sexual history can be collected over several meetings, especially when the woman is anxious. Continually monitoring one's own responses for negative or embarrassed feelings is essential because these are easily conveyed to the client. Usually more information is obtained if the nurse begins with open-ended questions and allows the woman to tell her story in the way most comfortable for her. Closed questions generally follow to facilitate gathering specific information such as medical history, menstrual history, and drug reactions. Women should be told why questions are being asked. The nurse can set limits if a woman offers excessive or irrelevant information, can redirect the client if information becomes tangential, and can encourage the client if progress is slow.

Beginning with the least threatening material, such as the woman's obstetrical history or childhood sexual education, and moving to more sensitive topics, such as her current sexual practices, is best. A general guide is to begin with questions about the woman's sexual education history (how did you learn about sex?) and proceed to personal attitudes and beliefs about sexuality and finally to assess actual sexual behaviors.

The nurse should avoid using excessive medical terminology during an interview; the nurse and the woman need to know the meaning of terms used. Euphemisms such as "slept with" should not be used. Only one question should be asked at a time, with the being given enough time to answer. Statistical questions such as "How many times a week do you have sexual intercourse?" are not helpful because normal practices vary among individuals. Rather than asking about a particular sexual experience that one may tend to deny, asking how many times the experience has occurred is better. This technique suggests that the experience is normal. Techniques such as "universalizing" or prefacing questions by comments such as "Many people [blank]" or "Other women I have talked with have said [blank]" may make the client feel more comfortable when answering sensitive questions.

A sexual history can be incorporated into a total health history or can be more formal and inclusive. A number of formats are available for use, and the reader is referred to other authors (Fogel, 1998; Fogel & Lauver, 1990; Heiman, 1995; MacLauren, 1995; and Zwelling, 1997). In most cases, sexual problems can be uncovered by asking a few questions such as the following:

- Are you sexually active? Are you sexually involved? Are you having sexual relations?
- Are you having any sexual difficulties or problems at this time? Do you have any pain?
- Has [illness, pregnancy, surgery] interfered with your being a partner? Has any [illness, surgery, medication, treatment] changed how you feel about yourself as a woman? Has any [disease, surgery, medication, treatment] altered your ability to function sexually?
- Is sex pleasurable for you? (Desire) Are you having difficulty with lubrication during sex? (Arousal) Are you able to have an orgasm or climax? (Orgasm) Do you have any pain or discomfort during sexual activity? (Pain).
- Are you satisfied with your sexual activity? Is it satisfactory? Are you happy with it?
- Do you have any sexual problems or questions?

Other components of the usual history can be significant for a sexual history. A woman's menstrual history, including age at menarche, characteristics of menstrual cycle (length, duration of flow, any associated premenstrual symptoms, ovulatory discomfort, and dysmenorrhea), should be obtained. The nurse should ask about the presence of vaginal discharge, discomfort, itching, and the woman's method of sanitary protection and level of satisfaction with the chosen method. If a woman is beyond her childbearing years, the nurse should ask if menopause has occurred or when it did and whether the woman experienced any difficulties such as vaginal dryness with sexual functioning. If problems have occurred, the nurse should ask how the woman dealt with them.

A woman's obstetrical history, including number of pregnancies, deliveries, and spontaneous and induced abortions, may be important. Any difficulties she had conceiving and any history of infertility should be noted. The nurse should ask about the woman's contraceptive history, including methods used, the woman's satisfaction or dissatisfaction with and confidence in each method, and partner participation when appropriate. Any history of sexually transmitted diseases, including pelvic inflammatory disease, must be recorded.

The nurse should ask a client to give a brief description of her sexual response cycle. Clarifying degree of lubrication present during sexual arousal or whether pain occurs during sexual intercourse is important. The nurse should ask the woman to provide a brief description of her present relationship and to rate her relationship with respect to communication, affection, sexual needs met, and sexual communication.

Physical Examination

When such is indicated by history or by the reason for seeking care, treatment goals, or the need for referral, the nurse may perform a physical examination. The examination may include determination of vital signs and aspects of a general physical examination, particularly an abdominal and pelvic exam. The pelvic exam should include inspection of the external genitalia and internal genitalia using a speculum and bimanual techniques.

Diagnostic Studies

Although no studies are specific to sexual assessment, often the history and physical examination may suggest a specific laboratory test. For example, an assay for prolactin levels would be appropriate if the physical examination reveals galactorrhea. Furthermore, tests are indicated when infection is suspected. Cultures for sexually transmitted diseases may be obtained if the woman has a history of purulent discharge or the nurse notes a discharge at the time of the physical examination. If a bladder infection is suspected when a woman complains of dyspareunia, a clean catch urine specimen for culture and sensitivity should be collected.

SEXUAL HEALTH CARE

General principles of sexual health care for all nurses include the following:

- Prevention of illnesses that can adversely affect sexuality and sexual functioning and reduction of violence, coercive sexuality, and behaviors that place women at risk for sexually transmitted diseases and unintended pregnancy
- Education, including provision of sexual information and resources
- Nonjudgmental, open, and direct communication regarding sexual matters
- Counseling to improve or sustain current sexual relationships or to solve a particular problem

Model for Intervention

A simple but effective method for providing sexual health care interventions is the PLISSIT model developed by Annon (1974; 1976). This approach, most used by nurses for sexual counseling, is made up of four levels of intervention: **P**ermission, **L**imited **I**nformation, **S**pecific **S**uggestions, and **I**ntensive **T**herapy. As the complexity of intervention levels increases, additional knowledge and skills are needed. All nurses should be able to provide *permission* and *limited information* related to many of the sexual concerns of clients. Many nurses and all advanced practice nurses should be able to intervene at the *specific suggestion* level. However, *intensive therapy* requires that nurses have special training in sexuality and sex therapy or that the client be referred to experts in the field of sex therapy.

The *permission* level is simple and involves the nurse giving permission to the client to function sexually as she usually does (with reassurance that such behaviors are normal), to talk with her partner, and to accept herself and her desires. Permission is given if the behavior is realistic, something with which both partners are comfortable, involves no danger or coercion, and causes no harm. Permission involves answering questions about sexual fantasies, feelings, and dreams and may include permission for things such as self-exploration (self-masturbation), initiation of sexual encounters, and using fantasy, erotica, and sexual aids such as oils, vibrators, and feathers. Asking about the effect of developmental changes, illness, or lifestyle alterations on sexuality may be ways of giving the woman permission to be a sexual being. Permission giving is particularly helpful for the client who is anxious about her sexual adequacy or the client with sexual dysfunction related to guilt over enjoyment of sexual practices.

Examples of interventions at this level are permission to be sexually aroused by normal feelings; to engage in safe activities that arouse sexual feelings, such as masturbation and fantasizing; and to have sexual intercourse as often as desired.

Limited information is often the solution when permission is not enough. The purpose of providing the information is to open topic(s) of sexual health for a client so that she then can discuss her specific concerns with the nurse. The information given at this level involves specific facts that relate directly to the woman's area of sexual concern. This level is helpful in changing potentially negative thoughts and attitudes about specific areas of sexuality and in refuting sexual myths. Any information offered should be immediately relevant and limited in scope. To provide this level of sexual health care, nurses need to be familiar with a range of sexual behaviors, norms, and forms of expression. This level is particularly useful when women have a sexuality knowledge deficit or anxiety associated with sexual misinformation.

Specific suggestions are useful when permission and limited information fail to improve the problem. The suggestions do not need to be exotic, complex, or imaginative; usually they will be apparent by the situation. The nurse gives direct behavioral suggestions to relieve a sexual problem that is limited in scope or of brief duration. The nurse and client agree on specific goals, and the nurse offers specific behavioral suggestions that are followed up after a brief time.

Numerous suggestions can be made to clients but always are tailored to an individual's needs and particular situation. For example, the nurse might suggest to the woman who is concerned because her husband's penis bumps her cervix with penetration, causing discomfort, that she try using a position that gives her more control over penetration such as the woman on top. Additional examples of specific suggestions are using a water-soluble lubricant to relieve vaginal dryness and prevent dyspareunia in postmenopausal women; sensate-focused exercises (mutual stimulation of erotic areas excluding the genitals); medication specific to an organism causing a vaginal infection; and alternative ways of sexual pleasuring (oral-genital contact, mutual masturbation, cuddling, holding, and massage).

Intensive therapy is used when the client's problems are not relieved with interventions from the first three levels or when the problems are personal and emotional difficulties interfere with sexual expression. This level of intervention is the most complex and should be offered only by professionals with advanced training in sexual counseling and therapy. Nurses must recognize the limits of their own knowledge and expertise and refer clients appropriately.

Dyspareunia

Too often women do not seek care for dyspareunia; thus the number of women who suffer from this disorder is unknown. Estimates of the prevalence in the general population are about 20% with a range of 4% to 40%. Some authorities suggest that as many as 60% of women experience dyspareunia at some time in their lives (Glatt, Zinner, & McCormack, 1990). Furthermore, the incidence appears to be increasing; however, what is not clear is whether the increase results from the increasing incidence of sexually transmitted diseases, changes in sexual behavior, or women's increased willingness to talk about sexual matters (Sarazin & Seymour, 1991). Most couples experience one or more mild, transient episodes with only minor interruption in sexual function. Almost 15% of women experience dyspareunia one or more times a year (Smith, 1997). As women age they also report more dyspareunia associated with changes in the urogenital system after menopause.

Dyspareunia may be classified as primary (pain experienced from the first attempt at intercourse) or secondary (pain developing after pain-free intercourse). Causes of dyspareunia are many and diverse (Table 14-4). Physical causes are most common and numerous (Fogel, 1998) and include sexually transmitted diseases, bladder disease, diabetes, anatomical defects, and decreased estrogen because of aging. Mechanical causative agents may be excessive douching or using irritating soaps or sprays. Dyspareunia also may develop from psychological factors related to family religious taboos or teachings that the vagina should not be touched; traumatic factors such as rape, incest, or previous painful intercourse; or factors such as a lack of complete arousal and inadequate vaginal lubrication, personal problems, or negative feelings toward one's partner (Heiman, 1995; Lazarus, 1989, Steege & Ling, 1993).

Table 14-4　**POSSIBLE CAUSES OF DYSPAREUNIA**

WHEN PAIN OCCURS	WHERE PAIN OCCURS	CONSIDER	MANAGEMENT
Precoital foreplay	External genitalia	Vulvovaginitis	Treat organism
		Inept male technique	Education and communication
		Vulvodynia	Treatment
		Arthritis in adjacent structures	Treatment
		Associated with abuse	Therapy (individual or group)
As penis enters	Introitus	Lack of lubrication	Education, water-soluble lubricant
		Infection/vaginitis	Treatment
		Position/angle of penis	Education and communication
		Urethritis/cystitis	Treatment
		Scar tissue	Medical/surgical intervention
		Rigid hymen	Education, surgical intervention
		Postmenopausal changes	Education, hormone replacement therapy, water-soluble lubricant
Penis in midvagina	Vaginal canal and adjacent structures	Cystitis	Treatment
		Vaginitis	Treatment
		Postmenopausal changes	Education, hormone replacement therapy, water-soluble lubricant
		Scars	Medical/surgical intervention
		Position of penis	Education
		Anorectal problems	Medical/surgical intervention
Deep penetration with thrusting	Lower back	Endometriosis	Medical (hormonal) or surgical intervention
	Lower abdomen	Related to pelvic inflammatory disease	Medical/surgical treatment
	Deep in pelvis	Position of penis	Education
		Arthritic/orthopedic problems	Medical/surgical intervention
		Posttrauma scars	Medical/surgical intervention
		Broad ligament varices	Medical/surgical intervention
During orgasm	Lower back	Endometriosis	Medical (hormonal) or surgical intervention
	Deep in pelvis	Scars at vaginal vault or abdomen	Medical/surgical intervention
	Lower abdomen	Broad ligament varices	Medical/surgical intervention
Post-coitus	Lower back	Endometriosis	Medical (hormonal) or surgical intervention
	Lower abdomen	Broad ligament varices	Medical/surgical intervention
	Deep in pelvis	Scars at vaginal vault or abdomen	Medical/surgical intervention

Sources: Ayers, A. (1995). Sexual dysfunction. In W. L. Star, L. L. Lommel, & M. T. Shannon (Eds.), *Women's primary health care: Protocols for practice.* Washington, DC: American Nurses Publishing. Fogel, C. I. (1998). Women and sexuality. In E. Q. Youngkin & M. S. Davis (Eds.), *Women's health: A primary care clinical guide* (2nd ed.). Upper Saddle River, NJ: Prentice Hall.

The diagnosis of dyspareunia usually is established by the woman's testimony. Thus obtaining a careful, accurate history is critical. General points to include in the history are these:

- Sexual response cycle and any alterations in phases of sexual response cycle the woman has noticed
- Attempts to conceive, previous high-risk pregnancy, postpartum difficulties, and contraceptive choices and problems associated with them
- Past and present illness, surgery, or medications
- Client's self-concept and body image
- Client's view of herself as a sexual being and level of confidence in ability to function sexually
- Past and current psychiatric problems or illnesses, including anxiety and depression and use of psychotrophic medications
- Client's satisfaction with current relationship
- Any history of sexual abuse
- Perceptions of sex-appropriate roles for men and women in relationships
- Perception regarding client's ability to fulfill these roles competently
- Sexual education, when received, and reactions to this information; assessing whether the information received was correct and accurate is important
- A woman's religious affiliation and beliefs and ethnic and cultural belief system also should be noted

In addition, a dyspareunia-specific history should include information about the pain: quality, quantity, location, duration, and aggravating and relieving factors. A complete medical, surgical, obstetrical, gynecological, and contraceptive history is collected and should include questions about previous vaginal or pelvic surgeries and pelvic trauma such as rape or sexual abuse. Finally, the nurse asks the woman about medications, douching, and the use of perineal products such as sprays, deodorants, and minipads.

Physical examination is necessary to determine the cause of dyspareunia and may include vital signs, a general physical examination, and an abdominal examination. A pelvic examination always is performed with special attention paid to the external genitalia, observing for irritation, lesions, and discharge. During the bimanual examination, the nurse should note any tenderness in the introitus, vagina, or pelvis and the presence of an unstretched or rigid hymen (Ayers, 1995). During the speculum examination, the nurse obtains cultures, when indicated.

The history and physical examination suggest which diagnostic tests are indicated. No tests are specific to sexual assessment. Laboratory studies may be indicated when evidence of infection exists.

Treatment for dyspareunia should address the specific cause of dyspareunia; for example, suggesting a water-soluble vaginal lubricant for the menopausal woman, treating the sexually transmitted disease, or providing information about techniques for sexual arousal. Although most physical conditions that result in dyspareunia can be managed on an outpatient basis, at times more extensive treatment is warranted. For example, a woman who has pain with deep pelvic thrusting and other symptoms associated with extensive endometriosis may require a hysterectomy for relief. Emotional care of women and their partners centers on support and specific treatment. Whenever possible, a woman should be reassured as to the normalcy of her anatomy, the frequency of this problem in other women, the likelihood of successful therapy, and the probable reason for her problem. Permission may be given not to have intercourse if painful and also to try a variety of positions and techniques for stimulation. Limited information and specific suggestions may be given to reduce or eliminate the pain and can be used to address the emotional component of the problem. Referral to mental health professionals may be indicated. Additionally, nurses and particularly advanced practice nurses may act as consultants to mental health professionals who are referring a client with dyspareunia for a physical and gynecological examination (Ayers, 1995).

SUMMARY

Sexuality begins with conception and develops throughout a woman's life. Sexual problems are among the most common of human concerns and are experienced by most women, if only briefly, at some point in their lives. Having a working knowledge of sexual functioning, sexual problems and dysfunctions, and how they are managed is essential for nurses caring for women. Central to nurses capably caring for women with sexual concerns or disorders is a nonjudgmental, supportive approach so that women are comfortable discussing sexual concerns. Nurses can promote healthy sexual functioning by fostering communication, providing accurate information and counseling, and, when needed, giving appropriate referrals to other health professionals.

REFERENCES

Alexander, B. A. (1997). Women's sexuality: A paradigm shift. In J. A. Rosenfeld (Ed.), *Women's health in primary care*. Baltimore: Williams & Wilkins.

Alexander, L. L., & LaRosa, J. H. (1994). *New dimensions in women's health*. Boston: Jones and Barlett.

Alteneder, R. R., & Hartzell, D. (1997). Addressing couples' sexuality concerns during the childbearing period. *Journal of Obstetric, Gynecologic, and Neonatal Nursing, 26*(4), 651–658.

American Psychiatric Association. (1994). *Diagnostic and statistical manual of mental disorders* (4th ed., revised). Washington, DC: American Psychiatric Press.

Andersen, B. L., Anderson, B., & DeProsse, C. (1989). Controlled prospective longitudinal study of women with cancer. I. Sexual functioning outcomes. *Journal of Consulting and Clinical Psychology, 57*, 683–691.

Annon, J. S. (1974). *The behavioral treatment of sexual problems*. Honolulu: Enabling Systems.

Annon, J. S. (1976). *The behavioral treatment of sexual problems: brief therapy*. New York: Harper & Row.

Ayers, A. (1995). Sexual dysfunction. In W. L. Star, L. L. Lommel, & M. T. Shannon (Eds.), *Women's primary health care: Protocols for practice*. Washington, DC: American Nurses Publishing.

Bachmann, G. A., Coleman, E., Driscoll, C. E., & Renshaw, D. C. (1999, April). Patients with sexual dysfunction: Your guidance makes a difference. *Patient Care for the Nurse Practitioner*, 14–25.

Bernhard, E. J. (1989). The sexuality of spinal cord injured women: Physiology and pathophysiology—A review. *Paraplegia, 27*(2), 99–112.

Bernhard, L. (1995). Sexuality in women's lives. In C. I. Fogel & N. F. Woods (Eds.), *Women's health care*. Thousand Oaks, CA: Sage Publications.

Bernhard, L. A. (1992). Consequences of hysterectomy in the lives of women. *Health Care for Women International, 13*, 281–291.

Blackwell-Stratton, M., Breslin, M. L., Mayerson, A. B., & Bailey, S. (1988). Smashing icons: Disabled women and the disability women's movements. In M. Eine & A. Asch (Eds.), *Women with disabilities: Essays in psychology, culture, and politics*. Philadelphia: Temple University Press.

Butcher, J. (1999). ABC of sexual health: Female sexual problems—Loss of desire, What about the fun? *British Journal of Medicine, 318*, 41–43.

Chalker, R. (1994). Updating the model of female sexuality. *SIECUS, 22*, 1-6.

Coker, A. L., Richter, D. L., Valois, R. F., McKeown, R. E., Garrison, C. Z., & Vincent, M. L. (1994). Correlates and consequences of early initiation of sexual intercourse. *Journal of School Health, 64*(9), 372–377.

Comfort, A. (1975). The normal in sexual behavior: An ethnological view. *Journal of Sex Education Therapy, 1*, 1–7.

Darling, C. A., Davidson, J. K., & Jennings, D. A. (1991). The female sexual response revisited: Understanding the multiorgasmic experiences in women. *Archives of Sexual Behavior, 20*, 535.

Davidson, J. K., & Darling, C. A. (1989). Self-perceived differences in the female orgasmic response. *Family Practice Journal, 8*(2), 75–84.

DeHaan, C. B., & Wallander, J. L. (1988). Self-concept, sexual knowledge and attitudes, and parental support in the sexual adjustment of women with early- and late-onset physical disability. *Archives of Sexual Behavior, 13*, 233–245.

Doress-Worters, P., & Ditzion, J. (1998). Women growing older. In Boston Women's Health Collective, *Our bodies, ourselves for the new century*. New York: Simon & Schuster.

Ellis, D. J., & Hewat, R. J. (1985). Mother's postpartum perceptions of spousal relationships. *Journal of Obstetric, Gynecologic, and Neonatal Nursing, 14*(2), 140–146.

Fischman, S. H., Rankin, E. A., Socken, K. L., & Lenz, E. R. (1986). Changes in sexual relationships in postpartum couples. *Journal of Obstetric, Gynecologic, and Neonatal Nursing, 15*(1), 58–63.

Fogel, C. I. (1995). Sexually transmitted diseases. In C. I. Fogel & N. F. Wood (Eds.), *Women's health care*. Thousand Oaks, CA: Sage Publications.

Fogel, C. I. (1998). Women and sexuality. In E. Q. Youngkin & M. S. Davis (Eds.), *Women's health: A primary care clinical guide* (2nd ed.). Stamford, CT: Appleton & Lange.

Fogel, C. I., & Lauver, D. (Eds.). (1990). *Sexual health promotion*. Philadelphia: W. B. Saunders.

Glatt, A. E., Zinner, S. H., & McCormack, W. M. (1990). The prevalence of dyspareunia. *Obstetrics and Gynecology, 75*, 433–436.

Heiman, J. R. (1995). Evaluating sexual dysfunction. In D. P. Lemke, J. Pattison, L. A. Marshall, & D. S. Cowley (Eds.), *Primary care of women*. Norwalk, CT: Appleton & Lange.

Henderson, D. J., Boyd, C. J., & Whitmarsh, J. (1995). Women and illicit drugs: Sexuality and crack cocaine. *Health Care for Women International, 16*, 113–124.

Johnson, B. K. (1996). Older adults and sexuality: A multidimensional perspective. *Journal of Gerontological Nursing, 22*(2), 6–15.

Johnson, C. L. (1996). Regaining self-esteem: Strategies and interventions for the infertile woman. *Journal of Obstetric, Gynecologic, and Neonatal Nursing, 25*(4), 291–295.

Kaplan, H. (1979). *Disorders of sexual desire and other new concepts and techniques in sex therapy*. New York: Brunner/Mazel.

Kaplan, H. S. (1983). *The evaluation of sexual disorders: Psychological and medical aspects*. New York: Brunner/Mazel.

Kasl, C. D. (1989). *Women, sex, and addiction: A search for love and power*. New York: Harper & Row.

Kelly, J. A., & Kalichman, S. C. (1995). Increased attention to human sexuality can improve HIV-AIDS prevention efforts: Key research issues and directions. *Journal of Consulting and Clinical Psychology, 63*(6), 907–918.

Kettl, P., Zarefoss, S., Jacoby, K., German, C., Hulse, C., Rowley, F., et al. (1991). Female sexuality after spinal cord injury. *Sexuality and Disability, 9*, 287–295.

Klock, S. (1999). Psychological aspects of women's reproductive health. In K. J. Ryan (Ed.), *Kistner's gynecology and women's health* (7th ed.) (pp. 534–536). St. Louis: Mosby.

Lamb, M. A., & Sheldon, T. A. (1994). The sexual adaptation of women treated for endometrial cancer. *Cancer Practice, 2*(2), 103–113.

Laumann, E., Paik, M., & Rosen, R. (1997). Sexual dysfunction in the United States: Prevalence and predictors. *Journal of the American Medical Association, 281*, 537–544.

Lauver, D., & Welch, M. B. (1990). Sexual response cycle. In C. I. Fogel & D. Lauver (Eds.), *Sexual health promotion*. Philadelphia: W. B. Saunders.

Lazarus, A. A. (1989). Dyspareunia: A multimodel perspective. In S. R. Leiblum & R. C. Rosen (Eds.), *Principles and practices of sex therapy*. New York: Guilford Press.

LeMone, P. (1993). Human sexuality in adults with insulin-dependent diabetes mellitus. *IMAGE, 25*(2), 101–105.

MacLauren, A. (1995). Comprehensive sexual assessment. *Journal of Nurse-Midwifery, 40*(2), 104–119.

Masters, W. H., & Johnson, V. E. (1966). *The human sexual response cycle.* Boston: Little, Brown.

Masters, W. H., Johnson, V. E., & Kolodney, R. C. (1995). *Human sexuality* (5th ed.). New York: Harper-Collins.

Morrison, J. (1995). *DSM-IV made easy.* New York: Guilford Press.

Murray, W. (2000). Decreased libido in postmenopausal women. *Nurse Practitioner Forum, 11*(4), 219–224.

Nelson, M. R. (1995). Sexuality in childhood disability. *Physical Medicine and Rehabilitation: State of the Art Reviews, 9*(2), 451–462.

Nosek, M. A., Howland, C. A., Young, M. E., Georgiou, D., Rintala, D. H., Foley, C. C., et al. (1994). Wellness models and sexuality among women with physical disabilities. *Journal of Applied Rehabilitation Counseling, 25*(1), 50–58.

Roberts, L. W., Fromm, L. M., & Bartlik, B. D. (1998). Sexuality of women through the life phases. In L. A. Wallis & A. S. Kasper (Eds.), *Textbook of women's health.* Philadelphia: Lippincott-Raven.

Rynerson, B. (1990). Sexuality throughout the life cycle. In C. I. Fogel & D. Lauver (Eds.), *Sexual health promotion.* Philadelphia: W. B. Saunders.

Sang, B., Warshow, J., & Smith, A. J. (1991). *Lesbians at midlife: The creative transition.* Minneapolis: Spinster's Ink.

Sarazin, S. K., & Seymour, S. F. (1991). Causes and treatment options for women with dyspareunia. *Nurse Practitioner, 16*(10), 30, 35–36, 38, 41.

Sawin, K. J. (1998). Health care concerns for women with physical disability and chronic illness. In E. Q. Youngkin & M. S. Davis (Eds.), *Women's health: A primary care clinical guide* (2nd ed.). Stamford, CT: Appleton & Lange.

Sayle, A. E., Savitz, D. A., Thorp, J. M., Hertz-Picciotto, I., & Wilcox, A. J. (2001). Sexual activity during late pregnancy and risk of preterm delivery. *Obstetrics & Gynecology 97*(2), 283–289.

Schover, L. R., Fife, M., & Gershenson, D. M. (1989). Sexual dysfunction and treatment for early stage cervical cancer. *Cancer, 63*, 204–212.

Seagraves, R. T. (1988). Psychiatric drugs and inhibited female orgasm. *Journal of Sex and Marital Therapy, 15*, 202–207.

Seidman, S. N., & Reider, R. O. (1994). A review of sexual behavior in the United States. *American Journal of Psychiatry, 151*(3), 330–341.

Sheaham, S. L. (1989). Identifying female sexual dysfunction. *Nurse Practitioner, 14*, 25–26, 28, 30, 32, 34.

Smith, R. P. (1997). *Gynecology in primary care.* Baltimore: Williams & Wilkins.

Steege, J. F., & Ling, F. W. (1993). Dyspareunia: a special type of pelvic pain. *Obstetric & Gynecological Clinics of North America, 20*(4), 779–793.

Steinke, E. E. (1988). Older adults' knowledge and attitudes about sexuality and aging. *IMAGE, 20*(2), 93–95.

Steinke, E. E. (1994). Knowledge and attitudes of older adults about sexuality in aging: A comparison of two studies. *Journal of Advanced Nursing, 19*, 477–485.

Taylor, D., & Sumral, A. C. (1993). *The time of our lives: Women write on sex after 40.* Freedom, CA: Crossing Press.

Teets, J. M. (1990). What women talk about: Sexuality issues of chemically dependent women. *Journal of Psychosocial Nursing, 28*(12), 4–7.

Warner, P. H., Rowe, T., & Whipple, B. (1999). Shedding light on the sexual history. *American Journal of Nursing, 99*(6), 34–40.

Watts, R. J. (1994). Sexual functioning of diabetic and non-diabetic African-American women: A pilot study. *Journal of the National Black Nurses Association, 7*(1), 60–69.

White, M. J., Rintala, D. H., Hart, K., & Fuhler, M. J. (1994, Summer). A comparison of the sexual concerns of men and women with spinal cord injuries. *Rehabilitation Nursing Research*, 55–61.

Wilkerson, N. N., & Shrock, P. (2000). Sexuality in the perinatal period. In F. H. Nichols & S. S. Humenick (Eds.), *Childbirth education: practice, research, and theory.* Philadelphia: W. B. Saunders.

Woods, N. F. (1995). Women's bodies. In C. I. Fogel & N. F. Woods (Eds.), *Women's health care.* Thousand Oaks, CA: Sage Publications.

World Health Organization. (1975). Education and treatment in human sexuality: The training of health professionals—Report of WHO meeting. *Technical Report Series*, 572.

Young, E. W., Koch, P. B., & Bailey, D. (1989). Research comparing the dyadic adjustment and sexual function-ing concerns of diabetic and non-diabetic women. *Health Care for Women International, 10,* 377–394.

Zwelling, E. (1997). Sexuality during pregnancy. In F. H. Nichols & E. Zwelling (Eds.), *Maternal-newborn nurs-ing: theory and practice.* Philadelphia: W. B. Saunders.

RESOURCES

The American Association of Sex Educators, Counselors, and Therapists: *www.aasect.org*

American Medical Association. Talking to Patients about Sex: Training Program for Physicians:
www.ama-assn.org/mem-data/joint/sex001.html

PLISSIT: *www.cchs.usyd.edu.au/bio/sex2000/plissit.html*

Questions and Approaches in Specific Areas of Sexuality:
www.cchs.usyd.edu.au/bio/sex2000/specifics.html

Pervin, L. *Sexuality and Disability*: *www.onlineece.net/courses.asp?course=55&action=view*

Chapter 15

Adolescent Women's Health Care

Leslie Skillman-Hull

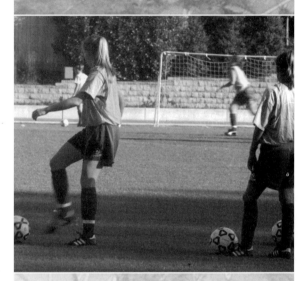

. . . . And I, for glee,

Took Rainbows, as the common way,

And empty Skies

The Eccentricity . . . .

Emily Dickinson

INTRODUCTION

This chapter describes the normal stages of pubertal growth, normal stages of adolescent psychosocial development, and major risk factors during adolescence. A significant transition in a young woman's health care is that from pediatrics to gynecology. Readiness, confidentiality, family involvement, and patient rights are discussed. The chapter then describes techniques for taking an adolescent history and performing a physical examination, with emphasis on performing a thorough and sensitive first pelvic examination. Young women's first experience with an advanced practice nurse and with her first pelvic examination can influence the way she seeks care for the rest of her life and is a foundation of preventive health care.

The final section of this chapter presents foundational information about specific conditions affecting the physical and emotional well-being of female adolescents. Providing health care to adolescents requires sensitivity and a thorough knowledge of medical and psychosocial conditions and pathological conditions arising in gynecological care. The approach to the specific conditions includes health-promoting actions, such as exercise and nutrition, disease prevention, diagnoses and treatments, and health restoration activities. The specific conditions covered are contraception, adolescent dermatology, eating disorders, menstrual concerns (amenorrhea, dysmenorrhea, dysfunctional uterine bleeding, premenstrual syndrome, and pelvic pain), sexually transmitted diseases (STDs), genital-urinary health, breast changes, adolescent pregnancy, and mood disorders. The goal of this chapter is to present an overview of the most salient health concerns of adolescent women and provide resources for more in-depth coverage of the specific conditions.

Adolescent women's health care, a specialty within women's heath, is a challenging field, given the complexity of adolescent physical and developmental issues and family dynamics. Not every health care provider is a good match for this age group. One might reflect on his or her own preferences and knowledge base to determine if one is best suited to care for adolescent women.

Adolescence is the dramatic process of physical, cognitive, and psychosocial changes generally starting and finishing in the second decade of life. The transformation of a dependent child into a self-sufficient adult is the favored outcome. According to Bragg (1997) "it is a time of intense preoccupation with the self, which is growing and changing daily, and represents a period during which women make important choices about life-style behaviors, including the use of tobacco, alcohol, and other drugs and sexual activity" (p. 577). Health care providers need to be able to appreciate differences between normal variations and abnormalities in growth and pubertal development (Neinstein & Kaufman, 1996).

Contextual Impact of Adolescence

A context exists for every experience in which an adolescent does or does not thrive. All human beings exist within a context, and, if understanding is to occur, then the experiences need to be in context or context-driven (Dewey, 1934; Gadow, 1994). For example, pelvic pain in a 12-year-old girl in the absence of an organic pathological condition might be linked to a history of physical abuse and associated emotional pain. This diagnosis can only be made once this link has been articulated to and confirmed by the adolescent. The approach to this patient depends on age: Concrete thinkers need a different kind of explanation than abstract thinkers (refer to the section on the emotional self). Part of treatment is understanding and giving meaning to things that happen to and in the body. Giving a symptom context is more likely to affect an adolescent's choice to comply with treatment and follow-up than when factual information is given out of context. The context of this section is presented in three contextual perspectives, that of the environment that encompasses the whole self, the physical self, and the emotional self and intellectual self.

Environment

The contextual impact of an adolescent on the environment or the environment on the adolescent generally is discussed in terms of educational and socioeconomic factors. Although these categories provide important data, the concept of an environmental context is more expansive. The theoretical perspectives of nursing describe environment as an array of qualities. Using a nursing theory to frame the relationships of client and clinical environments, adolescent women's health needs, access to information, and the overall dynamic conditions inherent in being human guides the nurse to maintain a receptive place from which to provide care.

Previously identified was the notion that adolescence is a time of self-exploration and other exploration. The process of testing one's self with internal quests and "other" driven experiences is natural for teenagers, is played out in the clinical setting as well, and is commonly seen by advanced practice nurses through the teen's hidden agenda. The presenting chief complaint may have something to do with the current clinical visit but is often not the major and only concern. In assuming a receptive quality in her interview, medical assessment, and evaluation, the advanced practice nurse invites the teen to trust and consequently share the most pressing concerns of the visit that day. Combining a nursing theoretical framework with the clinical knowledge an advanced practice nurse brings to the clinical setting enhances the possibilities for a more thorough diagnostic outcome.

For example, the nurse theorist Martha Rogers describes the relationships of human and environments in the language of Field Theory (1970, 1990a, 1990b). Terms such as *energy fields, integrality, pandimensionality*, and *irreducible wholes* provide the lens that focuses the advanced practice nurse's caregiving to offer a safe and open environment that supports the comfort of the adolescent to receive the help and guidance she seeks. Specifically, in the case of a 16-year-old woman's first pelvic examination, the teen's needs often extend beyond the surface reason for the appointment, the need for a Papanicolaou (Pap) smear. The array of concerns may include a desire for contraception and for information about the normal menstrual cycle and abnormal alterations, vaginitis, and consequences of sexual activity (for example, pregnancy, STDs, and human immunodeficiency virus [HIV]). The women's health care advanced practice nurse who provides (1) a safe and non-threatening examination room, (2) a personal style toward care that views self and other as integral in the quest for health-related knowledge, and (3) an opportunity for the unlimited pandimensional possibilities for achieving healing and health offers the adolescent a context conducive for information concerning the adolescent's physical and emotional health.

Physical Self

Puberty is not a single event in time but an evolution of changes, the juvenile transitioning into the adult. Although the physiological sequence of events is not well understood, what is known is that the hypothalamic-pituitary-gonadal axis begins operating in fetal life and is repressed by the central nervous system during the first decade of life. Neinstein and Kaufman (1996) state that "the exact trigger of puberty is unknown; however, it is known that puberty is associated with three distinct changes in the hypothalamic-pituitary unit, as follows:

1. A nocturnal sleep-related augmentation of pulsatile luteinizing hormone (LH) secretion begins as a result of the increase in the pulsatile release of gonadotropin releasing hormone (GnRH) (Marshall & Kelch, 1986).
2. The sensitivity of the hypothalamus and the pituitary to estradiol and testosterone decreases so that the gonadotropins, LH and follicle stimulating hormone (FSH),

begin to increase. This is probably the result of sequential maturation of the central nervous system.

3. In the female, a positive feedback system develops. Critical levels of estrogen trigger a large release of GnRH, stimulating LH to initiate ovulation" (p. 4).

Maturational phases in puberty are known as milestones: thelarche, the development of the breast; adrenarche, the development of pubic and axillary hair; peak growth velocity; and menarche, the first menstrual period. Table 15-1 summarizes the developmental milestones of normal puberty.

The timing of puberty is controlled primarily by genetic makeup. Other factors include general health and nutrition, race, geographic location, exposure to light, and psychological reasons (Tanner, 1962). A strong correlation has been identified among female family members' menarche (Speroff, Glass, & Kase, 1994). A decline in age of onset in females in developing countries may suggest the effect of improved nutrition and living conditions. One study suggests that menses will not start before a critical body mass (47.8 kg) is reached (Frisch & Revelle, 1970). Yet other studies indicate that body composition (the percentage of body fat) rather than total body mass is a crucial factor in the timing of pubertal events (Frisch, 1985; Maclure, Travis, Willett, & MacMahon, 1991).

For most adolescent females the sequence of pubertal changes begins with accelerated growth, followed by breast development, adrenarche, and menarche. The growth spurt for girls (11 to 12 years) occurs 2 years earlier than for boys. The typical adolescent female reaches her peak height velocity about 2 years after breast budding and 1 year before menarche (Speroff et al., 1994). The average pubertal growth spurt continues for 24 to 36 months and accounts for 20% to 25% of an adult's final height and 50% of an individual's ideal adult body weight (Neinstein & Kaufman, 1996). In females the peak weight velocity happens 6 to 9 months after the peak height velocity.

Another measure of puberty is secondary sexual characteristics. Marshall and Tanner (1969) identified characteristics of physical development of the breast and patterns of pubic hair growth that have become known as Tanner stages. Tanner staging is a sexual maturity rating scale that compares physical changes at five stages. Chapters 7

Table 15-1   MATURATIONAL MILESTONES OF NORMAL PUBERTY

STAGE OF PUBERTY	AGE OF ONSET (YEARS)		
	MEAN	MEDIAN	RANGE
Thelarche	10.9	9.8	7.8-13.5
Adrenarche	11.2	10.5	8.0-14
Peak growth velocity	11.5	11.4	9.0-14
Menarche	12.7	12.8	9.0-16

Sources: Laufer, M. R., & Goldstein, D. P. (1995). Pediatric and adolescent gynecology. In K. J. Ryan, R. S. Berkowitz, & R. L. Barbieri (Eds.), *Kistner's gynecology: Principles and practice* (6th ed., pp. 571–632). St. Louis: Mosby. Speroff, L., Glass, R. H., & Kase, N. G. (1994). *Clinical gynecologic endocrinology and infertility* (5th ed). Baltimore: Williams & Wilkins.

and 11 give more details of Tanner staging. Charting the sexual maturity rating in an adolescent's personal health record assists the practitioner in monitoring normal and abnormal sexual development patterns during puberty (Speroff et al., 1994, p. 377).

In U.S. females the normal age range of menarche is 9.1 to 17.7 years with a median of 12.8 (Speroff et al., 1994). The reproductive system in women, triggered by the events of puberty, reaches maturity when a positive feedback of estrogen on the pituitary and hypothalamus stimulates the midcycle luteinizing hormone surge necessary for ovulation. Menstruation usually begins with anovulatory cycles characterized by irregular and heavy bleeding. Anovulation may occur up to 12 to 18 months after menarche, and even as many as 50% of all adolescent females still may be anovulatory at 4 years after menarche (Vuorento & Huhtaniemi, 1992).

Emotional and Intellectual Self

Adolescents' psychosocial development occurs in an asynchronous style and creates an abundance of self-concerns. With that in mind, three phases of adolescent psychosocial development have been articulated by Neinstein, Juliani, and Shapiro (1996a) and serve as a practical guide for the nurse. These phases are described with the understanding that adolescents are not a homogeneous group and have individual responses to the demands and choices presented to them. Further integral to the psychosocial development is adolescent sexual preference development. Chapter 14 provides a more comprehensive discussion of female sexuality.

Table 15-2 compares the three phases of adolescent psychosocial development with four developmental tasks through which females must mature in adolescence to achieve adult qualities.

Early Adolescence

Early adolescence (approximately 10 to 13 years of age) is characterized by the most rapid physical changes, fostering a preoccupation with self and the body and initiating the separation from parents and the struggle toward independence. Wide mood swings and extreme emotional responses to seemingly ordinary events occur. A same-sex friend or peer group becomes the source for testing and expressing feelings. The early teen also has increased aptitude to reason abstractly, which supports the ability to daydream and fantasize about one's identity potentials. Emergence of sexual feelings, an increased need for privacy, and the self-construction of a value system are also characteristics of this phase. Risks are related to the teen's lack of impulse control.

Middle Adolescence

During middle adolescence (approximately 14 to 17 years of age), the rapid pubertal changes are waning and the focus on bodily changes become directed toward appearance. Clothes and the use of makeup are often totally consuming. Conflicts with parents increase as the time devoted to peers increases (Newman, 1989). Involvement with peers in clubs, team sports, gangs, and other groups intensifies as does conforming to peer values and dress. Sexual experimentation is initiated. Through exploration of

Table 15-2	PSCYHOSOCIAL DEVELOPMENT OF ADOLESCENTS		
TASK	**EARLY ADOLESCENCE**	**MIDDLE ADOLESCENCE**	**LATE ADOLESCENCE**
Independence	Less interest in parental activities Wide mood swings	Peak of parental conflicts	Reacceptance of parental advice and values
Body image	Preoccupation with self and pubertal changes Uncertainty about appearance	General acceptance of body Concern over making body more attractive	Acceptance of pubertal changes
Peers	Intense relationships with same-sex friends	Peek of peer involvement Conformity with peer values Increased sexual activity and experimentation	Peer group less important More time spent in sharing intimate relationships
Identity	Increased cognition Increased fantasy world Idealistic vocational goals Increased need for privacy Lack of impulse control	Increased scope of feelings Increased intellectual ability Feeling of omnipotence Risk-taking behavior	Practical, realistic vocational goals Refinement of moral, religious, and sexual values Ability to compromise and to set limits

From Neinstein, L. S., Juliani, M. A., & Shapiro, J. (1996a). Psychosocial development in normal adolescents. In L. S. Neinstein (Ed.), *Adolescent health care: A practical guide* (3rd ed., pp. 40–45). Baltimore: Williams & Wilkins.

heterosexual, bisexual, and/or lesbian relationships, sexual identities are started. The feelings of self and others are starting to be examined. Cognitive abilities and creativity are increasing, usually as idealistic future aspirations are diminishing. Risk-taking behaviors (accidents, tobacco and drug use, STDs, pregnancies, and suicides) escalate, stemming from feelings of immortality, omnipotence, and narcissism.

Late Adolescence

In late adolescence (approximately 18 to 21 years of age) begins the integration of identity and separation (Marcia, 1980). For teens who have progressed emotionally through the first two phases of psychosocial development, this phase is more tranquil and supports the acquisition of adult skills. The teens who have become stuck in either of the first two phases of adolescent psychosocial development often are challenged by emotional disorders, depression, and suicide as the responsibilities of adulthood increase (Bragg, 1997). Typically in late adolescence, relationships with parents improve and peer group values become less consuming (O'Koon, 1997). Now that pubertal development is completed, body image becomes less captivating. Cognitive development supports a more rational and realistic conscience that also begins to appreciate the art of compromise and the use of setting limits. Career planning and financial independence are important. Moral and sexual values may be integrated into less risky behaviors.

Additional Theories of Development

Gilligan's research (1982) in the 1970s challenged previous theories on psychosocial development as being male-focused, not viewing the female as having a different process, and as a result women's development was considered deviant. Gilligan's book *In a Different Voice* is based on the findings from three research projects and describes the participant's responses to questions about conceptions of self and morality and about experiences of conflict and choice. The main assumptions of her work are "that the way people talk about their lives is of significance, that the language they use and the connections they make reveal the world that they see and in which they act" (Gilligan, 1982, p. 2). Chapter 6 highlights more of the unique considerations of psychosocial development for women in addition to the more traditional approaches to human psychosocial development (Piaget & Inhelder, 1958; Erickson, 1959; Ginsberg & Opper, 1969).

Prevention: The Cornerstone to Healthy Adolescence

The experiences adolescents have in the health care system influence the knowledge and values of future adult populations about health care. The preventive health care approach has proved its long-term benefits (American Medical Association, 1991). The Writing Group of the 1996 Expert Panel on Women's Health (1997) recommends a health promotion and disease prevention approach to care of the adolescent. Development of health promotion and disease prevention behaviors may be influenced by relationships with health care providers.

Trust is a key component in any relationship between a health care provider and client. For adolescents who are in a stage of their lives when they have struggles with authority, are adjusting to a self-identity, and are influenced greatly by their peers and not their parents, developing a trusting relationship with a health professional is not easy and is nearly impossible in a 10-minute clinical appointment. Preserving a clinical appointment schedule that honors the extra needed time to establish a relationship and examining and diagnosing a physical or emotional problem of a client who may or may not have formal operational skills of cognition takes a longer time than an appointment with an adult who has the same condition. If time is not allotted, the adolescent may learn at a young age to avoid going to a clinic or health care provider because the teen thinks that "they [the health care provider] can't really help me, they don't have the time or the interest." This attitude is common and unfortunate, for it deprives the adolescent, and soon to be young adult, of experiences with health care providers at a time when preventive health knowledge is needed and a place is needed to obtain help when the home environment is not viewed as a resource. As the adolescent becomes adept at cognitive formal operations, approximately by age 18 to 20, adjusting appointment times to an adult standard seems reasonable (Sawyer, Blair, & Bowes, 1997).

In recent years, health care providers for geriatric clients have lobbied successfully to have longer appointment times for their clients (M. Crowley, personal communication, March 1996). Longer appointments are based on the physical restrictions and slower speech and thought processes in the geriatric patient. Many health care practices now allot greater time for geriatric appointments, especially for women requiring a pelvic examination or procedure. For the community of health care providers for adolescents to conduct a similar campaign to extend the standard amount of time allotted for treatment of their clients is crucial.

ADOLESCENT HEALTH HISTORY AND INTERVIEW

Adolescent women see health care providers for a variety of developmental concerns and experiences. Maintaining a high level of sensitivity to the uniqueness of each adolescent and the family she is part of brings the provider respect from the adolescent and her family while facilitating opportunities for enhancing diagnostic accuracy. Discussing in detail the unique focus of the adolescent history and physical examination is warranted because the discussion may lay the foundation for positive experiences for engagement with health care providers and systems in the future.

Although adolescents want to be approved and accepted by others, and this includes health care providers, they also want the health care provider to be someone to whom they can look up and who maintains a position of authority without judgment. Offering a friendly, sincere approach to an adolescent and demonstrating shared knowledge (the adolescent knows herself and the provider knows her profession) helps achieve the common goal of meeting the needs of the adolescent.

Provider-Client Relationship

Establishing Rapport

Establishing eye contact facilitates the accuracy of the data to be collected in the interview and health history. Eye contact may be offered easily by some young women and may be a major challenge to obtain with others. When eye contact is given cautiously or not at all, the provider must first identify what would make the teen feel safer and able to share her concerns. Safety needs may arise from physical concerns ("If my family knows I'm here, I'll be beaten"), psychological concerns ("If I wasn't a bad girl, I wouldn't have to be here"), cultural concerns ("My friend's grandpa died when he went to the clinic"; "Mama says if we pray, we will be healed"; "I don't want to die, but praying doesn't help the pain"), or a random misconception ("I've heard that 'the clamp' can squeeze your guts out"). Moving teens through their concerns and offering reassurance and accurate information is usually enough to bring a reticent teen to make eye contact and begin to feel safe with the provider. When a teen refuses to make any eye contact, the provider needs to negotiate with the teen how best to proceed with the visit and offer a follow-up visit to complete the total evaluation.

When eye contact is established easily, progress toward data collection and the physical examination can move swiftly, although not without consistent evaluation of the teen's comprehension of the examination process and health information.

Confidentiality

The U.S. Preventive Services Task Force (1989) recommends that health care providers for adolescents take a sexual history, discuss risk prevention, and provide confidential care (within legal limits) for all adolescent patients (Schuster, Bell, Peterson, & Kanouse, 1996). A policy of confidentiality that respects the privacy of the teen yet provides a mechanism for disclosure of information about self-harm or harm to others is standard practice in adolescent health care (Hoffman, 1990; Purcell, Hergenroeder, Kozinetz, O'Brien Smith, & Hill, 1997). Lack of private and confidential health services are barriers to adolescents' access to health care. Establishing the principles of privacy and confidentiality early in the interview lays the ground rules for all to comply (Becker, 1995).

When a parent accompanies a teen for a gynecological visit, the rules of confidentiality need to be stated and agreed on. The parent is to be informed that after the initial segment of the interview, the parent will be asked to step out of the examination room. The teen then has the rest of the interview and examination in privacy. Some teens may request to have the parent return to the room during the pelvic examination for comfort. What is important is to state specifically to the parent and teen that, except for a disclosure by the teen of abuse or suicide or homicidal ideation, the content of what the teen says is confidential unless she chooses to share it (Becker, 1995). When a parent seeks the opportunity to speak to the provider alone, permission should be sought from the adolescent.

Setting Limits and Role Modeling

Adolescents by nature of their developmental stage are challengers. Approaching the teen with a genuine, sincere interest and a matter-of-fact attitude helps the teen know the limits of acceptable behavior. Serving as an appropriate role model comes not only from one's appearance and how one conducts oneself as a practitioner but also in the language one chooses to use. From the onset of the relationship with the adolescent, the provider should call the woman by her name and not a pseudonym such as *sweetie, honey, pumpkin, doll,* or *baby-dear.* Using the teen's name offers her respect and unique identification, empowering her to use her own voice. Pseudonyms are demeaning and keep a power advantage on the side of the provider. The goal of any provider-client relationship is for egalitarian use of knowledge to move toward a common goal: the health maintenance of the client.

Interview and Health History

On entering an examination room where the teen and her parent await, the provider needs to introduce herself to the teen first and allow the teen to introduce her family member. This form of introduction, along with asking the question "Why are you seeking health care today?" establishes that the primary relationship is with the adolescent and often empowers her. Although focusing on the adolescent is important, it is also important to avoid an adversarial relationship with the parent.

Adolescent and Family Member

During the joint interview, parents are usually helpful in giving a medical history and their perspective on the concern of the immediate visit. To help parents feel included, the health care provider should focus them on data collection. Avoiding personal questions aids in identifying for the parent that the visit is for the teen yet includes the parent in a useful way. Information regarding the adolescent's perinatal events, developmental stages, immunization record, family history, allergies, and health maintenance can serve to supplement the teen's knowledge and the provider's. The joint interview also provides an opportunity to observe the relationship between the adolescent and her parent. After identifying the process of the remainder of the visit, the parent is told she will be excused from the room and may return for the summation if the adolescent so chooses.

Adolescent Only

For an adolescent to give a different reason for the appointment in private with the provider is not unusual. Anticipating this, the provider begins the construction of the diagnostic puzzle from several perspectives. Verbal communication depends on the developmental level of the teen. Understanding that open-ended questions may pose difficulty for the less advanced teen, the practitioner needs to be versed in alternative ways for collecting medical information. Nonverbal communication, observation of appearance, and listening to the adolescent's speaking language serve in opening discussion further. As a general rule the time spent interviewing and taking a health history with the teen and parent and then with the teen alone sets the stage for a successful examination and diagnosis. The interview phase of the appointment should not be dictated by a 15-minute schedule.

Different styles of information gathering are used. Written health history forms can be useful for literate and older teens. Verbal question-and-answer interviews are the most common but also are time consuming. The following discussion outlines two approaches for collecting biopsychosocial information. Perhaps a combination of these approaches would best serve the needs of the adolescent.

Traditional approach. First, a health history is collected that addresses medications, allergies, immunizations, past illnesses, past surgeries, and a review of systems similar to that collected from an adult woman. With teens, for the provider to assess issues about weight and exercise and menstrual, genitourinary, abdominal, respiratory, and visual changes is imperative. Often an eating disorder may be the basis for physical or emotional symptoms such as headaches, and visual problems arise when the nutrient levels in the body are diminished or depleted. The health care provider should always gather a menstrual history that includes the onset of menses (menarche), frequency of menstrual periods (in days), length of flow (in days), quality of flow (identified as light, moderate, or heavy by assessing the number of tampons or pads used in a day or hour), discomfort and actions taken for relief, intermenstrual spotting, vaginal discharge, breast symptoms, and any emotional changes during the cycle.

Concurrent with the health history or immediately following, psychosocial information is imperative to address. Because the most common causes of adolescent morbidity and mortality are social morbidities (accidents, substance abuse, and sexual behaviors), this portion of the interview cannot be overlooked. The acronym HEADSS, developed by Dr. Eric Cohen at Children's Hospital in Los Angeles, is used to organize the psychosocial interview in an efficient manner. HEADSS refers to **H**ome, **E**ducation/employment, **A**ctivities, **D**rugs, **S**ex, and **S**uicide/depression. The first three areas of questions are less sensitive topics and are a good place to begin this aspect of the interview. When progressing to the more sensitive topics, using the third person or past tense often helps. Box 15-1 gives some suggested questions for each category.

Alternative approach. An alternative approach to collecting the biopsychosocial information is by using a risk screening inventory. An example of such a tool is the West Virginia University Adolescent Risk Score by Perkins, Ferrari, Rosas, Bessette, Williams, and Omar (1997). This is a single-sheet grid with a row of 15 biopsychosocial categories followed by three columns of phrases that the provider circles indicating no risk, moderate risk, and high risk. Although all possibilities could not be stated, moderate risk is identified when no risk or high risk are not appropriate categories. Scoring is simple; no risk values are 0, moderate risk, 1, and high risk, 2. Table 15-3 shows the form of the West Virginia University Adolescent Risk Score.

Examination Room Environment

Care in the decor and arrangement of the clinic waiting room and examination rooms is important. In the waiting room appropriate posters about the harmful effects of drugs, family violence, and unintended pregnancy help to identify that the clinic and its providers are aware of these issues. Providing access to free pamphlets and brochures on topics of risk is helpful, such as for STDs and HIV, pregnancy and contraception, health for gay teens, cigarette smoking, and drugs and alcohol; safety issues such as seat belts, bike helmets, guns, domestic violence, and date rape; and how to avoid life-threatening accidents.

The practitioner may not have control over the physical size and shape of the examination room, but some principles apply to any women's gynecological setting. The examination table should be placed so that when a woman is in stirrups on the table, she is facing away from an opening door. If this is not possible, then a curtain should be installed to serve as a barrier between the woman receiving the examination and the hallway beyond the door, no matter who has access to the hall. Aesthetically pleasing art on the ceiling or the wall next to the examination table is helpful in eliciting a sense of serenity. This sense may work on a nonconscious level and help to reduce anxiety in a client.

If the examination room is only to be used by adolescent women, then posters appropriate to issues of this age and development may be useful: contraception options, oral contraceptive pill choices, breast self-examination, and the phases of the menstrual cycle. Visual aids like pelvic models are a must in the examination room of a teen, even if the teen has had a previous pelvic examination. Pamphlets addressing specific adolescent issues such as date rape, anorexia and bulimia, contraception, and STDs need to be easily accessible.

Box 15-1 SUGGESTED QUESTIONS FOR THE PYSCHOSOCIAL INTERVIEW USING HEADSS

Home
Who lives with you?
Where do you live?
Do you have any privacy?
How do family members get along?
Have you ever considered running away?

Education/Employment
Are you attending school and where?
Which subjects do you like most?
Which do you like least?
Are you involved in extracurricular activities?
How many schools have you attended in the past 3 years?
Do you work?
What are your goals and future plans after school?

Activities
What do you do for fun?
Tell me about some of your friends.
What safety precautions do you take when riding a bike or driving a car?

Drugs
Some teens smoke cigarettes: Do your friends or you smoke? How often and how much?
Some teens drink alcohol: Do any of your friends drink? Do you drink alcohol? Do you ever drive during or after drinking?
Some teens use drugs: Do any of your friends use drugs? What drugs do they use? What drugs have you used? Where do you use them and how frequent is your use?

Sex
(Make questions direct and specific. Some teens choose to be sexually active; others choose not to be.)
Have you ever had sex?
What did you use for protection against sexually transmitted diseases and pregnancy?
Have you ever had a sexually transmitted disease?
Have you ever been pregnant?
Have you ever had your body touched when you did not want to be touched?

Suicide/Depression
Tell me about your moods.
Do you often feel sad or angry?
What do you do when you feel this way?
Have you ever thought about hurting or killing yourself?
Tell me about your sleeping habits.
Do you have trouble sleeping at night?
Do you have trouble staying awake during the day?
Are you bored easily?
Does anyone in your family use drugs or alcohol?
Are there guns in your home?

| Table 15-3 | PERKINS' ADOLESCENT RISK SCREEN (PARS) | |

If patient is High Risk, circle right column; if Low Risk, circle left column.
If undecided, circle center column.
Date _____ Zip code _____ Insurance Type _____

	LOW RISK	MODERATE RISK	HIGH RISK
Body mass index (BMI)	Between 15% to 85% (Normal weight/ height per the growth chart)	Between 5% to 15%/85% to 95% (Just over or just under the normal range)	<5%/>95% (Much over or much under normal weight)
Weight perception	BMI normal and patient is satisfied	BMI normal and patient wants to lose	BMI <15% and patient wants to lose
Nutrition	Eats 3 meals/day and eats fruits, vegetables, and foods with fiber	Eats less than 3 meals/day or vegetarian without milk or eggs	Snacks a lot, eats fats and sugar, vomits or takes medication for weight loss
Exercise	5 times/week for at least 20 min each, with increased heart rate and sweating	Exercises less than 5 times/week, not strenuously	No regular exercise to increase heart rate; excessive exercise
Tobacco use	No smoke or chew	Smoke or chew less than daily; or stopped less than 6 weeks ago	Smoke or chew regularly
Drug use	Never used	Previously used; not in the past 3 months	Recently used or currently uses marijuana, huffing, LSD, cocaine, heroin, etc.
Alcohol use	Has only tasted it, or used for religious purpose	Social only, not more than once/week; less than 3 beers or 2 liquor drinks at a time	Drunkenness, blackouts; drinking interferes w/ school, family, etc.; 4 or more drinks at a time
Sexual activity	Never; or is married *and* faithful	Not in last 6 months; safe sex with condoms	Sex *without* regular use of condoms; first intercourse before age 16
School	B/C average or better; steady improvement in grades	Grades slipping; detention problem	Failing grades; suspension; often skips school
Depression	Usually happy	Often feels discouraged or down; cries a lot	Unhappy *most* of the time; feels hopeless; thoughts of suicide
Abuse	No physical or sexual abuse	Abuse reported and counseling received	Abuse still occurring or not treated with counseling
Safety	Uses seat belt/helmet; never rides with drunk driver	Usually uses seat belt/ helmet; rarely rides with drunk driver	Does not use seat belt/ helmet; has driven drunk; sometimes rides with drunk driver

Table 15-3	PERKINS' ADOLESCENT RISK SCREEN (PARS)—CONT'D		
	LOW RISK	**MODERATE RISK**	**HIGH RISK Violence**
Violence	No fights, no threats; does not carry a knife, gun, or rifle; no legal troubles	Threatens others; previous illegal acts (stealing, etc.) but not in past 3 months	Damages own or others' property; carries a gun, knife, or rifle; physical fights with peers; has had contact with police
Family relationships and responsibility	Gets along with family; completes chores or work duties	Often argues with family; does not complete chores or work duties	Physical and/or intense verbal fights with family
Friends and recreation	Has male and female friends; involved in clubs, activities, or hobbies	Has few friends; does things alone; has friends who often get into trouble	Has no friends, or belongs to gang or cult
Good qualities and future plans	Can name three good qualities about self; has plans for the future	Hard to think of good qualities about self; has few interests; does not have future plans	No good qualities about self; no interests or activities
Immunizations	Has received second MMR, tetanus within 10 years, hepatitis series, and has had varicella or been vaccinated	Lacks one item	Lacks two or more items
Main Diagnosis: _____		High risk:	_____
Provider Initial: _____		Moderate risk:	_____
		Low risk:	_____

Copyright K. C. Perkins, M.D.

PHYSICAL EVALUATION

Only after establishing a relationship with the young woman through the interview and history taking is beginning the physical evaluation appropriate. If during this process, the health care provider determines that the teen has never had a pelvic examination, has had a difficult experience with previous pelvic examinations, or is apprehensive about the examination, reviewing the process of the pelvic examination with the teen before initiating the physical examination is imperative.

A demonstration of the pelvic examination with a plastic model and speculum is helpful and offers a time when the teen can ask questions and admit concerns. Research (Johnson, 1980) has supported giving information as a sensory experience to a person before that person undergoes a potentially noxious procedure so as to better prepare the individual. For example, the health care provider may say, "When it is time for the pelvic examination, I will tell you everything that I am about to do before touching you." Next, the health care provider should indicate that the examination has two parts: first, the speculum examination and, second, the bimanual examination. Demonstrating how a speculum works, how a Pap smear or cervical culture is collected, and how the provider's hands will touch the patient, in particular during a bimanual examination, will assist the teen in coping with her first pelvic examination.

Physical Examination

The health care provider should have the teen sit on the side of the examination table and inform her of the sequence of the examination. The examination begins with evaluations of the visual fields, scalp and hair condition, skin conditions, ears, mouth for any obvious dental caries, thyroid, chest and lungs, deep tendon reflexes and with the sitting portion of the breast examination. Next, the health care provider assists the teen in lying comfortably in a supine position on the examination table and continues with the breast examination and assessing the adolescent's knowledge of breast self-examination. By first demonstrating a technique and then assisting the teen to touch her own breast and learn the proper technique, the practitioner is setting the stage for a lifelong healthy habit. Giving the teen breast self-examination literature to take home with her after the visit helps to reinforce the technique.

The health care provider then evaluates the heart, abdomen, and pulses. This part of the examination offers another opportunity for teaching. Tanning marks serve as a reminder to educate about exposure to the sun and ultraviolet light. The teen can be given accurate information about sunscreens and the effects of too much ultraviolet light exposure. Examining the torso also provides an opportunity to discuss weight, diet, and exercise. Determining if the teen is happy with her current weight and identifying what her desired ideal weight is helps the practitioner decide if diet and exercise guidelines need to be offered or if screening for anorexia nervosa or obesity are needed (see section on eating disorders in this chapter).

Finally, the health care provider assesses the extremities for mobility, bruises, and varicosities. If bruises appear suspicious, the health care provider should question the teen further about physical or sexual abuse. Abuse of a minor is a reportable offense, and knowing the laws of the state in which the practitioner works is now mandatory for nursing licensure in most states.

First Pelvic Examination

The central and most delicate part of the physical examination of the adolescent is the first pelvic examination. The health care provider introduces the teen to the stirrups and indicates that they are for correct positioning of the body for a comfortable and thorough examination. Next, the health care provider assists the teen in putting the heel of her foot in the base of the stirrup and relaxing her back against the examination table. The head of the table can be raised 30 to 40 degrees so that the patient is not flat. From the end of the examination table, the health care provider helps the teen move her buttocks close to the edge of the table, reassuring her that she will not slip off the end of the table. When a drape or sheet is used to cover the adolescent's lower body (with adolescents a drape is recommended), the cloth should be brought together between the knees and slid back toward the lower abdomen so that the legs are completely covered and only the genital area is open to observation. Talking with the patient and making eye contact during this preparation time helps keep the patient connected and gives the provider information about how the teen is progressing in anticipation of the examination.

In addition to positioning the patient, having a tray prepared with all the things required for a thorough examination aids in an efficient examination. Having alternative speculum and gynecological instruments accessible in the examination table drawers also aids in the ease of the examination. Having the examination table placed in a position that allows easy access to a call bell for emergencies or technical help is also important. Once all these things are verified, then the provider may commence with the actual pelvic examination.

A gentle and thorough first pelvic examination can be performed in several ways. The following is a procedure that has worked well for this author.

A bright light properly positioned illuminates the external genitalia well. The health care provider dons gloves and sits down on the stool at the end of the examination table, checks with the teen to see how she is doing, and then indicates the examination is about to begin. With the speculum in the nondominant hand, the health care provider begins by telling the teen that she will feel a touch on the inside of her leg by the back of the dominant gloved hand (for example, "Katie, you will feel me touch your left leg now"). The health care provider then slides the back of the gloved hand down the inside of the leg and gently but firmly touches the labia major; presses the skin firmly against the bony structure, checking for any palpable lumps or bumps on the right and left labia and escutcheon areas; and next separates the lips of the labia major and inspects the labia minora, making sure to inspect and palpate the clitoral area and urethral area through to the base of the vaginal opening. During this inspection, the health care provider assesses the condition of the hymen and vaginal opening. Conditions do exist that prevent further internal evaluation, and medical consultation is necessary before a speculum examination can be preformed.

When no prohibiting conditions exist, the health care provider should tell the patient and introduce the index finger of the dominant hand into the opening of the vagina and palpate around the opening, pressing the thumb toward the index finger and checking for any lumps or unusual findings in the Bartholin or Skene glands. If the muscle tone intensifies, the health care provider can work with the teen to relax the pubococcygeus muscle by putting a slight bit of pressure on the lower vaginal opening. As the muscle tone relaxes, the health care provider then indicates that she will be touching the leg with the speculum, which helps with temperature desensitization. Next, the health care provider touches the vulva with the tip of the speculum blades and slowly, firmly, and gently advances the speculum blades until they are in position to be opened. When using a narrow Pederson blade, the provider can attain greater distance into the vagina and closer approximation to the cervix than with a regular Pederson blade (which may be too wide) or a pediatric speculum (which has short blades) that may not reach far enough into the vagina to provide a good view of the cervix.

Once the speculum is in place, the health care provider opens the blades gently and as narrowly as permits good visualization of the cervix. The trick is to hold the speculum steady while moving one's head and body about so as to see adequately. With a first examination, the goal is to maximize the possibility of a positive experience. Being efficient, having the speculum inside the vagina for as short a time as is reasonable, maintaining communication about activities with the patient, and ensuring comfort adds to the success of a first pelvic examination. Some patients may be interested in looking and can be given a hand mirror.

At this stage the provider needs to observe the cervix and vaginal walls for normal (shape, color, and presence of the squamocolumnar junction) or abnormal (discharge, strawberry spots, Naboth cysts, bleeding, plaques, blisters suggestive of herpes, granular appearance suggestive of condylomata, etc.) conditions. Next the Pap smear can be taken along with any cultures suggested from the history and interview or because of visual findings on examination.

At the completion of the speculum examination, the health care provider inspects the walls of the vagina for any unusual findings as the speculum is retracted. Once the speculum is out, the health care provider praises the teen for accomplishing a major event in a young woman's life and assuages her anxieties and continues with the bimanual examination.

The bimanual examination allows for the evaluation of the pelvic organs through palpation. Generally for right-handed practitioners the index and middle finger of the gloved right hand are introduced into the vagina of the woman, and the internal hand is placed such that it supports the internal structures while the external hand sweeps over the lower abdomen and pelvis, palpating for any structural abnormalities and tender or painful areas. With the first pelvic examination the teen may be more comfortable with the practitioner using only one finger. For the young adolescent whose hymen is intact, or if speculum examination was not performed, or when structural problems are found, a rectal examination may be preferred. Once the internal examination route is chosen, the position, shape, contour, size and texture of the uterus and ovaries are noted and later documented. The bimanual examination typically concludes the physical examination.

Teaching Opportunities

As noted already, the physical examination serves as an opportunity to give the adolescent health maintenance information. Assessing the teen's knowledge about breast self-examination, maintaining healthy skin, and nutrition assists the practitioner in providing appropriate teaching. In addition, preparation for and performance of the pelvic examination are times when the health care provider can discuss menstrual concerns, pregnancy risk and intervention, sexually transmitted disease risk, and other gynecological health risks.

Breast Self-Examination

One teaching opportunity already mentioned is breast self-examination. Figure 15-1 is a visual description of the procedure and a convenient handout for the adolescent. The health history and physical examination provide an opportunity to have a comprehensive health assessment database for lifelong prevention and health promotion activities.

RISK FACTORS

Cognizance of adolescent risks is important as the health care provider assesses the adolescent's health status. Table 15-4 lists the leading causes of death among 15- to 24-year-olds in the United States in 1992.

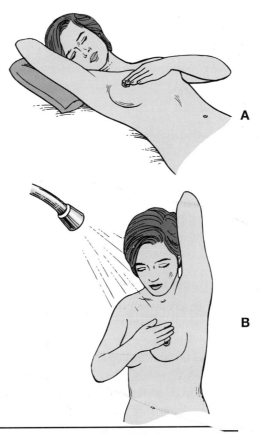

Figure **15-1** Breast self-examination. **A,** Lying down. **B,** In the shower. (From Lowdermilk, D. L., Perry, S. E., & Bobak, I. M. [2000]. *Maternity ana women's health care* [7th ed.]. St. Louis: Mosby.)

Table 15-4	LEADING CAUSES OF DEATH AMONG 15- TO 24-YEAR-OLDS FOR HISPANIC, WHITE NON-HISPANIC, AND AFRICAN-AMERICAN YOUTH: UNITED STATES, 1992

HISPANIC	NUMBER	WHITE NON-HISPANIC	NUMBER	AFRICAN-AMERICAN	NUMBER
Homicide	1732	Accidents and adverse effects	9528	Homicide	4652
Accidents and adverse effects	1624	Suicide	2154	Accidents and adverse effects	1684
Suicide	425	Homicide	1412	Suicide	536
Malignant neoplasms	216	Malignant neoplasms	1195	Diseases of heart	305
Human immuno-deficiency virus	91	Diseases of heart	529	Human immuno-deficiency virus	286
Diseases of heart	83	Congenital anomalies	315	Malignant neoplasms	276
Congenital anomalies	44	Human immuno-deficiency virus	193	Anemias	86
Cerebro-vascular diseases	27	Pneumonia and influenza	134	Chronic obstructive pulmonary disease	80
Pneumonia and influenza	24	Cerebrovascular diseases	117	Congenital anomalies	70
Complica-tions of pregnancy, childbirth	20	Chronic obstructive pulmonary disease	90	Pneumonia and influenza	57

Modified from Centers for Disease Control and Prevention & National Center for Health Statistics. (1994, December 8). Advance report of final mortality statistics, 1992. *Monthly Vital Statistics Report, 43*(Suppl. 6).

Accidents and Unintentional Injuries

In the United States, unintentional injuries are the leading cause of death among 15- to 24-year-olds, with motor vehicle crashes leading and with males being more at risk than females. Comparing three demographic groups—Hispanic, white non-Hispanic, and African-American—homicide is the leading cause of death for Hispanic and African-American 15- to 24-year-olds.

Asynchronous changes in physical development and cognitive development are thought to contribute to adolescent injuries. In the presence of alcohol and drugs, teens challenge authority or rules, desire more peer approval, and experiment with risky behaviors or situations (Neinstein & MacKenzie, 1996).

The following is the prevention strategy recommended in the *Guidelines for Adolescent Preventive Services* (American Medical Association, 1991):

Annual health guidance should be directed at helping adolescents to: abstain from use of alcohol and other drugs when impaired judgement can lead to injury (i.e., while driving a motor vehicle or swimming); use safety devices—including seat belts, motorcycle and bicycle helmets, and appropriate athletic protective gear; identify nonviolent ways to resolve interpersonal conflict; avoid use of handguns and other weapons; achieve physical conditioning before engaging in vigorous exercise and undergo proper rehabilitation before resuming athletic participation (p. 29).

Although use of seat belts in automobiles has reduced the number of fatalities greatly, adolescent seat belt usage is low. Ten percent of college students nationwide rarely or never used safety belts while riding in a car (Centers for Disease Control and Prevention [CDC], 1997d). Also, 56% of students had not used a seat belt the last time they rode in a car, truck, or van (CDC, 1989).

Substance Abuse

Bragg (1997) offers three motives related to drug use. The first is the desire to increase sensitivity and insight or to expand awareness. The second is the desire to have new experiences with peers and seek thrills. The third is for the drug effect, to get high. Teenagers want to fit in, and drug use often allows them to feel good and enhance their position with peers.

Because alcohol and psychoactive drug use among adolescents is illegal, caring for the adolescent who identifies herself as a user may be challenging morally for some professionals. Common guidelines for the role of the adolescent health care provider are to give "(a) general health guidance to all parents regarding the need to monitor their adolescent's social and recreational activities for alcohol and drug use; (b) general health guidance to all adolescents, which includes information on the hazards of using alcohol, other psychoactive drugs, and anabolic steroids; and (c) screening and early intervention" (American Medical Association, 1991, p. 117). Distinctions the health care provider can use in classifying the extent of substance abuse are "(a) casual, experimental or recreational use, which is driven by social factors and occurs within a context of relatively healthy psychosocial adjustment; (b) abuse, which is associated with underlying emotional distress, involves heavy and multiple drug use and has adverse consequences for interpersonal relationships and social functioning; and (c) physical and psychological dependency" (American Medical Association, 1991, p. 118).

Alcohol

Alcohol is the most widely used psychoactive substance by adolescents and in the United States. Inexpensive and easily available, 80% to 90% of adolescents by age 18 have used alcohol. In a 1995 national college health risk behavior survey (CDC, 1997d), 68.2% of college students had had at least one drink of alcohol during the 30 days before the survey, 4.2% had drunk alcohol on 20 or more of the 30 days preceding the survey, and 34.5% had five or more drinks of alcohol (binge drinkers) on at least one occasion during the 30 days preceding the survey. Binge drinkers are

3 times as likely as nonbinge drinkers to engage in unplanned sexual activity, 6 times as likely to drive after consuming large amounts of alcohol, and twice as likely to ride with an intoxicated driver (Neinstein & Pinsky, 1996a). Although more men develop alcoholism, women remain at risk.

Diagnosing an adolescent with a drinking problem vs. alcoholism is not simple. Alcoholism is defined as a primary, chronic disease with genetic, psychosocial, and environmental factors influencing its development and manifestations. Several screening instruments exist and have been assembled in the *NIAAA Treatment Handbook* (Lettieri, Nelson, & Sayers, 1987).

Consequences of alcohol use are associated with other drug use, unplanned sexual encounters, accidents, and physical changes (intoxication, gastritis, blackouts, cirrhosis, and decreased sexual functioning) (Bragg, 1997). Pregnant women who drink risk the fetus developing fetal alcohol syndrome, which is associated with mental retardation and other teratogenic affects. Adolescent women need to be informed early of the risks associated wih alcohol use and abuse. Further, counseling and referring to treatment programs may be necessary.

Other Psychoactive Drugs

The most popular of the illegal drugs in the United States is marijuana. During 1980 to 1990 the use of marijuana declined, but toward the end of that decade the trend changed and marijuana use now is increasing (American Medical Association, 1991). In 1992, 22% of high school seniors reported marijuana use in the past year, and by 1995 this percentage had increased to 34.7% (Neinstein, Heischober, & Pinsky, 1996). A 1995 study of college students found that 48.7% had used marijuana during their lifetime (CDC, 1997d). Although once felt to be a benign drug, marijuana does have negative physical and psychological health effects. Use in early adolescence is especially serious because of the negative affect on academic performance and family harmony (Schwartz, Hoffman, & Jones, 1987).

Hallucinogenic drugs include lysergic acid diethylamide (LSD), mescaline, peyote, psilocybin, morning glory seeds, 3-4 methylenedioxymethamphetamine (MDMA, Ecstacy), 2,5-dimethoxy-4-methamphetamine (STP), phencyclidine hydrochloride (PCP), jimsonweed, and dimethyltryptamine (DMT). Although these drugs traditionally are known as hallucinogens, the name is misleading. These drugs produce illusions or distortions of perceived reality rather than hallucinations (Neinstein & Heischober, 1996a).

Hallucinogens have other major health consequences, including cardiovascular neurological damage, psychological dependence, flashbacks, bad trip emotional responses triggered by one's feelings or the environment (which leave the drug user in panic), and long-term personality changes, depression, and psychosis. On the whole, hallucinogenic drug use decreased in the late 1970s, remained so until the late 1980s, and increased steadily into the mid 1990s (Neinstein & Heischober, 1996a). Approximately 12.7% of high school seniors in 1995 had used hallucinogens (Johnston, O'Malley, & Bachman, 1995). Twenty percent of college students nationwide reported using hallucinogens in their lifetime (CDC, 1997d). Distributing accurate information about the drugs and the associated risk behaviors (increase in injuries and accidents) with drug use may help lead the teen to experiment in a safe environment with drugs of lower dosage or choose not to use these drugs at all.

Stimulant illegal drugs such as cocaine and amphetamines increase the sensitivity of the postsynaptic receptor sites in the central nervous system and leave the user alert and full of confidence (Neinstein & Heischober, 1996b). For high school seniors the rate of use decreased from 17.3% in 1985 to 6% in 1995 (Johnston et al., 1995). Nationwide, 14.4% of college students had used some form of cocaine during their lifetime, and 4.0% had used crack or freebase forms of cocaine (CDC, 1997d). Stimulants have high addictive potentials, and cocaine is a powerful euphoriant with a short half-life, leading to a rapid development of tolerance. A user can progress from small doses to large daily quantities in a short period of time (Neinstein & Heischober, 1996b). Crack cocaine is a more concentrated form of cocaine with a shorter time to get its peak effect. Complications from cocaine abuse and overdose include cardiovascular conditions such as arrhythmias, hypertension, myocardial infarctions, and stroke; neurological conditions such as headaches, seizures, and cerebral hemorrhage; psychiatric changes such as toxic delirium, depression, paranoia, and suicide; obstetrical complications such as placental abruption, prematurity, and low-birth-weight infants; and other complications such as pulmonary edema, chronic rhinitis, erosion of the dental enamel, hyperprolactinemia, malnutrition, and sexual dysfunction. Supporting the respiratory and circulatory systems with treatment of arrhythmias and hypertension while maintaining a calm and reassuring environment is key for treating overdoses.

The last category of illegal drugs to be covered is the opioids. Crude opium is obtained from the seed pods of the poppy plant, from which morphine, codeine, and heroin are produced. Generally, opioids (natural and synthetic) are not popular drugs with adolescents. However, a recent increase in use of heroin probably is related to the trend of smoking heroin. The health care practitioner needs to disseminate the message that regardless of the route of administration, heroin dependence creates an intensely addictive disease with a difficult treatment and poor prognosis.

Anabolic Steroids

Anabolic steroids are synthetic derivatives of testosterone (Neinstein & Heischober, 1996b). Although anabolic steroid users do not have a *Diagnostic and Statistical Manual of Mental Disorders* classification, the drugs are addictive and users require detoxification and rehabilitation to suspend use. Like other abuse substances, steroid addicts may use up to 10 times the therapeutic dose.

The use of anabolic steroids is a growing problem among adolescents. Approximately 5% to 11% of high school students have used anabolic steroids (Komorowski & Richer, 1992; Terney & McLain, 1990). Steroid use among athletes is twice the use of nonathletes, and among intercollegiate athletes use has been reported at 20%. Anabolic steroids are taken to increase muscle mass and incite an aggressive emotional state. Despite the fact that males have a 2 to 7 times more frequent use of steroids than do their female counterparts, adolescent girls are also at risk.

Adverse health consequences of anabolic steroid use and abuse are changes in the serum lipid profile and increases in systolic blood pressure, along with effects on psychological, hepatic, and gonadal functioning. Deaths of professional athletes from cancer and suicide have increased awareness of the health hazards of steroid use (Komorowski & Richer, 1992). Prevention and accurate information given to potential users such as adolescent athletes is key to limiting steroid abuse.

Tobacco

Although somewhat different in its effect than the substances already mentioned, tobacco is a drug with major health consequences. Nicotine is highly addictive and affects neuronal pathways involved in behavioral reward and arousal processes. Cigarette smoking has been listed as the most important source of preventable morbidity and premature death in every report by the Surgeon General of the United States since 1964 (Neinstein & Pinsky, 1996b).

The prevalence of cigarette use is astounding. A study of college students in 1995 (CDC, 1997d) reported that 32.4% of college students nationwide currently used cigarettes or smokeless tobacco. Similarly, 21.6% of high school seniors were daily smokers (Johnston, O'Malley, & Bachman, 1995). In both groups the risks of cigarette smoking were underestimated greatly. Although in past decades the rate of male smokers has been considerably higher than the rate of female smokers, since the late 1980s the rates are comparable.

Other health consequences that have been correlated with cigarette smoking and adolescents are these:

- *Pubertal development*: Patterns of pubertal changes—faster and earlier pubertal development—are associated with girls and the age they start smoking cigarettes and drinking alcohol (Wilson, Killen, & Hayward, 1994). Wilson's study (1994) of 1463 females ages 10 to 18 found that girls with earlier puberty (less than 12.2 years of age) first reported smoking cigarettes at a median of 12.8 years, and this was 0.6 years younger than females with later puberty.
- *Academic performance*: Tobacco use has a negative affect on academic performance (Johnston et al., 1995).
- *Other substance abuse*: A positive association exists between smoking cigarettes and using alcohol and other illicit drugs. Statistics have shown that an adolescent who smokes a pack per day has a 95% association with other drug use, has an 81% association of use of a drug besides marijuana, and a 26% association with daily use of some illicit drug (Neinstein & Pinsky, 1996b).

These social associations with adolescent tobacco use are not the only negative side effects. Health consequences include a multitude of cardiovascular changes that are precursors for premature coronary artery disease; oral, lung, and genitourinary cancers; chronic obstructive pulmonary disease; peptic ulcers; premature wrinkling of the skin; and an increased rate of complications in pregnancy.

Treatment starts with prevention. One of the strongest and best understood messages comes from parents who demonstrate an interest in this issue and help their teen to make an informed choice. Parental role modeling, making the choice not to smoke or indicating the negative affects of smoking with emphasis on how difficult quitting is, is effective. Identifying high-risk groups, pregnant adolescents, oral contraceptive users, and hypertensive adolescents is important in addressing the need for healthy life-style choices. However, when the adolescent has chosen to be a smoker, information and support to engage in a cessation program can help and is the responsibility of all care providers.

Depression and Suicide

Some adolescents respond to the tumultuous physical and psychosocial changes inherent in this phase of growth and development with behaviors identified as out-of-control or acting-out. Often unrecognized, a common underlying condition is depression. In the National Adolescent Student Health Survey (CDC, 1989) of 8th and 10th graders, 61% reported feeling hopeless and sad, 45% reported difficulty coping with home and school, 36% declared having nothing to which to look forward to, and 34% expressed serious thoughts of attempting suicide. These rates did not vary by school grade, but females did report greater levels of emotional distress than did males. The challenge for the practitioner is to differentiate normal depressive mood swings from more serious depressive disorders. In general the adolescent with a depressive disorder is more likely than other adolescents to use and abuse alcohol or other drugs, smoke cigarettes, attempt suicide, have academic difficulties, change performance in school, and display other behavioral problems and psychosocial difficulties (American Medical Association, 1991; Wren, 1997). For more information about diagnosis and treatment of depression, refer to the section on mood disorders.

Although adolescents ages 15 to 24 years are a healthy group, their rate of mortality has not decreased significantly since 1960. Responsible for this statistic is the persistent significant death rate from violent causes: accidents, homicides, and suicides. For males 14 to 24 years of age, suicide is the third leading cause of death. For females in the same age group, suicide is the fourth leading cause of death (Neinstein, Juliani, & Shapiro, 1996b). About 2000 adolescents ages 15 to 19 and more than 3000 persons ages 20 to 24 commit suicide each year (American Medical Association, 1991). Suicide rates are highest for white adolescent males. Males outnumber females in completed suicides by 3:1, and females outnumber males in attempts by the same degree of 3:1. African-American males ages 10 to 19 years are the fastest changing group, increasing more than 200% between 1980 and 1992 (National Center for Health Statistics, 1994). Suicide is least common in all adolescents less than 14 years of age. In a nationwide study of college students, 10.3% seriously had considered attempting suicide, and 6.7% had made a specific plan to attempt suicide (CDC, 1997d).

Seasonal variations in suicide rates have been documented and show increases in the fall and spring. Regional variations in suicide rates for the United States from 1990 to 1994 found that the highest number of suicides (37%) were in the South (Alabama, Arkansas, Delaware, District of Columbia, Florida, Georgia, Kentucky, Louisiana, Maryland, Mississippi, North Carolina, Oklahoma, South Carolina, Tennessee, Texas, Virginia, and West Virginia). However, when state-specific crude suicide rates for the United States were ranked by quartiles, the rate for 10 of the 13 Western states (Alaska, Arizona, California, Colorado, Hawaii, Idaho, Montana, Nevada, New Mexico, Oregon, Utah, Washington, and Wyoming) ranked in the highest quartile. Furthermore, firearms were the leading method in all regions (CDC, 1997a).

In adolescents the firearm-related suicide death rate in 1992 was 65% among persons less than 25 years of age. Although the use of a firearm is more common in male suicides, the rate of firearm use is increasing significantly in female suicides. Other methods used for a completed suicide include poisoning (15% to 20% in males and 25% to 30% in females); suffocation by hanging, strangulation, or drowning (15% to 20% in males and 10% in females); and methods such as piercing with a sharp object or jumping from a high place (Neinstein, Juliani, & Shapiro, 1996b).

Risk factors associated with adolescent-attempted suicide include the following:

- Abuse of alcohol or other psychoactive drugs with depressive actions (Crumley, 1990)
- Feelings of hopelessness, helplessness, or low self-esteem (Swedo et al. 1991).
- Presence of firearms in the house (Brent, Perper, & Moritz, 1993)
- History of prior physical or sexual abuse (Riggs, Alario, & McHorney, 1990)
- Recent behavioral changes
- Alcoholic parents
- History of suicide in the family
- Recent loss of relationship (friend or relative)
- Poor school record
- Prior attempt and intention to repeat

One estimate suggests that at least 30% of adolescents with one suicide attempt will make another attempt within a 2-year period (McIntire & Angel, 1977).

Neinstein, Juliani, and Shapiro (1996b) identified a four-step process through which many adolescents progress on the way to attempted suicide. The first step is a sustained history of problems: suicide is a deficiency disease from lack of social connections or an underlying vulnerability. The second step is an escalation phase of the feelings of vulnerability established in childhood and brought out in the conflicts inherent in adolescence. The third step is a progression of social isolation stemming from traditionally poor communication with parents and manifestations of depression in substance abuse, delinquency, sexual promiscuity, and boredom. The fourth step is a precipitating event that capsulates the prolonged vulnerability and intensified despair (e.g., loss of a significant relationship, pregnancy, school problem, or a family fight).

Primary efforts at suicide prevention (e.g., school-based intervention programs) have not been wholly successful, so secondary efforts by health care practitioners focused on reducing self-destructive behaviors by those most at risk are imperative.

Maltreatment of Adolescents

Adolescent maltreatment is a reportable offense for which the health care provider needs to screen carefully and to refer to the appropriate child protection authorities. Adolescent maltreatment includes neglect, physical abuse, emotional abuse, and sexual abuse. The *Guidelines for Adolescent Preventive Services* of the American Medical Association (1991) use the following definitions:

- **Neglect** implies the failure of the caretaker to provide minimally adequate food, shelter, clothing, education, and health care (Richarson, 1992).
- **Physical abuse** implies injury of a nonaccidental nature with significant risk of death, disfigurement, or prolonged disability. In contrast to assault, the injury must have been inflicted by the parent, caretaker, or legal guardian (Richarson, 1992).
- **Emotional abuse** may include acts of omission, such as rejection or lack of discipline, or of commission, such as degrading comments or public humiliation (Richarson, 1992).
- **Sexual abuse** can be defined as the involvement of dependent, developmentally immature children and adolescents in sexual activities that they do not understand, to which they are unable to give informed consent, or that are inappropriate for family roles (Hibbard, 1992).

Maltreatment of adolescent females is reported more frequently than maltreatment of males. In general, maltreatment in adolescents is underreported compared with maltreatment of younger children (American Medical Association, 1991). Adolescent maltreatment is believed to be more difficult to substantiate because of less severe physical injuries sustained by the adolescent and the perceived concern that the adolescent is partially responsible for the assault.

Adolescents who were abused during early childhood have different characteristics than those who experienced maltreatment during adolescence. Adolescent-onset abuse appears to be related to parental inability to change patterns of discipline as the child develops. Maltreatment is most likely to occur during times of high stress and family crisis (Velsor-Friedrich, 1994).

Health consequences of abuse relate to the onset and character of the abuse. For example, when sexually abused children become adolescents, they are more likely than other adolescents to have major mood disorders, attempt suicide, and to engage in premature sexual activity, substance and alcohol abuse, and delinquency (American Medical Association, 1991). Associations exist between sexually abused female adolescents and the risk for emotional and sexual abuse in adulthood as well as the health risk behaviors of prostitution and intravenous drug abuse, putting the adolescent at risk for HIV infection.

Early identification of abuse is necessary to protect the physical and emotional well-being of the adolescent (American Medical Association, 1991). Clinical interview and physical examination corroboration are used to diagnose abuse. Because the health care provider is legally responsible for reporting abuse, sensitive handling of the adolescent before and after obtaining the information is paramount to the future health of the adolescent. A primary prevention strategy is to provide parents with skills to cope with the changing needs of the adolescent and the adolescent's affect on the family.

Negative Health Consequences of Sexual Behaviors

Experimentation is a natural consequence of the physical and psychosocial changes in adolescence. However, adolescents are at greater risk than adults for the negative consequences of sexual activity because they often lack information and because they perceive themselves to be invulnerable. Adolescents are less likely to use a method of contraception with all acts of intercourse, thus putting them more at risk for unintended pregnancy, STDs, and HIV (Neinstein & MacKenzie, 1996; Hatcher et al., 1994). These three risks are addressed next.

Unintended Pregnancy

More than 1 million adolescents in the United States conceive each year. Of the 1,040,000 teen pregnancies in 1990, 35% were aborted, 14% miscarried, and 51% were delivered (Alan Guttmacher Institute, 1994). Of the 51% of teens who delivered, 37% were unintended births. The timing of adolescent pregnancies has a relation with contraceptive use in that 20% of all premarital pregnancies occur within the first month after initiating sexual intercourse, and 50% occur in the first 6 months (Zelnick & Kantner, 1980).

The cost of adolescent unintended pregnancies is high. Societal costs have been estimated at more than $22 billion, of which 50% of the costs are for Aid to Families with Dependent Children, 35% are for food stamps, and 15% are for Medicaid (American Medical Association, 1991). A more subtle yet extremely high emotional and financial cost is the risk from poor weight gain (less than 20 lb) and delivering a low-birth-weight infant (less than 2500 g). Poor nutrition, late prenatal care, physical abuse during pregnancy, STD during pregnancy, and unplanned pregnancy are determinants of low-birth-weight infants, rather than physiological immaturity.

Although births to mothers under 20 (505,514 in 1996) have declined, the rate of adolescent pregnancies in the United States continues to be significantly higher than the rates in other countries with similar levels of teen sexual activity (CDC, 1997b). The discrepancy accents the importance of making effective contraception available to U.S. teens and actively supporting its use.

Sexually Transmitted Diseases

Each year adolescents account for an estimated 3 million to 6 million cases of STDs (American Medical Association, 1991). From studies of sexually active adolescent females the prevalence rates are 8% to 25% for *Chlamydia trachomatis*, 3% to 18% for

Neisseria gonorrhoeae, up to 48% for *Trichomonas vaginalis*, and 3% to 33% for human papillomavirus infection (Braverman & Strasberg, 1994; CDC, 1993b; Edet, 1993; Evander et al., 1995; Graves & Gardner, 1993; Millstein & Moscicki, 1995; Neinstein, 1996a; Quinn, 1994; Zenilman, 1990). "Although the actual numbers of many STDs are highest in the 20- to 24-year-old age group, adolescents still have the highest risk if these rates are corrected to include only those who are sexually active" (Neinstein, 1996a, p. 853).

Female adolescents are at greater risk because the adolescent use of barrier methods is not always correct or consistent; the adolescent cervix has a greater affinity for cervical ectopy that consists of a greater number of columnar epithelium present on the ectocervix, which attracts *N. gonorrhoeae* and *C. trachomatis*; and adolescents have immature immune systems. Adolescents may be less protected against STDs because they have had less previous exposure (Neinstein, 1996a).

When counseling the adolescent about STD prevention, reviewing condom and other contraceptive method use, the relation between multiple sexual partners and reinfection, and the risk of HIV with unprotected sexual intercourse, oral sex, and rectal sex is paramount.

Human Immunodeficiency Virus/Acquired Immunodeficiency Syndrome

HIV infection is one of the largest epidemics to affect modern society, and acquired immunodeficiency syndrome (AIDS) is the leading cause of death in women 25 to 34 years of age. Adolescent rates of HIV infection are increasing, and women are the fastest growing group infected with HIV (CDC, 1995). An estimated 25% of individuals who are infected with HIV contracted the virus before the age of 22 (National Institutes of Health, 1997). The danger of contracting HIV in adolescence is from risky sexual behaviors and drug use or both. The source of HIV infection in women 13 to 24 years of age is 40% to 50% by heterosexual contact and 22% by injection drug use (CDC, 1995). Prevention efforts must be community based to have the greatest impact; school-based clinics, condom access, and health education in lower grades combined with the efforts of health care educators have worked in some cities.

Box 15-2 summarizes health promotion and disease prevention activities for the adolescent. It outlines history, physical exam, laboratory tests, risk assessment, and immunizations specific for the adolescent woman.

HEALTH ASSESSMENT, PROMOTION, RESTORATION, AND DISEASE PREVENTION: COMMON ADOLESCENT CONCERNS

Patterns of good health start in youth, mature with age and experience, and need to be assessed by skilled health professions during the process of maturation. Inspired by advances in adolescent health research and the recommendations for clinical preventive services developed in the national health objectives by the U.S. Preventive Services Task Force and the Public Health Service for the year 2000, an increasing number of health professionals are supporting the development of clinical strategies aimed at improving adolescent health and well-being through primary and secondary prevention

Box 15-2 SUMMARY OF HEALTH PROMOTION AND DISEASE PREVENTION ACTIVITIES IN ADOLESCENT WOMEN

History	Physical Exam	Laboratory Tests	Risk Assessment	Immunizations
Medical history: Includes childhood illnesses, immunizations, visual changes, respiratory, abdominal, genitourinary, obstetrical/gynecological history; age of menarche; and menstrual history	Height and weight	Tuberculosis skin test in high-risk persons	Scholastic performance	Tetanus and diphtheria booster once during adolescence
Age of first coitus, consensual/nonconsensual sexual practices, safe sex practices, and STDs*	Visual acuity	Sexually transmitted disease (STD)* screening, gonorrhea, chlamydia, VDRL,* and HIV* counseling and testing	Tobacco, alcohol, and drug use	Measles/mumps/rubella once during adolescense
Contraception, number of partners, and sexual orientation	Oral cavity exam	Pap smear	Symptoms of physical and emotional abuse	Hepatitis B
Surgical history	Palpation of thyroid	Vision screening	Symptoms of depression and suicide	Influenza annually if high risk
Family history	Cardiovascular assessment	Pregnancy test if indicated	Evidence of social isolation	Pneumococcal vaccine if high risk
Current medications, steroid use, prescriptions, and over-the-counter drugs	Respiratory assessment		Symptoms of increased stress	
Self-care	Skin exam		Risk factors for STDs* and unintended pregnancy	
Weight history	Lymph node exam		Driving motor vehicle	
Dietary intake	Breast exam		Lack of regular exercise	
Regular exercise	Pelvic exam		Excessive dietary intake or lack of dietary intake	
Tobacco, alcohol, and drug use	Rectal exam		Sunlight or ultraviolet light exposure	
Psychosocial history	Scoliosis screen		Evidence of increased stress	
Home life	Tanner staging		Accident and injury avoidance	
			Parental involvement	
			Prevention strategies	
			Use of seat belts in motor vehicles; use of helmets for skateboarding	
			Prevention and cessation of tobacco, alcohol, and drug use	
			Avoiding being a passenger in a car driven by someone under the influence of alcohol	

Box 15-2 SUMMARY OF HEALTH PROMOTION AND DISEASE PREVENTION ACTIVITIES IN ADOLESCENT WOMEN —CONT'D

History	Physical Exam	Laboratory Tests	Risk Assessment	Immunizations
Education and employment Daily activities, history of child abuse or neglect, domestic violence, emotional or physical abuse by parents, history of depression, and suicide risk			Regular exercise program Dietary plan: restriction of fat and cholesterol; adequate intake of iron and calcium; maintenance of balanced diet Avoiding bingeing or purging for weight control Teaching breast self-exam Discussing contraception and STD* risk reduction Discussing violent behavior and ways to reduce risk Available resources Discussing stress reduction	

*STDs, sexually transmitted diseases; VDRL, Venereal Disease Research Laboratory; HIV, human immunodeficiency virus.

endeavors. This strategy is addressed by the *Guidelines for Adolescent Preventive Services* (American Medical Association, 1991), which recommends clinical criteria not only for treating physical disease and the medical consequences of adolescent health risk behaviors but also for actively attempting to prevent or modify these behaviors. Further, the strategy of the guidelines is predicated on the concern for long-term health outcomes of health behaviors that begin during adolescence and for the immediate health and well-being of adolescents. The success of this strategy is believed to depend on the partnership of the community, parents, adolescents, and health professionals.

This section focuses on clinical concerns of adolescent women. Prevention is the preferred approach, achieved primarily through teaching skills that adolescents can use to avoid risky behaviors. Improved nutrition and consistent healthful exercise solidify the mind, body, and soul and increase receptivity for healthful choices (McKay & Diem, 1995). For adolescent women, avoiding unintended pregnancy ensures greater opportunities in life (American Medical Association, 1991; Becker, 1995; Bragg, 1997; Forrest, 1994; Goldberg & Klerman, 1995; Neinstein, Rabinovitz, & Schneir, 1996; Reeder, Martin, & Koniak-Griffin, 1996). The mystery of the menstrual cycle needs to be grounded in the physiological facts and personalized to allay the young woman's fears and concerns and to meet her needs. Adolescents now deal with life-threatening diseases and harmful outcomes from sexual choice consequences. Information about STDs and genital-urinary disorders and their prevention and treatment is crucial. The psychological well-being of the adolescent female needs to be evaluated for potentially life-threatening depression and suicidal ideation while teaching improved self-esteem through self-affirming practices.

EXERCISE AND NUTRITION

In all areas of women's health, good standards of care include proper nutrition and exercise. These guidelines should be offered in written form, reviewed, and later followed up to ensure healthful behaviors. Guidance about adolescent nutrition can be found in Chapter 11.

Standards of exercise for adolescents have not been established, but planned, structured, repetitive, and purposeful activity leading to health-related physical fitness needs to be encouraged. Two recommendations for adolescents from a panel of experts for physical activity are these (*Physical Activity Guidelines for Adolescents,* 1994, p. 301):

1. All adolescents should be physically active daily or nearly every day as part of play, games, sports, work, transportation, recreation, physical education, or planned exercise in the context of family, school, and community activities.

2. Adolescents should engage in three or more sessions per week of activities that last 20 minutes or more at a time and that require moderated to vigorous levels of exercise exertion.

The four principal components of fitness are body composition, strength, flexibility, and cardiovascular fitness. Over the past 3 decades obesity in adolescents and young adults has increased (Hergenroeder & Neinstein, 1996). The recommendation to decrease caloric consumption and increase energy expenditure is important in reducing the rate of obesity. Strength can be improved safely by resistance training. Before initiating this kind of strength-training program, developing a customized plan with a trainer is recommended. Flexibility is important for indicating weakness and asymmetry of muscle and joint health. For athletes who have had sports injuries, a combination program of building strength and increasing flexibility decreases the probability of a subsequent injury. Cardiovascular fitness is best achieved through aerobic exercises, lasting 20 to 25 minutes, three to four times per week. To prevent injuries and promote continuity with aerobic exercise, adolescents should be evaluated for their current level of fitness and given direction to achieve the desired level of fitness.

The greatest documented health risk for lack of physical fitness and a sedentary lifestyle is the risk of cardiovascular disease and premature death. "The level of fitness influences heart disease both directly and indirectly through its effect on blood pressure, serum lipid levels, and obesity" (American Medical Association, 1991, p. 62).

The number of female athletes has been increasing and so have their injuries. Female rates of injury are similar to male rates of injury in the same sport. Prevention of injuries is best achieved by all-around physical training. When injuries do occur to female athletes, access to qualified sports medicine personnel should not be limited because of sex.

Although breast injuries are rare, sore and tender breasts from vigorous exercise are common. The best preventive measure is use of a sports bra to support and protect breast tissue.

As mentioned previously, a special concern for female athletes is osteopenia. This condition is the consequence of extensive athletic training, amenorrhea, and degeneration of bone density. Female athletes with amenorrhea have higher rates of stress fractures and a greater potential for osteoporosis after menopause. To prevent these potentially crippling conditions, female athletes need to maintain a certain level of body weight composition, consider taking exogenous hormones, ingest 1500 mg of elemental calcium daily, and obtain psychological counseling for any eating disorders (Chapman, Toma, Tuveson, & Jacob, 1997).

CONTRACEPTION

Preparing adolescents to cope with the issue of becoming sexually active is the combined responsibility of the family, school, community, and health care professions. Diagrams of genital differences with physical descriptions of reproductive organs and functions are necessary for dispelling false information. Role playing about choosing to abstain from or engage in sexual activities, when done in a safe environment, is a helpful way to enlighten a teen.

Although the availability of contraception has improved over the last century, misunderstandings about efficacy, safety, and use persist. According to Letterie and Royce (1995), a 1993 survey of females from 15 to 45 years found that "only 73% of those who wished to avoid pregnancy used contraception. The remainder, primarily adolescent and women older than 40 years, stated that they did not use any contraception because of fears regarding side effects and health risks." Promoting accurate information about methods of contraception is the role of the health care practitioner. Together, adolescent and practitioner can work to match the right contraception to the unique needs of each adolescent. A counseling session that demonstrates some and reviews all contraceptive options best facilitates this goal. In some facilities, education also is accomplished by a family planning counselor.

Understanding efficacy is essential in the process of making a contraceptive choice. Efficacy is reported in terms of method effectiveness (the theoretical or lowest expected percentage) and use effectiveness (the usual field experience or typical use percentage). Table 15-5 compares the effectiveness of contraceptives by method and pregnancy rate. All methods of contraception should be reviewed, even when a teen seems to know precisely what she wants. She may not know all her options.

Oral Hormonal Contraception

The oral contraceptive pill (OCP) was approved by the Food and Drug Administration (FDA) in 1960. Since then the pill has become one of the most popular forms of reversible contraception. More than 30 combination pills are on the market worldwide,

Table 15-5 | **EFFECTIVENESS OF CONTRACEPTIVE METHODS**

METHOD	PREGNANCIES PER 100 WOMEN YEARS ALL AGES	
	LOWEST PER METHOD	TYPICAL PER USER
No contraception	85	85
Combination oral contraceptive	0.1	3
Progestin-only oral contraceptive	0.5	3
Progestin injections		
Medroxyprogesterone acetate	0.3	0.3
Norethindrone enanthanate	0.4	0.4
Progestin implants		
Levonorgestrel	0.3	0.3
Intrauterine device		
Progestasert	2	3
Copper T 380A	0.8	3
Barrier methods		
Diaphragm and cerival cap	6	18
Condoms	2	12
Aerosol foam, jelly, cream, tablets	3	21
Sponge		
Parous women	9	28
Nulliparous women	6	18
Periodic abstinence		
Rhythm method	1-9	20
Surgical sterilization		
Tubal ligation	0.2	0.4

Modified from Dickey, R. P. (1994). *Managing contraceptive pill patients* (pp. 129–129, 8th ed.). Durant, OK: Essential Medical Information Systems.

along with five progestin-only pills (Table 15-6). The wide array of different products and formulations has kept practitioners challenged as to the best match of OCP and woman.

Oral contraceptives are also one of the most researched pharmaceuticals ever prescribed. The improved safety of OCPs since the 1960s has been associated with the decreased amount of estrogen and newer formulations of progestin. In the 1970s and 1980s, research supported decreasing the concentration of estrogen (ethinyl estradiol or mestranol) by 2 to 4 times. Today the range of ethinyl estradiol is 20 to 50 µg per tablet. In the 1980s and 1990s, research focused on changes in the concentration and types of progestin. First-generation progestins (norethindrone, norethindrone acetate, norethynodrel, ethynodiol diacetate, and norgestrel) are derivatives of 19-nortestosterone and have adverse androgenic side effects (acne and adverse affects on the cholesterol-lipoprotein profile). Today, second-generation progestins (norgestimate, desogestrel, and gestodene) are available and have reduced

Table 15-6	ORAL CONTRACEPTIVE TYPES, DOSAGES, AND PHYSIOLOGY				
ORAL CONTRACEPTIVE	ESTROGEN DOSAGE	PROGESTERONE DOSAGE	PROGESTA-TIONAL	ANDRO-GENIC	ENDO-METRIAL
Low Dose Monophasics					
Brevicon (Syntex) 21 to 28 day	0.035 mg ethinyl estradiol	0.5 mg norethindrone	L	L	I
Demulen 1/35 (Searle) 21 or 28 day	0.035 mg ethinyl estradiol	1 mg ethynodiol diacetate	I/H	L	L
Desogen (Organon) 28 day	0.03 mg ethinyl estradiol	0.15 mg desogestrel	I/H	L	L/I
Genora 1/35 (Rugby) 28 day	0.035 mg ethinyl estradiol	1 mg norethindrone	I	L/I	I
Levlen (Berlex) 21 or 28 day	0.03 mg ethinyl estradiol	0.15 mg levonorgestrel	L/I	I	L
Loestrin 1/20 (Parke-Davis) 21 day	0.02 mg ethinyl estradiol	1 mg norethindrone acetate	I	I/H	
Loestrin 1.5/30 (Parke-Davis) 21 day	0.03 mg ethinyl estradiol	1.5 mg norethindrone acetate	I	I/H	L
Loestrin Fe 1/20 (Parke-Davis) 28 day 7 pills 75 mg ferrous fumarate	0.02 mg ethinyl estradiol	1 mg norethindrone acetate	I	I/H	L
Loestrin Fe 1.5/30 (Parke-Davis) 28 day 7 pills 75 mg ferrous fumarate	0.02 mg ethinyl estradiol	1 mg norethindrone acetate	I	I/H	L
Lo-Ovral (Wyeth) 21 or 28 day	0.03 mg ethinyl estradiol	0.3 mg norgestrel	L/I	I	L/I
Modicon (Ortho) 21 or 28 day	0.035 mg ethinyl estradiol	0.5 mg norethindrone	L	L	I
Nelova 1/35E (Warner-Chilcott)	0.035 mg ethinyl estradiol	1 mg norethindrone	I	L/I	I
Nelova 0.5/35 E (Warner-Chilcott)	0.035 mg ethinyl estradiol	0.5 mg norethindrone	L	L	I
Nordette (Wyeth) 21 or 28 day	0.03 mg ethinyl estradiol	0.15 mg levonorgestrel	L/I	I	I
Norethin 1/35 E (Schiapparelli Searle) 28 day	0.035 mg ethinyl estradiol	1 mg norethindrone	I	L/I	I

Modified from Dickey, R. P. (1993). *Managing contraceptive pills* (7th ed.). Durant, OK: Essential Medical Information Systems.
L, low; *H*, high; *I*, intermediate.

Continued

Table **15-6** ORAL CONTRACEPTIVE TYPES, DOSAGES, AND PHYSIOLOGY—CONT'D

ORAL CONTRACEPTIVE	ESTROGEN DOSAGE	PROGESTERONE DOSAGE	PROGESTA-TIONAL	ANDRO-GENIC	ENDO-METRIAL
Norinyl 1+35 (Syntex) 21 or 28 day	0.035 mg ethinyl estradiol	1 mg norethindrone	I	L/I	I
Ortho-Cept (Ortho) 21 or 28 day	0.03 mg ethinyl estradiol	0.150 mg desogestrel	I/H	L	I
Ortho-Cyclen (Ortho) 21 or 28 day	0.035 mg ethinyl estradiol	25 mg norgestimate	L	L	L/I
Ortho-Novum 1/35 (Ortho) 21 or 28 day	0.035 mg ethinyl estradiol	1 mg norethindrone	I	L/I	I
Ovcon 35 (Mead Johnson) 21 or 28 day	0.035 mg ethinyl estradiol	0.4 mg norethindrone	L	L	I
Triphasics					
Ortho-Novum 7/7/7 (Ortho) 21 or 28 day	7 days: 0.035 mg ethinyl estradiol 7 days: 0.035 mg ethinyl estradiol 7 days: 0.035 mg ethinyl estradiol	7 days: 0.5 mg norethindrone 7 days: 0.75 mg norethindrone 7 days: 1 mg norethindrone	L/I	L/I	I
Tri-Levien (Berlex) 21 or 28 day	6 days: 0.03 mg ethinyl estradiol 5 days: 0.04 mg ethinyl estradiol 10 days: 0.03 mg ethinyl estradiol	6 days: 0.05 mg levonorgestrel 5 days: 0.075 mg levonorgestrel 10 days: 0.125 mg levonorgestrel	L	L/I	I
Tri-Cyclen (Ortho) 21 or 28 day	7 days: 0.035 mg ethinyl estradiol 7 days: 0.035 mg ethinyl estradiol 7 days: 0.035 mg ethinyl estradiol	7 days: 0.18 mg norgestimate 7 days: 0.215 mg norgestimate 7 days: 0.25 mg norgestimate	L	L	L/I
Tri-Norinyl (Syntex) 21 or 28 day	7 days: 0.035 mg ethinyl estradiol 9 days: 0.035 mg ethinyl estradiol 5 days: 0.035 mg ethinyl estradiol	7 days: 0.5 mg norethindrone 9 days: 1 mg norethindrone 5 days: 0.5 mg norethindrone	L/I	L/I	I
Triphasil (Wyeth) 21 or 28 day	6 days: 0.03 mg ethinyl estradiol 5 days: 0.04 mg ethinyl estradiol 10 days: 0.03 mg ethinyl estradiol	6 days: 0.05 mg levonorgestrel 5 days: 0.075 mg levonorgestrel 10 days: 0.125 mg levonorgestrel	L	L/I	I

| Table 15-6 | ORAL CONTRACEPTIVE TYPES, DOSAGES, AND PHYSIOLOGY—CONT'D | | | | |

ORAL CONTRACEPTIVE	ESTROGEN DOSAGE	PROGESTERONE DOSAGE	PROGESTA-TIONAL	ANDRO-GENIC	ENDO-METRIAL
Biphasics					
Jenest (organon) 28 day	7 days: 0.035 mg ethinyl estradiol 14 days: 0.035 mg ethinyl estradiol	7 days: 0.5 mg norethindrone 14 days: 1 mg norethindrone	L/I	L/I	I
Ortho-Novum 10/11 (Ortho) 21 or 28 day	10 days: 0.035 mg ethinyl estradiol 11 days: 0.035 mg ethinyl estradiol	10 days: 0.5 mg norethindrone 11 days: 1 mg norethindrone	L/I	L/I	I
Moderate Dose Monophasics					
Demulen 1/50 (Searle) 21 or 28 day	0.050 mg ethinyl estradiol	1 mg ethynodiol diacetate	I/H	L	I
Genora 1/50 (Rugby) 28 day	0.05 mg mestranol	1 mg norethindrone	I	L/I	I
Norethin 1/50 M (Schiapparelli Searle) 28 day	0.05 mg mestranol	1 mg norethindrone	I	L/I	I
Norinyl 1 + 50 (Syntex) 21 or 28 day	0.05 mg mestranol	1 mg norethindrone	I	L/I	I
Norlestrin 1/50 (Parke-Davis) 21 day	0.05 mg ethinyl estradiol	1 mg norethindrone acetate	I	I	I
Norlestrin FE 1/50 (Parke-Davis) 28 day 7 pills 75 mg ferrous fumerate	0.05 mg ethinyl estradiol	1 mg norethindrone acetate	I	I	I
Norlestrin 2.5/50 (Parke-Davis) 21 day	0.05 mg ethinyl estradiol	2.5 mg norethindrone acetate	H	H	H
Norlestrin Fe 2.5/50 (Parke-Davis) 28 day 7 pills 75 mg ferrous fumerate	0.05 mg ethinyl estradiol	2.5 mg norethindrone acetate	H	H	H
Ortho-Novum 1/50 (Ortho) 21 or 28 day	0.05 mg mestranol	1 mg norethindrone	I	L/I	I
Ovcon 50 (Mead Johnson) 21 or 28 day	0.05 mg ethinyl estradiol	1 mg norethindrone	I	L/I	I

Continued

Table 15-6   ORAL CONTRACEPTIVE TYPES, DOSAGES, AND PHYSIOLOGY—CONT'D

ORAL CONTRACEPTIVE	ESTROGEN DOSAGE	PROGESTERONE DOSAGE	PROGESTA-TIONAL	ANDRO-GENIC	ENDO-METRIAL
Ovral (Wyeth) 21 or 28 day	0.05 mg ethinyl estradiol	0.5 mg norgestrel	H	H	I/H
Progestin Only Micronor (Ortho) 28 day		0.35 mg norethindrone	L	L	L
Nor-QD (Syntex) 42 day		0.35 mg norethindrone	L	L	L
Ovrette (Wyeth) 28 day		0.075 mg norgestrel	L	L	L

androgenicity and may even have beneficial effects on the cholesterol-lipoprotein profile. Box 15-3 lists the contraindications to using OCPs.

In the clinical management of oral contraceptives the first consideration is the choice of contraceptive pill. Speroff, Glass, and Kase (1994) suggests that "the best choice is the lowest dose at the lowest cost." In general, this approach is sound advice; however, listening to the adolescents' unique needs ultimately will guide the practitioner to the best choice.

Combination Pills

Combination OCPs contain estrogens and progestins and can be differentiated into three groups: monophasic, biphasic, and triphasic. *Monophasic* refers to the amount and type of estrogen and progestin being the same for 21 days followed by 7 days of no hormonal ingestion. *Biphasic* refers to the amount and type of estrogen being consistent for 21 days, whereas the amount of progestin changes after 7 days and the type is consistent, followed by 7 days of no hormonal ingestion. *Triphasic* refers to the type of estrogen being the same for 21 days, but the amount may vary with the progestin. The type of progestin also remains consistent, although the amount changes 3 times in 21 days, followed by 7 days of no hormonal ingestion.

The mechanism of action is the prevention of pregnancy through the suppression of ovulation by inhibiting gonadotropin secretion at the level of the pituitary-hypothalamic axis. Estrogen works to suppress follicle stimulating hormone secretion, thus preventing selection and emergence of a dominant follicle, and progestin works primarily to suppress luteinizing hormone secretion, thus preventing ovulation (Speroff, Glass, & Kase, 1994, p. 723). Progestins also have several direct effects on the reproductive organs by thickening cervical mucus, influencing peristalsis within the fallopian tubes, and rendering the endometrium hostile to implantation.

Although the combination OCP has a method effectiveness of 0.1%, the user rate falls to 3.0% (see Table 15-5). Part of the reason for this decrease is from poor

---

Box 15-3 ABSOLUTE AND RELATIVE CONTRAINDICATIONS FOR USE OF ORAL CONTRACEPTIVE PILLS

Absolute Contraindications

1. Undiagnosed abnormal vaginal bleeding
2. Known or suspected pregnancy
3. Thrombophlebitis, thromboembolic disorders, cerebral vascular disease, coronary occlusion, a history of these conditions, or conditions predisposing to these problems
4. Greatly impaired liver function. Steroid hormones are contraindicated in patients with hepatitis until liver function test results are normal.
5. Known or suspected breast cancer
6. Smokers over the age of 35

Relative Contraindications

1. *Migraine headaches.* Research has drawn the association between high-dose pill use and an increased risk of stroke in migraine sufferers; however, some women report an improvement in their headaches (using monophasic oral contraceptive pills).
2. *Hypertension.* A woman under 35 who is otherwise healthy and whose blood pressure is controlled by medication can elect to use oral contraceptives.
3. *Gestational diabetes.* Low-dose formulations do not produce a diabetic glucose intolerance response in women with previous gestational diabetes, and no evidence indicates that oral contraceptives increase the incidence of diabetes mellitus. Speroff and others (1994) support the belief that women with previous gestational diabetes can use oral contraceptives with annual assessment of the fasting glucose level.
4. *Diabetes mellitus.* Effective prevention of pregnancy outweighs the small risk in diabetic women who are under age 35 and otherwise healthy.
5. *Epilepsy.* Oral contraceptives do not exacerbate epilepsy, and, in some women, improvement in seizure control has occurred. Antiepileptic drugs, however, may decrease the effectiveness of oral contraceptives.
6. *Sickle-cell disease or sickle cell–hemoglobin C disease.* Patients with sickle-cell trait can use oral contraceptives. The risk of thrombosis in women with sickle-cell or sickle cell–hemoglobin C disease is theoretical and has medical-legal implications. Speroff and others (1994) believe that effective protection against pregnancy in these patients warrants the use of low-dose oral contraceptives.
7. *Gallbladder disease.* Generally, most clinicians do not prescribe oral contraceptives for patients with active disease.
8. *Obstructive jaundice in pregnancy.* Not all patients with this history develop jaundice while using oral contraceptives, especially with the low-dose formulations.
9. *Uterine leiomyoma.* This condition is not a contraindication with the low-dose formulations.
10. *Elective surgery.* The recommendation that oral contraception should be discontinued 4 weeks before elective surgery to avoid the increased risk of postoperative thrombosis is based on data derived from high-dose pills. Following this recommendation is safer, if possible, but is probably less critical with low-dose contraceptives.

Modified from Speroff, L., Glass, R. H., Kase, N. G. (1994). *Clinical gynecologic endocrinology and infertility* (5th ed.). Baltimore: Williams & Wilkins.

instruction about how to take the pill or what to do if a side effect occurs. One cannot stress enough in counseling adolescents that instructions need to be given clearly, simply, and repetitively. A written handout about OCPs that the teen can take home with her provides a helpful resource she can use anytime. The handout on OCPs should include the mechanism of action, side effects, advantages and disadvantages, how to initiate use, identification of a backup method, medication interactions, how to discontinue the method, and important resources such as the clinic name and practitioner's name and phone number. Once the specific oral contraceptive has been selected, a hands-on experience with the packaging (e.g., removing the pill from the packaging) is invaluable to concrete thinkers, which most teens are.

In prescribing an OCP, first taking a thorough history and performing a physical examination with a pelvic examination and Pap smear is customary. If the adolescent is sexually active already, the history and physical examination provide an opportunity to evaluate for pregnancy and sexually transmitted diseases. Once pregnancy is ruled out and any STD is diagnosed and treatment prescribed with education, then the focus may shift to which contraceptive pill should be given.

Initiating OCP use occurs in two ways. Traditionally, the first pill is taken the first Sunday after menses begins, or, if menses begins on a Sunday, the first pill is taken that day. Newer pills have an any-day start, meaning that the day of the week one's menses begins is the day one takes the first pill. This any-day start approach is easy for the adolescent but challenges the practitioner in solving problems when side effects occur.

Generally, contraceptive pill packages are arranged with 3 weeks of the active hormone and 1 week of a nonhormonal pill, totaling 28 pills. During the week of nonhormonal pills, the woman can expect her menses. With a 21- day pill package the woman does not take any pills for 1 week, has her menses, and resumes taking pills 7 days after the last pill (not at the end of her menses). The 21- and 28-day packaged OCPs maintain the woman's natural cycle, which is comforting to many women. An alternative approach is to delete the pill-free interval and maintain the active pills for up to 3 cycles and then have a withdrawal bleed. This approach works well for athletes who want to avoid menses during times of competition.

The majority of women, and especially adolescents, have the best oral contraceptive results with a combination low-dose monophasic pill (Hatcher et al., 1994; Moriarty, 1997; Nelson & Neinstein, 1996). Rarely prescribed for teens, the progestin-only pill has advantages for women who need to avoid exogenous estrogen exposure.

Progestin-Only Pills

Also known as the minipill, the progestin-only pill is best prescribed for women who should not take exogenous estrogens or who are lactating. The pill must be taken at the same time each day. The progestin-only pill is not the method of choice for most adolescents and women lacking organization or who have compulsive tendencies.

The mechanism of action depends on small amounts of circulating progestins having an influence on cervical mucus and the endometrium. Although the increase in progestins thickens the cervical mucus and the endometrium involutes and becomes inhospitable for implantation, the gonadotropins are not suppressed consistently, so ovulation can occur. Because of the primary effect of the minipill on the cervix and endometrium, if and when a failure occurs and the woman becomes pregnant, the incidence of ectopic implantation is higher. Efficacy depends on regularity, and no pill-free interval occurs. The effect of the minipill on the cervical mucus is such that after 22 hours permeability starts to diminish, and replenishing its effect takes 2 to 4 hours (Speroff, Glass, & Kase, 1994, p. 749).

The woman begins taking the minipill on the first day of menses. A backup method needs to be used for at least 7 days. Identifying a time of day that a routine activity happens is the best time to take the minipill. The hormonal influence is so sensitive that if the minipill is taken more than 3 hours late, a backup method should be used for 48 hours.

The most reported side effect of the minipill is irregular menstrual bleeding. This bleeding may take the form of unpredictable spotting, frequent and short cycles, or amenorrhea. This side effect is the main reason a woman may discontinue the method.

Barrier Methods

The barrier methods of contraception include the male condom, the female condom, a variety of spermicidal preparations (vaginal inserts, films, foams, jellies, and creams), the contraceptive sponge, the diaphragm, and the cervical cap. All these methods work on the principle that a physical barrier or spermicide prevents sperm from reaching the upper reproductive tract in women. Each method has its own rate of effectiveness (see Table 15-5).

In general, adolescents are counseled to be familiar with and to use barrier methods for STD and pregnancy prevention. Barrier methods are easy to obtain and initially less expensive than prescribed methods. Because of the climbing rates of HIV infection and the already high rates of other STDs in the adolescent population, condoms are promoted for each act of intercourse.

Condoms

The male condom is a sheath that covers the erect penis and provides two forms of protection: pregnancy and STDs (Figure 15-2). Traditionally the condom has been used as a contraceptive device to prevent the passage of semen into the female genitalia, thus decreasing the possibility of pregnancy. Since the mid-1980s and the discovery of the AIDS virus, latex condoms have been recommended to prevent infection with HIV and other STDs.

Condoms come in a variety of colors, textures, shapes, sizes, and thicknesses. Condoms for oral sex are now flavored. Other names for condoms are rubbers, prophylactics, or skins. Natural skins or processed collagenous tissue condoms are an alternative to the latex condom, but these do not protect against HIV and some STDs. Spermicidal condoms offer an added benefit of nonoxynol 9 to immobilize and kill ejaculated sperm and inhibit the transmission of STDs to the female's upper genital tract. For individuals who have an allergy to latex, a new material, tactylon (a synthetic thermoplastic elastomer), is now available. The tactylon condom also protects against STDs and HIV.

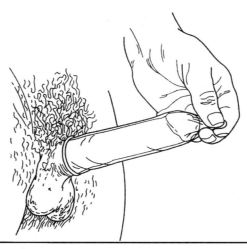

Figure 15-2 Male condom. (From Hatcher, R. A., Trussell, J., Stewart, F., Stewart, G. K., Kowal, D., Guest, F., et al. [1994]. *Contraceptive technology* [16th ed.]. New York: Irvington.)

One of the greatest advantages of the condom is its low cost and easy accessibility. Condoms can be purchased for as little as 50 cents each, and many clinics distribute them for free. Condoms can be purchased by men or women from a variety of places: pharmacies, grocery stores, public restrooms, restaurants, family planning clinics, and mail order services to name a few. Other advantages of condoms include the following:

■ Condoms are easily portable.
■ Condoms encourage male participation in contraception and prevention of STDs.
■ Condoms enhance hygiene by containing the postcoital discharge in the condom and away from the vagina.
■ Condoms are reversible contraception without adverse effects on fertility.
■ Condoms prevent allergic reactions for women who are sensitive to their partner's semen.
■ Condoms enhance erections and help prevent premature ejaculation.
■ Condoms may be used during lactation.
■ Condoms are available without a prescription or examination.

The following are disadvantages of condoms:

■ Condoms possibly cause a change in the male glans sensitivity.
■ Condom use interrupts foreplay.
■ Condoms challenge sexual spontaneity.
■ Condoms may prove to be expensive for frequent use.
■ The man may not want to be involved with the responsibility for contraception or infection prevention.
■ Condoms decrease sensation for some women.
■ Condoms potentially are embarrassing to purchase.
■ Condom breakage may occur for a variety of reasons.

Clinical management focuses on the appropriate use of condoms. Demonstrating how to unroll and secure the condom in place, making sure the tip has enough room to collect the ejaculate, is invaluable to inexperienced potential users. If extra lubrication is necessary, the health care provider should recommend water-based lubricants or spermicidal creams or gels. Oil- or petroleum-based products should never be used because these deteriorate the quality of the condom. The health care provider should instruct the adolescent that if during coitus she becomes concerned about slippage or a tear, she should stop coitus and investigate. The male should withdraw the penis while holding onto the rim of the condom as one would after coitus. If the condom has slipped or is torn, the male should replace it with a new condom before resuming intercourse. To minimize the risk of pregnancy, the woman should insert a spermicidal gel or foam immediately after withdrawal. If this action does not seem satisfactory, then the woman should obtain a postcoital contraceptive within 72 hours. The health care provider needs to advise the woman that condoms are not reusable and a new one needs to be placed on the erect penis before each act of intercourse.

All pharmaceutical products have an expiration date. The health care provider should encourage the adolescent to read about the product before she buys it and make sure that the product has not reached the expiration date. Condoms keep for a long time if stored in a cool, dry, and dark place. Condoms carried in a wallet have a much shorter life span and should be replaced after a month.

Female Condom

The Reality Female Condom (Female Health Company, Chicago, Illinois) was approved for use by the FDA in 1993. The condom is a polyurethane sheath with a ring at either end. The closed end and smaller ring are inserted into the vagina, and the larger ring at the open end remains outside the vaginal opening.

Although the typical first-year failure rate of the female condom has been reported to be as high as 25%, the condom also has a 5% perfect use failure rate. Practicing insertion of the female condom before actual use is important for successful use. The lubrication on the female condom and the insertion process of the inner ring of the female condom (similar to a diaphragm insertion) contribute to the difficulty in using this method. This method may not be the best for young teens and teens uncomfortable with touching their bodies.

Protection from STDs is an advantage of latex male condoms and is envisioned to be an advantage of the female condom, especially for women whose partners refuse to use latex condoms. Male and female condoms are not recommended for simultaneous use. The female condom, similar to the male condom, is a single-size disposable item that is sold over the counter. The female condom may be inserted up to 8 hours before coitus. Care must be taken during insertion to prevent tearing by a fingernail or other sharp object. At the time of intercourse, it is important for the woman to guide the penis in place and then be attentive to the position of the outer ring, ensuring that the ring does not slide into the vagina. The male partner needs to know that if the sheath should begin to adhere to the penis that an increased risk of breakage exists. Figure 15-3 is an example of a female condom and the directions for use.

Spermicides

Spermicides have been available in a variety of consistencies for many years. Some of the earliest spermicides were natural acids, for example, lemon juice. Today spermicides come packaged in foam containers, tubes of jelly or cream, vaginal suppositories and vaginal film, and in condoms. The main ingredient in all spermicides found in the United States is nonoxynol 9 or octoxynol 9. The spermicide is a surfactant that works by destroying the sperm cell membrane. Although spermicides are effective when used alone (3% perfect use and 21% typical use), their efficacy increases when used with a barrier method or with a condom. Spermicides also have been effective against organisms that cause STDs, and are free from systemic side effects. As a method of contraception for adolescents, spermicides are popular simply because they can be obtained without prescription or the need first to have a pelvic examination.

Table 15-7 compares the different types of spermicides, their actions, and brand names. The duration of activity is approximately 1 hour unless used with the cervical cap or diaphragm. The onset of activity is immediate except for suppositories, tablets, and film, which take 10 to 15 minutes to dissolve and cover the cervix effectively.

Although contraindications to spermicides are few, allergy and sensitivity to the spermicide or inert base (cream, jelly, or foam) can occur. Other disadvantages include a relatively high failure rate (18% to 21% typical first-year failure rate), a short time interval between placement in the vagina and intercourse but a delay in timing of 10 to 15 minutes for activation of suppositories and film, and an undesirable taste with oral-genital sex. Some teenagers have identified spermicides as too messy or unpleasant because they are not comfortable touching their genitalia.

The advantages to teen users of spermicides are the easy accessibility without prescription, ease of learning their use, and ability to use with or without the involvement of a partner. Other advantages include no proven side effects, a useful backup method with other contraceptives, and extra lubrication.

When instructing adolescents on the use of spermicides, the health care provider should be sure to emphasize the importance of using the spermicide *every time* one has intercourse and before penis penetration of the vagina. The health care provider should provide the adolescent with the following instructions:

- Remind the adolescent that sperm can be in the preejaculate fluid, and so any penile contact with the vagina puts the woman at risk.
- Make sure the adolescent knows how to use the specific spermicide of choice (e.g., with film, insertion needs to be with a dry finger and at least 5 minutes before coitus).
- Encourage the adolescent to prepare beforehand so that one has everything ready before intercourse (such as an applicator for additional applications of cream, jelly, or foam).

THE FEMALE CONDOM

What is the female condom?

The female condom is a thin, soft, loose-fitting pouch with two flexible rings at either end. One ring helps hold the device in place inside the woman's vagina over the end of the womb (cervix), while the other ring rests outside the vagina.

Outer ring lies against the labia

Inner ring is used for insertion; helps hold female condom in place

How does it work?

The female condoms made of polyurethane, a type of plastic. The plastic condom covers the inside of the vagina, cervix, and perineum (outer lips). The device acts as a barrier to help prevent pregnancy and the transmission of germs that can cause sexually transmitted diseases (STDs), including human immunodeficiency virus (HIV) and acquired immunodeficiency syndrome (AIDS). The device can be inserted by the woman up to 8 hours before sex.

How to insert the female condom

1. Find a comfortable position. You may want to stand up with one foot on a chair, squat with knees apart, or lie down with legs bent and knees apart.
2. Hold the female condom with the open end hanging down. Squeeze the inner ring with your thumb and middle finger.
3. Holding the inner ring squeezed together, insert the ring into the vagina and push the inner ring and pouch into the vagina past the pubic bone.
4. When properly inserted, the outer ring will hang down slightly outside the vagina. During intercourse, when the penis enters the vagina, the slack will lessen.

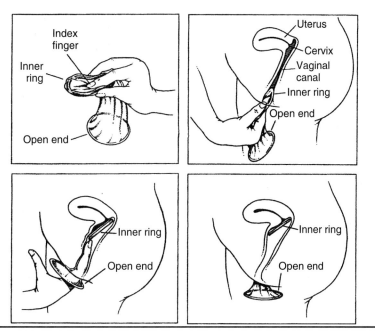

Figure 15-3 Female condom. (From Neinstein, L. S., & Nelson, A. [1996]. In L. S. Neinstein [Ed.], *Adolescent health care: A practical guide* [3rd ed.]. Baltimore: Williams & Wilkins.)

Table 15-7   SPERMICIDES

INERT BASE AND VEHICLE	ONSET OF ACTION	DURATION OF ACTION	SPERMICIDE	BRAND NAME
Foam Aerosol large	Immediate	>60 minutes	Nonoxynol 9	Delfen, Emko, and Koromex
Aerosol small	Immediate	>60 minutes	Nonoxynol 9	Emko, Because, and Emko Prefil
Creams and Jellies Reusable applicator	Immediate	>60 minutes	Nonoxynol 9	Conceptrol, Delfen, Koromex Jel, Ortho-Gynol II, and Ramses
Reusable applicator	Immediate	>60 minutes	Octoxynol 9	Koromex cream, Ortho-Gynol
Single-use packets	Immediate	>60 minutes	Nonoxynol 9	Conceptrol Jel and Milex Shur Seal Jel
Suppositories and Tablets	10-15 minutes	<60 minutes	Nonoxynol 9	Encare, Intercept, Prevent, Koromex inserts, and Semicide
Vaginal Contraceptive Film	15 minutes	<60 minutes	Nonoxynol 9	Film

Modified from Hatcher, R. A., Trussell, J., Stewart, F., Stewart G. K., Kowal, D., Guest, F., et al. (1994). *Contraceptive technology* (17th rev. ed., p. 180). New York: Irvington. Neinstein, L. S., & Nelson, A. (1996). Barrier contraceptives. In L. S. Neinstein (Ed.), *Adolescent health care: A practical guide* (3rd ed., pp. 720–736). Baltimore: Williams & Wilkins.

■ Remind the adolescent to avoid douching after intercourse for at least 8 hours to ensure the effectiveness of the spermicide.

Contraceptive Sponge

The vaginal sponge was first made available in the United States in 1983. Although a relatively expensive method, the sponge grew in popularity among young contraception users because of its easy insertion and aesthetic appeal. The contraceptive sponge is a "small pillow-shaped polyurethane sponge that contains 1 gram of nonoxynol-9 spermicide. The sponge has a concave dimple on one side that is intended to fit over the cervix and decrease the chance of dislodgment during intercourse" (Hatcher et al., 1994, p. 194). It also has a woven polyester string loop that helps with removal.

Before inserting the sponge, the woman holds it under running water to moisten and activate the spermicide. The woman then places the sponge high in the vagina. The sponge may be left in place for up to 24 hours, after which the risk of toxic shock syndrome increases. During the 24 hours, contraceptive coverage is continuous no matter how many acts of intercourse are performed. The sponge should be left in place for 6 hours after the last act of intercourse and before removal.

In early 1995 the only manufacturer of the sponge in the United States discontinued production. Although the method had no safety problems, the manufacturer voluntarily stopped production because of quality control problems involving health standards at the factory. Currently, the sponge is being manufactured for sale outside the United States.

Diaphragm

The diaphragm is a dome-shaped cup made of flexible rubber latex (Figure 15-4) that fits anatomically in the vagina from the posterior fornix to the anterior vaginal wall behind the pubic bone, completely covering the cervix. The woman places the diaphragm in the vagina manually or with an introducer for certain types of diaphragms. The diaphragm is used with a spermicidal gel or cream, which is placed in the dome before insertion and comes in contact with the cervix. The diaphragm is fit professionally and is available only by prescription. Diaphragms range in size from 50 to 105 mm in increments of 5 mm. The four types of diaphragms, which vary primarily by rim and seal, are these:

■ *Arcing-spring rim*: The arcing spring has a double spring and is strong and firm. The arc shape when the diaphragm is folded facilitates placement over the cervix. Two types of arcing-spring rims are one that folds only in one direction and one that folds in all directions. This diaphragm is suited especially for women with less vaginal muscle tone, although all women can use this style.

■ *Coil-spring rim*: The coil spring is an intermediate spring strength and is suitable for women with average vaginal muscle tone. This diaphragm has no arc, and an introducer is helpful in accurately placing it over the cervix.

■ *Flat-spring rim*: The flat spring has a thin rim with gentle spring strength. The diaphragm folds flat on insertion and may be placed with an introducer. This

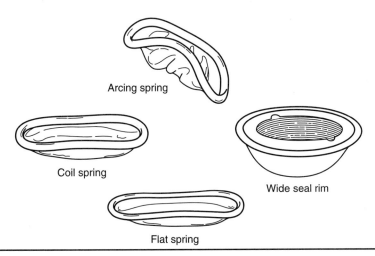

Arcing spring

Coil spring

Wide seal rim

Flat spring

Figure **15-4** Diaphragms. (From Hatcher, R. A., Trussell, J., Stewart, F., Stewart, G. K., Kowal, D., Guest, F., et al. [1994]. *Contraceptive technology* [16th ed.]. New York: Irvington.)

diaphragm is an appropriate choice for women with excellent vaginal muscle tone or a shallow pubic arch.

■ *Wide-seal rim*: The wide seal has a flexible flange attached to an inner edge of the rim to hold spermicide in place and to maintain a better seal. The diaphragm is available with the arcing- and coil-spring rims.

The diaphragm is used in combination with a spermicidal gel or cream. The spermicide is placed on the inside of the dome, the surface that touches the cervix. Debate has risen about the use of spermicide on the rim and whether this can increase the possibility for slippage (Craig & Hepburn, 1982). Avoiding the rim and covering the entire surface of the dome with spermicide is probably the best choice. The wide-seal rim diaphragm is designed to hold the spermicide in place and seal the rim more effectively (Hatcher et al., 1994, p. 192). In the early 1980s the issue was raised of safety from birth defects in subsequent pregnancies after spermicide use. Two separate research studies by Jick and others (1981, 1982) found that the incidence of birth defects increased among babies whose mothers had obtained and possibly used a vaginal spermicide within 600 days preceding delivery or abortion and that an association existed between spermicide use and miscarriage. These reports brought major concerns to the women who had chosen diaphragm and spermicide methods of contraception for their relative lack of medical side effects. Later studies (Mills et al., 1985; Shapiro, Slone, & Heinonen, 1982; Warburton, Neugut, & Lustenburger, 1987), however, did not support the original findings, and the FDA determined that the evidence did not necessitate a warning on spermicide labels regarding use and pregnancy (Lemberg, 1984).

The placement of the diaphragm by the adolescent is crucial for contraceptive efficacy. The arcing diaphragm aids in positioning because of its curved shape. The flat and coil spring lie in a straight plane and need more checking to ensure proper placement. These two diaphragms come with an introducer that may assist some women in proper placement.

When a practitioner fits a diaphragm, she first educates the woman about the process for fitting. Then using fitting diagrams to assist in teaching, the practitioner demonstrates the process of insertion and removal. Once the practitioner decides on the diaphragm size and type that offers the best fit, she then allows the woman to practice insertion and removal several times until the woman feels confident and demonstrates appropriate technique.

Determining the appropriate diaphragm begins with choosing a type and then size. Most women can use the arcing diaphragm, which slips into place easier and is more difficult to insert incorrectly. The flat- and coil-spring diaphragms have a more gentle rim, which is often more comfortable, and can be assisted into place by an introducer. Once the type of diaphragm is selected, a size can be estimated in the following way:

■ With a gloved hand, the health care provider inserts the index and middle fingers into the vagina until the middle finger reaches the posterior wall of the vagina.

■ The health care provider uses the tip of the thumb to mark the point at which the index finger touches the pubic bone.

- The health care provider extracts the fingers.
- The health care provider places the diaphragm rim on the tip of the middle finger.

The opposite rim should lie just in front of the thumb (Hatcher et al., 1994, p. 211). Next, the practitioner inserts the corresponding fitting diaphragm into the woman and checks the fit. The diaphragm should fit snugly and also comfortably. An appropriate level of comfort is indicated if the diaphragm allows one finger tip to be between the inside of the pubic arch and the anterior edge of the diaphragm rim. The correct fit is the largest diaphragm size that is comfortable for the woman. Typically the health care provider tries more than one size to determine the best fit. The health care provider should avoid choosing a diaphragm too small because vaginal depth increases during sexual arousal, and the diaphragm may move and not completely cover the cervix. Similarly, a diaphragm too large may produce increased vaginal pressure, causing abdominal pain or cramping, vaginal ulcerations, or recurrent urinary tract infections. Scheduling a follow-up visit and having the adolescent return with the diaphragm in place for a recheck of the fit is often helpful.

Box 15-4 contains instructions for the woman on inserting the diaphragm. The time parameters influencing the diaphragm use are suggested as insertion with a spermicide no longer than 1 hour before intercourse and removal no sooner than 6 hours after the last act of intercourse. The longest time a diaphragm should be inserted is 24 hours. In addition, with each new act of intercourse, an additional applicator full of spermicide needs to be inserted into the vagina.

The following are the advantages of the diaphragm:

- Sensible form of temporary and long-term contraception
- No systemic effects or change in a woman's hormone pattern

Box 15-4 INSTRUCTIONS FOR WOMEN ON INSERTING A DIAPHRAGM

Always check the diaphragm for holes, tears, or weakening areas by holding it up to the light, stretching the rubber, and gently pulling the dome away from the rim. Then fill the diaphragm cup with a teaspoon to a tablespoon of contraceptive cream or jelly, and spread it evenly over the inside surface of the dome and to the rim. Avoid getting the spermicide on the fingers that will hold the diaphragm for insertion, so as to have better control.

To insert the diaphragm, fold the edges together and hold firmly with one hand. With the other hand spread the labia and insert the diaphragm. The best position to do this is the most comfortable one and may include standing with one leg lifted (i.e., on a toilet seat or chair), squatting, and lying on one's back. Push the diaphragm back and downward along the posterior wall of the vagina as far as it will go. Next, tuck the front rim up and behind the pubic bone. Finally check to make sure the cervix is behind the dome of the diaphragm.

When using an introducer, the diaphragm is stretched over the device and then is guided into the vagina in the same manner as in hand manipulation. Once the anterior rim of the diaphragm is behind the cervix, the diaphragm is released from the introducer, which then is retracted. The posterior rim then is checked for its position behind the pubic bone and adjusted if necessary.

■ Protection against the spread of STDs
■ Protection against cervical neoplasms

The reasons for not prescribing a diaphragm include the following:

■ Allergy to spermicide, rubber, or latex
■ Inability to learn correct placement technique
■ Interference with an acceptable fit because of abnormalities in vaginal anatomy
■ Recurrent urinary tract infections despite a satisfactory fit
■ A history of toxic shock syndrome
■ Lack of a trained practitioner to fit the diaphragm

Cervical Cap

The cervical cap is a thimble-shaped latex rubber contraceptive device (Figure 15-5). The Prentif Cavity Rim Cervical Cap (Prentif Cervical Cap) has a groove just under the rim on the inside of the cap that assists in maintaining the fit of the cap over the cervix by suction. The Prentif Cervical Cap comes in four sizes (22 mm, 25 mm, 28 mm, and 31 mm) and is measured by the internal rim diameter. The Prentif Cervical Cap is manufactured in England and distributed in the United States by Cervical Cap Ltd., Los Gatos, California. Before years of investigational research and the 1988 approval by the FDA, no cervical cap was available in the United States.

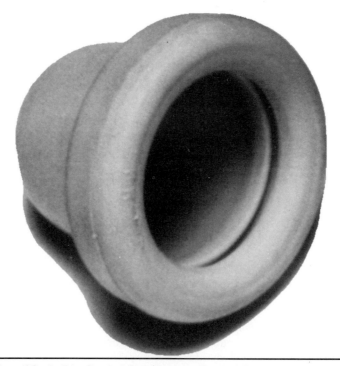

Figure 15-5 Prentif Cavity Rim Cervical Cap. (Courtesy Cervical Cap Ltd., Los Gatos, Calif.)

The cervical cap is similar to the diaphragm in that it acts as a mechanical barrier preventing sperm from passing from the vagina through the cervix into the uterus and tubes. Approximately 80% of women can be fitted with a cervical cap. The cervical cap generally cannot be fit if the cervix is too long, too short, or too small. The cap fit is critical to contraceptive effectiveness. The effectiveness is enhanced with the use of a spermicide. Use of a spermicide at every insertion is recommended. The cap may be kept in place for up to 48 hours but then should be removed so that the body has a chance to excrete its natural cleansing mucus. The cervical cap may be inserted long before the act of intercourse but is recommended to be in place for 30 minutes before intercourse to enhance the suction. As with the diaphragm, the recommendation is to leave the cap in place for 8 hours after the last act of intercourse.

The theoretical effectiveness is similar to the diaphragm. Data show that pregnancies are caused primarily by faulty technique; for example, incorrect placement, no use of spermicide, or inconsistent use (Sprik & Skillman, 1986). The cap has a potential use effectiveness of 96% when used correctly and consistently with every act of intercourse.

The advantages of the cervical cap include the following:

- The cap can be inserted into place long before the act of intercourse and can stay in place for up to 48 hours.
- The cap uses less spermicide than the diaphragm and does not require additional spermicide with each act of intercourse.
- The cap fits differently than the diaphragm, so women with poor muscle tone or a history of bladder infections can be fitted.
- The cap has fewer known side effects than the pill or IUD.
- The cap is not a systemic form of contraception.
- The cap is not associated with irregular bleeding or pelvic infections as is the IUD.
- The cap offers some reduction of STD risk.

The disadvantages of the cervical cap include the following:

- The cap is not appropriate for all cervix types (position, shape, and size determine a good fit).
- The cap requires a prescription and must be fitted professionally.
- The cap requires teaching in placement, removal, cleaning, and storage.
- For some the cap may be more difficult to insert or remove than a diaphragm.
- The cap can be dislodged from the cervix during intercourse.
- A Pap smear is recommended 3 months after initiation of use and then annually, monitoring for dysplasia.
- The cap may become malodorous (especially if used longer than 48 hours) and needs special attention in cleaning.
- The cap must be replaced every 2 to 3 years and refitted after each pregnancy.

The cervical cap has more user restrictions than the diaphragm. These restrictions include women who have an unusually short or long cervix, an unusually shaped or asymmetrical cervix, a history of cervical laceration or scarring, a history of toxic shock syndrome, an abnormal and unresolved Pap smear, a current cervicitis or vaginal infection, or a current pelvic, tubal, or ovarian infection.

The practitioner must have formal training to obtain the skill and understanding of fitting a cervical cap best. In assessing the woman, the health care provider first performs a speculum examination and obtains a Pap smear if one is not current and also evaluates the health, contour, and size of the cervix. Then on bimanual examination the health care provider assesses the size, position, and any surface irregularities of the cervix and surrounding vaginal wall. A fitting cap is chosen and placed on the cervix. If the cap fits snugly around the cervix and produces a seal that allows rotation but resists removal on tugging, then the cap has a good fit. After instructing the woman how to insert and remove the cap, the health care provider has her practice the process several times for dexterity and confidence and then rechecks the cap for accurate placement by the woman and compares the cap chosen with the next size up or down to ensure the most appropriate fit (Summerhayes, 1995). The optimum time to fit a cervical cap is in the middle of the woman's menstrual cycle. Box 15-5 contains instructions for inserting the cervical cap.

To ensure the effectiveness and safety of the cervical cap, the health care provider instructs the woman *not* to do the following:

- Wear the cap longer than 48 hours or remove it sooner than 8 hours after intercourse.
- Overfill the cap with spermicide, which interferes with the seal.

Box 15-5 INSTRUCTIONS FOR WOMEN ON INSERTING A CERVICAL CAP

1. Hold the cap up to the light and check for holes and turn the cap inside out looking at the outside surface and inside surface for any irregularities.
2. Fill the cap dome one third full with spermicide.
3. If unfamiliar with the location of the cervix, check its location before inserting the cap.
4. Take a comfortable position for insertion, squeeze the cap rim together with forefinger, middle finger, and thumb and insert the cap into the vagina.
5. Once the cap is through the introitus, it may try to adhere to the anterior vaginal wall, so continue exerting gentle pressure and guide the cap in place over the cervix.
6. Put some additional pressure on the dome of the cap to help set up the seal.
7. With the forefinger check that the placement of the cap is on the cervix and that the rim of the cap is touching the vaginal wall evenly.
8. Check the fit by wiggling and tugging on the dome. If the cap remains in place, it is on the cervix properly. To remove the cervical cap, first insert the forefinger and put pressure against the side of the cap. Then when the cap has tilted away from the vaginal wall and cervix, slip the finger over the rim and gently pull the cap down and off the cervix and out of the vagina. Clean the cap with warm, soapy water, making sure to clean well the inside groove. If an odor persists, the cap may be soaked for 15 minutes in vinegar, alcohol, or spirits of wintergreen. Allow the cap to dry and store it in a container that can be open to air, but out of direct sunlight. Keep the cervical cap away from high heat, which hastens deterioration of the latex rubber.

- Wear the cap during menses.
- Use the cap when using a vaginal medication.
- Douche when the cap is in place.

During the first month of cervical cap use, a backup method of contraception should be used. During this time, different positions for intercourse should be used to test if the cap remains in place with each position. If dislodgement occurs more than once, the woman should use an alternative contraception method and contact the practitioner who fit the cap for a reevaluation. For each new sexual partner, using a backup method and retesting the cap for dislodgment in various positions is important. The health care provider should remind the woman always to bring the cap to her annual gynecological appointment so that the size can be rechecked.

If the woman cannot be fitted for a cervical cap, she may need support in accepting this. The cap may have been identified as her best option, so the woman may be devastated if she is unable to manage the cap or if an appropriate anatomical fit cannot be obtained. The practitioner needs to be sensitive, offering support and another opportunity for meeting her contraceptive needs.

Historically, cervical caps are the oldest contraceptive and have been made out of metal, bees-wax, rubber, wood, etc. Continued research on the cervical cap has attempted to create a cap with a one-way valve, a cap that can remain in place for longer than 48 hours, a cap made of a different and more pliable material than latex rubber, and a custom-fit cap.

Long-Acting Hormonal Contraception

Two long-acting forms of hormonal contraception, Norplant and Depo-Provera, are currently available in the United States. The Norplant System was approved by the FDA in December 1990 after almost 30 years of research into the possibility of an implantable contraceptive (Letterie & Royce, 1995). The Norplant System involves surgical insertion of six flexible nonbiodegradable silicone capsules (34 mm long and 2.4 mm in diameter) that emit levonorgestrel subcutaneously for up to 5 years. The mechanism of action is similar for all progestin-only forms of contraception. The constant serum level of progestin serves to inhibit ovulation (50%), thicken cervical mucus, and make the endometrium uninhabitable. The failure rate in the first year of use is 0.09%, with an overall failure rate of 3.7% for the 5 years.

Depo-Provera, also known as depo medroxyprogesterone acetate (DMPA), is a deep intramuscular injectable contraceptive given every 12 weeks, with more "forgiveness" in terms of exact timing than most other hormonal contraception. Although DMPA has been available for clinical uses other than contraception (i.e., it helps to control menorrhagia) for many years, it was approved finally for use as a contraceptive method in the United States in late 1992. The delay in FDA approval was based on concern over a DMPA study using beagles that associated DMPA use with an increased number of mammary gland tumors, with some becoming malignant. Subsequent studies have not supported this original finding, but the relationship of long-term DMPA use and later breast cancer development bears noting.

The mechanism of action for DMPA is through the suppression of follicle stimulating hormone and luteinizing hormone levels in the hypothalamus and elimination of the luteinizing hormone surge. When DMPA is given in 150 mg per 1-mL injections every 3 months, then the failure rate is 0.3% (Hatcher et al., 1994, p. 290). This low rate makes DMPA an effective contraceptive, especially for adolescents and their ever-changing life patterns.

The major drawback to the long-acting progestin method of contraception includes its affect on the menstrual cycle. Unpredictable irregular bleeding is the most reported side effect and should be considered during the counseling session before choice of these methods. Acne and weight gain are among some of the more frequently reported lesser side effects and are to be considered as possible reasons for discontinuance in the adolescent population.

Intrauterine Device

The IUD was popular in the late 1960s and early 1970s, used by 10% of women in the United States who were using contraception. One particular design, the Dalkon shield, was responsible for increased numbers of infections, pregnancies, and maternal deaths (Hatcher et al., 1994; Nelson & Neinstein, 1996). With these events and a more litigious climate in the United States, all designs of IUD came under scrutiny and eventually were removed from the market in the early 1980s. Two IUDs currently are available in the United States: the CopperT 380A (Paragard) and the Progesterone T (Progestasert). A third IUD, the Levonorgestrel-IUD (LNg-20 IUD) is soon to be marketed in the United States (Hatcher et al., 1994, p. 348). Although the favorability of the IUD is increasing, fewer than 2% of contraceptive users in the United States use this method (Letterie & Royce, 1995, p. 489). Those women who do choose the IUD are usually in their 30s and 40s (Hatcher et al., 1994, p. 347). This method rarely is recommended for adolescents because of the high-risk nature of their sexual practices (such as higher incidences of STDs and multiple sexual partners).

The mechanism of action is not well understood. Apparently the IUD affects the prevention of fertilization in two ways: by interfering with the migration of sperm from the vagina to the fallopian tubes (immobilization of sperm) and by speeding transport of the ovum through the fallopian tubes. Other enzymatic and biochemical processes are believed to occur as well as local effects on the endometrium, but their contributions to the IUD function are unclear (Hatcher et al., 1994, p. 348).

IUDs are a one-decision method in that once the device has been inserted, the woman does not need to decide when and what about contraception. Insertion of an IUD can be any time during the menstrual cycle, given the woman is not already pregnant. Possibly the best time for insertion is the last day of menstrual flow when the cervical os is still slightly open. The duration of recommended use differs between the types of IUDs. The Paragard is approved for up to 8 years of use, and the Progestasert needs to be replaced annually. Knowing when to replace the IUD is crucial to its effectiveness.

Cost is another inhibiting factor for IUD use in adolescents. Generally the cost for insertion in a family planning clinic is between $200 and $300, whereas costs in a private office often are higher. Other disadvantages include pelvic inflammatory disease (the greatest risk of which is at the time of insertion), menstrual problems (such as dysmenorrhea and menorrhagia), expulsion, and pregnancy.

Postcoital Options

Postcoital contraception, also known as emergency contraception and the morning after treatment, has improved significantly since the 1960s when high doses of diethylstilbestrol (25 to 50 mg/day) were prescribed. The intention of an emergency form of contraception is a one-time protection treatment. This option is important especially in the situation of sexual assault, contraceptive failure (a condom breaks or a diaphragm or cervical cap dislodges), or failure to use a method of contraception.

The mechanism of action is not understood clearly but is thought to interfere with implantation. Efficacy is based on ingesting the treatment within 72 hours and results in a 2% failure rate with the combination OCP. The following are documented and effective treatment regimens (Fasoli, Parazzinni, Cecchetti, & La Vecchia, 1989; Speroff et al., 1994):

■ *Lo Ovral or Levelen*: Eight tablets given in a split dose (four) 12 hours apart
■ *Ovral*: Four tablets given in a split dose (two) 12 hours apart
■ *Ethinyl estradiol*: 2.5 mg twice daily for 5 days
■ *Conjugated estrogens*: 15 mg twice daily for 5 days, or 50 mg intravenously on each of 2 consecutive days

Alternative methods of emergency postcoital contraception include copper IUD insertion and oral RU-486, 600 mg in a single dose. The copper IUD can be inserted up to 5 days after unprotected intercourse and has a low failure rate of 0.1% (Fasoli et al., 1989). However, this method is not to be offered to women who are at risk for infection, as in the case of rape or multiple sexual partners. Mifepristone (RU-486) is appearing to be the best option of the future, with less gastrointestinal side effects and a zero rate of failure (Glasier, Thong, Dewar, & Baird, 1992). Menstrual cycles usually are delayed after oral mifepristone, so starting hormonal contraception immediately after treatment is recommended so as to prevent another pregnancy while the woman waits for menses to begin. Patients can expect irregularity in their next menses and should return for a pregnancy test in 2 to 3 weeks.

Adolescents requesting emergency postcoital contraception should be instructed about all of their options. The practitioner needs to review the side effects and offer reassurance. Adolescents should be informed that this method of contraception exists and is available to them.

Abstinence

The option of abstinence is generally not easy for a practitioner to present to an adolescent having a clinic appointment with the specific intention of obtaining information about contraception. Abstinence is best presented during routine health care visits, *before* a young woman is sexually active. Clarifying the two types of abstinence, total abstinence and periodic abstinence, also is important. Total abstinence refers to never having sexual intercourse, and periodic abstinence refers to abstaining from sexual intercourse during the fertile days of the menstrual cycle.

The woman's health nurse practitioner is not likely to see the adolescent using periodic abstinence unless she has had a failure with this method. If per chance an adolescent does want to use periodic abstinence for contraception, then she can be instructed in fertility awareness. The methods of fertility awareness include calendar charting, cervical mucus charting, basal body charting, and symptothermal charting. For more specific instruction in these methods, the reader is referred to Varney (1997, pp. 73-82) and Hatcher and others (1994, pp. 327-340). In general, the teen should be dissuaded from periodic abstinence unless the teen is exceptionally mature, has regular menstrual periods, is knowledgeable about reproduction and the menstrual cycle, and can conceptualize what she would do if the method failed and she became pregnant.

If a teen chooses total abstinence, the health care provider should support her decision and help her to be effective. The health care provider can suggest that she be clear about her intentions not to have sex and avoid situations that could endanger her choice. She needs to decide in advance what presexual activities she will allow and which ones she will avoid. She needs to avoid situations that increase the pressure for sexual relations by staying sober and avoiding places where no one else knows where she is. The adolescent should continue to seek information and learn about her body, what safe sexual practices are, and how to obtain contraception. Making condoms available and free to adolescents during their clinic visits helps reiterate the importance of being safe and being responsible.

GENERAL HEALTH CONCERNS

Dermatology

Dissemination of accurate information about the consequences of prolonged and increased ultraviolet light exposure is important for preventive health measures. Advising adolescents of the risks of ultraviolet light exposure and the benefits of protection are relevant to teaching health promoting behaviors.

Healthy skin begins with common sense skin care. Identifying what type of skin a woman has, oily, normal, dry, or combination aids in choosing the soap and moisturizer to use. Protecting the skin from the sun with sunscreen products and proper clothing such as hats and beach wear coverups helps prevent premature aging. Maintaining a healthy diet and hydration with plenty of water ensures the turgor and suppleness of the skin.

In addition to teaching healthy skin habits, respecting adolescents' sensitivity to their own self-image is relevant to helping teens seek help for all dermatological conditions. Acne is the most common dermatological concern during adolescence, is reported to affect 85% of the adolescent population to some degree, and has psychological and physical ramifications.

Acne appears early in puberty during the preteen years, generally before menarche in girls (Lucky et al., 1994). The appearance of acne usually coincides with adrenarche, the rise of adrenal androgens, specifically dehydroepiandrosterone sulfate. Sebaceous glands are androgen-sensitive aspects of hair follicles, the function of which is secretion of lipids to lubricate the skin and hair (Pakula & Neinstein, 1996, p. 349). Acne affects the sebaceous glands of the face, neck, and upper trunk. Androgens are cited as decreasing the linoleic acid concentration in the sebum of acne patients, contributing to abnormal keratinization and obstruction of the pilosebaceous ducts (Pakula & Neinstein, 1996; Speroff et al., 1994). Abnormal keratinization of the sebaceous and follicular ducts results in retention hyperkeratosis and microcomedo formation (comedogenesis). The excessive sebum and the anaerobic environment created by the plugged follicle results in the colonization and proliferation of the anaerobic diphtheroid *Propionibacterium acnes* (Pakula & Neinstein, 1996). The bacteria trigger immune and nonimmune inflammatory reactions by several mechanisms that irritate the sebaceous and follicular ducts.

The clinical appearance of acne includes comedones, pustules, inflammatory papules, nodules, cysts, and scars, which are defined as follows (Pakula & Neinstein 1996):

- **Comedones** have three variations and may appear 2 years before the onset of puberty. Microcomedones are the precursors to all acne lesions and are microscopic congregations of keratin, lipids, bacteria, and rudimentary hair below the skin surface. Open comedones (blackheads) are epithelium-lined sacs filled with keratin and lipids, black in appearance from melanin pigment and without inflammation unless traumatized. Closed comedones (whiteheads) are lesions, palpable at 1 to 3 mm, with a microscopic opening that prevents the escape of contents and can resolve spontaneously unless traumatized, in which case the comedone becomes inflamed.
- **Pustules** are lesions with a visible central core of purulent material.
- **Papules** are inflammatory lesions measuring less than 5 mm in diameter.
- **Nodules** are inflammatory lesions measuring 5 mm or greater and can result when pustules rupture and form abscess.
- **True cysts** are the rare residual lesions of healed pustules or nodules and are lined by epithelium.
- **Scars** include depressed scars, perifollicular fibrosis, and hypertrophic scars and keloids.

The grading of acne is not standardized but generally is classified as mild, moderate, and severe with descriptions of lesion type, distribution, morphology, complications, therapeutic responses, and the overall affect on the person. During the physical examination, observation of the combined presence of hirsutism, alopecia, or virilization affects the choice of therapeutic approach.

The differential diagnosis includes gram-negative folliculitis, cosmetic acne, drug-induced acne, acne mechanica, acne conglobata, and nonacne lesions (flat warts, perioral dermatitis, adenoma sebaceum, and hidradenitis suppurativa) (Pakula & Neinstein, 1996).

Acne may have a social and negative psychological affect on the adolescent. Addressing the meaning of acne for each adolescent is crucial for compliance with the treatment regimen, psychological support, and follow-up. Taking a thorough history assists in identifying contributing factors such as menstrual cycle variations and the use of oral contraceptives or other medications (drugs or cosmetics) that affect acne. Educating the adolescent regarding the importance of the timing and consistency of her treatment and the delay in treatment response (improvements may take more than a month of therapy) is also advantageous for good compliance.

Treatment is determined by the severity of the adolescent's acne. Table 15-8 provides descriptions by which the severity of the acne is determined.

A list of the topical medications for acne therapy appears in Box 15-6. Nurse practitioners need to know topical therapies and feel comfortable with recommending them. Systemic antibiotic therapy (Table 15-9) may be maintained after consultation with a physician or dermatologist. Systemic hormonal therapy such as OCPs with less androgenic progestins (desogestrel or norgestimate) helps lessen the effects of acne. When prescribing an OCP to an adolescent with acne, the health care provider needs to evaluate the acne in follow-up appointment.

Common sense advice to practitioners is to use a few drugs and know them well. An important consideration is to ask the adolescent what drugs she has already tried and what drugs her friends are using. Clarifying a choice of medication different from a peer also may aid in compliance.

Other Skin Conditions

Warts

Warts are skin eruptions and are classified by where they occur on the body. The cause of warts is the human papillomavirus (HPV), which has been categorized by several different deoxyribonucleic acid (DNA) types. Common warts are a cosmetic concern for

Table 15-8   ACNE SEVERITY DETERMINATION

SEVERITY OF ACNE	TREATMENT
Mild comedonal acne	May respond to topical over-the-counter or prescription preparations such as salicylic acid, sulfur, or benzoyl peroxide.
Moderate to severe comedonal acne	May respond to the treatment regimen for mild acne with the addition of retin-A at bedtime.
Mild inflammatory acne	May respond to the addition of a topical antibiotic or a combination form of benzoyl peroxide and antibiotic such as Benzamycin gel (5% benzoyl peroxide and 3% erythromycin).
Unresponsive moderate to severe inflammatory acne	Requires a systemic antibiotic.
Nodular/nodulocystic acne	When unresponsive to systemic antibiotics, requires treatment with isotretinoin (Accutane) by an experienced practitioner.

Modified from Pakula, A., & Neinstein, L. S. (1996). Acne. In L. S. Neinstein (Ed.), *Adolescent health care: A practical guide* (3rd ed., pp. 349–359). Baltimore: Williams & Wilkins.

Box 15-6 TOPICAL THERAPY FOR ACNE

Benzoyl peroxide
  2.5%, 4%, 5%, and 10%
  5% benzoyl peroxide and 3% erythromycin
  Benzoyl peroxide-sulfur
Tretinoin (retin-A)
  0.025%, 0.05%, and 0.1% cream
  0.01% and 0.025% gel
  0.05% liquid
Peeling agents
Salicylic acid
Alpha-hydroxy acids
Resorcinol
Resorcinol-sulfur
Sulfacetamide-sulfur
Topical antibiotics
  Clindamycin (Cleocin T solution, C/T/S)
  Erythromycin (A/T/S solution, T-Stat solution, Erygel, Akne-mycin)
Metronidazole
Tetracycline (Topicycline)

Modified from Pakula, A., & Neinstein, L. S. (1996). Acne. In L. S. Neinstein (Ed.), *Adolescent health care: A practical guide* (3rd ed., pp. 349–359). Baltimore: Williams & Wilkins.

Table 15-9 SYSTEMIC ANTIBIOTIC THERAPY FOR ACNE

DRUG	DOSE	ADVANTAGES	DISADVANTAGES
Tetracycline	250-1500 mg/day	Inexpensive	Poor compliance and gastrointestinal upset; teeth discoloration
Doxycycline	50-200 mg/day	Inexpensive and improved compliance	Photosensitivity and esophageal ulceration
Minocycline	50-200 mg/day	Low resistance and low photosensitivity	Expensive; vertigo-like symptoms, lupuslike reaction, and rare teeth and skin discoloration
Erythromycin	500-1000 mg/day	Inexpensive	Gastrointestinal upset and frequent resistance
Clindamycin	300-450 mg/day	Effective	Limited to short-term use; pseudomembranous colitis
Trimethoprim-sulfamethoxazole	1-2 double-strength tablets per day	Effective in gram-negative folliculitis	Bone marrow suppression

Modified from Pakula, A., & Neinstein, L. S. (1996). Acne. In L. S. Neinstein (Ed.), *Adolescent health care: A practical guide* (3rd ed.). Baltimore: Williams & Wilkins.

most teens (the peak prevalence being between ages 10 to 20 years). Data show a more serious connection between HPV and cervical cancer.

Four types of warts are flat warts, planter warts, common warts, and genital warts. *Flat warts* (verruca vulgaris) are less than 5 mm, slightly raised, smooth, skin-colored lesions. Usually located on the dorsa of the hands, face, and knees, they can appear as small colonies that spread in the direction of irritation, by scratching or shaving. *Planter warts* (verruca plantaris) are single or grouped lesions even with the surface of the skin and having a hyperkeratotic covering, with scattered pinpoint black dots (thrombosed blood vessels). These lesions appear on the plantar surface of the feet. *Common warts* (verruca vulgaris) have distinct margins and are firm and raised papules measuring 1 to 5 mm. These lesions generally are located on the hands and fingers, especially near the nails but also can be found on other parts of the body. *Genital warts* (condyloma acumintum) appear on and in the genital area and have four subgroupings. More details are provided in the section on STDs.

Molluscum Contagiosum

Molluscum contagiosum is considered a sexually transmitted infection caused by one of the poxviruses. Infection is located in the genital area as well as the legs, arms, and chest. The lesion is a skin-colored, raised dome with a characteristic central depression. The lesions generally appear in clusters and are asymptomatic unless directly irritated. Transmission occurs through direct human contact and incubation is 1 to several months. Diagnosis is by clinical appearance, Pap smear, or microscopic evaluation for molluscum inclusion bodies. Treatment choices include liquid nitrogen applied directly to the lesion, podophyllin or trichloroacetic acid applied to the excised base of the lesion, and light electrodesiccation. Counseling the woman about transmission and the need to have her partner evaluated is important for successful therapy. The health care provider should educate the adolescent, indicating that the infection is not associated with systemic disease and is prevented by safe sex practices and not sharing intimate items and towels. Follow-up evaluation is recommended within 1 month.

Sunburn

Prevention is the best recommendation for sunburn. Acclimating to the sun gradually may be helpful, but only for those who do not have a skin type that burns. Avoiding the exposure of the sun during the midday hours (10 AM to 3 PM) is paramount for shielding the skin from the harmful ultraviolet rays of the sun. When avoiding exposure is not possible, especially on summer beach days or during snow recreation on sunny days, a sunscreen with a sun protection factor of 15 or greater allows for tanning without the severity of burning. Two kinds of ultraviolet radiation affect the skin, A and B. Sunburns and all three types of skin cancer—melanoma, basal cell, and squamous cell—are activated by ultraviolet B rays. Ultraviolet B has intense rays and is most active midday and diminishes in the evening. Alternately, ultraviolet A has longer rays that penetrate deep into the skin and are responsible for the aging of skin (wrinkles, spotting, and loss of tone). Ultraviolet A is constant thoroughout the day (Freyer, 1998).

Educating adolescents about the long-term consequences of sunburns, prolonged exposure to the sun, and not having adequate sunscreen and hydration is imperative to maintaining healthy skin and avoiding skin alterations such as skin cancer. In addition, practitioners need to identify for the adolescent any medications that increase photosensitivity. Some known medications are oral contraceptive pills, tetracycline, diphenhydramine, sulfonamides, phenothiazines, psoralen, and tranquilizers.

Tattoos

Tattoos are becoming more popular with a broader segment of society. Adolescents may choose to have a tatoo for personal reasons, but too often tattoos are chosen because of peer pressure or gang participation. The medical consequences of having a tattoo include infections (hepatitis, syphilis, tuberculosis, and potentially HIV), adverse reaction to the dye, and scarring and keloid formation. Although techniques in the removal of tattoos are improving (e.g., laser surgery), the cost and physical discomfort are significant considerations.

MENTAL HEALTH CONCERNS

Growing up psychologically healthy is a cumulative process influenced by temperament, parents, significant others, and environmental conditions. Siegler (1997) has identified five developmental tasks and suggests that these usually are accomplished in the following sequence (p. 16):

1. Separating from old ties
2. Creating new attachments
3. Establishing a mature sexual identity and a mature sexual life
4. Formulating new ideas and new ideals
5. Consolidating character

As the adolescent progresses through these stages, communication with parents and professionals may become strained. As a professional, for the health care provider to know ways to reach a struggling teen and assist parents with better patterns of communication is important. One approach is to use the four *Cs*: compassion, communication, comprehension, and competence (Seigler, 1997). *Compassion* is empathy that shows the adolescent that the health care provider genuinely is concerned and wishes to connect with rather than criticize her problem. *Communication* begun in a compassionate tone offers the teen an opportunity to share and begin to resolve small and large issues. Communication also allows for mutuality and intimacy to be nurtured while parents and professionals confirm important realities and offer significant information. *Comprehension* puts into meaning the thoughts and behaviors a troubled adolescent displays. Comprehension allows for parents and professionals to share their perspective, indicate that the teen's situation is not intimidating, and continue to look for hidden meanings. Finally, *competence* demonstrates a variety of ways to solve problems and assist the teen to develop her own repertoire of responses. Instilling the teen with hope motivates the adolescent to continue to struggle with the developmental challenges that lead the way toward adulthood.

The following sections address the mental health concerns of women with eating disorders and mood disorders. Although these issues necessitate the assistance and evaluation of a professional, the use of the four *Cs* is valuable in uncovering the possible reasons for these behaviors.

Eating Disorders

One of the more frustrating clinical issues for adolescent providers is that of influencing healthful eating habits. Eating habits are developed long before the teen begins her process of self-identity and making individual choices. Practitioners providing care to all family members can instruct about healthful eating habits. Practitioners caring for adolescents need to provide annual counseling about the benefits of proper diet, ways to achieve it, and suggestions for safe weight management. An annual assessment of the weight-to-height ratio (body mass index; Figure 15-6), body image statements, and patterns of dieting aid in early detection and prevention of eating disorders.

Although the causes of the different eating disorders are not well understood, the disorders are thought to evolve from a combination of sociocultural, physiological, and psychological factors. In the United States the sociocultural factors include media standard of thin, model-type body characteristics not consistent with the medical ideal weight parameters. This pervasive media image coupled with extreme dieting to obtain the unrealistic goal, the physiological devastation of a starving body, and the psychological pain of failing to achieve the goal no matter how unrealistic the goal set the stage for a woman to begin a pattern of disordered eating. Although external factors contribute heavily to disordered eating, an underlying psychopathological condition will always exist that requires the practitioner's attention.

Overeating

Compulsive overeating is diagnosed when uncontrolled eating is not related to hunger and is followed by guilt and shame about the behavior and a consequent weight gain (Harris & Seimer, 1995). For the compulsive overeater a cyclic pattern develops: "binging, rigid dieting, feelings of deprivation and increasing anxiety, followed by binging again in response to anxiety or feelings of failure and despair due to inability to maintain diet" (Harris & Seimer, 1995, p. 687). For the compulsive overeater, food is used to cope with stress, boredom, depression, emotional conflicts, anxiety, loneliness, anger, and daily problems. Compulsive overeating behaviors begin in childhood when a pattern develops of responding to external cues of hunger (smell or sight of food) rather than internal cues of hunger and satiation. Compulsive overeating is one means to obesity for adolescents.

Obesity and overweight are defined as body weight or excess body fat above an arbitrary standard often defined in relation to height. Unlike with minimum weight standards, maximum weight standards are less fixed and deserve more flexibility in interpretation because of the nature of adolescent growth spurts. Many scales have been developed that offer a method for determining the range of ideal to nonideal body

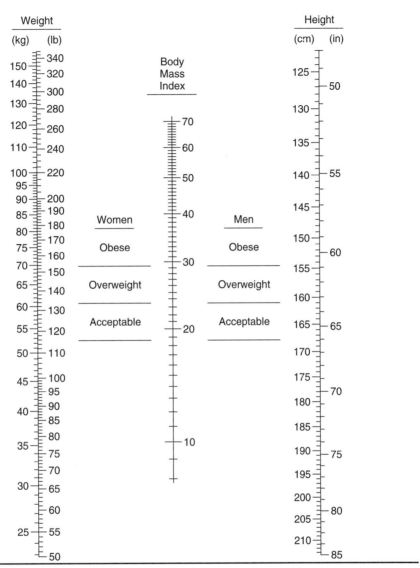

Figure **15-6** Body mass index.

weight. Himes and Dietz (1994) recommend screening adolescents by using the Quetelet's Index or body mass index (see Figure 15-6). The calculation of the body mass index is body mass in kilograms divided by height in meters squared.

Obesity in adolescents is not easy to diagnose appropriately. Adolescence is a time of rapid body changes when the proportion of body fat in females increases from 19% to approximately 23% by age 20 (American Medical Association, 1991). A 1987 report by Gortmaker, Dietz, Sobel, and Wehler shows that among adolescents ages 12 to 17, approximately 26% of white females and 25% of black females were obese as defined by a skinfold thickness greater than the 84th percentile. Table 15-10 reviews the 5th, 50th, and 95th percentile of body mass index for children and adolescents.

Obesity has a number of subtypes and is considered a multifactorial chronic disease. Because the cause of obesity is not certain, many theories describe this phenomenon. A familial or genetic component has been substantiated through research on twins, but environmental factors are difficult to control and thus cannot be ignored. The fat cell theory notes that three times in life fat cells rapidly increase (gestation, first year of life, and adolescence). Overeating during these times increases the number of fat cells, which cannot be lost later in life but only reduced in size. Other theories describe behaviors of overeaters (such as skipping breakfast and eating larger quantities later in the day, eating fast, eating when not hungry, eating when depressed or anxious, and underestimating the number of calories consumed). Still other theories focus on activity levels, internal regulatory mechanisms, and hormone imbalances. Obesity probably never is caused by just one factor, and the combination of factors is unique to each woman (Edwards, 1993).

Prevention is the way to approach overweight and obesity. Teaching good nutrition to pregnant mothers so that excessive weight gain in the third trimester is avoided starts the child out in the best of circumstances. During the first year of life, mothers should be encouraged to breast-feed the baby and wait to introduce cereals until 3 to 4 months of age. Later during puberty and adolescence, the health care provider and parents can encourage and demonstrate healthy lifestyle choices. These choices include developing regular physical activity, eating at appropriate meal times, not bingeing late in the day,

Table 15-10	FEMALE PERCENTILE VALUES OF BODY MASS INDEX		
	PERCENTILE		
AGE (YEARS)	**5TH**	**50TH**	**95TH**
10	14.3	17.1	24.2
11	14.6	17.8	25.7
12	15.0	18.3	26.8
13	15.4	18.9	27.9
14	15.7	19.4	28.6
15	16.1	19.9	29.4
16	16.4	20.0	30.0
17	16.9	20.7	30.5
18	17.2	21.1	31.0
19	17.5	21.4	31.3

Modified from Neinstein, L. S. (Ed.). (1996). *Adolescent health care: A practical guide* (3rd ed., p. 142). Baltimore: Williams & Wilkins; originally modified from Hammer, L. D., Kraemer, H. C., Wilson, D. C., et al. (1991). Standardized percentile curves of body-mass index for children and adolescents. *American Journal of Diseases of Children 145*, 260.

and avoiding sedentary activities (e.g., watching television) that entice one to engage in nonnutritive eating and less activity.

Weight reduction is difficult at any age, but the adolescent's belief in her invincibility makes recognition and treatment of the problem all the more challenging. During adolescence, weight reduction needs to be avoided when growth spurts are occurring. However, when a teen is morbidly obese, restricted caloric intake and increased activity need to be initiated when obesity is first diagnosed and modified if a growth spurt starts. The health consequences of obesity are rarely a concern to the adolescent; however, obesity begun in adolescence is known to be more severe than obesity in adulthood. Further, the health consequences of hypertension, serum lipid changes, cardiovascular disease, cerebrovascular disease, gallbladder disease, diabetes mellitus, cancer (in particular gallbladder, biliary duct, breast, ovarian, and uterine cancers), arthritis, and psychological issues (depression, low self-esteem, disturbed body image, and social solitude) have an earlier onset in the obese adolescent who becomes an obese adult compared with her thinner counterparts (Harris & Seimer, 1995; MacKenzie & Neinstein, 1996).

Therapeutic methods to assist in weight reduction in obese adolescents require a combination of approaches. Nutrition counseling (see Chapter 11), exercise (see Chapter 12), behavior modification, and support group participation have potential benefits. Basic recommendations for a balanced weight reduction diet are including foods from the five food groups (milk, meat, bread, fruits, and vegetables), eating at least three meals per day, limiting the caloric value of food and and reducing caloric intake, and preparing foods in a less caloric manner (e.g., baking instead of frying). More accurate assessment of actual caloric intake can be determined through the use of a diet diary. When the diet diary is reviewed with a health professional, specific foods and behaviors are identified and consequently can be adjusted for more successful weight reduction. Increasing physical activity has emotional and physical benefits and can be accomplished through establishing a weekly exercise regimen (walking for a half hour daily, participating in aerobics 3 times a week, always using the stairs at work or school, etc.). Support groups address the psychological issues motivating weight reduction and are often helpful for women who need a social outlet for identification with their problem. Support groups that attend to the issues of obesity and weight reduction are Teenage Obesity Programs, Weight Watchers, or any structured group that focuses on the concerns of diet, exercise, and weight management.

Anorexia Nervosa

Anorexia nervosa is a malingestion syndrome affecting 9 to 10 times more females than males. The worldwide incidence is reported at 1 per 100,000 and in some cultural groups (white, pubertal females in Western countries) is as high as 1 per 200. The mean age of onset is 13.75 years with a range from 10 to 25 years (American Medical Association, 1991; American Psychiatric Association, 1994; MacKenzie & Neinstein, 1996).

The diagnostic criteria include the following (American Psychiatric Association, 1994):

- Unwillingness to maintain a minimal normal weight for age and height (weight less than 85% of recommended level because of weight loss or failure to make expected weight gain during a period of growth)
- Extreme fear of gaining weight or becoming fat
- Dissonance in the experience of one's own body image and the seriousness of the current low body weight
- Absence of at least three menstrual cycles in a postmenarchal female

The differential diagnosis must distinguish anorexia nervosa from other eating disturbances, which include a preoccupation with weight, food fads, fat phobia, and a finicky eater. Other possible causes to be differentiated are brain tumors, Crohn disease, cystic fibrosis, depression, early pregnancy, hyperthyroidism, mesenteric artery syndrome, sarcoidosis, tuberculosis, or weight loss from bodybuilding or sports. However, the diagnosis of anorexia nervosa needs to be considered carefully when unexplained weight loss and food avoidance are demonstrated together, especially in the presence of hyperactivity.

Evaluation begins with a thorough history and the option of selective screening tools. The history questions gather data about the following (Harris & Seimer, 1995):

- *Menstrual characteristics*: Age of menarche, regularity and pattern of cycles, sexual activity, and use of contraception
- *Social atmosphere*: Configuration of family of origin; current status of living and eating (alone or with others); number and characteristics of relationships; use of laxatives, diuretics, appetite suppressants, and syrup of ipecac (chronic use can lead to cardiomyopathy and sudden death); and history of psychological counseling
- *Attitude*: Body image and especially current weight (preferred ideal weight, method for achieving ideal weight, actual weight over past 6 months, highest and lowest weight ever, and family members' weight history)
- *Diet history*: A 24-hour recall dietary record including meals, snacks, caffeine, alcohol, recreational and prescription drug consumption; discussion of the woman's interpretation of what is a reasonable meal, a binge, and a feeling of satiation; having the woman keep a food and mood diary for several days that includes times of the day when foods were eaten, with whom they were eaten, activities while eating (such as sitting, walking, or lying down), and feelings before, during, and after eating
- *Exercise*: Type of exercise and frequency; determination of athletic or compulsive in nature (in particular evaluate for the female athlete triad: disordered eating, amenorrhea, and osteoporosis); whether purging behaviors accompany compulsive exercise; and also who is associated with exercise (coach, parents, friends)

Tools that assist in differentiating anorexia nervosa from bulimia or weight-preoccupied otherwise normal young women include the Eating Attitudes Test and Eating Disorders Inventory, bulimia tests, and Diagnostic Survey for Eating Disorders (Harris & Seimer, 1995; MacKenzie & Neinstein, 1996).

When anorexia is suspected, a complete physical examination is necessary and should focus on aspects of emaciation (e.g., skin turgor and color, lanugo on face and extremities, hair loss or thinning, brittle nails, dehydration, and a scaphoid abdomen) and dental changes associated with purging. Laboratory tests appropriate to determining the diagnosis include the following:

■ *Blood chemistries*: Complete blood count, platelet count, and erythrocyte sedimentation rate; electrolytes, blood urea nitorgen, and creatinine

■ *Urinalysis*: Carbohydrate metabolism (elevated protein and ketones indicate poor intake); specific gravity (elevated with dehydration and dilute with excess water intake to maximize a measured weight; urine pregnancy test when the woman is sexually active or has amenorrhea

■ *Endocrine studies*: Follicle stimulating hormone and luteinizing hormone (usually decreased); thyroid function studies (may be low although thyroid-stimulating hormone may be normal); prolactin level

■ *Electrocardiogram*: Evaluate for arrhythmias and bradycardia

■ *Liver function tests*: Other causes of unknown weight loss (influenced by malnutrition)

Advanced practice nurses should use a collaborative approach to the care of women with anorexia. A treatment plan needs to be multidisciplinary with medical and psychoactive consultation (Lyon et al., 1997; MacKenzie & Neinstein, 1996). MacKenzie and Neinstein (1996) recommend a staged intervention plan focusing first on determining a correct diagnosis, then on replenishing nutritional stores, and finally on engaging in long-term therapy. Once the diagnosis of anorexia nervosa is determined, the practitioner informs the young woman and her family, and they agree on a therapeutic plan. Attending to the nutritional status of the adolescent is crucial because many of her emotional and behavioral problems may result from malnutrition. When the adolescent is in physical danger from hypovolemia and hypertension or when the family is in crisis with an unstable home environment, a short-term hospitalization is recommended. The goals of this hospitalization should focus on weight gain (through nutrition counseling and oral modes of eating, or more invasive means such as a nasogastric tube or intravenous hyperalimentation) and a cognitive approach to psychotherapy. In addition to psychotherapy, behavioral contracts may be useful in hospital treatment and in outpatient therapy (Box 15-7). The concluding intervention stage, long-term therapy, begins at discharge from the hospital or after the initial diagnosis in the outpatient visit. Although commencement of individual and family sessions of psychotherapy is imperative, the progress of the adolescent in establishing a trusting relationship with the primary health care provider is vital. Role modeling healthful eating behaviors and satisfaction with one's own body image and weight may be significantly helpful to the teen. Setting goals that encourage self-control, self-definition, and self-esteem aid in progress toward recovery. Often anorexia nervosa is accompanied with an underlying depression, and antidepressant medication may be beneficial to these adolescents (Depression Guideline Panel, 1993b). Group therapy also has a place with this population and offers the advantage of having peers challenge one another about beliefs, maintaining appropriate weight, difficult peer relationships, and ways in which they try to fool themselves and their practitioners.

Box 15-7 SAMPLE OUTPATIENT CONTRACT FOR ADOLESCENTS WITH ANOREXIA NERVOSA

Initial weight:
Initial height:
Goal weight:

_____

Visits clinic twice weekly until_____lb
Visits clinic weekly until_____lb
Visits clinic every 2 weeks until_____lb
Visits clinic once a month until_____lb
Visits clinic every 3 months for 1 year after_____lb reached
—Hospitalization if weight or physical state does not improve over a 4-week period.
—No cooking or kitchen work until_____lb
—No ballet until_____lb
—No gymnastics until_____lb
—No participation in physical education classes at school until_____lb

_____
(Patient)

_____
(Physician)

Anorexia nervosa has a mortality rate up to 22%, with 5% being the most commonly reported rate. Generally, outcomes in the area of weight respond best to therapy, with mild improvement of menstruation and only fair results with psychological readjustment (Gillbert, Rastam, & Gillberg, 1994; Steinhausen & Seidel, 1993). Forty-five percent persist with depressive symptoms. Predictors of a good prognosis are high educational achievement, early age of onset, good educational adjustment, improvement in body image after weight gain, good initial ego strength, and a supportive family (MacKenzie & Neinstein, 1996, p. 577).

Bulimia

Although bulimia has its own definition and diagnostic criteria, the condition often is considered on the continuum with anorexia nervosa. Bulimia is an eating disorder distinguished by binge eating and activities associated with weight control, such as fasting, purging, excessive exercise, and laxative abuse. The individual with bulimia is usually of normal weight and aware of the abnormal eating behaviors.

The age range for women with bulimia is 13 to 58 years, in contrast to women with anorexia nervosa, 10 to 25 years. Bulimia prevalence rates are estimated at 1% to 3% of young women in Western industrialized countries and 95% of all affected are female.

Bulimic women also have an increased incidence of depression, affective disorders, and substance abuse (Depression Guideline Panel, 1993a).

The *Diagnostic and Statistical Manual of Mental Disorders,* fourth edition (American Psychiatric Association, 1994) criteria for bulimia are these:

■ Recurrent episodes of binge eating (rapid consumption of a large amount of food in a discrete period of time, usually less than 2 hours)

■ A sense of lack of control over eating during the episode (i.e., a fear of not being able to stop eating)

■ A regular cycle of self-induced vomiting, use of laxatives, or rigorous dieting or fasting to counteract the effects of binge eating

■ A minimum average of two binge-eating episodes per week for at least 3 months

Two types of bulimia have been identified:

■ *Purging type*: Individual regularly self-induces vomiting or abuses laxatives, diuretics, or enemas.

■ *Nonpurging type*: Individual uses other inappropriate compensatory behaviors such as fasting or excessive exercise but not purging.

The classic signs of bulimia are dental erosions (usually on the inner enamel of the teeth), skin changes on the dorsum of the hand related to self-induced vomiting (scarring, calluses, and ulceration), and parotid gland enlargement, usually bilateral and painless. Evaluation needs to include a complete history and physical examination. Laboratory studies are similar to those of anorexia with the addition of a serum amylase test (to confirm vomiting), urine tests to detect diuretic or laxative abuse, and a chest radiograph to rule out aspiration pneumonia.

Treatment focuses on the modification of attitudes toward self-image and the reduction of bulimic eating (Lipscomb & Agostini, 1995). Eating three meals a day is a major deterrent to the loss of control that leads to a binge. With the reduction in binge eating comes a decrease in purging, fasting, and compulsive exercise. With a more regular eating pattern the depression may be minimized because of better nutrition and less self-ridicule and anxiety that accompany a binge. Antidepressants have been helpful in controlling bulimia. The serotonin reuptake inhibitors or tricyclics are recommended for their stimulant and appetite-suppressant antidepressive qualities. Individual, family, or group therapy is a useful process alone or accompanying the use of antidepressant medication. Referral to a dentist for teeth enamel evaluation helps preserve what remains of the adolescent's adult teeth. The health care provider should recommend dietary modifications for women who have used diuretics (low-salt diet until fluid control normalizes) and a high-fiber diet for laxative users to reduce potential constipation problems and should follow-up weekly until bingeing subsides and healthful behaviors are demonstrated.

Mood Disorders

Primary mood disorders include depressive (unipolar) and manic-depressive (bipolar) conditions. These conditions have been and continue to be underdiagnosed and undertreated by primary care and nonpsychiatric practitioners. Mood disorders are common in primary care practices, and nurse-practitioners can gain confidence in making mood disorder diagnoses and offering proper treatment. Other major risk factors for depression are a family history of depressive disorder, female gender, prior attempted suicide, lack of social supports, stressful life events, postpartum period, medical comorbidity, and current substance abuse. Although the social stigma surrounding depression is waning, the stigma still prevents many from obtaining the health care they need. The cost of the illness in pain, suffering, disability, and death is high.

According to the Depression Guideline Panel (1993a):

Depressive disorders should not be confused with the depressed or sad mood that normally accompanies specific life experiences—particularly losses or disappointments. Mood disorders involve disturbances in emotional, cognitive, behavioral, and somatic regulation. A clinical depression or a mood disorder is a syndrome (a constellation of signs and symptoms) that is not a normal reaction to life's difficulties. A sad or depressed mood is only one of many signs and symptoms of a clinical depression. In fact, the mood disturbance may include apathy, anxiety, or irritability in addition to or instead of sadness; also, the patient's interest or capacity for pleasure or enjoyment may be markedly reduced. Not all clinically depressed patients are sad, and many sad patients are not clinically depressed.

The *Diagnostic and Statistical Manual of Mental Disorders,* fourth edition (American Psychiatric Association, 1994) defines a major depressive episode as having at least five of the following symptoms present for a 2-week period, and these moods represent a change from previous functioning. At least one of the symptoms is depressed mood or loss of interest or pleasure in most activities.

- Depressed or irritable mood most of the day nearly every day
- Greatly diminished interest or pleasure in all or most activities of the day nearly every day
- Significant weight loss or weight gain when not dieting or decrease or increase in appetite
- Insomnia or hypersomnia nearly every day
- Psychomotor agitation or retardation nearly every day
- Fatigue or loss of energy nearly every day
- Feelings of worthlessness or excessive or inappropriate guilt nearly every day
- Diminished ability to think or concentrate (indecisiveness) nearly every day
- Recurrent thoughts of death, suicidal ideation, or suicide attempt

Major depressive disorder usually begins in the mid-20s and 30s, although depression may begin at any age. Symptoms may develop over days or weeks. A major depressive episode may have only a single occurrence with a complete recovery; however, more than 50% of persons experiencing one episode eventually experience another (Depression Guideline Panel, 1993a).

Unipolar Forms

Three classifications make up the unipolar forms of primary mood disorders. *Major depressive disorder* consists of one or more episodes of major depression with or without full recovery between these episodes. *Dysthymic disorder* features a low-grade, more persistent, less episodic depressed mood and associated symptoms for at least 2 years, during which a major depressive episode has not occurred. Many patients with dysthymic disorder subsequently suffer superimposed episodes of major depression over the course of their illness. In such cases, dysthymic and major depressive disorders are diagnosed according to the *Diagnostic and Statistical Manual of Mental Disorders*, fourth edition. *Depression not otherwise specified* is a residual category reserved for patients with symptoms and signs of depression that do not meet the formal diagnostic criteria for dysthymic or major depressive disorders (Depression Guideline Panel, 1993a, p. 18).

Bipolar Forms

Bipolar mood disorders are recurrent, episodic conditions characterized by a history of at least one manic or hypomanic episode. Ninety-five percent of persons with bipolar disorder also have recurrent episodes of major depression (Depression Guideline Panel, 1993a). Bipolar disorders also are grouped into three types:

1. **Bipolar I disorder** requires at least one manic episode, along with (nearly always) major depressive episodes. A manic episode consists of a distinct period of elevated or irritable mood, along with several symptoms such as grandiosity, decreased need for sleep, pressured speech, and poor judgment.
2. **Bipolar disorder not otherwise specified** is a residual category that includes bipolar II disorder and is a condition characterized by recurrent episodes of major depression along with hypomanic (but not full-blown manic) episodes and other forms that do not meet formal criteria for bipolar I or cyclothymic disorder.
3. **Cyclothymic disorder** is characterized by numerous hypomanic episodes and numerous periods of mild depressive symptoms insufficient in duration or severity to meet the criteria for major depressive episodes. Cyclothymic disorder is typically chronic, lasting at least 2 years by definition (Depression Guideline Panel, 1993a, p. 19).

Diagnosis and Treatment

Adolescents with depressive disorders have not been well researched. Giles, Jarret, Biggs, Guzick, and Rush (1989) found that early onset of major depression (before age 20) was associated with a greater likelihood of a more recurrent pattern in adulthood. Comparisons of adult depression and adolescent depression show a similarity in mood changes, feelings of hopelessness, and feelings of worthlessness. Differences in manifestations of adult vs. adolescent depression include the following: depressed adolescents who act out receive angry responses, adolescent appearance is less depressed and more rebellious and angry, and acting-out behaviors, including suicide attempts, are more typical among adolescents (Neinstein & MacKenzie, 1996).

Figure 15-7 is a schematic of the differential diagnosis of primary mood disorders. The schematic includes the diagnostic criteria for depression (five out of nine symptoms) and the occurrence of a manic episode.

Other conditions associated with depression include the following (Neinstein & MacKenzie, 1996):

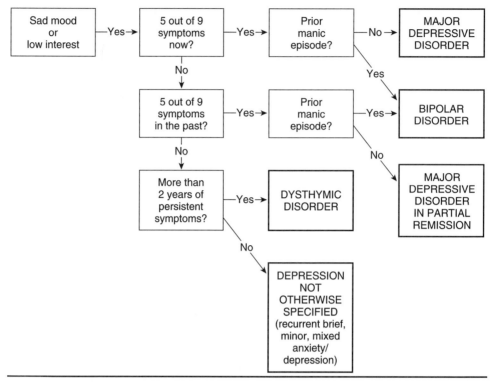

Figure 15-7 Differential diagnosis of primary mood disorders. (From Depression Guideline Panel. [1993]. *Depression in primary care, vol. 1, Detection and diagnosis: Clinical practice guideline number 5* [AHCPR Publication No. 93-0551]. Rockville, MD: U.S. Department of Health and Human Services, Public Health Service, Agency for Health Care Policy and Research.)

■ Uncomplicated bereavement (secondary to a stressful loss and usually starting within 2 to 3 months following the death and may last up to a year)

■ Organic affective syndrome (a persistent or pronounced depressed mood secondary to a physical diagnosis such as hyperthyroidism, pheochromocytoma, brain tumors, or collagen vascular disease)

■ Adjustment disorder with depressed mood (a depressive reaction to one or more identifiable psychosocial stressors that happens within 3 months of the initial stressor)

Nurse practitioners need to have astute diagnostic skills with mood disorders to refer the patient for psychopharmacological evaluation and psychiatric treatment. Management, however, requires consideration of the potential benefits and harm regarding all alternatives, including being involved with the adolescent as a support rather than as a primary care provider. Optimal treatment is treatment acceptable to the patient, predictably effective, and associated with minimal side effects.

According to the Depression Guideline Panel (1993b, p. 23),

Once major depressive disorder is diagnosed, interventions that predictably decrease symptoms and morbidity, earlier than would occur naturally in the course of the illness, are logically tried first. The key initial objectives of treatment, in order of priority, are (1) to reduce and ultimately to remove all signs and symptoms of the depressive syndrome, (2) to restore occupational and psychosocial function to that of the asymptomatic state, and (3) to reduce the likelihood of relapse and recurrence.

Treatment options include antidepressant medications, psychotherapy, a combination of medication and psychotherapy, or electroconvulsive therapy (Depression Guideline Panel, 1993b). Medication has the advantage of being easy to administer and is effective in treating mild, moderate, and severe forms of major depression. The disadvantages of medication are the potential for a suicide attempt, unwanted side effects, adherence to a strict medication schedule, and frequent visits to the health care provider. Psychotherapy has the advantage of no physiological side effects and acquisition of coping skills that may help the adolescent avoid recurrence. The disadvantages of psychotherapy are the expense, time commitment, finding a compatible and well-trained therapist, and delayed treatment effects that are measurable later than with medication. The combination of medication and psychotherapy offers a higher probability of response, a greater degree of response for individual patients, and a lower attrition rate from treatment. The disadvantages of the combination approach to treatment include all the disadvantages of each alone. Electroconvulsive therapy, although rarely used on adolescents, has proven efficacy in severely symptomatic patients who have failed to respond to one or more medication trials.

SPECIFIC MENSTRUAL HEALTH CONCERNS

Menstruation is the physiological phenomena of the uterus shedding its lining, approximately at monthly intervals from menarche to menopause. Traditionally, the first day of menstrual flow is identified as the first day of the menstrual cycle. The normal phases of the menstrual cycle are defined by the endometrial and ovarian patterns of change. The endometrium undergoes three distinct phases during the menstrual cycle. The first phase is the **menstrual** phase and corresponds with the first 5 days of the cycle. Second is the **proliferative** phase (days 6 through 14), and third is the **secretory** phase (days 15 through 28 or the last 14 days of the menstrual cycle). The ovarian pattern of change has two corresponding phases. The **follicular** phase starts on day 1 of the menstrual cycle and continues until ovulation or day 14 in a 28-day cycle. The **luteal** phase (day 15 or postovulation through day 28 or the last day of the cycle) follows the follicular phase and corresponds with the secretory phase of the endometrium. The time interval in the luteal phase is 14 days (±2) and is based on the life of the corpus luteum. The follicular phase is not as consistent in length. The differences in the menstrual cycle from 21 to 35 days are caused by the variations in follicular development.

Figure 15-8 illustrates the menstrual cycle dynamics. The typical 28-day cycle is used for purposes of illustration. Pattern variations can be compared easily. For example, on day 12 of the menstrual cycle, events at the ovarian level show that

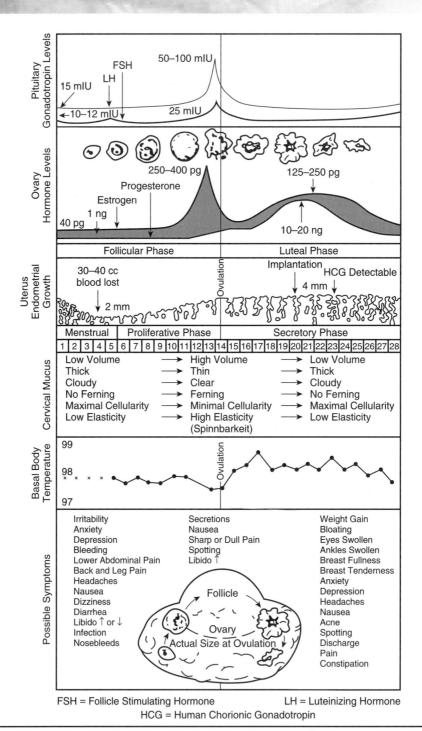

Figure 15-8 Menstrual cycle events: hormone levels, ovarian and endometrial patterns, and cyclical temperature and cervical mucus changes. (From Hatcher, R. A., Trussell, J., Stewart, F., Stewart, G. K., Kowal, D., Guest, F., et al. [1994]. *Contraceptive technology* [16th ed.]. New York: Irvington.)

estrogen is peaking, whereas on the gonadotropin level, luteinizing hormone is preparing to surge, and on the basal body temperature record the temperature is decreasing. All of these events prepare for ovulation on day 14 of the cycle. For more complete physiological information, see Chapter 7.

As stated previously, the onset of puberty is an evolving sequence of maturational phases known as milestones. The four maturational milestones of puberty for females are thelarche, the development of the breast; adrenarche, the development of pubic and axillary hair; peak growth velocity; and menarche, the first menstrual period. When these phases are not in synchronization, the events can lead to premature thelarche (neonatal breast hypertrophy commonly occurring in girls ages 1 to 4 years of age), premature adrenarche (the presence of virilization and the absence of breast development, or estrogenization of the labia and vagina), precocious puberty (secondary sex characteristics occurring before 8 years of age), or delayed puberty (lack of developed signs of puberty by age 17).

The clinician needs to understand several conditions affecting a woman's genital and reproductive health for proper evaluation and diagnosis once a woman has entered puberty and is ready for or is having menstrual periods. Six significant conditions are amenorrhea, dysfunctional uterine bleeding, dysmenorrhea, premenstrual syndrome (PMS), pelvic pain, and infections. These conditions are not exclusive but are the most common alterations in menstrual health presented to the practitioner.

Amenorrhea

According to Speroff and others (1994, p. 402), amenorrhea is diagnosed if the following criteria are fulfilled:

- No periods by age 14 in the absence of growth or development of secondary sexual characteristics
- No periods by age 16 regardless of the presence of normal growth and development with the appearance of secondary sexual characteristics.
- In a woman who has been menstruating, the absence of periods for a length of time equivalent to a total of at least three of the previous cycle intervals or 6 months of (no menses) amenorrhea

Traditionally, amenorrhea has been defined as *primary* or *secondary*. Primary amenorrhea is menarche that has not occurred by the age of 16. Secondary amenorrhea is the loss of menses for more than 6 months in a woman who has had previously normal cycles and who is not pregnant. Speroff and others (1994, p. 402) now believe that this dual form of categorization can lead to diagnostic omissions. To avoid such diagnostic errors, they offer instead the organizing schema that compartmentalizes the causes of amenorrhea (Box 15-8).

The normal physiological events of menstruation are outlined in Figure 15-9, with the four compartments superimposed so that visual recognition more easily distinguishes the relationships.

In diagnosing amenorrhea, one begins with a thorough history and physical examination. When amenorrhea presents in puberty, the practitioner needs to consider

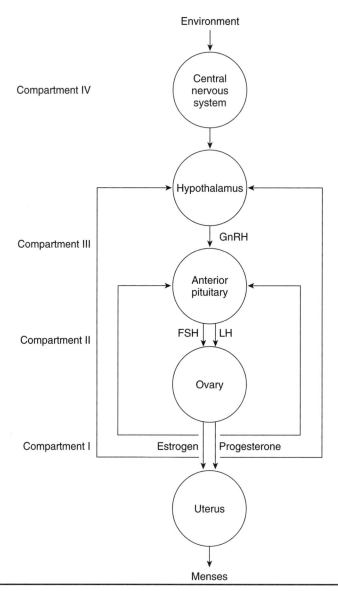

Figure 15-9 The basic principles underlying the physiology of menstrual function. (From Speroff, L., Glass, R. H., & Kase, N. G. [1994]. *Clinical gynecologic endocrinology and infertility* [5th ed.]. Baltimore: Williams & Wilkins.)

congenital abnormalities and the diagnosis of secondary amenorrhea of adult onset. During the evaluation of the external genitalia, specific attention to the vagina aids in determining the effects of estrogen. Well-cornified, rugated, vaginal epithelium suggests normal estrogen status, whereas poorly cornified vagina epithelium with scant cervical

---

Box 15-8 DISCRETE COMPARTMENTS ON WHICH MENSTRUATION DEPENDS

Compartment I	Disorders of the outflow tract or uterine target organ
Compartment II	Disorders of the ovary
Compartment III	Disorders of the anterior pituitary
Compartment IV	Disorders of central nervous system (hypothalamic) factors

From Speroff, L., Glass, R. H., & Kase, N. G. (1994). *Clinical gynecologic endocrinology and infertility* (5th ed.). Baltimore: Williams & Wilkins.

---

mucus suggests a low estrogenic state. Once the external genitalia are evaluated and found to have the effects of estrogen, to be patent and connected with the internal genitalia, then evaluations of the uterus, ovaries, pituitary, hypothalamus, and other central nervous system sources are required.

The workup for amenorrhea is initiated in a stepwise progression (Speroff et al., 1994). After pregnancy has been ruled out definitively, Step 1 includes measuring thyroid-stimulating hormone and prolactin, followed by a progesterone challenge test. If the thyroid-stimulating hormone is elevated, then the diagnosis of hypothyroidism is given and treated. Although only a small percentage of women with amenorrhea have this diagnosis, the evaluation is easy and the diagnosis is important to rule out. When the results of the progesterone challenge test are positive and the thyroid-stimulating hormone and serum prolactin are normal, then the diagnosis is **anovulatory amenorrhea**. When galactorrhea is absent and the prolactin level is normal (less than 20 ng/mL in most laboratories), no further evaluation of a pituitary tumor as the cause is needed so long as the response to the progesterone challenge test is positive. If galactorrhea is present with the amenorrhea and the serum prolactin level is elevated, then a coned-down view of the sella turcica by computerized tomography or magnetic resonance imaging is recommended.

The woman's health care nurse practitioner may choose to refer the patient to a specialist or proceed with the next step. In Step 2, estrogen and progesterone are given to stimulate the endometrium and differentiate the diagnosis of an inoperative end organ (uterus) outflow tract from the diagnosis of preliminary estrogen proliferation of the endometrium that has not occurred. If the response is a negative withdrawal, then the diagnosis of end organ problem is given. If, however, the response to the oral estrogen and progesterone prescription is positive, then Step 3 is warranted. In Step 3, the assay levels of gonadotropins are evaluated and further studies are determined by the resulting values (Speroff et al., 1994).

The workup can take some time before a definitive diagnosis can be made. The consequences of this delay usually are not worrisome to the adolescent; however, a parent may be anxious. Giving information and reassurance to the teen and her family in a way that acknowledges their concerns and fears is important.

The specific disorders of secondary amenorrhea are listed in Box 15-9 and are grouped according to the compartment with which they correlate.

In adolescents the most likely diagnosis of amenorrhea is anovulation. Treatment options for anovulation include no initial intervention and allowing the teen to monitor the regularity of her cycles by a monthly calendar, with a 3-month follow-up appointment for another progesterone challenge test if menses has not occurred; administration of cyclical progesterone at 10 mg medroxyprogesterone daily for the first 10 days of the month; or administration of a low-dose oral contraceptive for menstrual regulation.

Monthly menstruation in an adolescent is an important part of her identity development. Because of the social and psychological benefits associated with a regular menstrual pattern and the importance of avoiding a prolonged state of unopposed estrogen effect on the endometrium, initiation of a therapeutic regimen is encouraged. Research is showing that young women who have prolonged periods of hypoestrogen are at risk for osteoporosis. Athletes and dancers who would prefer not to have their periods can use a continuous hormone therapy of 0.625 mg conjugated estrogens and 2.5 mg medroxyprogesterone acetate taken daily. An alternative therapy that helps in preventing osteoporosis is a low-dose oral contraceptive taken every day without a pill-free interval. In the rare case, when a hypoestrogenic woman cannot use hormone therapy, supplemental calcium (1000 to 1500 mg daily) needs to be strongly advised. High calcium combined with exercise is a most effective means to protect bone density.

Dysfunctional Uterine Bleeding

Dysfunctional uterine bleeding is defined as a variety of bleeding manifestations of anovulatory cycles without other medical illness or pathological findings (Speroff et al., 1994). The qualities of menstruation are noted as flow duration and amount. The usual duration of flow is 4 to 6 days, with a range of 2 to 8 days. The normal volume of

---

Box 15-9 SPECIFIC DISORDERS OF SECONDARY AMENORRHEA WITHIN COMPARTMENTS

Compartment I	Asherman syndrome
Compartment II	Ovarian disorders
	Abnormal chromosomes
	Normal chromosomes
Compartment III	Prolactin tumors
Compartment IV	Anovulation
	Weight loss or anorexia
	Hypothalamic suppression
	Hypothyroidism

From Speroff, L., Glass, R. H., & Kase, N. G. (1994). *Clinical gynecologic endocrinology and infertility* (5th ed.). Baltimore: Williams & Wilkins.

menstrual blood loss is 30 to 40 mL, and greater than 80 mL is considered abnormal (Speroff et al., 1994). The amount of normal blood loss corresponds to 10 to 15 moderately soaked pads or tampons. Other definitions that characterize deviations in menstruation include these:

- *Oligomenorrhea:* Intervals greater than 35 days
- *Polymenorrhea:* Intervals less than 21 days
- *Menorrhagia:* Regular, normal intervals with excessive flow and duration
- *Metrorrhagia:* Irregular intervals with excessive flow and duration

Although oligomenorrhea has some of the same clinical properties of amenorrhea, the menstrual flow may be normal or irregularly heavy or light.

Menorrhagia

Acute menorrhagia in adolescents causes a spectrum of complaints varying from minor pattern changes in menstruation to life-threatening hemorrhage. The condition, no matter how modest, deserves attentive consideration by the practitioner because menorrhagia is a great concern to the teen and parent. In cases of minor variation, after confirmation through physical examination and blood work, the timing is ripe for the practitioner to educate the teen and family member about the normal menstrual cycle and its variations.

When the adolescent with acute menorrhagia presents in the clinic or emergency room, she usually has been bleeding heavily for several days or even weeks. She is generally pale, anxious, and admits to low energy. Typically the teen is within the first year of her menarche and has not established ovulatory cycles. Although the majority of teens experiencing acute menorrhagia have a diagnosis of anovulatory uterine bleeding, the differential diagnosis is summarized in Box 15-10.

The differential diagnosis of dysfunctional uterine bleeding is one of exclusion. A common cause of dysfunctional uterine bleeding is pregnancy and related complications. Pregnancy needs to be considered even if the teen denies sexual activity. The local genital tract conditions are diagnosed by a thorough pelvic examination and microbial assessment. Systemic causes are diagnosed through personal and family history and blood tests. Hormonal causes are evaluated by chart review and history of contraceptives or hormonal prescriptions.

Management includes the following laboratory studies: hematocrit, hemoglobin, platelet count, blood type and cross match, clotting studies (prothrombin time, partial thromboplastin time, and a bleeding time), serum beta-human chorionic gonadotropin, and cervical cultures for *Neisseria gonorrhoeae* and *Chlamydia trachomatis* (Laufer & Goldstein, 1995).

Treatment is determined by the diagnosis. In the case of anovulatory uterine bleeding, the immediate treatment regimen is to give intense estrogen-progestin therapy for 7 days using a low-dose monophasic oral contraceptive twice a day. At the end of the week the teen again will bleed. On the fifth day of bleeding the teen resumes hormonal treatment with a cyclic oral contraceptive for 3 months. At the end of the 3 months, if contraception is desired, then the oral contraceptive is continued, and if contraception is

Box 15-10 DIFFERENTIAL DIAGNOSIS OF ADOLESCENT MENORRHAGIA

Anovulatory Uterine Bleeding

Pregnancy-Related Complications
Spontaneous abortion
Complications of pregnancy termination procedures
Ectopic pregnancy
Gestational trophoblastic diseases
Bleeding in the third trimester of pregnancy

Local Genital Tract Conditions
Benign and malignant tumors (vaginal, cervical, uterine, or ovarian)
Infection
Intrauterine contraceptive devices
Trauma
Intravaginal foreign bodies

Systemic Causes
Coagulation disorders
Thyroid dysfunction
Diabetes mellitus
Nutritional disorders and iron deficiency
Hepatic diseases
Renal diseases

Hormonal Causes
Oral contraceptives
Intramuscular
Subcutaneous

From Laufer, M. R., & Goldstein, D. P. (1995). Pediatric and adolescent gynecology. In K. J. Ryan, R. S. Berkowitz, & R. L. Barbieri (Eds.), *Kistner's gynecology: Principles and practice* (6th ed., pp. 571–632). St. Louis: Mosby.

not desired, then the treatment switches to 10 mg of medroxyprogesterone for 10 days each month to ensure therapeutic effect. When the bleeding is more severe, the practitioner needs to consult with the physician and plan for hospitalization and a potential dilatation and curettage.

Follow-up includes physical evaluation of anemia, nutrition, and the occurrence of ovulatory cycles. The psychosocial impact of the event of acute adolescent menorrhagia needs to be explored with the teen, so positive attitudes regarding future reproductive health are sustained.

Anovulatory Hypermenorrhea or Metrorrhagia
Chronic heavy menses, whether cyclical or at irregular intervals, is a frequent complaint in adolescents. Differentiation between possible causes of heavy menses such as anovulation and uterine pathological conditions, systemic diseases, and coagulation defects is important.

Management of anovulatory hypermenorrhea includes evaluation of the same laboratory studies listed for menorrhagia, with the addition of thyroid function tests. Adolescents without anemia and not in need of contraception can be managed by verifying anovulation through the charting of a basal body temperature (Speroff et al., 1994). Prostaglandin inhibitors may help reduce menstrual flow. When excess menstrual flow also is combined with anemia, treatment with 10 mg medroxyprogesterone acetate daily for 10 days in a month is an option. An alternative that is necessary for adolescents desiring a method of contraception is low-dose monophasic oral contraceptive pills.

Anovulatory Polymenorrhea

The complaint that menstrual periods are occurring too frequently may be caused by physiological events or the misinformed adolescent. Through a history the practitioner may discover that the teen is counting her interval from the last day of her menses to the first day of the next menses. Using a menstrual calendar and providing information about normal menstrual physiology helps to inform and ease the concerns of these adolescents. Management of true polymenorrhea is attained by monthly treatment with 10 mg medroxyprogesterone acetate for the first 10 days of the month. Treatment is for 3 to 6 months, followed by observation for the occurrence of ovulatory cycles. If this treatment plan fails, then a dilatation and curettage is indicated (Speroff et al., 1994).

Dysmenorrhea

Dysmenorrhea is pain with menstruation in the lower abdomen with cramping. The severity of dysmenorrhea relates the duration and amount of menstrual flow (Andersch & Milsom, 1982). Studies about dysmenorrhea are rare, so data are limited regarding the population affected. Up to 72% of adolescents are reported to be affected, and a proportion of these missed school or work with every menses (Sanfillipo, 1993).

Two kinds of dysmenorrhea are distinguished. Primary dysmenorrhea, a condition associated with ovulatory cycles, is due to myometrial contractions induced by prostaglandins originating in secretory endometrium (Speroff et al., 1994, p. 524). Secondary dysmenorrhea is associated with pathological conditions (e.g., endometriosis, obstructing müllerian anomalies, and other pathological pelvic conditions). Dysmenorrhea in adolescents is usually primary.

Dysmenorrhea generally begins 1 to 3 years after menarche. The pain typically begins 1 to 4 hours after the onset of menses and continues for 24 to 48 hours. In some cases the pain can last as long as 4 days or start up to 2 days before the onset of menses. Other associated symptoms include headache, dizziness, lower back pain, thigh cramps, nausea and vomiting, fatigue, nervousness, diarrhea, and syncope.

Before deciding on appropriate treatment of dysmenorrhea, a thorough history and physical examination are performed. In assessing the teen's response to her cramps and menstrual characteristics, some key questions to ask are these:

■ Does the pain interfere with activities of daily living (e.g., school, intramural activities, sports, family dynamics)?

■ What associated symptoms are experienced (e.g., nausea, dizziness, or lethargy)?

■ Do other family members (e.g., sister or mother) have similar symptoms?

■ Is there a family history of endometriosis?

■ What medications have been tried, and what has been their effectiveness?

Interpreting a previous response to an over-the-counter medication such as ibuprofen may be crucial when trying to convince a teen who has tried a nonsteroidal antiinflammatory drug (NSAID) that a similar drug taken in a more specific way will be effective.

Women with primary dysmenorrhea have greater production of endometrial prostaglandins. The agent responsible for dysmenorrhea is prostaglandin $F_{2\alpha}$. Antiprostaglandin agents (NSAIDs) have been successful in relieving the painful effects of prostaglandin $F_{2\alpha}$. The carboxylic acid NSAID agents frequently used for treating dysmenorrhea are divided into four groups: **acetic acids** (indomethacin, sulindac, and tolmetin) were once popular but have many side effects; **salicylic acids** and **esters** (aspirin and diflunisal) inhibit cyclooxygenase but may increase menstrual flow and definitely have less potency than other NSAIDs; **propionic acids** (ibuprofen, naproxen, fenoprofen, ketoprofen, and flurbiprofen) are recommended most commonly; and **fenamates** (mefenamic acid, meclofenamate, tolfenamic acid, and flufenamic acid) are more recent drugs and are the most effective in relieving pain (Laufer & Goldstein, 1995; Speroff et al., 1994). Although analgesics are not helpful to all women suffering from dysmenorrhea, some NSAIDs and oral contraceptives assist in decreasing the severity. Women also report a decease in the severity of dysmenorrhea after a vaginal delivery.

Treatment regimens begin with the onset of menses and include a choice of one of the following prescriptions:

■ *Naproxen sodium:* 550 mg initially and then 275 mg every 6 hours

■ *Ibuprofen:* 400 mg every 4 to 6 hours to 800 mg 3 times a day with a loading dose of 800 to 1200 mg

■ *Mefenamic acid:* 500 mg initially and then 250 mg every 6 hours or 100 mg 2 to 3 times a day

■ *Meclofenamate:* 100 mg initially and then 50 to 100 mg every 6 hours

Medication is prescribed for two or three cycles and then evaluated. Before changing the type of medication, the health care provider should first increase the dosage and have the teen keep a menstrual calendar to see if any improvement has occurred.

The contraindications to NSAID use are known or suspected ulcer disease, gastrointestinal bleeding, renal disease, clotting disorders, preoperative patients, and patients with allergies to aspirin and NSAIDs or who have aspirin-induced asthma. Gastric upset is common with NSAIDs, so patients should be informed to take them with food.

Alternative therapy for dysmenorrhea includes low-dose oral contraceptives and comfort measures (hot-water bottle, warm baths, soothing warm herbal teas, and massage) in mild cases or with NSAIDs for more severe cases. Reassurance and education about the physiology of the menstrual cycle aid the adolescent in coping with her condition. When dysmenorrhea persists and the adolescent has tried NSAIDs and oral contraceptives, further evaluation and consideration of a laparoscopy for diagnosis are warranted.

Premenstrual Syndrome

Premenstrual syndrome is defined by Speroff and others (1994, p. 515) as follows:

The cyclic appearance of one or more of a large constellation of symptoms (over 100) just before menses, occurring to such a degree that lifestyle or work is affected, followed by a period of time entirely free of symptoms. The most frequent encountered symptoms include the following: abdominal bloating, anxiety, breast tenderness, crying spells, depression, fatigue, irritability, thirst and appetite changes, and variable degrees of edema of the extremities—usually occurring in the last 7 to 10 days of the cycle. The exact collection of symptoms in an individual is irrelevant; the diagnosis is made by prospectively and accurately charting the cyclic nature of the symptoms.

The cyclical nature of symptoms is what is underscored in making the diagnosis of PMS. The American Psychiatric Association has established guidelines for diagnosing PMS under the designation of luteal phase dysphoric disorder (American Psychiatric Association, 1987). These criteria are as follows:

A. Symptoms are related temporarily to the menstrual cycle, beginning during the last week of the luteal phase and remitting after the onset of menses.

B. The diagnosis requires at least five of the following, and one of the symptoms must be one of the first four:

1. Affective lability; for example, sudden onset of being sad, tearful, irritable, or angry
2. Persistent and marked anger or irritability
3. Marked anxiety or tension
4. Markedly depressed mood or feelings of hopelessness
5. Decreased interest in usual activities
6. Easily fatigued or marked lack of energy
7. Subjective sense of difficulty in concentrating
8. Marked change in appetite, overeating, or food craving
9. Hypersomnia or insomnia
10. Physical symptoms such as breast tenderness, headaches, edema, joint or muscle pain, and weight gain

C. The symptoms interfere with work or usual daily activities or relationships.

D. The symptoms are not an exacerbation of another psychiatric disorder.

The cause of PMS has not been supported scientifically, but biological theories abound. A few of these theories include low progesterone levels, high estrogen levels, changes in estrogen-to-progesterone ratios, increased aldosterone activity, increased adrenal activity, subclinical hypoglycemia, vitamin deficiencies, and excess prolactin secretion.

Adolescents tend to have mild cases of PMS. Charting a menstrual calendar, with physical and emotional changes, for three cycles is helpful not only to the clinician for appropriate diagnosis but also to the adolescent for reassurance and identification of her most troublesome symptoms. The calendar serves as a source of data for the Daily Rating Form (DFR) from which information gaps can be identified (Figure 15-10). The DRF uses a 6-point Rating Scale where 1 = not at all, 2 = minimal, 3 = mild, 4 = moderate, 5 = severe, and 6 = extreme. The mood symptoms increase premenstrually and decrease after the onset of menses. A PMS pattern can be interpreted after 2 to 3 menstrual cycles.

Once PMS has been diagnosed, management starts with counseling about alterations in diet and exercise. Most women find lifestyle changes challenging and adolescents more so. A persuasive technique an understanding practitioner can use is offering examples of other adolescents who have made healthful choices and their experiences. Another benefit for the teen when she makes a healthful lifestyle choice is a greater sense of control over her life. Recommendations for diet changes include avoiding salty foods, caffeine, alcohol, chocolate, and concentrated sweets and adding complex carbohydrates (brown rice, multigrain breads, and pasta), fruits and vegetables, high-fiber foods, low-fat meats, and low-fat milk products. Eating smaller, more frequent meals (4 to 6) per day during the premenstrual phase helps avoid hypoglycemic responses. Aerobic exercise and stress reduction activities during this time aid in establishing a sense of well-being.

Pharmacological therapies are considered only for specific symptoms when lifestyle changes have not been effective. Spironolactone, 25 to 50 mg once a day for 10 days before the onset of menses, is a diuretic effective when symptoms of edema and weight gain from fluid retention exist. Symptoms of fatigue, headache, and general aches and pains are helped with mefenamic acid (Ponstel), 250 mg every 8 hours starting on day 18 of the cycle and increased to 500 mg every 8 hours on day 19 of the cycle but not to be taken for more than 1 week (Laufer & Goldstein, 1995). Some adolescents find relief when they use oral contraceptives. The appropriate selection of an oral contraceptive for this use needs to be individualized, and generally a monophasic pill is a better choice because of less fluctuation in hormone amounts.

PMS is a complex condition. The practitioner needs to offer long-term support to women with this diagnosis. Explorations into relationships, family dynamics, and self-image help unravel the underlying issues that are producing the conflict, lack of control, and overriding symptoms. Helping the adolescent come to terms with the subtle nature of the problem, the fundamental psychological response involved, and the opportunity to take hold of one's life illustrates the kind of commitment a practitioner involved with PMS patients needs to have.

Pelvic Pain

Pelvic pain for most women is associated with their menses, is likely dysmenorrhea, and can be relieved by the previously mentioned treatment options. Pelvic pain that has not improved with the use of antiprostaglandin medication necessitates a physical examination with a pelvic examination. Pelvic pain traditionally is differentiated as acute and chronic.

Date	Menstru-ating?	Active, restless	Mood swings	Depressed, sad, low, blue, lonely	Anxious, jittery, nervous
2/26	N	1 (2) 3 4 5 6	(1) 2 3 4 5 6	1 2 (3) 4 5 6	(1) 2 3 4 5 6
2/27	N	(1) 2 3 4 5 6	(1) 2 3 4 5 6	(1) 2 3 4 5 6	(1) 2 3 4 5 6
2/28	N	1 2 (3) 4 5 6	(1) 2 3 4 5 6	(1) 2 3 4 5 6	(1) 2 3 4 5 6
2/29	N	1 (2) 3 4 5 6	(1) 2 3 4 5 6	(1) 2 3 4 5 6	(1) 2 3 4 5 6
3/01	N	1 (2) 3 4 5 6	1 2 (3) 4 5 6	1 (2) 3 4 5 6	1 (2) 3 4 5 6
3/02	N	1 2 3 (4) 5 6	1 2 3 (4) 5 6	1 2 3 (4) 5 6	1 2 3 (4) 5 6
3/03	N	1 2 3 (4) 5 6	1 2 3 4 5 (6)	1 2 3 4 5 (6)	1 2 3 4 5 (6)
3/04	N	1 2 3 (4) 5 6	1 2 3 4 5 (6)	1 2 3 4 5 (6)	1 2 3 4 5 (6)
3/05	N	1 2 3 (4) 5 6	1 2 3 4 5 (6)	1 2 3 4 5 (6)	1 2 3 4 5 (6)
3/06	N	1 2 3 (4) 5 6	1 2 3 4 5 (6)	1 2 3 4 5 (6)	1 2 3 4 5 (6)
3/07	N	1 2 3 4 (5) 6	1 2 3 4 5 (6)	1 2 3 4 5 (6)	1 2 3 4 5 (6)
3/08	Y	1 2 (3) 4 5 6	1 (2) 3 4 5 6	(1) 2 3 4 5 6	(1) 2 3 4 5 6
3/09	Y	(1) 2 3 4 5 6	(1) 2 3 4 5 6	(1) 2 3 4 5 6	(1) 2 3 4 5 6
3/10	Y	(1) 2 3 4 5 6	(1) 2 3 4 5 6	(1) 2 3 4 5 6	(1) 2 3 4 5 6
3/11	Y	(1) 2 3 4 5 6	(1) 2 3 4 5 6	(1) 2 3 4 5 6	(1) 2 3 4 5 6
3/12	Y	(1) 2 3 4 5 6	(1) 2 3 4 5 6	(1) 2 3 4 5 6	(1) 2 3 4 5 6
3/13	Y	(1) 2 3 4 5 6	(1) 2 3 4 5 6	(1) 2 3 4 5 6	(1) 2 3 4 5 6
3/14	Y	(1) 2 3 4 5 6	(1) 2 3 4 5 6	(1) 2 3 4 5 6	(1) 2 3 4 5 6
3/15	N	(1) 2 3 4 5 6	(1) 2 3 4 5 6	(1) 2 3 4 5 6	(1) 2 3 4 5 6
3/16	N	(1) 2 3 4 5 6	(1) 2 3 4 5 6	(1) 2 3 4 5 6	(1) 2 3 4 5 6
3/17	N	(1) 2 3 4 5 6	(1) 2 3 4 5 6	(1) 2 3 4 5 6	(1) 2 3 4 5 6
3/18	N	(1) 2 3 4 5 6	(1) 2 3 4 5 6	(1) 2 3 4 5 6	(1) 2 3 4 5 6
3/19	N	(1) 2 3 4 5 6	(1) 2 3 4 5 6	(1) 2 3 4 5 6	(1) 2 3 4 5 6
3/20	N	(1) 2 3 4 5 6	(1) 2 3 4 5 6	(1) 2 3 4 5 6	(1) 2 3 4 5 6
3/21	N	(1) 2 3 4 5 6	(1) 2 3 4 5 6	(1) 2 3 4 5 6	(1) 2 3 4 5 6
3/22	N	(1) 2 3 4 5 6	(1) 2 3 4 5 6	(1) 2 3 4 5 6	(1) 2 3 4 5 6
3/23	N	(1) 2 3 4 5 6	(1) 2 3 4 5 6	(1) 2 3 4 5 6	(1) 2 3 4 5 6
3/24	N	(1) 2 3 4 5 6	(1) 2 3 4 5 6	(1) 2 3 4 5 6	(1) 2 3 4 5 6
3/25	N	1 (2) 3 4 5 6	1 (2) 3 4 5 6	(1) 2 3 4 5 6	(1) 2 3 4 5 6
3/26	N	(1) 2 3 4 5 6	1 (2) 3 4 5 6	1 (2) 3 4 5 6	1 (2) 3 4 5 6
3/27	N	(1) 2 3 4 5 6	(1) 2 3 4 5 6	(1) 2 3 4 5 6	(1) 2 3 4 5 6
3/28	N	1 2 3 (4) 5 6	1 2 3 4 (5) 6	1 2 3 4 (5) 6	1 2 3 (4) 5 6
3/29	N	(1) 2 3 4 5 6	1 2 3 4 (5) 6	1 2 3 4 5 (6)	1 2 3 4 5 (6)
3/30	N	1 2 3 (4) 5 6	1 2 3 4 (5) 6	1 2 3 4 5 (6)	1 2 3 4 5 (6)
3/31	N	1 2 3 (4) 5 6	1 2 3 4 (5) 6	1 2 3 4 5 (6)	1 2 3 4 5 (6)
4/01	N	1 2 3 (4) 5 6	1 2 3 4 (5) 6	1 2 3 4 5 (6)	1 2 3 4 5 (6)
4/02	N	1 2 (3) 4 5 6	1 2 3 4 (5) 6	1 2 3 4 5 (6)	1 2 3 4 5 (6)
4/03	N	1 2 (3) 4 5 6	1 2 3 4 (5) 6	1 2 3 (4) 5 6	1 2 3 (4) 5 6

Figure 15-10 Premenstrual syndrome daily charting: premenstrual pattern. (From Gise, L. H. [1991]. Premenstrual syndrome: Which treatments help? *Medical Aspects of Human Sexuality, 66.*)

Acute Pelvic Pain

Acute pelvic pain demands immediate response, predominately affects women of reproductive years, and is associated with sexual activity or ovarian ovulatory function. The differential diagnosis is outlined in Box 15-11.

After taking a thorough history, the physical examination starts with observation of the patient's posture and mobility and a set of vital signs. In assessing the abdomen, the health care provider first has the patient point to the area of pain, observes for any distention or guarding, assesses bowel tones, and palpates for rigidity, rebound, and masses. In assessing the pelvis, the speculum examination allows for visual and culture evaluation of vaginal and cervical surfaces. The bimanual examination facilitates the location of masses or the site of pain: cervical or uterine motion tenderness. A rectovaginal examination is performed to evaluate the posterior pelvis. In the age group

---

Box 15-11 DIFFERENTIAL DIAGNOSIS OF ACUTE PELVIC PAIN IN ADOLESCENT FEMALES

Gynecological Causes
Adnexal torsion
Endometriosis
Infection
   Pelvic inflammatory disease
   Tuboovarian abscess
Ovarian
   Corpus luteum cyst
   Endometrioma
   Mittelschmerz
   Neoplasm
   Ruptured cyst
Uterine
   Fibroids
   Dysmenorrhea

Pregnancy-Related Causes
Abortion: septic or spontaneous
Ectopic pregnancy

Gastrointestinal Causes
Appendicitis
Constipation
Diverticulitis
Gastroenteritis
Inflammatory bowel disease

Urological Causes
Acute cystitis
Renal calculi

From Klotz, M. M. (1995). Dysmennorrhea, endometriosis, and pelvic pain. In D. P. Lemcke, J. Pattison, L. A. Marshall, & D. S. Cowley (Eds.), *Primary care of women* (pp. 420–432). Norwalk, CT: Appleton & Lange.

15 to 19 years, pelvic inflammatory disease is the most frequently identified gynecological cause of acute pelvic pain.

Pelvic inflammatory disease. Pelvic inflammatory disease (PID) is an infection affecting the upper reproductive tract of women and especially young women under the age of 25 (Ivey, 1997). PID usually is localized in the fallopian tubes, in which case the name is *salpingitis.* PID is caused by a combination of mixed aerobic and anaerobic organisms, of which *N. gonorrhoeae* and *C. trachomatis* are the most prevalent (Soper, 1995).

Risk factors for PID include having multiple sexual partners, intercourse without the use of a barrier method of contraception, intercourse with a male partner with untreated urethritis, a history of PID or sexually transmitted disease, nulliparity, and recent insertion of an IUD. Among adolescents are three additional risk factors: an immature immune system, a larger zone of cervical ectopy, and thinner cervical mucus, all allowing for easier transmission of the infecting organism from lower reproductive tract to upper reproductive tract.

More than 1 million new episodes of PID occur annually in the United States (Ivey, 1997; Laufer & Goldstein, 1995). Although the overall incidence of PID has declined in the past decade, the incidence in adolescents has increased. Adolescents are particularly susceptible to asymptomatic forms of PID and thus long-term sequelae are more devastating.

The classic symptoms are lower abdominal pain, vaginal discharge, and fever and chills. These symptoms begin or worsen with the onset of the menstrual period. Diagnosis is made when the woman is febrile (temperature greater than 38°C [100.4°F]); pelvic findings are purulent cervical discharge, uterine tenderness, adnexal fullness, and cervical motion tenderness; and abdominal findings are distention, rebound tenderness, guarding, or hypoactive bowels. Clinical laboratory findings show an elevated white blood cell count, an elevated estimated sedimentation rate, and positive cervical cultures for *C. trachomatis* or *N. gonorrhoeae.*

Treatment for PID can be offered in outpatient facilities, but recurrent or severe first cases usually require hospitalization. Outpatient antibiotic therapy is (1) a 14-day treatment of 400 mg ofloxacin twice daily with 500 mg metronidazole twice daily or 450 mg clindamycin 4 times a day or (2) ceftriaxone (250 mg intramuscularly) and 100 mg doxycycline orally twice daily for 14 days. A more recent and costly approach is azithromycin given in a single dose at the time of diagnosis.

Once outpatient treatment is initiated, close supervision is essential for complete recovery. A revisit within 48 to 72 hours offers the opportunity to check for improvement of symptoms. When no improvement occurs or the condition worsens, an early revisit assists in the evaluation and change in treatment plan, which is crucial for adolescents, because their future fertility is compromised more easily with incomplete or conservative treatment plans.

Mittelschmerz. Mittelschmerz is the midcycle, unilateral pain associated with follicular rupture during ovulation. The pain is intermittent, and vaginal spotting may occur. Treatment options include reassurance and information about the normal menstrual cycle or a form of ovulation suppression.

Ovarian cysts. Ovarian growths are benign 90% of the time. The most common is the ovarian cyst, which most frequently is functional (follicular or corpus luteum cysts). Diagnosis is enhanced by pelvic ultrasound and aids in treatment decisions. A cyst measuring less than 8 cm is followed for two to three cycles and is expected to resolve. Approximately 25% to 35% of the functional cysts persist. These functional cysts and cysts measuring greater than 8 cm usually do not resolve spontaneously and are more apt to rupture, infarct, or torse. Surgery is necessary when the cyst is multilocular or septate or is an endometrioma. When an adolescent has had a functional cyst resolve or rupture, oral contraceptive pills are an appropriate treatment for suppression of the ovary and follicular development.

Ectopic pregnancy. Although not a common occurrence in adolescents, ectopic pregnancy is part of the differential diagnosis, especially if the teen admits to being sexually active and has a history of PID or using an IUD. Ectopic pregnancy is the second leading cause of pregnancy-related mortality. Symptoms vary significantly and may present as mild, unilateral, pelvic discomfort to severe, diffuse pain in a hemodynamically unstable patient. Examination may yield a normal-sized uterus or an appropriately enlarged uterus with or without cervical motion tenderness. The adnexa may be tender, but often a mass is not palpated.

Because the diagnosis is not evident initially but the consequences of missing the diagnosis can be fatal, evaluating for pregnancy is important. Albeit taking a thorough menstrual and pregnancy history is essential, a beta-human chorionic gonadotropin level that can be quantified if necessary is the minimal standard of care for any woman of reproductive age. Vaginal probe ultrasound can differentiate an ectopic from an intrauterine pregnancy with an adnexal mass, an abscess or PID after a spontaneous or therapeutic abortion, or causes unrelated to pregnancy such as appendicitis.

Acute cystitis. The most common urinary tract infection in women of reproductive age is acute, uncomplicated cystitis. Factors affecting the risk of infection include poor hygiene, sexual intercourse, intravaginal contraceptives, stress, and poor hydration. Women complain of dysuria, urgency, frequency, and low suprapubic pain. Urine characteristics consist of bacteriuria with or without hematuria, pyuria, and often a concentrated odor. Wet preparations or leukocyte esterase dipsticks confirm the diagnosis. Urinary cultures are appropriate for pregnant women and recurrent cases or treatment failures. Treatment antibiotics are given in a 3-day regimen, which has been shown clinically to have comparable outcomes to the 7-day regimen, at lower cost and decreased drug side effects. The initial drug of choice is trimethoprim-sulfamethoxazole 160/800 mg twice daily. Emphasis on improved hygiene and hydration assist the positive outcome of treatment.

Constipation. Although constipation is generally not a life-threatening health risk, the condition is common among teens and a real source of discomfort. Constipation is characterized by dense, hard stool, with or without flatulence, and straining with defecation. The usual pattern of bowel movements is interrupted and often is accompanied by edema, bloating, headache, tender abdomen, and back pain. Chronic constipation increases the risk of irritable bowel syndrome. Treatment usually consists of increasing the fluids and fiber in the diet and developing a regular exercise regimen. Reviewing with the adolescent what good bowel habits are also is effective. In acute cases an enema or stool softener is appropriate.

Appendicitis. Although usually affecting women ages 20 to 40 years, appendicitis affects enough teens to be a worthy differential diagnosis in acute pelvic pain. Pain is typically moderate to severe and constant and increases with movement. Pain that may present as diffuse eventually localizes to the right lower quadrant. Loss of appetite and vomiting accompany the pain. Voluntary guarding, rebound tenderness, and an elevated white blood cell count are also highly suspicious for appendicitis. Treatment is surgical by laparotomy or laparoscopy with appendectomy. The prognosis is excellent if surgery is uncomplicated and occurs before the appendix ruptures.

Chronic Pelvic Pain

Chronic pelvic pain has no specific definition but can be considered as 3 or more months of constant or intermittent, cyclical or acyclical pain that has not been given a definitive diagnosis after several visits to the practitioner. Chronic pelvic pain frequently is a source of frustration, anger, and disillusionment to the adolescent, parents, and practitioner. Patience and perseverance are qualities that the practitioner needs during the typically long process of determining the appropriate diagnosis and treatment.

The differential diagnosis includes many organ systems that can be the source of the symptoms or an aspect of referred pain. The cause can be functional or psychogenic. Box 15-12 lists the differential diagnosis of chronic pelvic pain.

The diagnostic approach to the patient with chronic pelvic pain includes a thorough history and chart review, specifically noting the description, location, and radiation of the pain, exacerbating events, relieving factors, and associating factors with urinary, gastrointestinal, musculoskeletal symptoms, or with the menstrual cycle. Evaluation of stress and the adolescent's responses to stressful events aids in identifying social and familial effects on the problem. A complete physical examination including a pelvic examination is necessary. In the abdominal examination the health care provider should identify carefully areas of tenderness (deep from abdominal wall tenderness), organomegaly, and masses. The pelvic examination aids in evaluating vaginal and cervical anomalies and the collection of cultures and cytological specimens. The bimanual and rectal examinations (including the evaluation of the cul-de-sac) allow palpation of structures for any abnormalities and areas of tenderness.

The initial laboratory workup includes a complete blood count with differential and erythrocyte sedimentation rate, urinalysis and culture, cervical cultures for *N. gonorrhoeae* and *C. trachomatis*, and beta-human chorionic gonadotropin. Other studies include pelvic ultrasonography (to assess genital tract anomalies or masses or for when an adequate pelvic examination cannot be performed), radiological examination (not recommended in adolescents), and laparoscopy. Recommendations for laparoscopy in adolescents include (1) dysmenorrhea unresponsive to the usual therapy with prostaglandin inhibitors and ovulation suppression and (2) confirmation or exclusion of clinically suspected endometriosis, chronic pelvic inflammatory disease, pelvic adhesions, appendiceal fecalith, ovarian cysts, and pelvic serositis.

Box 15-12 DIFFERENTIAL DIAGNOSIS OF CHRONIC PELVIC PAIN IN ADOLESCENT FEMALES

Gynecological Causes
Chronic pelvic inflammatory disease
Dysmenorrhea
Endometriosis
Mittelschmerz
Ovarian cyst
Genital tract malformation
Pelvic congestion
Pelvic stenosis

Gastrointestinal Causes
Appendiceal fecalith
Constipation or bowel spasms
Dietary intolerance (lactose)
Inflammatory bowel disease

Urinary Causes
Hydronephrosis
Urethral stricture
Urethral caruncle
Urinary retention
Urinary tract infection

Orthopedic Causes
Herniation of intervertebral disk
Lordosis, kyphosis, or scoliosis

Adhesions
Postoperative
Pelvic infection

Psychogenic Causes

From Laufer M. R., & Goldstein, D. P. (1995). Pediatric and adolescent gynecology. In K. J. Ryan, R. S. Berkowitz, & R. L. Barbieri (Eds.), *Kistner's gynecology: Principles and practice* (6th ed., pp. 571–632). St. Louis: Mosby.

Research (Emans & Goldstein, 1989; Goldstein, DeCholnocky, & Emans, 1980; Laufer, 1992) has shown that endometriosis is the most frequent finding, almost 50% of the cases, followed by postoperative adhesions secondary to appendectomy or ovarian cystectomy.

Treatment of chronic pelvic pain is based on the diagnosis. When the diagnosis is endometriosis, all medical and surgical options should be reviewed despite the fact that endometriosis can reoccur. Early treatment aids not only in the comfort of the patient but also in the preservation of her reproductive potential. Hormone therapy creates a low-estrogen environment, minimizing the bleeding of the endometrial implants and preventing further spread of the tissue in the pelvis or abdomen during retrograde menstruation. Gonadotropin-releasing hormone agonists are an option, but the side effect of decreased bone density is a major problem. Another approach is using synthetic progestin or androgens to create a high-androgen environment that causes the endometriotic implants to atrophy. Danazol currently is the drug of choice and is given for 6 months. The side effects from an androgenic drug include lowering of the high-density lipoproteins, irregular menses, weight gain, edema, acne, oily skin, voice changes, and hirsutism. Another option is the use of noncyclic oral contraceptive pills, which have moderate benefits and side effects (nausea and break-through bleeding).

INFECTIONS

The changing climate of adolescent sexuality has increased the incidence of STDs, vaginal infections, and toxic shock syndrome in younger women. Early adolescents (10 to 13 years of age) and middle adolescents (14 to 17 years of age) are less likely to initiate a visit to a health care provider for preventive information, condoms, or treatment. Consequently, younger women are being introduced to potentially harmful reproductive infections and receiving delayed treatments out of ignorance or difficulty in obtaining appropriate health care. The education of young women about the choices and consequences of their sexual behaviors is essential to the reproductive health of our society.

Sexually Transmitted Diseases

The term *sexually transmitted diseases* or *sexually transmitted infections* has evolved from its historical reference as venereal disease or morbus venereus. The 20- to 24-year-old age group has the highest actual numbers of STDs. However, when the group numbers are adjusted to include only the sexually active, then adolescents age 12 to 19 years old are at greatest risk for STDs (Neinstein, 1996).

Neisseria gonorrhoeae

A bacterial infection, *N. gonorrhoeae,* was first distinguished from *Treponema pallidum* (syphilis) in 1879 (Kampmeier, 1984). The organism is a gram-negative, spherical or oval cocci seen in pairs and located within polymorphonuclear leukocytes. Several strains of *N. gonorrhoeae* exist, and growth of the bacteria depends on a rich culture media and a carbon dioxide environment such as a candle jar.

Symptoms. Often *N. gonorrhoeae* is asymptomatic in females, or the teen may complain of vaginal discharge, dysuria, or urinary frequency. Asymptomatic urethral and cervical infections may endure if untreated. Clinical manifestations are similar in *N. gonorrhoeae* and *C. trachomatis* (see next section) and in the same person frequently occur together. Mucosal columnar epithelial cells are the most susceptible to infection, and both organisms produce cervicitis and dysuria-pyuria. Other conditions associated with *N. gonorrhoeae* and *C. trachomatis* infections are dyspareunia, labial swelling and tenderness, Bartholin gland infection, endometritis, salpingitis, and perihepatitis. Both organisms can cause systemic arthritis-dermatitis syndrome and conjunctivitis of the newborn. In addition, about 1% of persons with *N. gonorrhoeae* develop disseminated gonorrhea, and women with immune-altering diseases and pregnancy are at greatest risk (Neinstein, 1996).

Diagnosis. For a complete evaluation, cultures must be taken from all three sites of possible infection: the pharynx, endocervix, and rectum. The cultures are inoculated on individual modified Thayer-Martin medium culture plates. When collecting a culture, the health care provider should be sure not to use a lubricant in the genital area, for lubricants are often toxic to organisms and interfere with culture growth. To obtain an appropriate culture, the swab needs to be in contact with the orifice for 20 to 30 seconds and rotated. Cultures take 24 to 48 hours to grow and because of this, most practitioners treat presumptively. Two alternative and new diagnostic methods are becoming more available: detection of gonococcal enzymes and DNA probe assays.

Treatment. Over time strains of gonococci have become penicillin resistant, creating a universal problem and leading to the development of new antibiotics to treat *N. gonorrhoeae* in general. The treatment regimen of choice is one of the following antibiotic drug therapies:

- *Ceftriaxone:* 125 mg intramuscularly
- *Ciprofloxacin:* 500 mg orally in a single dose
- *Cefixime:* 400 mg orally in a single dose
- *Ofloxacin:* 400 mg orally in a single dose in combination with one of the following:
- *Doxycycline:* 100 mg twice a day for 7 days
- *Azithromycin:* 1 g in a single dose

The combination treatment is effective against *N. gonorrhoeae* and *C. trachomatis*, which has been identified as a coinfection in a majority of cases. The cure rate is greater than 95% for anal and genital infections and 90% for pharyngeal infections (U.S. Preventive Services Task Force, 1996). Quinolones (e.g., ciprofloxacin and ofloxacin) are contraindicated for pregnant women, nursing mothers, and patients under 18 years of age.

Sexual activity is to be discontinued until the course of treatment is finished and all sexual partners also have received treatment. Adolescents with a documented STD and no history of sexual activity should be evaluated for sexual abuse. The follow-up culture is a good time to discuss safer sex again. Patients with one STD should be tested for others.

Chlamydia trachomatis

C. trachomatis genital infection is the most commonly reported infectious disease in the United States (CDC, 1997c). The prevalence of *C. trachomatis* in sexually active adolescents is 5% to 15%, regardless of socioeconomic status (Mosure et al., 1997). Because of the asymptomatic nature of *C. trachomatis* infections, prolonged exposure to untreated infections can cause inflammation and scarring to a woman's reproductive tract. Furthermore, *C. trachomatis* infections have been found to facilitate HIV transmission (Wasserheit, 1992). Based on the risks and complications of *C. trachomatis*, the recommendation is that all sexually active adolescent women having a pelvic examination should receive routine screening for this infection (CDC, 1993a; U.S. Preventive Services Task Force, 1996).

Symptoms. *Chlamydia* manifests similar to *N. gonorrhoeae*, infecting columnar epithelium to cause a mucosal infection. The most likely location for a *C. trachomatis* infection is on the cervix but also may be found in the urethra and rectum. *C. trachomatis* may reside in the cervix for greater than a year and be asymptomatic (Cates, 1990). To emphasize the asymptomatic nature of this organism, 70% of adolescent females reported as having *C. trachomatis* infections are asymptomatic. All sexually abused adolescents should be screened for *C. trachomatis*.

Other infections associated *C. trachomatis* include urethritis, PID, bartholinitis, Fitz-Hugh-Curtis syndrome (perihepatitis), and infections of the neonate.

Diagnosis. *Chlamydia* is an obligate intracellular organism, with viruslike characteristics, infecting columnar epithelium. *Chlamydia* is isolated in the laboratory only by cell culture from urethral or endocervical columnar cell specimens. The endocervical culture has been the gold standard for identifying *Chlamydia*. Cultures for this organism have shown high sensitivity and specificity, which is ideal for diagnosis. However, *Chlamydia* cultures are costly and have a 48-hour incubation period. Other nonculture tests that distinguish *Chlamydia* are these (Biro, Reising, Doughman, Kollar, & Rosenthal, 1994; Loeffelholz, Lewinski, & Silver, 1992; Schubiner, Lebar, & Jemal, 1990):

- Direct immunofluorescence assay tests detect the presence of major outer membrane protein or lipopolysaccharide by rolling a swab on a slide, dry fixing it, staining the slide, and examining the slide with fluorescent microscopy (time: less than 1 hour).
- Enzyme immunoassay tests detect chlamydial lipopolysaccharide and quantitate the presence of an enzyme reaction with a spectrophotometer. The specimen is collected on a swab and placed in a tube for transport (time: 3-4 hours).
- Nucleic acid hybridization tests (DNA probe) use a chemiluminescent DNA probe to detect the presence of *C. trachomatis* ribosomal RNA from an endocervical swab specimen (time: 2-3 hours).
- Leukocyte esterase test is a urine dipstick test used for screening for urinary tract infections or urethritis. The accuracy of these tests has shown high specificity (97% to 100%) and more variability in sensitivity (58% to 88%).

Treatment. Because testing is not available at all clinical settings, treatment is advised for all persons with the following characteristics:

- A positive result from a *Chlamydia* culture or test
- The presence of mucopurulent cervicitis, PID, gonorrhea, or nongonococcal urethritis
- Exposure to a sexual partner with *Chlamydia* symptoms or a positive culture

The recommended course of treatment is 100 mg doxycycline orally twice daily for 7 days, or 1 g azithromycin orally in a single dose. Alternative treatments include 500 mg erythromycin base orally 4 times a day for 7 days, 300 mg oflaxacin orally twice daily for 7 days, or 500 mg sulfisoxazole orally 4 times a day for 10 days (least effective). Azithromycin and oflaxacin are not approved for use during pregnancy and have adolescent age restrictions.

Mucopurulent Endocervicitis

Mucopurulent endocervicitis is not a diagnosis based on a single organism. The condition can be caused by *C. trachomatis, N. gonorrhoeae,* mycoplasmata, or even possibly herpes simplex virus.

Symptoms. Often women report mucopurulent endocervicitis as asymptomatic discharge. The mucopurulent discharge is perceived as a normal vaginal discharge.

Diagnosis. A presumptive diagnosis is made when one of the following criteria is found:

- Mucopurulent or yellow-green secretions from the endocervix. The secretions appear yellow or green on a white cotton swab (positive swab test)
- Cervical friability
- Edema or erythema in the zone of cervical ectopy
- Microscopic evaluation identifying 30 or more polymorphonuclear leukocytes per high-power field magnification or greater than 10 polymorphonuclear leukocytes per oil immersion field of a Gram-stained smear.

Treatment. When *N. gonorrhoeae* is identified on Gram stain, then the treatment regimen effective for gonococcal and chlamydial infections is advised. When only chlamydial infection is identified or suspected, then a chlamydial treatment regimen should be used. These treatments must take into account the local prevalence rates for *N. gonorrhoeae* and *C. trachomatis* and be adjusted as indicated.

Pelvic Inflammatory Disease

The section on chronic pelvic pain includes a discussion of PID.

Syphilis

The organism responsible for syphilis is *Treponema pallidum,* a slender spirochete with regular spirals and a length of 6 to 20 µm. Transmission is through sexual contact, including sexual intercourse and kissing. Although rare, transmission from infectious cutaneous or mucous membrane lesions has occurred. Although the incidence of syphilis in the United States peaked in 1948 at 70,000 reported cases, rates again began to rise in the 1970s and 1980s, peaking again in 1990 at 50,000 reported cases (CDC, 1987; CDC, 1993b). In 1995 the incidence of primary and secondary syphilis had fallen to 15,027 (CDC, 1997c). The microorganism *T. pallidum* enters the body through abrasions in mucous membranes and spreads by the lymphatic system and blood vessels. The spirochetes cause cellular infiltrates that necrose and form ulcers. By the time of tertiary syphilis the scarring is widespread. Reinfections of syphilis are possible.

Symptoms. Chancre characterizes the **primary** phase of syphilis and is found at the site of inoculation approximately 10 to 90 days after exposure. The most common location of the chancre is on the external genitalia and measures from several millimeters to 1 cm. The chancre appears as a papule that erodes to an indurated, painless ulcer with slightly elevated edges, and has a thin, yellow serous discharge. Painless regional lymphadenopathy is usually present. The chancre generally heals in 4 to 6 weeks (Neinstein, 1996).

Symptoms of **secondary** syphilis vary and usually appear 6 weeks to 6 months after initial exposure, with an average of 3 weeks after the chancre appears. During this phase, infectious lesions appear on the skin, and *T. pallidum* can be isolated from them and in body fluids. The most common skin eruption is a papulosquamous rash on the palms of the hands and soles of the feet. Mucous membrane lesions are also common, appearing as shiny, round, flat, grey to pinkish-white patches with a red outer edges. Condylomata lata are found on the vulva and perineum, look like a moist wart, and are highly contagious. Lymphadenopathy may be general or regional and is characterized by discrete, firm, nonpainful nodes. Often secondary syphilis is accompanied by systemic flulike symptoms including low-grade fever, headache, sore throat, hoarseness, weight loss, myalgia, and arthralgia. Even when untreated, the manifestations of secondary syphilis improve within 2 to 10 weeks. Relapse of secondary syphilis symptoms may occur up to 2 years later (CDC, 1987).

Latent syphilis has two phases. The first phase, or early latent syphilis, is the first year of infection and includes primary and secondary syphilis. The second phase, or late latent syphilis, refers to time after the first year and before the onset of late syphilis. The manifestations of latent syphilis are a lack of clinical symptoms, continued positive serological tests (Venereal Diseases Research Laboratory [VDRL] and fluorescent treponemal antibody absoprtion [FTA-ABS]), and a negative spinal fluid serum test.

The symptoms of **tertiary (late)** syphilis may occur as early as 1 year after initial exposure or as late as 30 years in the untreated or inadequately treated individual. Late syphilis in the adolescent population has not been reported (Neinstein, 1996). The common characteristics of late syphilis are gummata and cardiovascular effects. Gummata are cutaneous lesions affecting the bone, soft tissue, skin, or viscera. Although not contagious, gummata are indolent, asymmetric, few in number, and amenable to treatment. Cardiovascular syphilis generally occurs after 10 years and is characterized by aortitis.

The onset of **neurosyphilis** may occur at any time during the progress of syphilis and affects 10% to 20% of individuals with untreated syphilis after a year (Neinstein, 1996). Adolescents rarely have neurological involvement. Three types of neurosyphilis have been identified: asymptomatic neurosyphilis (identified by an abnormal cerebrospinal fluid), acute syphilis meningitis, and meningovascular syphilis.

Although the description of **congenital syphilis** is beyond the scope of this chapter, mentioning the condition is relevant because a pregnant teenager possibly can transmit the disease to her fetus. Understanding that the fetus becomes susceptible to the illness after the fourth month of gestation underscores the importance of providing adequate detection and treatment for the mother before the sixteenth week of gestation. The rate of congenital syphilis is nearly 90% for untreated maternal cases (CDC, 1993b).

Diagnosis. The diagnosis of primary syphilis includes differentiation from herpes simplex virus (HSV), chancroid, lymphogranuloma venereum, granuloma inguinale, and trauma. The differential diagnosis in secondary syphilis focuses on dermatological changes.

A sexual history revealing the number of partners and sexual contacts of each partner is important data to obtain when identifying any STD in a woman. Also, any painless lesion on the genitalia, undiagnosed rash, or patchy hair loss should prompt suspicion of syphilis. The physical examination verifies the presence of symptoms and further differentiates an STD. Adolescents often present without symptoms, so laboratory evaluation is essential and the adjunct to diagnosis for adults as well.

Laboratory evaluation includes darkfield examination, direct fluorescent antibody, and serological tests. The darkfield examination is the definitive diagnosis for primary syphilis, and the specimen is acquired by the following technique (Neinstein, 1996, p. 930).

1. Clean the lesion with saline and gauze.
2. Abrade the lesion with dry gauze.
3. Squeeze the lesion (with gloved fingers) to express serous transudate. The practitioner should avoid causing bleeding because blood makes darkfield examination more difficult.
4. Place a drop of transudate on a slide.
5. Place a drop of saline on transudate and cover with a cover slip.
6. Examine the specimen under a darkfield microscopy.
7. The procedure must be repeated on 3 successive days before the test is considered negative.
8. For internal lesions a bacteriological loop can be used to transfer the fluid to a slide.
9. For lymph node aspiration: Clean skin, inject 0.2 mL or less of sterile saline, and aspirate the node. Place fluid on the slide.

This technique also may be used for specimen collection for direct fluorescent antibody staining. The specimen is obtained from a primary lesion in the same manner as for a darkfield slide only without the use of saline, and the slide is air dried. The slide then is transported to a laboratory or state health department that performs direct fluorescent antibody staining.

The third means for testing is serological examination. Such tests are only presumptive in primary syphilis but definitely diagnostic in secondary syphilis. The two most common and least expensive tests are nontreponemal antibody tests: the rapid plasma reagin (a qualitative test) and the VDRL (a quantitative test). Once a rapid plasma reagin is positive, a VDRL is obtained to correlate with the amount of disease activity. VDRL titers are followed over time to identify a response to treatment.

Other serological tests specific for treponemal antibodies include FTA-ABS, used to confirm a positive result from a VDRL or rapid plasma reagin test; micro-hemagglutination *T. pallidum* test, also a test to confirm a positive result from a VDRL; and *T. pallidum* immobilization, used to prove a past or present infection but because of its cost is controlled for research and difficult cases. Testing for neurosyphilis requires cerebrospinal fluid (CSF) and interpretation of the results is more cumbersome. Although the standard CSF test is the VDRL, this test is not sensitive for active disease. The FTA-ABS test is sensitive but not specific for neurosyphilis. However, if the FTA-ABS test is negative, the probability of neurosyphilis is small.

For latent and late syphilis the testing depends on the VDRL and the FTA-ABS. Because the VDRL is only 70% sensitive in latent and late syphilis, obtaining an FTA-ABS is imperative (Neinstein, 1996).

Treatment. Although the specific treatment regimen for syphilis depends on the phase of the disease, penicillin is the drug of choice and the only proven therapy for neurosyphilis, congenital syphilis, and syphilis during pregnancy (CDC, 1998).

The treatment regimen for *primary* and *secondary syphilis* is as follows:

■ *For nonallergic patients:* Penicillin G benzathine, 2.4 million units in a single dose

■ *For penicillin-allergic nonpregnant patients:* Doxycycline 100 mg orally twice a day for 2 weeks or 500 mg tetracycline orally 4 times a day for 2 weeks. When compliance with therapy and follow-up can be ensured, treatment of 500 mg erythromycin orally 4 times a day for 2 weeks may be considered.

■ *For penicillin-allergic pregnant patients:* Patients should be desensitized and then treated with penicillin.

Follow-up includes clinical and serological examination at 6 months and 12 months. If titers fail to decline fourfold within 6 months, the person is at risk for treatment failure. Evaluation of HIV status and CSF to identify neurosyphilis, as well as appropriate retreatment (the late syphilis regimen in the absence of neurosyphilis), is recommended (CDC, 1998).

The treatment regimen for *latent syphilis* is as follows:

■ *Early latent syphilis:* Penicillin G benzathine, 2.4 million units administered intramuscularly in a single dose

■ *Late latent syphilis:* Penicillin G benzathine, 7.2 million units total administered in three doses of 2.4 million units intramuscularly at 1-week intervals

The CDC (1998) recommends repeating nontreponemal serological testing at 6, 12, and 24 months. The health care provider should evaluate for neurosyphilis and appropriately retreat when titers increase fourfold, an initially high titer (greater than 1:32) fails to decline fourfold within 12 to 24 months, or clinical symptoms develop.

The treatment regimen for *tertiary syphilis* is as follows:

■ CDC-recommended treatment: Penicillin G benzathine, 7.2 million units total administered in three doses of 2.4 million units intramuscularly at 1-week intervals (CDC, 1998). Follow-up depends partially on the clinical response of the lesions. Treatment should be referred to and managed by an expert.

The treatment regimen for *neurosyphilis* is as follows:

■ *CDC-recommended treatment:* Aqueous crystalline penicillin G, 18 million to 24 million units a day, administered as 3 million to 4 million units intravenously every 4 hours for 10 to 14 days

■ *Alternative treatment* (when compliance can be ensured): Penicillin G procaine, 2.4 million units intramuscularly each day and 500 mg probenecid orally 4 times a day for 10 to 14 days

Follow-up evaluation of CSF pleocytosis is recommended every 6 months until normal, along with CSF-VDRL and CSF protein after treatment. When the cell count has not returned to normal after 6 months or the CSF is not completely normal by 2 years, retreatment is necessary.

Syphilis in HIV-infected persons follows the same diagnostic and treatment guidelines for patients without HIV infections. Neurosyphilis needs to be considered in the differential diagnosis of neurological disease in HIV-infected persons. Clinical and serological evaluation for treatment failure is advised at 3, 6, 9, 12, and 24 months after therapy. Treatment failures are managed the same way as for non-HIV infected persons.

Chancroid

Commonly called *soft chancre* to differentiate it from hard chancre (syphilis), chancroid once was considered rare in the United States but now has become endemic in certain regions. A cofactor for HIV transmission, chancroid also appears as a coinfection with *T. pallidum* and HSV (CDC, 1998). Diagnosis is suspected when the presence of a genital ulcer and painful inguinal lymphadenopathy are not accompanied by a positive *Gonorrhea* or *Chlamydia* culture or a positive darkfield examination for *T. pallidum*. Definitive diagnosis is made by the detection of *Haemophilus ducreyi* on a special culture media, but this media is not widely available. Polymerase chain reaction testing may soon become available.

The treatment regimens recommended by the CDC (1998, p. 19) include the following:

- *Azythromycin:* 1 g orally in a single dose
- *Ceftriaxone:* 250 mg intramuscularly in a single dose
- *Ciprofloxacin:* 500 mg orally twice daily for 3 days
- *Erythromycin base:* 500 mg orally 4 times a day for 7 days

Follow-up examination in 3 to 7 days after the onset of therapy is recommended to evaluate the progress of the ulcer and the need for needle aspiration of any buboes. Patients with chancroid also should be retested 3 months after diagnosis for HIV and syphilis if the initial tests were negative.

Herpes Simplex Virus

Genital herpes is caused by a large DNA virus and is recurrent and incurable. Two types of virus have been identified, HSV-1 and HSV-2, the latter being responsible for approximately 90% of the genital infections (Schack & Neinstein, 1996). The virus enters the body through mucosal contact or small abrasions in the skin and makes its way to the nervous system where it lies latent. Transmission occurs only in humans and mostly through sexual contact: genital to genital or oral to genital. Not all persons affected are aware they carry the virus because symptoms are mild or unrecognizable. In contrast, most primary infections are severe enough that a clinic visit or even hospitalization is necessary.

Symptoms. Primary or first clinical episodes of genital herpes have an incubation period of 1 to 40 days, and symptoms may last up to 3 weeks, with viral shedding occurring most of that time. Prodromal symptoms of burning, aching, heat, or itching precede the small vesicles (1 to 2 mm) that erupt on the genitalia. The lesions are painful in nearly 100% of the cases in women and may be extensive, including the perineum, vagina, and cervix. The vesicles break down into pustules that ulcerate, crust, and eventually heal. Labial edema, dysuria, and inguinal lymphadenopathy are common and often interfere with the ability to sit comfortably.

HSV lies dormant in the sensory neurons and may never be reactivated or may become expressed frequently or irregularly. Stressors that are thought to play a role in the activation of HSV are ultraviolet light exposure, times of extreme emotional stress, fever, heat, moisture, oral contraceptives, pregnancy, and trauma (Corey, 1990).

Recurrent episodes last from 7 to 12 days, with viral shedding averaging 4 days (Lichtman & Papera, 1990). Prodromal symptoms occur in about 50% of infected persons, and, as in primary episodes, symptoms are worse for women (Schack & Neinstein, 1996). The vesicles are similar to those that appear in primary episodes although smaller and affecting less tissue.

Diagnosis. Diagnosis is determined in part by history of contact with a sexual partner with known infection, recurrence of infection, or culture. During the ulcerative stage, diagnosis includes a syphilis serological test and darkfield examination. In general, laboratory testing can include the following:

- Pap smear (inexpensive but not sensitive)
- Tzanck smear (also inexpensive, but sensitivity depends on progression of the lesion)
- Viral culture (the expected means for diagnosis with the ability to differentiate HSV1 from HSV2)
- Serological titers (used for research purposes)
- Immunofluorescence techniques (differentiate between the HSV types and have a high sensitivity level)
- Enzyme-linked immunosorbent assay (sensitive but not able to differentiate HSV types).

The collection procedure for smears and cultures necessitates intense swabbing of the lesion using a cotton or Dacron swab. The best source for obtaining a viral culture is from the base of the lesion in the pustule and ruptured vesicle or ulcer phase. Specimens obtained during the pustular phase are the most sensitive and reliable.

Treatment. To be effective, treatment must be started quickly. The earlier a primary clinical episode is diagnosed, the earlier the treatment can begin and help minimize the severity and duration of the episode. When a woman has six or more recurrent episodes, she will need a prescription with a refill so that self-initiation of treatment is possible during the prodrome or presence of the first lesion. When recurrences are frequent and are not affected by early initiation of treatment, then suppressive treatment is recommended. The choice of treatment is determined by the kind of clinical episode. The CDC (1998) recommends the following treatments according to the clinical episode.

A. Primary first clinical episode (one of the following):
  1. *Acyclovir:* 400 mg orally 3 times a day for 7 to 10 days
  2. *Acyclovir:* 200 mg orally 5 times a day for 7 to 10 days
  3. *Famciclovir:* 250 mg orally 3 times a day for 7 to 10 days
  4. *Valacycolvir:* 1 g orally twice daily for 7 to 10 days
B. Episodic recurrent infections (one of the following):
  1. *Acyclovir:* 400 mg orally 3 times a day for 5 days
  2. *Acyclovir:* 200 mg orally 5 times a day for 5 days

    3. *Acyclovir:* 800 mg twice daily for 5 days
    4. *Famciclovir:* 125 mg orally twice daily for 5 days
    5. *Valacyclovir:* 500 mg orally twice daily for 5 days
C. Daily supressive therapy:
    1. *Acyclovir:* 400 mg orally twice daily
    2. *Famciclovir:* 250 mg orally twice daily
    3. *Valacyclovir:* 250 mg orally twice daily
    4. *Valacyclovir:* 500 mg orally once a day
    5. *Valacyclovir:* 1 g orally once a day
D. Severe disease necessitating hospitalization:
    1. *Acyclovir:* 5 to 10 mg/kg body mass intravenously every 8 hours for 5 to 7 days or until clinical resolution

Management of the primary clinical episode includes acquiring a culture or smear; screening for other STDs; suggested pain relief options (tap water sitz bath, oatmeal bath, analgesics, topical protection for deep fissures such as petrolatum, rest, and avoidance of ultraviolet light and heat); a prescription for acyclovir or valacyclovir if seen within the first week of symptoms; oral and written information about the virus, how it is transmitted, abstinence from sex during the presence of lesions, and other sources of information (e.g., National Herpes Hotline at 919-361-8488); good hygiene practices pertaining to lesion care and hand washing techniques; and a follow-up visit.

The follow-up visit allows the practitioner to confirm the diagnosis, assess the status of the infection, and determine the need for further treatment and also provides an opportunity for the partner to attend with the woman and address the specific concerns of the couple. The health care provider and patient also should review the process of transmission, the possibility for recurrence, and the need to use safe sex practices for preventing the spread of herpes and the acquisition of other STDs.

Special considerations. When pregnant women have a known history of HSV, cultures should be acquired during the first prenatal visit and again near term. Treatment with acyclovir has not shown to increase risk for major birth defects (CDC, 1998). The greatest concern is transmission of HSV to the newborn during labor. The CDC (1998) recommends that "all women should be examined and carefully questioned regarding whether they have symptoms of genital herpes. Infants of women who do not have symptoms or signs of genital herpes infection or its prodrome may be delivered vaginally. Abdominal delivery does not completely eliminate the risk for HSV infection in the neonate." In addition, suppressive therapy is not recommended to be given routinely in the last month of pregnancy.

Human Papillomavirus (HPV)

HPV, otherwise known as *genital warts*, *condylomata accuminata*, or *venereal warts*, is the most predominant viral STD. HPV is a small, slow-growing DNA virus and is part of the papovavirus family that produces eruptions on the perineum, anus, vulva, vagina, cervix, and larynx. Approximately 70 different genotypes of HPV have been identified, and of these, 22 types affect the genital tract, of which the most common types are numbers 6, 11, 16, 18, 31, 33, and 35 (Nelson & Neinstein, 1996). HPV types 6 and 11 have not been associated with invasive squamous cell carcinoma; however, the other listed types have had associations with dysplasia and squamous cell carcinoma. Multiple HPV types may coexist.

Transmission is usually by sexual contact, but the disease has been known to occur from formites (e.g., underwear, examination gloves, tanning beds, sauna benches, and biopsy forceps) or in nonsexually active individuals. On average, incubation is 3 months, with a range of 3 weeks to 9 months or more.

Symptoms. Genital warts are usually asymptomatic, but sensations of burning, pruritus, and pain have accompanied eruptions. Four different types of genital warts occur (Nelson & Neinstein, 1996, p. 956):

■ *Classic soft sessile or pedunculated growths*: These are usually 2 to 3 mm in diameter and 10 to 15 mm in height, with multiple fingerlike projections, and occur most frequently in moist areas such as the vaginal introitus and vagina.

■ *Small flat-topped warts*: These are usually 1- to 4-mm papules, often located at the transformation zone of the cervix, and may be all but invisible without colposcopy or acetic acid staining, which causes them to have a blanched white appearance.

■ *Squared-off keratotic papules*: These papules are usually 4 to 10 mm in diameter and typically occur in nonmucosal dry skin areas.

■ *Giant condylomata acuminata*: These are larger, rounded, soft papules and nodules with a pebbly, strawberry-like surface

Diagnosis. The differential diagnosis of HPV is made at the exclusion of condylomata lata, molluscum contagiosum, granuloma inguinale, seborrheic keratosis, and invasive or benign neoplasms. Pap smear, colposcopy, and punch biopsy aid in the determination of HPV infection.

Treatment. Treatment regimens for HPV must be tailored to the individual and the experience of the health care provider. No one treatment is better than another unless a treatment has failed. First treatments of external HPV can be accomplished by the individual or practitioner. *Internal* genital warts, vaginal and cervical, require consultation and referral for treatment by an expert.

For **external** genital warts, the CDC (1998) recommends the following treatment:

A. Patient-applied treatment
   1. Podofilox 0.5% solution or gel. Apply with a cotton applicator to visible warts twice a day for 4 days, followed by 4 days of no therapy. This treatment cycle may be repeated 4 times only. The initial application is best applied by the health care provider with instructions as to how to apply the medication and the location of the warts. Safety of this drug during pregnancy has not been established.
   2. Imiquimod 5% cream. Apply with a finger at bedtime for 3 times in 1 week for up to 16 weeks. The treatment site should be washed 6 to 10 hours after application. Safety of this drug during pregnancy has not been established.

B. Provider-administered treatment
   1. Cryotherapy with liquid nitrogen or cryoprobe. Repeat applications every 1 to 2 weeks.
   2. Podophyllum resin, 10% to 25% in a compound tincture of benzoin. A small amount of the drug is applied to each wart, making sure none is dripped on

unaffected skin, and air dried before the woman gets up from the treatment table. To reduce local irritation, the drug is washed off 4 hours after application. Repeat weekly if necessary. Safety of this drug during pregnancy has not been established.

3. Trichloroacetic acid and bichloroacetic acid, 80% to 90%. Apply a small amount to each wart and allow to air dry. Repeat weekly if necessary.

4. Surgical removal by tangential scissor excision, tangential shave excision, curettage, or electrosurgery: LEEP or laser ablation.

C. Alternative treatments

1. Intralesional interferon

2. Laser surgery

For **internal** genital warts, the CDC (1998) recommends the following treatment:

A. Vaginal warts

1. Cryotherapy with liquid nitrogen (application with a cryoprobe is not recommended because of the increased risk of perforation)

2. Trichloroacetic acid and bichloroacetic acid, 80% to 90%

3. Podophyllum, 10% to 25% in compound tincture of benzoin applied to a treated area that must be dry before the speculum is removed

B. Urethral meatus warts

1. Cryotherapy with liquid nitrogen

2. Podophyllum, 10% to 25% in compound tincture of benzoin. The treatment area must be dry before contact with normal mucosa. Applications may be done weekly if necessary.

C. Anal warts

1. Cryotherapy with liquid nitrogen

2. Trichloroacetic acid and bichloroacetic acid, 80% to 90%, applied to warts

3. Surgical removal

D. Oral warts

1. Cryotherapy with liquid nitrogen

2. Surgical removal

E. Cervical warts

1. Consultation with an expert is necessary for women with exophytic cervical warts. High-grade squamous intraepithelial lesions must be excluded before treatment begins. Other treatment regimens have had mixed results. Combined therapies such as liquid nitrogen followed by podophyllum are not found to be more effective but may increase complications.

2. The use of interferons systemically is not effective. Interferon used intralesionally has comparable efficacy and recurrence rates to other therapies. However, the CDC (1998) does not recommend this therapy for routine use because of inconvenient routes of administration, frequent office visits, and association with adverse systemic effects.

Follow-up depends on the type of treatment. An important adjunct to therapy is the education that annual Pap smears are necessary to maintain one's health, that HPV is communicable and so safe sex practices should be used, and that the viral manifestations may recur.

Ectoparasitic Infections

Pediculosis pubis. Pediculosis pubis is a sexually transmitted infection caused by *Phthirus pubis*, a pubic crab louse 1 to 4 mm in length. Initial contact is usually asymptomatic until after a week or so, when bites cause pruritus and secondary infections from scratching. The lice and nits generally can be found in pubic hair, axillary hair, abdominal and thigh hair, and sometimes in the hair of eyebrows, eyelashes, and beards. Clinical diagnosis is based on history and the presence of nits (small, shiny, yellow, oval, dewdrop-like eggs) affixed to hair shafts or lice (yellowish, oval, wingless insect).

CDC (1998) treatment recommendations include:

■ *Permethrin:* 1% cream rinse applied to affected areas and washed off after 10 minutes
■ *Lindane:* 1% shampoo applied for 4 minutes to the affected area and then thoroughly rinsed off (this regimen is not recommended for pregnant or lactating women or for children less than 2 years old)
■ *Pyrethrins with piperonyl butoxide:* Applied to the affected area and washed off after 10 minutes

If symptoms persist after 1 week, a retreatment with an alternative medication is recommended. For pediculosis of the eyelashes, occlusive ophthalmic ointment needs to be applied to the eyelid margins twice a day for 10 days. Bedding and affected clothes should be washed in hot water and dried in a high-heat dryer or dry-cleaned.

Scabies. Scabies is a sexually transmitted disease caused by the parasite *Sarcoptes scabiei*. The small adult mite, approximately 0.2 mm, is round and has eight legs. The female lays eggs in the epidermis, and the eggs develop into adults in 10 days. Scabies are host-specific for humans (Nelson & Neinstein, 1996).

The primary symptom of scabies is pruritus that increases at night. The lesion starts as a small papule that reddens, erodes, and sometimes crusts. Generally what appears next is a burrow: a dark, dotted line 2 to 12 mm long that is straight or wavy. Lesions are found most commonly on the finger webs, flexor surfaces of the wrists, extensor surface of the elbows, axillary folds, nipples, abdominal girth, buttocks, thighs, and the male penis. Scabies is rarely seen on the face, scalp, and neck except in children.

Diagnosis is made by clinical observation of the distinctively characteristic burrow. In addition, a shave biopsy or lesion scrape onto a slide and examination with oil emersion may show ova, organisms, or feces.

Treatment regimens recommended by the CDC (1998) include the following:

■ *Permethrin:* 5% cream applied to all areas of the body from the neck down and washed off after 8 to 14 hours
■ *Lindane (1%):* 1 ounce of lotion or 30 g of cream applied thinly to all areas of the body from the neck down and thoroughly washed off after 8 hours
■ *Sulfur (6%) precipitate in ointment:* Applied thinly to all areas nightly for three nights. Previous applications should be washed off before new applications are applied. The

patient should thoroughly wash 24 hours after the last application. Lindane is not recommended for use after a bath or by pregnant or lactating women, persons with extensive dermatitis, or children less than 2 years old.

Counseling about decontamination of clothing and bedding by machine-washing or machine-drying on the hot cycle, dry-cleaning, or removal from body contact for greater than 72 hours is important for complete treatment. A 1-week follow-up appointment helps to evaluate any remaining symptoms of pruritus or the need for an alternative therapy.

HIV and AIDS

HIV is a retrovirus that causes AIDS. AIDS was first identified in 1981, and the virus was discovered in 1983 (Minkoff, 1986). The untreated infection progresses from asymptomatic to the manifestation of AIDS in a period of 1 month to 17 years (CDC, 1998). Research continues to track cases in an effort to identify factors influencing the AIDS-free periods.

HIV is an infection of global concern because on almost every continent AIDS is the leading cause of death among young women (Hatcher et al., 1994). Improved awareness about the risk factors for HIV infection transmission has led to increased testing and earlier diagnosis. Early diagnosis is important because medications are available that slow the decline of the immune system and in some cases keep the virus dormant. Treatment interventions also can be initiated to prevent other opportunistic infections, such as tuberculosis, *Pneumocystis carinii* pneumonia, and toxoplasmosis encephalitis. The earlier diagnosis of HIV also allows the health care provider an opportunity to educate about transmission prevention and health promoting options.

Transmission of the HIV virus is known to occur in the following ways (Hatcher et al., 1994; Lichtman & Papera, 1990):

- Sexual contact: vaginal and anal intercourse
- Sharing of needles and syringes
- Transfusion of infected blood or blood products
- Transplacentally via mother to child
- Postnatally via breast milk
- Artificial insemination
- Transplantation of an infected organ
- Exposure of health care providers to infected blood by needles, etc.

Diagnosis. The diagnosis of HIV infection is made by clinical evidence and serological testing for HIV-1 antibody. An initial screening test is the enzyme immunoassay. When the enzyme immunoassay is reactive, confirmation of the positive result is made by another test, the Western blot or an immunofluorescence assay. A negative result only confirms that the individual was HIV negative 6 months before the test. Given the lag time in verification of the disease, taking a complete sexual history, counseling on the need for a second test in 6 months, and providing a safe environment for the individual for follow-up is imperative. When an HIV-1 test is negative and the individual has clinical symptoms suspicious for HIV infection, an HIV-2 test needs to be conducted.

HIV-2 is not common in the United States but is endemic in West Africa and has shown increasing prevalence in France, Portugal, Angola, and Mozambique (CDC, 1998).

An adjunct to serological testing is the manner in which the clinic attends to the privacy issues of the individual and the importance of data collection for sexually transmitted diseases. Informed consent is required before testing, and in some states written consent is required. Counseling in person before and after testing is critical for the psychological and physical health of the individual. These counseling sessions provide an opportunity for the individual to express concerns and health care providers to educate about transmission, prevention, and the disease itself.

Symptoms of acute retroviral syndrome are characterized by fever, malaise, lymphadenopathy, diarrhea, weight loss, night sweats, and skin rash. Sexually active persons with acute retroviral syndrome should have an HIV test done. The syndrome usually occurs before HIV testing is positive and within a few weeks of HIV infection. Data suggest that the initiation of antiretroviral therapy at this early phase of the disease may influence the prognosis. Two approaches to therapy include (1) zidovudine or (2) two nucleoside reverse transcriptase inhibitors and a protease inhibitor (CDC, 1998).

Treatment. If the diagnosis is made at a facility that does not provide comprehensive HIV services, the HIV-infected individual must be referred to such a facility. An initial evaluation includes the following (CDC, 1998):

- A medical history, detailing sexual practices, substance abuse, previous STDs, and HIV-related symptoms
- Physical examination
- STD testing and a Pap smear for women
- Complete blood and platelet counts and blood chemistry profile
- Hepatitis A testing CD4+ T-lymphocyte analysis
- Purified protein derivative
- Viral load test
- Chest radiograph
- Psychological evaluation

Vaginal Infections

Infections of the vagina with lesser consequences than STDs include bacterial vaginosis, *Candida albicans*, and trichomoniasis. Often the symptoms associated with these infections are more bothersome to youth than an actual STD. Although acquisition of such vaginal infections may not be by sexual means, much confusion exists over this notion. Denial of symptoms can occur when a teen fears admitting to a problem even when she has not been sexually active. Getting information to adolescents and their parents about vaginal changes not associated with sexual intercourse is an important step in educating women in general to obtain early evaluation of any vaginal change.

Diagnosing a vaginitis has four components:

1. Observation of vaginal secretions and the condition of cervical and vaginal tissue
2. Measurement of the pH of the vaginal secretions

3. Microscopic evaluation
4. The whiff test

Vaginal secretions are characterized by color, quality (homogenous or clumpy), and odor. The pH varies by diagnosis. When a microscope is available, diagnosis becomes more exact. Microscopic evaluation begins with the collection of a sample of vaginal discharge during the pelvic examination. A cotton-tipped swab collects the vaginal secretions and is placed in a test-tube with a small amount of saline solution or is applied directly to a slide in a drop of saline solution. If a test tube is not used, then a second slide is prepared immediately. This slide has a drop of potassium hydroxide solution on it, and when the swab of vaginal secretions is mixed into it, an acrid odor (fishy smell) is released. This odor is considered a positive whiff test. The swab should always be mixed in the saline solution first. This prevents lysis of the living cells that are necessary for accurate diagnosis. Cover slips are then placed on top of the samples, which are then ready for microscopic evaluation.

Bacterial Vaginosis

Bacterial vaginosis appears as a milky white, homogenous discharge with a pH greater than 4.5. Under microscopy, bacterial vaginosis is diagnosed positively when clue cells are present. Clue cells appear as small circles, clustered at the borders of epithelial cells (Figure 15-11, *A*). The whiff test also is positive.

Candida Albicans (Yeast)

Candida albicans—also referred to as yeast, monilia, and fungus—appears as a clumpy discharge with a range of coloration from white to cream to yellow to greenish-yellow. The pH is normal, less than 4.5. Under microscopy, *Candida* presents as buds of yeast usually accompanied by hyphae (Figure 5-11, *B*). The whiff test is negative.

Trichomoniasis

Trichomoniasis is diagnosed by the presence of trichamonads, a one-celled organism with a flagellum (Figure 5-11, *C*). The discharge is homogenous and often accompanied with strawberry spots that are visible on the cervix and vaginal lining. This microbe is diagnosed easily under microscopy because of its motility. The whiff test is negative unless also accompanied by the presence of bacterial vaginosis.

Management

Bacterial vaginosis is treated with metronidazole 500 mg orally twice daily for 7 days or with clindamydin cream 2%, one full applicator (5 g) intravaginally at bedtime for 7 days or with metranidazole gel 0.75%, one full applicator (5 g) intravaginally twice a day for 5 days. The CDC (1998) recommends that pregnant women receive treatment and that sexual partners do not need to be treated.

The treatment for *Candida albicans* is topical azole medications, such as clotrimazole, miconazole, tiocanazole, or teracanazole. These are used intravaginally in the form of cream, tablet, ointment, or suppositories, and the treatment ranges from 3 to 7 days. There is an effective oral agent which is fluconazole (Diflucon) 160-mg oral

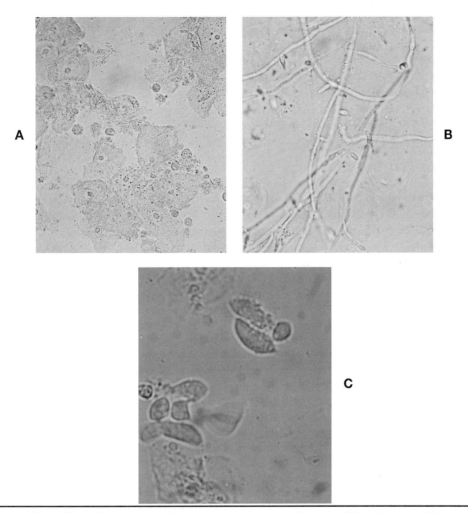

Figure 15-11 Vaginal infections. **A,** Bacterial vaginosis: clue cells. **B,** *Candida albicans:* budding, branching hyphae. **C,** Trichomoniasis: motile trichomonads. (From Zitelli, B. J., & Davis, H. W. [1994]. *Atlas of pediatric physical diagnosis* [4th ed.]. St. Louis: Mosby.)

tablet, one tablet in a single dose. Pregnant women should be treated with topical medications only and treatment of sexual partners is not recommended.

Trichomoniasis is treated with metronidazole 2 g orally in a single dose or metranidzole 500 mg orally twice daily for 7 days. It is recommended that sex partners and pregnant women receive the 2 g of metronidazole in a single dose (CDC, 1998).

Toxic Shock Syndrome

Toxic shock syndrome (TSS) is a potentially lethal condition that affects men and women, but predominantly young menstruating women (15 to 19 years of age) who use tampons (Broome, 1989). TSS was diagnosed initially in the early 1980s as occurring with one specific type of tampon. Since the removal of that tampon and implementation of mandatory labeling with standardized absorbency ratings (regular, super, super plus) for each tampon, the incidence of TSS has decreased.

The disease in menstruating young women is associated with the development of an exotoxin (toxic shock toxin 1) by *Staphylococcus aureus*. Cultures from the vagina have grown *S. aureus* in 98% of women with TSS and only 7% in controls (Laufer & Goldstein, 1995). TSS has been associated with continuous tampon use and peak occurrences are on day 4 of the menses.

TSS also has been associated with use of the contraceptive sponge and diaphragm. All patients who are prescribed barrier methods of contraception should be informed of the relative risks of TSS. Symptoms of diarrhea, vomiting, and rash that occur with tampon use during menstruation should be evaluated for TSS.

Variations in severity of TSS symptoms occur. The CDC has set criteria to study the epidemiology of TSS based on the more severe manifestations of the syndrome. These criteria include the following (Laufer & Goldstein, 1995, p. 601):

A. Fever (temperature greater than 102° F [38.8° C])
B. Rash (diffuse, macular erythroderma that looks like sunburn)
C. Desquamation 1 to 2 weeks after the onset of the illness, particularly of palms and soles
D. Hypotension (systolic blood pressure less than 90 mm Hg for adults, or orthostatic syncope)
E. Involvement of three or more of the following organ systems:
   1. Gastrointestinal (vomiting or diarrhea)
   2. Muscular (severe myalgia or creatinine phosphokinase level greater than twice the upper limit of normal)
   3. Mucous membranes (vaginal and oropharyngeal, or conjunctive hyperemia)
   4. Renal (blood urea nitrogen or creatinine greater than twice the upper limits of normal)
   5. Hepatic (total bilirubin, aspartate aminotransferase, alanine aminotranferase greater than twice the upper limits of normal)
   6. Hematological (platelet count less than 100,000/mm^3)
   7. Central nervous system (disorientation or alterations in consciousness when fever and hypotension are absent)
F. Negative results on the following tests, if obtained:
   1. Blood, throat, or CSF cultures
   2. Serological tests for Rocky Mountain spotted fever, leptospirosis, or measles

Adolescents with any of these symptoms should be instructed to remove a tampon if during menstruation or remove a contraceptive sponge or diaphragm if present and go to the emergency room. Management of patients with TSS is the same as for any person in shock. After fluid administration has begun, a pelvic examination is done to remove any remaining tampon or sponge and to obtain cultures. In addition, collection of blood, rectum, oropharynx, anterior nares, and urine cultures enhances management. Antistaphylococcal antibiotics such as nafcillin sodium, cephalosporins, or vancomycin hydrochloride are given for 7 to 14 days. Vaginal irrigation with saline or an antibiotic solution may be performed, although no scientific evidence supports the benefits of this action.

Because of the high rate of reoccurrence (approximately 30%), tampon use should be avoided for at least 8 months (Ciesielski & Broome, 1986). Compliance with the antibiotic regimen and avoidance of tampons and vaginal contraceptives help minimize the potential for reoccurrence. If the adolescent chooses to use tampons, the health care provider should inform her that a maximum frequency rate for changing tampons has not been established and that using the smallest appropriate-sized tampon while alternating with pads, especially during sleep, helps prevent TSS.

Breast Masses

The breast tissue of adolescents is typically dense. Findings in the breasts of adolescent females are usually normal physiological tissue changes or fibrocystic changes. Physiological changes are varied sets of complaints, commonly differing from month to month, and can be managed clinically. Fibrocystic changes are described as a tender, swollen, lumpy breast and are most bothersome the week before menses. Adjusting dietary influences such as restricting sodium intake and avoiding caffeine products (cola, chocolate, tea, and coffee) and wearing a good, supportive bra help to minimize the discomforts.

The majority of true breast masses in adolescents, when excised, are fibroadenomata. Goldstein and Pinsonneault (1990) found that in a study of 100 breast biopsy specimens, 83% were fibroadenomata (adult, 58; juvenile, 19; and giant, 2), 8% were fibrocystic mastopathies, and 9% were other masses. Breast cancer is rare in adolescents. The breast tumor, juvenile papillomatosis, also is rare. Often mistaken for a fibroadenoma, the tumor qualities are atypical papillary duct hyperplasia and multiple cysts. Juvenile papillomatosis has been associated with the development of breast cancer and requires careful surveillance.

After thorough inspection and palpation of the breasts, the mass should be measured and the teen instructed to return after her next menstrual period. If the mass enlarges or persists after several menstrual cycles, referral for a fine-needle aspiration or ultrasound is appropriate. Fine-needle aspiration will obtain a specimen that can be fixed to a slide and sent for cytological review, collapse a cystic mass with or without specimen, or obtain no specimen, in which case an excisional biopsy is recommended.

Adolescents are generally self-conscious of any bodily change. Issues dealing with the breast are particularly tricky. Adolescents often express a preference to deny any breast problem whether or not it causes discomfort. Assisting the teen to feel comfortable about touching her own breasts and having a practitioner examine her breasts is a key to obtaining a complete evaluation. The importance of teaching breast self-examination during an adolescent's first gynecological physical examination cannot be stressed enough.

A final area of alteration in breast health includes trauma injuries. A mass from a contusion generally takes several weeks to resolve. More severe traumas can take up to several months to resolve and may leave palpable scar tissue indefinitely. If at the site of a trauma a palpable mass is delineated and nontender, a preexisting condition may be indicated. Follow-up with trauma cases is important in maintaining an accurate diagnosis.

ADOLESCENT PREGNANCY AND PREMATURE PARENTING

Scope of the Problem

Teenage pregnancy is a public health concern of major proportion. The United States has the highest adolescent pregnancy rate of any developed country. More than 1 million teenage girls become pregnant annually (Henshaw, 1993). Another way to say this is that one in every 10 teenagers in the United States gets pregnant every year. The majority (85%) of these pregnancies are unintended (Alan Guttmacher Institute, 1994; CDC, 1997). Contraception usage remains low: only one third of sexually active female adolescents uses a contraceptive method regularly. The gap in timing between the initiation of sexual activity and use of contraception, approximately 6 to 12 months, is a well-studied and yet puzzling statistical phenomenon (Alan Guttmacher Institute, 1994).

Although the trend in pregnancy rate (defined as the rate of live births plus the rate of induced abortions per 1000 females) from 1970 to 1986 has been declining slightly for all women aged 15 to 19, the birth rate trend since 1986 has been increasing. Although adolescent pregnancy rates are high, preventive measures appear to be having a positive effect, for the increase in pregnancy rate has not kept pace with the increase in sexual activity rate. The statistical analysis reported in the September 1997 issue of *Mortality and Morbidity Weekly Report* has identified a decline in birth rate for teenagers 15 to 19 years of age from 1991 to 1996. In 1991 the birth rate was 62 per 1000 women 15 to 19 years of age. From 1995 to 1996 the preliminary birth rate, expressed as 54.7 per 1000 women 15 to 19 years of age, decreased 4%. The decline in birth rate was reported in all age, racial, and ethnic groups (CDC, 1997b). Although some progress appears to have been made, the factors contributing to this trend have not been definitively identified.

The abortion rate since the late 1970s in sexually experienced women 15 to 19 years of age has declined. Teens account for about one quarter of all abortions in the United States. A majority of unintended pregnancies in adolescents (53%) ends in abortion (Alan Guttmacher Institute, 1994). Other factors that correlate with a teen choosing to have an abortion include higher income status, parents with higher education, being white, and having a younger partner (Pakula & Neinstein, 1996, p. 660).

In comparison with abortion, adoption is a less popular choice. Although adoption has never been a popular choice among African-American youths (1%), it has declined in preference in white teens from 19% in 1972 to 3% in 1988 (Pakula & Neinstein, 1996).

One of the most significant statistics is the nonmarital birth rate. In teens less than 20 years of age the total number of nonmarital births has quadrupled since 1960 for a total of 69% of all teen births in 1991. As alarming as the nonmarital birth rate statistic is, so is the repeat birth rate. Approximately 25% of adolescent mothers age 16 and younger and 20% of adolescent mothers 17 to 18 have a second child within 2 years of their first child (Mott, 1986).

Developmental Issues of Pregnant Adolescents

Depending on the age of the pregnant teen, she may be engaged in the challenges of early, middle, or late adolescence (see the section on the emotional and intellectual self for a review of these stages). The developmental issue most affected by the condition of pregnancy and parenthood is that of developing an identity. Identity development is compromised or halted as the teen integrates the tasks of pregnancy, bonding, and preparing to care for another with the tasks of developing self-identity and independence. The process of learning how to separate from parents while learning how to bond and attach to a newborn has substantial conflict. Practitioners working with pregnant teens need to acknowledge this conflict in the adolescent's development and help foster ways of positive growth and attainment of these conflicting goals.

Process of Becoming Pregnant

Decision making is a task learned over time and through experience with consequences of actions. Along the route to pregnancy and parenthood are several decision points concerning choices about sexuality. Reeder and others (1995) modified the work of Flick (1986) to identify four decision points in teen sexuality that can lead to parenthood (Box 15-13). Anticipatory guidance from health care providers, parents, and teachers regarding the types of questions encountered at each decision point is helpful in the process of making informed decisions. Acquiring information before an experience is a valuable form of preventive health care.

Decision 1

The practitioner's role in helping the teen to make healthy decisions is through role modeling and fostering responsible decision making. Confronting the teen in a genuine manner about how she is taking responsible steps to cope with the consequences of her decisions is appropriate. Framing questions in a nonthreatening way is advantageous to good communication. For example, the following are two approaches to obtaining information about the youth's sexual activity and preparation to avoid an unintended pregnancy.

Box 15-13 DECISION POINTS LEADING TO PARENTHOOD

Decision 1	Sexual activity	To become sexually active or to remain sexually inactive
Decision 2	Contraception	To use or not to use contraception appropriately
Decision 3	Pregnancy	To deliver the child or to abort the pregnancy
Decision 4	Parenthood	To rear the child or to place the child formally or informally for adoption

Modified from Reeder, S. J., Martin, L. L., & Koniak-Griffin, D. (1995). *Maternity nursing* (18th ed., pp. 931–954). Philadelphia: J. B. Lippincott.

Scenario One

Practitioner:	"Are you currently sexually active? (Are you having sex with boys, girls, or both?)"
Teen:	"No."
Practitioner:	"What do you know about contraception, and have you thought about which method you would use when you do become sexually active?"
Teen:	"No, I'm not going to get pregnant."

Scenario Two

Practitioner:	"Ann, my next set of questions is more personal. The questions are, however, important to your health. Again, let me remind you that I will keep this information confidential. I would now like to talk with you about relationships. Are you presently going out with anyone?"
Teen:	"Yes."
Practitioner:	"What is this person's first name?" (Seeking sexual orientation)
Teen:	"Jules."
Practitioner:	"Excuse me, did you say *his* name is Jules?" (Clarify when the name is genderless.)
Teen:	(a) "No, *her* name is Jules." (The practitioner focuses on issues of lesbian sexual health and social acceptance.)
	(b) "Yes." (The practitioner proceeds with questioning that elicits information regarding the use of contraception and the consequences of unintended pregnancy.)
Practitioner:	"Some teens your age choose to be sexually active, that is, they have sexual intercourse. Other teens choose not to have sexual intercourse. What have you and your partner decided."
Teen:	"Jules and I are not sexually active, but we might be. What shall I do?"

The teen's last question is vague and needs further clarification before an answer is offered. Furthermore, some teens look to authority figures for permission and how to make the right choice. Again, the practitioner needs to know her own personal biases and share them with the teen but then be neutral and encourage the teen to think through what will be the best choice for her. In the latter case, finding out exactly what advice the teen is seeking is a start. Does she want information about sex, about contraception, about how to talk with her partner, or about how to make a difficult decision and when to make it? As a practitioner, making assumptions about the nature of a question is easier, but this may close the discussion prematurely, before the teen is able truly to get her real question asked and answered.

Decision 2

The choice to use contraception is a major step in the process of decision making to prevent pregnancy and STDs. Once the decision to use contraception has been made, usually taking much time and deliberation, then the challenge of how to obtain the desired contraceptive method follows. Condoms and spermicides are the most convenient because they can be purchased over the counter, but the public conditions surrounding such a purchase may be prohibiting. Other barrier methods, the OCP, IUD, Norplant, and Depo-Provera all require a health care practitioner visit. The process of obtaining an appointment also may be a point of difficulty if transportation is needed, the appointment time is not convenient, or insurance coverage requires a parent signature, etc. Eventually the adolescent will prevail in her attempt to acquire contraception, or she will make an alternate decision.

Decision 3

The teen who has not chosen to use contraception or who has a contraceptive failure should be interviewed before having a pregnancy test to determine the affect of receiving news of a pregnancy. Then when the practitioner has the test results, she is better equipped to support the adolescent's response and help the teen to address her next set of decisions.

When an adolescent is diagnosed with a pregnancy, her choices are to maintain or to terminate the pregnancy. The number of weeks of gestation passed is a factor in how many options she has. When the pregnancy is diagnosed in the first 12 weeks (the first trimester), the adolescent has three choices: to maintain the pregnancy and become a parent, to maintain the pregnancy but give up the child to foster care or adoption, or to terminate the pregnancy. When the pregnancy is beyond the first trimester, the third option, to terminate the pregnancy, is governed by the laws of the state and the number of weeks of gestation. In general, second trimester abortions have more risks and are performed before 22 weeks (see the section on abortion in Chapter 16).

If the adolescent chooses to continue the pregnancy, she would do well to seek prenatal care to sustain the health and safety of herself and the developing child. Attaining prenatal care forces other tasks that the adolescent may or may not be comfortable with; namely, telling her parents and boyfriend that she is pregnant. Typically, the teen's ability to communicate difficult information to parents, authority figures, and friends is not yet mature and often leaves the young teen denying the situation until late in the pregnancy. In most cases, prenatal care is not initiated until a parent or significant other or adult is apprised of the pregnancy.

Decision 4

When the adolescent has chosen to maintain a pregnancy, she needs to decide next whether she will keep the child and take on the tasks of parenthood or place the baby for adoption. The option of adoption is a less popular choice, mainly because the stigma associated with single parenthood has decreased since the 1970s. The choice of adoption needs to be offered at different times during the adolescent's pregnancy. At the pregnant adolescent's initial visit, the practitioner should review this option and give the teen a community resource handout to take home. In subsequent prenatal visits and early postpartum, the topic needs to be reconsidered, as appropriate. Each state has its own laws governing the process of adoption. Some states allow years for the biological parents to reclaim the parental rights of their child in adoption. State laws and the options of open or closed adoptions, confidentiality, and length of time for completion of the adoption process are important factors in facilitating a smooth transition when adoption is chosen.

Pregnancy Care

Prenatal care for adolescents and adults follows the same gestational schedule for physical changes and specific prenatal tests. The difference in caring for a pregnant adolescent is in the developmental and social needs of the individual (Baker, 1996). Extra time is needed for education and counseling and requires visits every 2 weeks through the eighth month and weekly thereafter. Participation in a group of pregnant peers is helpful for social support needs. Although adequate prenatal care usually can be offered to pregnant teens by a single provider or a general obstetrician/gynecologist group practice, specific adolescent clinics focused on the issues of prenatal care tend to offer more comprehensive care, including obstetrician/gynecologist physician care (attending to high-risk physical pregnancy needs), nurse practitioner care (attending to many physical care needs as well as education and counseling needs), social worker care (evaluating the home, community, and school resources), and a liaison or visiting nurse (monitoring the adjustments in the home of a high-risk pregnancy or the transition to parenthood during the immediate postpartum period).

Consistent attendance at groups or prenatal visits is another hurdle for providers of prenatal care to adolescents. Research has shown that when a pregnant adolescent's parent is involved with prenatal visits or prenatal group work, the adolescent responds better to the needs of her newborn and is less likely to have a repeat pregnancy within 2 years (McAnarney, 1983; Roye & Balk, 1996).

When a pregnant adolescent attends her prenatal visits and classes, the practitioner has the opportunity to educate the teen about her changing body, appropriate nutrition and weight gain, the growth of her baby, how to prepare for labor, and what considerations for newborn care should be anticipated before delivery. Assessing the developmental level of each teen helps the practitioner focus learning tasks. For example, the pregnant teen in late adolescence has a greater capacity to understand the consequences of her actions on her body and on the developing baby (e.g., poor nutrition causes greater personal fatigue and is a risk factor for low-birth-weight infants) (Berenson, 1997), whereas a pregnant teen in early adolescence is usually more defiant, influenced by her peers' choices, and concerned about her body image ("I can't eat all that food because it will make me fatter than I already am, and I'm only 22 weeks"). Although nutrition is a major concern for health care practitioners, body image is of greater concern for the adolescent. Encouraging the teen to adjust her body image standards during pregnancy and learning about good nutrition for her and her future newborn challenges the practitioner to use her knowledge of nutrition, development issues of adolescence, and prenatal care needs during the changes of gestation. Group work is often the best way to assist the pregnant teen in early and middle adolescence, for it provides a peer group that can offer support and identify common goals and specific concerns.

Engaging the father of the child in prenatal care visits educates him in the process of pregnancy, labor and delivery, and eventual parenting. Encouraging the couple to disclose their feelings (fears and desires) and knowledge deficits to each other in the presence of the health care practitioner allows for the opportunity to clarify expectations and to correct false knowledge. Just as with adult males involved with their wives' labor, including the adolescent male in the labor and delivery experience is important to the eventual bonding the father has with his child. Addressing the pregnant adolescent and the baby's father as a team or couple helps acknowledge the support roles they play in each other's life.

Prenatal visits for adolescents offer care similar to what is offered to adult pregnant women and is presented in Chapter 16. Labor preparation through childbirth education classes specifically for teens, although scarce, is available. When childbirth preparation is not given through the prenatal clinic or the teen chooses not to attend structured childbirth preparation classes, the health care practitioner needs to review this content, assess for learned information, and supplement the information as needed. An important, although often overlooked, aspect in the preparation is the teen's need, at the time of labor and delivery, to separate from the prenatal clinic health care provider and attach to and trust a new provider of care for her. Although all women are sensitive to this transference of care and relationship, adolescents are particularly vulnerable. Advanced preparation, through stating that the health care provider will or will not attend the birth, is crucial to the teen's emotional well-being. Teaching and role-modeling skills of assertiveness to meet her needs during labor and delivery is a critical behavior the practitioner can bestow on the pregnant teen. Insisting that a family member or significant other be with the adolescent at all times in labor also helps make sure that the needs of the teen are voiced.

Labor and delivery are a most profound experience. The prenatal health care provider who does not deliver her clients must know the staff and physical plant of the hospital or birthing center her clients will use. Follow-up with adolescents after delivery is important and often aids the adolescent in feeling that someone in the health care system really does care.

Postpartum Experience

For the women's health care nurse, adolescent needs during postpartum have changed incredibly since the decrease in number of hospital days. Although the physical needs of the adolescent may be attended to in a 48-hour postpartum stay, the emotional needs and child care needs require more attention. With early discharge, 48 hours, the adolescent needs a visiting nurse to come to the home to assess the mother and child. Return visits to the clinic generally are in 2 weeks for teens who have had cesarean sections or medical complications during pregnancy, labor and delivery, or postpartum, and in 6 weeks for teens who delivered vaginally without complications. The health care provider assessing a first-time adolescent mother needs to make telephone calls before the 6-week appointment or have a home health nurse communicate her intention to visit.

For evaluation of routine postpartum care, see Chapter 16. For initial evaluation of the newborn the women's health care practitioner should know newborn physical assessment. Knowing how to assess a newborn serves two purposes: first, the practitioner is better able to evaluate and interpret the consequences of an abnormality in the newborn and, second, the practitioner can better answer the new mother's questions about her newborn.

Adolescents as Parents

The transition to parenthood is filled with challenges. Adolescent mothers may be struggling with single parenthood and living with their family of origin, while other adolescent mothers may be adjusting to being part of a couple with a boyfriend and living together apart from or with the boyfriend's parents. Struggling with a variety of new identities—spouse, mother, single provider, and adolescent—may be a connecting and meaningful transition or one that predisposes the teen to emotional disharmony and postpartum depression (Paulson & Sputa, 1996).

In addition to struggling with identity, one's place in life, one's home, in general the environment that the mother enters with her new infant, and all the responsibilities of parenthood may not be compatible and thus may have various negative consequences. When a teen mother has difficulties identifying supports in the immediate and 6-week postpartum time, the practitioner needs to be alert to this and take action to assess for possible depression and adjustment problems. Panzerine, Slater, and Sharps (1995) found that depressed adolescent mothers displayed "less effective maternal-infant feeding interactions, less confidence in the ability to adequately care for the new baby, a reliance upon emotion-focused coping including emotional detachment and withdrawal, and less satisfaction with social supports" (p. 118).

Attachment and Infant Care

The process of bonding or attaching to one's baby may not happen automatically. Young adolescents and parents in unintended pregnancies have higher rates of nonbonding behaviors (Reis, 1989). Attachment is important for the survival of the infant. Infants whose mothers had difficulties demonstrating attachment had a higher incidence of sudden infant death syndrome (Horwitz, Klerman, Kuo, & Jekel, 1991) and other causes of postneonatal death, including abuse and infection (Roye & Balk, 1996).

A method of helping adolescent parents respond more sensitively to their newborn infant is interaction coaching for adolescent parents (Censullo, 1994). This intervention is designed for nurses and adolescent health care providers and is a three-part once-a-week support/education group that helps to identify normal newborn behaviors, observe infant cues and learn appropriate responses, and practice self-recognition of achievement. The fact that early adolescent parent-infant relationships place the child at risk because adolescent mothers respond less sensitively to their infants than older mothers is a compelling reason to know and offer interaction coaching for adolescent parents or a similar program (Arenson, 1994).

SUMMARY

In summary, the goal of this chapter was to present an overview of the most salient health concerns of adolescent women and to provide resources for more in-depth coverage of specific conditions. Adolescent women's health care is a challenging field that requires the integration of adolescent physical and developmental issues with changing family dynamics. Women's health providers serve in pivotal roles in caring for adolescent women, which impact their health across the life span.

REFERENCES

Alan Guttmacher Institute. (1994). *Sex and America's teenagers.* New York: Author.

American Medical Association, Department of Adolescent Health. (1991). *Guidelines for adolescent preventive services (GAPS).* Washington, DC: Author.

American Psychiatric Association. (1994). *Diagnostic and statistical manual of mental disorders* (4th ed.). Washington, DC: Author.

Andersch, B., & Milsom, I. (1982). An epidemiologic study of young women with dysmenorrhea. *American Journal of Obstetrics and Gynecology, 144,* 655.

Arenson, J. D. (1994). Strengths and self-perceptions of parenting in adolescent mothers. *Pediatric Nursing, 9*(4), 251–257.

Baker, T. J. (1996). Factors related to the initiation of prenatal care in the adolescent nullipara, *Nurse Practitioner, 21*(2), 26–42.

Becker, J. L. (1995). Adolescent medicine. In D. P. Lemcke, J. Pattison, L. A. Marshall, & D. S. Cowley (Eds.), *Primary care of women* (pp. 15–24). Norwalk, CT: Appleton & Lange.

Berenson, A. B. (1997). Inadequate weight gain among pregnant adolescents: Risk factors and relationship to infant birth weight. *American Journal of Obstetrics and Gynecology, 176,* 1220–1227.

Biro, F. M., Reising, S. F., Doughman, J. A., Kollar, L. M., & Rosenthal, S. L. (1994). A comparison of diagnostic methods in adolescent girls with and without symptoms of *Chlamydia* urogenital infection. *Pediatrics, 93,* 476.

Bragg, E. J. (1997). Pregnant adolescents with addictions. *Journal of Obstetric, Gynecologic, and Neonatal Nursing, 26*(5), 577–592.

Braverman, P. K., & Strasburger, V. C. (1994). Sexually transmitted diseases. *Clinical Pediatrics, 33,* 26.

Brent, D. A., Perper, J. A., & Moritz, G. (1993). Firearms and adolescent suicide: A community case-control study. *American Journal of Disabled Children, 147,* 1066.

Broome, C. (1989). Epidemiology of toxic shock syndrome in the United States: Overview. *Review of Infectious Disease, 11*(1), S14–S21.

Cates, W. (1990). The epidemiology and control of sexually transmitted diseases in adolescents. *Adolescent Medicine: State of the Art Review, 1,* 409.

Censullo, M. (1994). Strategy for promoting greater responsiveness in adolescent parent-infant relationships: Report of a pilot study. *Journal of Pediatric Nursing, 9*(5), 326–332.

Centers for Disease Control and Prevention. (1987). Increases in primary and secondary syphilis in the United States. *Morbidity and Mortality Weekly Report, 36,* 393.

Centers for Disease Control and Prevention. (1989). Results from the National Adolescent Student Health Survey. *Morbidity and Mortality Weekly Report, 38,* 147.

Centers for Disease Control and Prevention. (1993a). 1993 sexually transmitted diseases treatment guidelines. *Morbidity and Mortality Weekly Report, 42,* RR–14.

Centers for Disease Control and Prevention. (1993b). Surveillance for gonorrhea and primary and secondary syphilis among adolescents, United States: 1981-1991. *Morbidity and Mortality Weekly Report, 42,* 1.

Centers for Disease Control and Prevention. (1995). HIV/AIDS surveillance report. *Morbidity and Mortality Weekly Report, 7*(1), 13.

Centers for Disease Control and Prevention. (1997a). Regional variations in suicide rates: United States, 1990-1994. *Morbidity and Mortality Weekly Report, 46*(34), 789–793.

Centers for Disease Control and Prevention. (1997b, September 12). State-specific birth rates for teenagers: United States, 1990-1996. *Morbidity and Mortality Weekly Report, 46,* 837–842.

Centers for Disease Control and Prevention. (1997c). Summary of notifiable diseases in the United States, 1996. *Morbidity and Mortality Weekly Report, 45*(53), 1–15.

Centers for Disease Control and Prevention. (1997d). Youth risk behavior surveillance: National College Health Risk Behavior Survey: United States, 1995. *Morbidity and Mortality Weekly Report, 46*(SS-6), 1–56.

Centers for Disease Control and Prevention. (1998). 1998 Guidelines for treatment of sexually transmitted diseases. *Morbidity and Mortality Weekly Report, 47*(RR-1), 1–119.

Chapman, P., Toma, R. B., Tuveson, R. V., & Jacob, M. (1997). Nutrition knowledge among adolescent high school female athletes. *Adolescence, 32*(126), 435–446.

Ciesielski, C., & Broome, C. (1986). Toxic shock syndrome: Still in the differential. *Journal of Critical Illness 1*(6), 26.

Corey, L. (1990). Genital herpes. In K. K. Holmes, P. A. Mardh, P. F. Sparling, & P. J. Wiesner (Eds.), *Sexually transmitted diseases* (2nd ed.). New York: McGraw-Hill.

Craig, S., & Hepburn, S. (1982). The effectiveness of barrier methods of contraception with and without spermicide. *Contraception, 26*(4): 347.

Crumley, F. E., (1990). Adolescent suicide attempts. *Journal of the American Medical Association, 241,* 2404.

Depression Guideline Panel. (1993a). *Depression in primary care: vol. 1. Detection and diagnosis: Clinical practice guideline number 5* (AHCPR Publication No. 93-0550). Rockville, MD: U.S. Department of Health and Human Services, Public Health Service, Agency for Health Care Policy and Research.

Depression Guideline Panel. (1993b). *Depression in primary care: vol. 2. Treatment of major depression: Clinical practice guideline number 5* (AHCPR Publication No. 93-0551). Rockville, MD: U.S. Department of Health and Human Services, Public Health Service, Agency for Health Care Policy and Research.

Dewey, J. (1934). *Art as experience.* New York: Berkley Publishing Group.

Edet, E. E. (1993). The prevalence of *Chlamydia trachomatis* infection among gynecological patients. *British Journal of Clinical Practice, 47,* 21.

Edwards, K. I. (1993). Obesity, anorexia and bulimia. *Medical Clinics of North America, 77*(4), 899–909.

Emans, S. J., & Goldstein, D. P. (1989). *Pediatric and adolescent gynecology* (3rd ed.). Boston: Little, Brown.

Erikson, E. H. (1959). Identity and the life cycle (Monograph). *Psychological Issues, 1*(1), 1–71.

Evander, M., Edlund, K., Gufstafsson, A., Jonsson, M., Karlsson, R., et al. (1995). Human papillomavirus infection is transient in young women: A population-based cohort study. *Journal of Infectious Diseases, 171,* 1026.

Fasoli, M., Parazzinni, F., Cecchetti, G., & La Vecchia, C. (1989). Post-coital contraception: An overview of published studies. *Contraception, 39,* 459.

Flick, L. H. (1986). Paths to adolescent parenthood: Implications for prevention. *Public Health Reports, 101*(2) 132–147.

Forrest, J. D. (1994). Epidemiology of unintended pregnancy and contraceptive use. *American Journal of Obstetrics and Gynecology, 170,* 1485–1489.

Freyer, F. J. (1998, June). [Interview with Dr. Darrell Rigel, President of the American Academy of Dermatology]. *Providence Journal-Bulletin,* pp. B2–B3.

Frisch, R. E. (1985). Body fat, menarche, and reproductive ability. *Seminars in Reproductive Endocrinology, 3,* 45.

Frisch, R. E., & Revelle, R. (1970). Height and weight at menarche and a hypothesis of critical body weights and adolescent events. *Science, 169,* 397.

Gadow, S. (1994). Whose body? Whose story? The question about narrative in women's health care. *Soundings, 77*(3/4), 295–307.

Giles, D. E., Jarrett, R. B., Biggs, M. M., Guzick, D. S., & Rush, A. J. (1989). Clinical predictors of recurrence in depression. *American Journal of Psychiatry, 146,* 764–767.

Gillbert, I. C., Rastam, M., & Gillberg, C. (1994). Anorexia nervosa outcome: Six-year controlled longitudinal study of 51 cases including a population cohort. *Journal of the American Academy of Child and Adolescent Psychiatry, 33,* 729.

Gilligan, C. (1982). *In a different voice.* Cambridge, MA: Harvard University Press.

Ginsberg, H., & Opper, S. (1969). *Piaget's theory of intellectual development.* Upper Saddle River, NJ: Prentice-Hall.

Glasier, A., Thong, K. J., Dewar, M., & Baird, D. T. (1992). Mifepristone (RU-486) compared with high-dose estrogen and progestogen for emergency postcoital contraception. *New England Journal of Medicine, 327,* 1041.

Goldenberg, R. L., & Klerman, L. V. (1995). Adolescent pregnancy: Another look. *New England Journal of Medicine, 332*(17), 1161–1162.

Goldstein, D. P., DeCholnoky, C., & Emans, S. J. (1980). Adolescent endometriosis. *Journal of Adolescent Health Care, 1,* 37.

Goldstein, D. P., & Pinsonneault, O. (1990). Management of breast masses in adolescent females. *Clinical Practice Gynecology, 1,* 131.

Gortmaker, S. L., Dietz, W. H. Jr., Sobol, A. M., Wehler, C. A., et al. (1987). Increasing pediatric obesity in the United States, *American Journal of Diseases in Children, 141*(5), 535–540.

Graves, A., & Gardner, W. A. (1993). Pathogenicity of *Trichomonas vaginalis. Clinical Obstetrics and Gynecology, 36,* 145.

Grimwood, A. K., Burgess, M. A., Ferson, M. J., Gilbert, G. L., Hogg, G., Isaacs, D., et al. (1996). Acyclovir for the prevention and treatment of varicella zoster in children, adolescents, and pregnancy. *Journal of Paediatric Child Health, 32,* 211–217.

Harris, N. L., & Seimer, B. (1995). Psychosocial health concerns. In D. P. Lemcke, J. Pattison, L. A. Marshall, & D. S. Cowley (Eds.), *Primary care of women* (pp. 657–696). Norwalk, CT: Appleton & Lange.

Hatcher, R. A., Trussell, J., Stewart, F., Stewart, G. K., Kowal, D., Guest, F., et al. (1994). *Contraceptive technology* (16th ed.). New York: Irvington.

Henshaw, S. K., (1993). Abortion trends in 1987 and 1988: Age and race. *Family Planning Perspectives, 24,* 85–86.

Hergenroeder, A., & Neinstein, L. S. (1996). Guidelines in sports medicine. In L. S. Nienstein, *Adolescent health care: A practical guide* (3rd ed., pp. 304–346). Baltimore, MD: Williams & Wilkins.

Hibbard, R. A. (1992). Sexual abuse. In E. R. McAnarney, R. Kriepe, R. Orr, & G. Comerci (Eds.), *Textbook of adolescent medicine* (pp. 1123–1127). Philadelphia: W. B. Saunders.

Himes, J., & Dietz, W. H. (1994). Guidelines for overweight in adolescent preventive services from an expert committee. The Expert Committee on Clinical Guidelines for Overweight & Preventive Services. *American Journal of Clinical Nutrition, 59*(2) 307–316.

Hoffman, A. D. (1990). Legal issues in adolescent medicine. In A. D. Hoffman & D. E. Greydnaus (Eds.), *Adolescent medicine* (pp. 519–530). Norwalk, CT: Appleton & Lange.

Horwitz, S., Klerman, L., Kuo, H., & Jekel, J. (1991). School-age mothers: Predictors of long-term educational and economic outcomes. *Pediatrics, 87,* 862–868.

Ivey, J. B. (1997). The adolescent with pelvic inflammatory disease: Assessment and management, *Nurse Practitioner, 22*(2), 78–93.

Jick, H., Shiota, K., Shepard, T. H., Hunter, J. R., Stergachis, F., Madsen, S., et al. (1982). Vaginal spermicides and miscarriage seen primarily in the emergency room. *Teratogen, Carcinogen, and Mutagenesis,* 2(2), *105.*

Jick, H., Waler, A. M., Rothman, K. J., Hunter, J., Holmes, L. B., Watkins R. N., et al. (1981). Vaginal spermicides and congenital disorders. *Journal of the American Medical Association, 245*(13), 1329.

Johnson, J. (1980). Sensory experiences prior to noxious stimuli decreases the amount of perceived pain. *Nursing Research, 11,* 875.

Johnston, L. D., O'Malley, P. M., & Bachman, J. G. (1995, December 11). *Cigarette smoking among American teens rises again in 1995.* Ann Arbor: News and Information Services of the University of Michigan.

Kampmeier, R. H. (1984). Late benign syphilis. In K. K. Holmes, P. A. Mardh, P. F. Sparkling, & P. J. Weisner (Eds.), *Sexually transmitted diseases.* New York: McGraw-Hill.

Komorowski, E. M., & Richer, V. I. (1992). Adolescent body image and attitudes to anabolic steroid use. *American Journal of the Diseased Child, 146,* 823–828.

Laufer, M. R. (1992). Endometriosis in adolescents. *Current Opinion in Pediatrics, 4,* 58.

Laufer, M. R., & Goldstein, D. P. (1995). Pediatric and adolescent gynecology. In K. J. Ryan, R. S. Berkowitz, & R. L. Barbieri (Eds.), *Kistner's gynecology: Principles and practice* (6th ed., pp. 571–632). St. Louis: Mosby.

Lemberg, E. (1984). The vaginal contraceptive sponge: A new non-prescription barrier contraceptive. *Nurse Practitioner, 9*(10), 24.

Letterie, G. S., & Royce, R. (1995) Contraception. In D. P. Lemcke, J. Pattison, L. A. Marshall, & D. S. Cowley (Eds.), *Primary care of women* (pp. 484–498). Norwalk, CT: Appleton & Lange.

Lettieri, D. J., Nelson, J. E., & Sayers, M. A. (1987). *NIAAA treatment handbook: Series 2. Alcoholism treatment assessment research instruments* (DHHS Publication No. 87-1380). Washington, DC: U.S. Department of Health and Human Services.

Lewin, K. (1964). *Field theory in social science* (D. Cartwright, Ed.). New York: Harper.

Lichtman, R., & Papera, S. (1990). *Gynecology: Well woman care.* Norwalk, CT: Appleton & Lange.

Lipscomb, P. A., & Agostini, R. (1995). Disordered eating. In D. P. Lemcke, J. Pattison, L. A. Marshall, & D. S. Cowley (Eds.), *Primary care of women* (pp. 77–84). Norwalk, CT: Appleton & Lange.

Loeffelholz, M. J., Lewinski, C. A., & Silver, S. R. (1992). Detection of *Chlamydia trachomatis* in endocervical specimens by polymerase chain reaction. *Journal of Clinical Microbiology, 30,* 2847.

Lowdermilk, D. L., Perry, S., & Bobak, I. M. (2000). *Maternity and women's health care* (7th ed.). St. Louis: Mosby.

Lucky, A. W., Biro, F. M., Huster, G. A., Leach, A. D., Morrison, J. A., & Ratterman, J. (1994). Acne vulgaris in premenarcheal girls: An early sign of puberty with rising levels of dehydroepiandrosterone sulfate. *Archives of Dermatology, 130,* 308–314.

Lyon, M., Chatoor, I., Atkins, D., Silber, T., Mosiamann, J., & Gray J. (1997). Testing the hypothesis of the multi-dimensional model of anorexia nervosa in adolescents. *Adolescence, 32*(125), 101–111.

MacKenzie, R., & Neinstein, L. S. (1996). Anorexia nervosa and bulimia. In L. S. Neinstein (Ed.), *Adolescent health care: A practical guide* (3rd ed., pp. 564–583). Baltimore: Williams & Wilkins.

Maclure, M., Travis, L. B., Willett, W., & MacMahon, B. (1991). A prospective cohort study of nutrient intake and age at menarche. *American Journal of Clinical Nutrition, 54,* 649.

Marcia, J. E. (1980). Identity in adolescence. In J. Adelson (Ed.), *Handbook of adolescent psychology* (pp. 159–187). New York: Wiley & Sons.

Marshall, J. C., & Kelch, R. P. (1986). Gonadotropin-releasing hormone: Role of pulsatile secretion in the regulation of reproduction. *New England Journal of Medicine, 315,* 1459.

Marshall, W. A., & Tanner, J. M. (1969). Variations in pattern of pubertal changes in girls. *Archives of Disease in Childhood, 44,* 291.

McAnarney, E. R. (Ed.). (1983). *Premature adolescent pregnancy and parenthood.* New York: Grune & Stratton.

McIntire, M. S., & Angel, C. R. (1977). Recurrent adolescent suicide behavior. *Pediatrics, 60,* 605–608.

McKay, L., & Diem, E. (1995). Health concerns of adolescent girls. *Journal of Pediatric Nursing 10*(1), 19–27.

Mills, J. L., Reed, G. F., Nugent, R. P., Harley, E. F., & Barendes, H. W. (1985). Are there adverse effects of periconceptional spermicide use? *Fertility and Sterility, 43*(3), 442.

Millstein, S. G., & Moscicki, A. B. (1995). Sexually-transmitted disease in female adolescents: Effects of psychosocial factors and high risk behaviors. *Journal of Adolescent Health, 17*(2), 83–90.

Minkoff, H. (1986). Acquired immunodeficiency disease. *Journal of Nurse-Midwifery, 31*(4), 189–193.

Moriarty, A. L. (1997). Contraceptive options for adolescents. *Journal of Pediatric Health Care, 11*(3), 144–146.

Mosure, D. J., Berman, S., Fine, D., Delisele, S., Cates, W., & Boring, J. R., III. (1997). Genital *Chlamydia* infections in sexually active female adolescents: So we really need to screen everyone? *Journal of Adolescent Health, 20,* 6–13.

Mott, F. L. (1986). The pace of repeated childbearing among young American mothers. *Family Planning Perspectives, 18,* 5–12.

Neinstein, L. S. (1996). Overview of sexually transmitted diseases. In L. S. Neinstein (Ed.), *Adolescent health care: A practical guide* (3rd ed., pp. 853–874). Baltimore: Williams & Wilkins.

Neinstein, L. S., & Heischober, B. S. (1996a). Hallucinogens. In L. S. Neinstein (Ed.), *Adolescent health care: A practical guide* (3rd ed., pp. 1039–1059). Baltimore: Williams & Wilkins.

Neinstein, L. S., & Heischober, B. S. (1996b). Miscellaneous drugs: stimulants, inhalants, opioids, depressants, and anabolic steroids. In L. S. Neinstein (Ed.), *Adolescent health care: A practical guide,* (3rd ed., pp. 1052–1070). Baltimore: Williams & Wilkins.

Neinstein, L. S., Heischober, B. S., & Pinsky, D. (1996). Marijuana. In L. S. Neinstein (Ed.), *Adolescent health care: A practical guide* (3rd ed., pp. 1032–1038). Baltimore: Williams & Wilkins.

Neinstein, L. S., Juliani, M. A., & Shapiro, J. (1996a). Psychosocial development in normal adolescents. In L. S. Neinstein (Ed.), *Adolescent health care: A practical guide* (3rd ed., pp. 40–45). Baltimore: Williams & Wilkins.

Neinstein, L. S., Juliani, M. A., & Shapiro, J. (1996b). Suicide. In L. S. Neinstein (Ed.), *Adolescent health care: A practical guide* (3rd ed., pp. 1116–1123). Baltimore: Williams & Wilkins.

Neinstein, L. S., & Kaufman, F. R. (1996). Normal physical growth and development. In L. S. Neinstein (Ed.), *Adolescent health care: A practical guide* (3rd ed., pp. 3–39). Baltimore: Williams & Wilkins.

Neinstein, L. S., & MacKenzie, R. (1996). High-risk and out-of control behavior. In L. S. Neinstein (Ed.), *Adolescent health care: A practical guide* (3rd ed., pp. 1094–1106). Baltimore: Williams & Wilkins.

Neinstein, L. S., & Pinsky, D. (1996a). Alcohol. In L. S. Neinstein (Ed.), *Adolescent health care: A practical guide* (3rd ed., pp. 1008–1017). Baltimore: Williams & Wilkins.

Neinstein, L. S. & Pinsky, D. (1996b). Tobacco. In L. S. Neinstein (Ed.), *Adolescent health care: A practical guide* (3rd ed., pp. 1018–1031). Baltimore: Williams & Wilkins.

Neinstein, L. S., Rabinovitz, S. J., & Schneir, A. (1996). Teenage pregnancy. In L. S. Neinstein (Ed.), *Adolescent health care: A practical guide* (3rd ed., pp. 656–676). Baltimore: Williams & Wilkins.

Nelson, A., & Neinstein, L. S. (1996). Oral contraceptives. In L. S. Neinstein (Ed.), *Adolescent health care: A practical guide* (3rd ed., pp. 695–712). Baltimore: Williams & Wilkins.

Newman, B. (1989). The changing nature of the parent-child relationship from early to late adolescence. *Adolescence, 96*, 915–924.

O'Koon, J., (1997). Attachment to parents and peers in late adolescence and their relationship with self-image. *Adolescence, 32*(126), 473–482.

Pakula, A., & Neinstein, L. S. (1996). Acne. In L. S. Neinstein (Ed.), *Adolescent health care: A practical guide* (3rd ed., pp. 349–359). Baltimore: Williams & Wilkins.

Panzerine, S., Slater, E., & Sharps, P. (1995) Coping, social support, and depressive symptoms in adolescent mothers. *Journal of Adolescent Health, 17*(2), 113–119.

Paulson, S. E., & Sputa, C. L. (1996). Patterns of parenting during adolescence: Perceptions of adolescents and parents. *Adolescence, 31*(122), 369–381.

Perkins, K., Ferrari, N., Rosas, A., Bessette, R., Williams, A., & Omar, H. (1997). You won't know unless you ask: The biopsychosocial interview for adolescents. *Clinical Pediatrics, 36*(2), 79–86.

Physical activity guidelines for adolescents. (1994). *Pediatric Exercise Science, 6*, 299–463.

Piaget, J., & Inhelder, B. (1958). *The growth of logical thinking from childhood to adolescence* (A. Parsons & S. Seagrin, Trans.). New York: Basic Books. (Original work published 1955).

Purcell, J. S., Hergenroeder, A. C., Kozinetz, C., O'Brien Smith, E., & Hill, R. B. (1997). Interviewing techniques with adolescents in primary care. *Journal of Adolescent Health, 20*(4), 300–305.

Quinn, T. C. (1994). Update on *Chlamydia trachomatis* infections. *Infectious Medicine, 11*, 201.

Reeder, S. J., Martin, L. L., & Koniak-Griffin, D. (1995). *Maternity nursing* (18th ed., pp. 931–954). Philadelphia: J. B. Lippincott.

Reis, J. (1989). A comparison of young teenage, older teenage, and adult mothers on determinants of parenting. *Journal of Psychology, 123*, 141–151.

Richarson, A. C. (1992). Physical and emotional abuse. In E. R. McAnarney, R. Kriepe, R. Orr, & G. Comerci (Eds.). *Textbook of adolescent medicine* (pp. 1119–1122). Philadelphia: W. B. Saunders.

Riggs, S., Alario, A. J., & McHorney, C. (1990). Health risks and attempted suicide in adolescents who report prior maltreatment. *Journal of Pediatrics, 116*, 815.

Rogers, M. E. (1970). *The theoretical basis of nursing.* Philadelphia: F. A. Davis.

Rogers, M. E. (1990a). Nursing science and the space age. In V. A. Malinsky & E. A. M. Barrett (Eds.), *Martha E. Rogers: Her life and her work* (pp. 256–267). Philadelphia: F. A. Davis.

Rogers, M. E. (1990b). Nursing: Science of unitary, irreducible, human beings: Update 1990. In E. A. M. Barrett (Ed.), *Visions of Rogers' science-based nursing* (Publication No. 15-2285, pp. 5–11). New York: National League for Nursing.

Roye, C. E., & Balk, S. J. (1996). Evaluation of an intergenerational program for pregnant and parenting adolescents. *Maternal-Child Nursing Journal, 24*(1), 32–40.

Sanfillipo, J. S. (1993). Dysmenorrhea in adolescents. *Female Patient, 18*, 29.

Sawyer, S. M., Blair, S., & Bowes, G. (1997). Chronic illness in adolescents: Transfer or transition to adult services? *Journal of Paediatric Child Health, 33*, 88–90.

Schack, L. E., & Neinstein, L. S. (1996). Herpes genitalis. In L. S. Neinstein (Ed.), *Adolescent health care: A practical guide* (3rd ed., pp. 349–359). Baltimore: Williams & Wilkins.

Schubiner, H. H., Lebar, W., & Jemal, C. (1990). Comparison of three new nonculture tests in the diagnosis of *Chlamydia* genital infections. *Journal of Adolescent Health Care, 11*, 505.

Schuster, M. A., Bell, R. M., Peterson, L. P., & Kanouse, D. E. (1996). Communication between adolescents and physicians about sexual behavior and risk prevention. *Archives of Pediatric & Adolescent Medicine, 150*(9), 906–913.

Schwartz, R. H., Hoffman, N. G., & Jones, R. (1987). Behavioral, psychological, and academic correlates of marijuana usage in adolescence. *Clinical Pediatrics, 26*, 264.

Shapiro, S., Slone, D., & Heinonen, O. P. (1982). Birth defects and vaginal spermicides. *Journal of the American Medical Association, 247*(17), 2381.

Siegler, A. L. (1997). *The essential guide to the new adolescence: How to raise an emotionally healthy teenager.* New York: Dutton.

Soper, D. E. (1995). Sexually transmitted diseases and pelvic inflammatory disease. In D. P. Lemcke, J. Pattison, L. A. Marshall, & D. S. Cowley (Eds.), *Primary care of women* (pp. 339–347). Norwalk, CT: Appleton & Lange.

Speroff, L., Glass, R. H., & Kase, N. G. (1994). *Clinical gynecologic endocrinology and infertility* (5th ed.). Baltimore: Williams & Wilkins.

Sprik, M., & Skillman, L. (1986). *Cervical cap: Contraceptive research analysis of behaviors from self-reported contraceptive use—diaries.* Unpublished manuscript, University of Rochester School of Nursing, Rochester, New York.

Steinhausen, H. C., & Seidel, R. (1993). Outcome in adolescent eating disorders. *International Journal of Eating Disorders, 14*, 487.

Summerhayes, L. (1995). *The cervical cap.* Los Gatos, CA: Cervical Cap.

Swedo, S. E., Rettew, D. C., Kuppenheiner, M., Lum, D., Dolan, S., Goldberger, E. (1991). Can adolescent suicide attempters be distinguished from at-risk adolescents? *Pediatrics, 88*(3), 620–629.

Tanner, J. M. (1962). *Growth at adolescence* (2nd ed.). Oxford: Blackwell Scientific Publications.

Terney, R., & McLain, L. (1990). The use of anabolic steroids in high school students. *American Journal of the Diseased Child, 144*, 99–103.

U.S. Preventive Services Task Force. (1989). *Guide to clinical preventive services: An assessment of the effectiveness of 169 interventions.* Baltimore: Williams & Wilkins.

U.S. Preventive Services Task Force. (1996). *Guide to clinical preventive services: An assessment of the effectiveness of 169 interventions* (2nd ed.). Baltimore: Williams & Wilkins.

Varney, H. (1997). *Varney's midwifery* (3rd ed.). Boston: Jones and Bartlett.

Velsor-Friedrich, B. (1994). Family violence: A growing epidemic. *Journal of Pediatric Nursing, 9*(40), 272–274.

Ventura, S. J., Martin, J. A., Taffel, S. M., Mathews, T. J., & Clarke, S. C., (1994). Advance report of final mortality statistics, 1992. *Monthly Vital Statistics Report,* vol. 43, no. 5. Hyattsville, MD: National Center for Health Statistics.

Vuorento, T., & Huhtaniemi, I. (1992). Daily levels of salivary progesterone during the menstrual cycle in adolescent girls. *Fertility & Sterility, 58*, 685.

Warburton, D., Neugut, R. H., & Lustenberger, A. (1987). Lack of association between spermicide use and trisomy. *New England Journal of Medicine, 317*(8), 478.

Wasserheit, J. N. (1992). Epidemiological synergy: Interrelationships between human immunodeficiency virus infection and other sexually transmitted diseases. *Sexually Transmitted Diseases, 19*, 61–77.

Wilson, D. M., Killen, J. D., & Hayward, C. (1994). Timing and rate of sexual maturation and the onset of cigarette and alcohol use among teenage girls. *Archives of Pediatric & Adolescent Medicine, 148*, 789.

Wren, D. J. (1997). Adolescent female "voice" changes can signal difficulties for teachers and administrators. *Adolescence, 32*(126), 463–470.

Writing Group of the 1996 Expert Panel on Women's Health (1997). Women's health and women's health care: Recommendations of the 1996 AAN Expert Panel on Women's Health. *Nursing Outlook, 45*(1), 7–15.

Wulff, M. B., & Steitz, J. A. (1997). Curricular track, career choice, and androgyny among adolescent females. *Adolescence, 32*(125), 43–49.

Younkin, E., & Davis, M. (1994). *Women's health: A primary care clinical guide.* Norwalk, CF: Appleton & Lange.

Zelnick, M., & Kantner, J. E. (1980). Sexual activity, contraceptive use, and pregnancy among metropolitan area teenagers: 1971-1979. *Family Planning Perspectives, 12*, 230.

Zenilman, J. M. (1990). Gonococcal infections in adolescents. *Adolescent Medicine: State of the Art Review, 1*, 497.

RESOURCES

Adolescent Health Links: *www.nsl.memaster.CA/tomflem/tem/health.html*
AIDS Hotline: *(800) 342-2437 (24 hours/7 days a week)*
MSN Encarta—Adolescence: *http://encarta.msn.com*
Adolescence Directory: *http://education.indiana.edu*
AMA—Adolescence Health Online: *www.ama-assn.org*
1 up Health—Puberty & Adolescence Information: *www.1uphealth.com*

Chapter 16

Women During the Reproductive Years

Michelle Teschendorf

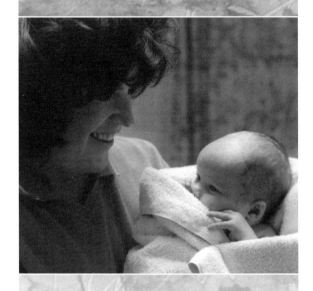

Taking joy in living is a woman's best cosmetic.

Rosalind Russell

INTRODUCTION

Women during their childbearing years are no longer restricted to a narrow range of lifestyle choices. The women's movement of the twentieth century expanded women's roles and removed role-limiting restrictions. The American family is ever evolving and changing, and at the core of most families are women (1996 American Academy of Nursing Expert Panel on Women's Health, 1997). Women are better educated and live longer, with their life expectancy at 76 years, compared with 62 years in 1940 (Peters, Kochanek, & Murphy, 1998). Women are experiencing rapidly expanding multiple roles with the ability to choose more than just a career or motherhood (Gramling, Lambert, & Pursley-Crotteau, 1998). Since 1950 the percentage of women's participation in the workforce has increased 170%, with more than half of adult women working (U.S. Department of Health and Human Services, 1998). Families are also changing and may include two parents with careers, single parenthood, mixed families, and a phenomenon known as the "sandwich generation": women who have children and older parents that need care. More options for planning reproductive choices are available. Delaying pregnancy or choosing never to have children is more common. Some life decisions can create issues in achieving and maintaining a pregnancy. Fortunately, new techniques in assistive reproductive therapies increase the ability of infertile couples to conceive. Each of these issues influences a woman's health and the health care system.

The 1994 International Conference on Population and Development in Cairo set a goal of changing the traditional biomedical view of women primarily in their reproductive role to one of women's general health needs. The expanded definition of women's health attempts to integrate health care throughout the life span, in the context of women's multiple roles and diverse social circumstances, instead of focusing on childbearing (Writing Group of the AAN Expert Panel on Women's Health, 1996). This biopsychosocial perspective broadens the view of women's health care to encompass health promotion, maintenance, and restoration rather than acute care. This chapter presents factors that influence women's health during their reproductive years from the perspective of health promotion and disease prevention.

Women ages 15 to 44 make up more than 44% of the female population in the United States, and 30% of that population is comprised of women in the older cohort, ages 20 to 44. The population of women in their reproductive years is estimated to continue to decline as the "boomers" reach mid-life (National Women's Law Center, 2000.)

A woman's age influences her ability to assimilate knowledge, adopt healthy behaviors, and access care. One of the largest health concerns for women in their reproductive years is reproductive control. Contraceptive choices vary as women move through different stages of their reproductive life. Although contraceptives protect women from pregnancy, many of them do not protect them against sexually transmitted diseases (STDs). The prevalence of STDs in reproductive women is increasing because of lifestyle choices of unprotected sex, multiple partners, and the early onset of sexual activity (Morin, 1998b). Other lifestyle choices that influence women's health are smoking, alcohol consumption, and use of illicit drugs, and, according to the Centers for Disease Control and Prevention (1998), these habits are increasing in young women.

The dramatic fall in maternal and infant mortality and morbidity rates over the past 100 years has been attributed to hospital births. However, women are increasingly unhappy with the medical model of childbirth (Craft, 1997). In response, most obstetrical units are open to family and friends, with deliveries occurring in homelike settings. Nurse practitioners and midwifery services are increasing. However, most of women's health care is still delivered by physicians.

Mortality rates for women have decreased significantly since the legalization of abortions in the United States in 1973, but problems continue to exist related to access to such services. Levels of public funding and interpretation of the law influence who can obtain an abortion. In the United States, federal funding for abortions is prohibited, affecting poor, young women in particular. Women are pursuing higher education and careers and delaying marriage and reproduction. Women in their reproductive years have more freedom and choices than ever before. The lifestyle choices made during the reproductive years definitely affect women's present and future health.

This chapter presents common options associated with reproductive choices, preconceptual planning for pregnancy, pregnancy, choosing to remain childless, choosing to terminate a pregnancy, choosing to pursue infertility work, and adoption. The last section covers the more common gynecological conditions affecting reproductive function. First, the chapter examines contextual issues influencing choices of family and single life from the perspective of health promotion and disease prevention.

HEALTH PROMOTION AND DISEASE PREVENTION

Social and economic influences are guiding health care to a community-based, preventative model. Other factors that influence preventative health care in women include age, environment, lifestyle, health behaviors, culture and ethnicity, and education.

Women may tend to ignore their own needs, placing others first. They may see the importance of changing unhealthy behaviors but may lack the skills and information to make these changes. Other barriers to change are limited time and willpower (Tessaro et al., 1998). Motivation and social support are important factors in changing lifestyle patterns. Nurses have a great opportunity to influence women's health because their focus is primarily on health care promotion, particularly for advanced practice nurses (Spatz, 1996).

Trying to juggle family and career responsibilities can lead to stress and sleep deprivation. Time management, proper nutrition, exercise, management of stress, and rest are the secrets to good health. Health care providers can foster health prevention and promotion through sensitivity to women's needs, education, and enhancement of access to care. Empowering women to be active participants in their care provides a sense of self-worth and self-esteem.

Access to health care is a problem for many women. Currently primary preventive services for women are below the recommended levels (Rafferty, 1998). Besides access, the cost of heath care may place some women in a position of economic distress, thus preventing them from seeking health care. Using advanced practice nurses as primary care providers can be effective in providing a variety of health care services for women at reduced cost.

Family Issues

General systems theory can be applied to families. A system can be defined as a complex of elements in mutual interaction. Each individual family member is a system and a subsystem (Wright & Leahey, 1994). Families are ever changing and dynamic. Therefore as families change, society changes because each is a system interacting with the other.

Today the many types of families can be classified into three groups: traditional, nontraditional, and high-risk. The traditional family has two parents that are married; however, within the last 50 years this type of family has been on the decline. Traditional families can be single or dual income. Nontraditional families include single parent, blended, adopted, unmarried couples with children, multigenerational, and homosexual parents. Healthy families are able to adapt to changes in the family unit. Those families that cannot change or are under severe stress are considered high-risk. Stress factors include divorce or marital conflict, adolescent parenting, violence, substance abuse, or a child with special needs.

Women in the reproductive years are also in their prime for establishing careers. They may have older parents that need attention and care beside their own immediate family. Having children at this stage may add stress and time management concerns. Balancing multiple roles is an issue for this age group. The nurse must be cognizant of assessing the role of family within a women's life and the role the woman plays in the life of the family. The two are highly interactive. Caregiving may at times be a welcomed or unwelcomed burden.

Single Women

Women today have a choice to remain single, and many become single after divorce. Although single women report contentment, many experience feelings of loss and grief (Lewis & Moon, 1997). They are aware of the advantages and the drawbacks of remaining single. Although enjoying the freedom to dictate their lifestyles, women trying to cope with a single household may face various stressors. Besides functioning as homemakers and caregivers, they may be the sole providers for the family's financial needs. Single-parent families are more likely to live below the poverty level, which places them at risk.

Single does not always mean being alone. Many single women have children or other family responsibilities. Single women make up 18% of the heads of household in the United States today (U.S. Census Bureau, 1999).

Childless by Choice

Being child-free is an alternative to the cultural belief of procreation. Many women are comfortable with their lifestyles and self-confident about the choice to remain childless. Besides lifestyle, overpopulation and its effects on the environment can be a concern to some individuals. Couples that choose to remain childless often are pressured by family and friends to become parents. Some of the issues with which they may be confronted are selfishness, loneliness in old age, and workplace conflicts such as taking up slack for parents (Heaton, Jacobson, & Holland, 1999).

Lesbians

Increasing numbers of women are identifying themselves as lesbians. Fear and unpleasantness are stumbling blocks to seeking obstetrical and gynecological care (Zeidenstein, 1990). Sensitive providers eliminate heterosexual assumptions when taking a health history. Typical questions such as marital status, sexual activity, and birth control may need to be eliminated.

Many lesbian couples desire children and seek assistance in obtaining them. Discrimination and insensitivity to their needs often leads to substandard care (Lucas, 1991). For the lesbian, attempting pregnancy can be accomplished through therapeutic donor insemination. The sperm can come from a sperm bank or a known donor.

Another choice is having intercourse with a male who is aware of the lesbian's desire to have children. As with heterosexual women, attempting to achieve pregnancy is characterized by stress. Support for these women tends to come from peers instead of family. Biopsychosocial support and guidance through this process allows the couple to achieve pregnancy and establish parenting roles.

COMPREHENSIVE ASSESSMENT

Assessments for reproductive age women are similar to assessments for adolescent, mid-life, and elder women. Pregnancy-related assessment is discussed in more detail in the following sections. Also refer to Chapter 8 on health history and Chapter 10 on physical assessment for information on a comprehensive assessment of women.

Box 16-1 presents key items for assessing women during their reproductive years.

Preconceptual Health

Preventive health care has been identified as an effective measure for improving health. The relatively new field of preconceptual health care focuses on women during their childbearing years who are not pregnant but desire pregnancy in the near future. In addition, men should be encouraged to seek assessment because male factors become intrinsic in pregnancy outcomes. Preconceptual health promotion focuses on identifying women's reproductive risks before pregnancy, whereas counseling provides the safest environment for discussing a developing fetus (Nasso, 1997). The purpose of preconceptual health promotion is to reduce pregnancy morbidity and poor outcomes, thereby improving infant morbidity and mortality rates. Preconceptual care has the potential to improve the overall health status of women and their families.

The basic components of preconceptual care are (1) appropriate and ongoing risk assessments, (2) health promotion and education, and (3) medical and psychosocial interventions and follow-up (Summers & Price, 1993). Prenatal care and interventions usually begin too late for the most critical period in fetal development, which is the first 60 days after conception. Some medical conditions, medicines, diets, occupational exposures, or social practices may have consequences in those early weeks of pregnancy. To maximize the opportunity for a healthy baby, women in the reproductive age group should receive the information necessary to make informed decisions about their reproductive futures.

All women who can become pregnant and present for care are candidates for preconceptual care, which is most effective as part of primary care visits for well-woman care or other conditions. At every visit a women of childbearing age should be screened for current or future pregnancies.

Preconceptual care begins with a basic history and physical examination that is the same standard of care for all adult women. Assessment of lifestyle risks is appropriate, with counseling for modification. Risks may include smoking, alcohol intake, lack of exercise, poor nutrition, use of illegal drugs, unprotected sex, and exposure to chemicals in the workplace and home. Medical conditions to be identified include diabetes, hypertension, anemia, sexually transmitted diseases, heart or kidney conditions, and

Box 16-1 ASSESSMENT DURING THE REPRODUCTIVE YEARS

History	*Physical Exam*	*Laboratory Tests*	*Risk Assessment*	*Immunizations*
Medical history: Diabetes, hypertension, anemia, and sexually transmitted diseases	Height and weight	Pap smear as indicated	Exposure to chemicals in workplace and at home; tobacco, alcohol, and drug use; illegal drug use	Tetanus/diphtheria booster every 10 years
Review of systems to determine signs or symptoms of cancer, heart disease, kidney disease, or chronic disease	Visual acuity	Mammogram as indicated	Symptoms of physical or emotional abuse	Rubella vaccine as indicated
	Oral cavity exam	Rubella titer as indicated; Rh factor, hematocrit, and hemoglobin	Symptoms of depression, suicide, and abnormal bereavement	Hepatitis B
	Palpation of thyroid and breast exam	Nonfasting total blood cholesterol every 5 years or more frequently as indicated	Evidence of social isolation	Influenza annually if high risk
	Cardiovascular and respiratory assessments	Fasting blood glucose as indicated	Symptoms of emotional abuse or physical abuse	Pneumococcal vaccine if high risk
Obstetrical/ gynecological history: Age of menarche, menstrual history, age of first coitus, consensual/ nonconsensual sex, sexual practices, safe sex practices, STDs*, contraception, number of partners, and sexual orientation	Skin exam	Urinalysis as indicated	Symptoms of increased stress	
	Lymph node exam	Pregnancy test as indicated	Risk factors of STDs; unintended pregnancy; high-risk pregnancy	
	Pelvic exam	Tuberculosis skin test in high-risk women	Driving a motor vehicle	
	Rectal exam	STD screening*: GC*, syphillis, chlamydia, VDRL*, HIV* counseling and testing, hepatitis B; urinalysis for protein and sugar	Regular exercise and dietary intake	
Surgical history		Pap smear	Excessive or deficient dietary intake; sun/ ultraviolet light exposure	
Family history: Breast and ovarian cancer, cardiovascular disease, diabetes, mental status, coping strategies, family assessment, and role assessment		Vision screening	Evidence of social isolation and increased stress	
		Pregnancy test	Prevention strategies	
			Use of smoke detector in home	
			Use of seat belts in motor vehicles; use of helmets on skateboards	
			Prevention or cessation of tobacco, alcohol, and drug use	

Box 16-1 ASSESSMENT DURING THE REPRODUCTIVE YEARS

History	*Physical Exam*	*Laboratory Tests*	*Risk Assessment*	*Immunizations*
Current medications, prescriptions, and over-the-counter drugs Self-care Dietary intake Regular exercise Tobacco, alcohol, or drug use Psychosocial history: History of child abuse or neglect, domestic violence, emotional or physical abuse by parents			Limiting alcohol intake Avoiding being a passenger in a car driven by someone under the influence of alcohol Regular exercise program Dietary plan: Restriction of fat, cholesterol; adequate intake of iron and calcium; maintenance of balanced diet Avoidance of bingeing and purging for weight control Teaching breast self-exam Teaching signs and symptoms of cancer and cardiovascular disease Discussing osteoporosis prevention Discussing contraception STD* risk reduction Violent behavior; ways to reduce risk Available resources Sunlight and ultraviolet light Discussing stress reduction in employment Assessing workplace environmental safety	

*STD, sexually transmitted disease; GC, gonorrhea culture; VDRL, venereal disease reference laboratory; HIV, human immunodeficiency virus.

any other chronic disease. Management of these problems improves pregnancy outcomes. The preconceptual period also is ideal for identifying genetic risks and counseling prospective couples. Routine laboratory testing includes Rh factor, rubella titer, hematocrit and hemoglobin, syphilis, hepatitis B, urine for protein and sugar,

Papanicolaou (Pap) smear, and gonococcal culture (Summers & Price, 1993). Human immunodeficiency virus testing and illicit drug screening may be offered. Other laboratory testing may be necessary for medical conditions or genetic screening.

A holistic approach to preconception care includes helping the women or couples to identify psychological readiness. Preconception care also educates couples about the average length of time to conceive and the optimal time to conceive. A general assessment of mental status, coping mechanisms, and stress management may be included with referrals to the appropriate resources. The timing of a pregnancy is a concern for some women. Family and work obligations can influence a woman's decision to attempt conception.

Cultural values and beliefs can guide health practices. By recognizing and understanding the differences and ethnic influences, appropriate care can be provided (Doswell & Erlen, 1998). Specific preconceptual care is based on the health beliefs of each culture. Strategies to promote culturally sensitive care encompass cultural assessments, education, and awareness regarding ethical issues of diversity.

All women of reproductive age should have access to prepregnancy assessment. Often the women with the greatest need for health care services have barriers in accessing care. Programs in women's shelters, youth centers, public clinics, and abuse treatment centers are providing alternatives to preconceptual care. Many health care organizations also offer educational programs focused on preconceptual care. The settings vary from hospitals and clinics to work and community sites.

Nutrition

Reproductive outcomes have been linked to women's nutritional status. A lower than recommended intake of essential nutrients during preconception and the prenatal period increases the incidence of major congenital anomalies (Hally, 1998). Often optimal nutritional well-being is difficult to maintain. Most American women do not obtain the Recommended Daily Allowance (RDA) of essential minerals and vitamins in their diets. Daily vitamin and mineral supplements have been suggested as a means to improve the health of some women.

Preconceptional folate supplementation has a strong protective effect against neural tube defects (Berry et al., 1999). If folic acid is started before pregnancy, the chances of a baby having a neural tube defect decrease by at least 50 percent. Increasing folate in the diet can be done with orange juice, leafy green vegetables, and beans. However, diet alone is not adequate enough to prevent neural tube defects. Therefore it is recommended that 400 µg of synthetic folic acid be taken daily. Unfortunately, not enough women of reproductive age are aware of the need for an increase in folate. As a public service, the March of Dimes launched a campaign in 1999 to increase public awareness of the need for folic acid preconceptually and during pregnancy. Neural tube defects can be serious birth defects that may be preventable with the intake of folic acid.

Weight

Neither an excessive or suboptimal amount of body fat appears to be healthy (Hally, 1998). Underweight women of reproductive age may have abnormal menstrual function or infertility. Inadequate nutrition during pregnancy has been associated with low-birth-weight infants (Doyle, Crawford, Srivastava, & Costeloe, 1999). Obese individuals are at risk for hypertension, diabetes, cardiovascular disease, reproductive cancers, and preeclampsia during pregnancy (Morin, 1998a).

The insurance industry has developed standard height and weigh charts to determine eligibility and coverage risks. These charts have become guidelines for normal weights (Table 16-1).

Although these tables have been revised, many diseases are too complex to use height and weight alone as determining health risk factors.

Body mass index (BMI), waist-to-hip ratio, and waist circumference are other measurements used to guide health care management. BMI is a ratio between weight and height and is a better predictor of disease. Calculating BMI is done by (1) multiplying weight (in pounds) by 703, (2) multiplying height (in inches) by height (in inches), and (3) dividing the product in (1) by the product in (2). An increase in BMI is associated with an increase in health risks (Table 16-2).

A waist-to-hip ratio greater than 0.8 in women and a waist circumference greater than 39 inches are significant for an increased risk. Individuals with an excessive accumulation of abdominal fat have been shown to have a significantly higher risk of coronary artery disease and type 2 diabetes (Pouliot et al., 1994).

Table **16-1** **HEIGHT AND WEIGHT TABLE FOR WOMEN**[*]

HEIGHT	SMALL FRAME[†]	MEDIUM FRAME[†]	LARGE FRAME[†]
4'10''	102-111	109-121	118-131
4'11''	103-113	111-123	120-134
5'0''	104-115	113-126	122-137
5'1''	106-118	115-129	125-140
5'2''	108-121	118-132	128-143
5'3''	111-124	121-135	131-147
5'4''	114-127	124-138	134-151
5'5''	117-130	127-141	137-155
5'6''	120-133	130-144	140-159
5'7''	123-136	133-147	143-163
5'8''	126-139	136-150	146-167
5'9''	129-142	139-153	149-170
5'10''	132-145	142-156	152-173
5'11''	135-148	145-159	155-176
6'0''	138-151	148-162	158-179

Source: Metropolitan Life Insurance Company, 1999.
[*]Weights at ages 25 to 59 are based on lowest mortality.
[†]Weight in pounds according to frame (indoor clothing weighing 3 pounds; shoes with 1-inch heels).

Table **16-2**   **HEALTH RISK ASSOCIATED WITH BODY MASS INDEX**

BMI CATEGORY	HEALTH RISK BASED SOLELY ON BMI	RISK ADJUSTED FOR THE PRESENCE OF COMORBID CONDITIONS OR RISK FACTORS
19-24	Minimal	Low
25-26	Low	Moderate
27-29	Moderate	High
30-34	High	Very High
35-39	Very High	Extremely High
40+	Extremely High	Extremely High

Source: Shape Up America! (1996). *Guidance for treatment of adult obesity*. Retrieved from *www.shapeup.org*.

Exercise

Exercise can have a positive influence on health promotion by increasing cardiovascular performance, strengthening the musculoskeletal system, and improving psychological status. Although physical and mental benefits of exercise are supported by health professionals, more than 60% of U.S. adults do not engage in the recommended amount of activity, with 25% not active at all (U.S. Department of Health and Human Services, 1996). Regular exercise patterns should be established at a young age and should continue throughout life; however, this is not currently the norm. Motivation to exercise comes from a belief that exercise is beneficial to one's health and a lack of perceived barriers to being physically active. Physical inactivity is more prevalent among women than men. Physical activity does not need to be vigorous or intense to improve health. However, benefits appear to be proportional to the amount of physical activity. An increase in activity adds benefits, so emphasizing the amount rather than the intensity of physical activity allows more options in selecting an activity that can be incorporated into women's daily lives.

Many young women cite a lack of personal time because of other obligations, such as work and family, as a hindrance to routine exercise. Women may be able to reach the recommended guidelines for physical activity with a combination of household, occupational, and leisure activities done in multiple short intervals rather than an intense daily workout (Wilbur, Miller, Montgomery, & Chandler, 1998). Because of current lifestyles, these frequent, short intervals of physical activity may be more appropriate for women. Through a modest increase in daily activity, most women can improve their health.

Current recommendations advise that physical activity should be an accumulation of moderate intensity totaling 30 minutes on most, if not all, days of the week (U.S. Department of Health and Human Services, 1996). Previously sedentary women should start with a short duration of physical activity (5 minutes) and build slowly to their desired level of exercise. Support from other persons may help to increase and maintain regular exercise. *Healthy People 2010* objectives encourage the individual and the community to be a part of improving the nation's overall health through physical activity (U.S. Department of Health an^d Human Services, 2000). Besides encouraging regular exercise, health care providers can establish exercise programs within health care settings and work sites.

During the reproductive years, women will have bone loss associated with osteoporosis beginning at age 30 (Wilbur, Miller, Montgomery, & Chandler, 1998). Resistance and endurance activities are recommended for cardiovascular and musculoskeletal health of this age group. Endurance activities are those in which bones and muscles work against gravity. Walking, stair climbing, bicycling, dancing, running, and racket sports are weight-bearing activities. Resistance exercises, such as lifting weight, are particularly effective for increasing muscle and bone strength. Both types of exercise increase bone density and should be alternated. Loss of bone mass can occur in pregnant women at risk who are placed on long-term bed rest. Returning to exercise reverses the effects of bed rest on bones. However, while on bed rest, these women need exercise to minimize bone loss.

Exercise during pregnancy and postpartum should be individualized according to each woman's health. Only obstetrical or medical complications prevent women from participating in an exercise program. Most guidelines of a general fitness program can be adapted for pregnant women (American College of Obstetricians and Gynecologists, 1994b). Mild to moderate regular exercise is preferred over intermittent activity with minimal risk for the woman or the fetus. Fetal heart rates rise 5 to 25 beats per minute during maternal exercise (Riemann & Kanstrup Hansen, 2000). Non–weight-bearing exercises rather than weight-bearing exercises seem better fitted to the physiological changes during pregnancy. After the first trimester, vigorous exercise, prolonged standing, and lying supine should be avoided because of changes in the circulatory system. Also maternal heart rate and body temperature may increase with exercise. However, a lack of evidence for any harmful effects of exercise on pregnancy indicates healthy women may exercise during pregnancy safely with few restrictions. During the 4-to 6-week postpartum period, prepregnancy exercise routines should be resumed gradually until normal physiological condition returns.

Immunizations

Preventable illnesses put a strain on the economy, medical resources, and work environment. Immunizations reduce the incidence of vaccine-preventable diseases. *Healthy People 2010* made immunizations one of the priority areas for national health promotion and disease prevention. Unfortunately, 60,000 to 80,000 Americans die every year from vaccine-preventable diseases (Droste, 1998). Advanced practice nurses providing primary care are in a position to decrease the spread of communicable diseases through vaccinations. Integrating immunization into women's health during the reproductive years is essential. Because of childhood immunizations, women in their reproductive years should be immune to measles, rubella, mumps, tetanus, diphtheria, hepatitis B, and polio (American College of Obstetricians and Gynecologists and American Academy of Pediatrics, 1997).

Routine use of immunizations during pregnancy is not recommended because of the low likelihood of exposure, the risk of disease to the woman or fetus, and risk from the vaccine itself (Hackley, 1999). Instead, preconceptional immunization of women to prevent disease during their pregnancy is preferred. Table 16-3 gives recommendations

Table 16-3 | **ADULT IMMUNIZATION SCHEDULE**

VACCINE	RECOMMENDED PRECONCEPTION	RECOMMENDED DURING PREGNANCY
Chickenpox (varicella)	Contraindicated 1 month before pregnancy	Contraindicated during pregnancy
Hepatitis A	—	Contraindicated during pregnancy
Hepatitis B	—	Data not available on the safety to fetus; however, vaccine contains only noninfectious hepatitis B surface antigen and should not be contraindicated if a woman is otherwise eligible
Influenza (flu)	—	Maybe given if woman is at risk
Mumps, measles, and rubella (MMR)	Contraindicated 3 months before pregnancy	Contraindicated during pregnancy
Pneumococcal	—	The safety for pregnant women has not been evaluated; vaccine should be given only if the risk of infection is high
Tetanus-diphtheria (Td)	—	Safe during first trimester; may be given during second and third trimesters if necessary

Modified from Centers for Disease Control and Prevention. (1997). *Recommendations of the Advisory Committee on Immunization Practices*. Washington, DC: Department of Health and Human Services.

for immunization preconceptionally and during pregnancy. Also Chapter 13 discusses immunizations.

Contraception and Family Planning

Reproductive control is an issue that has affected women for thousands of years; today women have a range of options that are safe and effective. No one method of contraception suits everyone, and all methods have advantages and disadvantages. Birth control methods range from over-the-counter condoms and vaginal spermicides to doctor-prescribed medication, devices, and surgical procedures (see Chapter 15).

Information about contraceptives is important for women for preventing unintended pregnancies and reducing the risk of sexually transmitted diseases. According to the National Women's Law Center (2000), 50% of pregnancies in the United States are unplanned. Women 20 to 24 years of age are no more likely to use contraceptives than adolescents and actually have a higher rate of unintended pregnancies and abortions (Abma, Chandra, Mosher, Peterson, & Piccinino, 1997). The tendency is to focus on teenagers while neglecting the concerns and experiences of young adult women. This age group needs guidance, support, and education to meet family planning needs.

Contraceptive practices during the reproductive years usually focus on the female or male partner. However, contraceptive use is influenced by the dynamics of each relationship (Glei, 1999). Women in unstable relationships and changing partners are less likely to plan contraceptive use. Another concern with long-term use of contraceptives is cost. Many women do not have health care insurance. Even for those who do, not all health care plans cover oral contraceptives. Out-of-pocket expenses for contraception are costly for women. A proposal titled Equity in Prescription Insurance and Contraceptive Coverage has been introduced in the U.S. Congress, but Congress has not acted on the bill.

HEALTH MAINTENANCE

At the beginning of the twentieth century women were viewed as an extension of men. "Female" problems were of little concern to the male-dominated medical field. Medical research was conducted on men, and the findings were applied to women. Women's health was equated to reproduction (Weisman, 1997). In 1920 women won the right to vote, but women did not become politically prominent until the women's movement reemerged in the late 1960s and early 1970s. The women's liberation movement helped to remove the barriers to education and jobs. The 1990s have been labeled the decade of women's health (Quimby, 1994). Women can admit freely that they are different and yet have overlapping qualities with men. They are taking charge of their medical care and have the ability, knowledge, and confidence to influence overall health care. Women consider family life, physical life, work life, psychological health, practical difficulties, and social life the components of health (Shaw, Brickley, Evans, & Edwards, 1998).

Women's health encompasses a broad spectrum of issues and is no longer focused solely on pregnancy. Many of those issues deal with the reproductive system and potential problems. It is essential that advanced practice nurses be knowledgeable and skilled in the care of women, ensuring care and enhancing the quality of women's lives. The role of advanced practice nurses varies depending on their education, clinical experience, and written practice agreements (Engstrom et al., 1999). Along with assessment, diagnosis, and treatment of various women's health conditions, an advanced practice nurse can manage or comanage treatment and follow-up care. The next section examines conditions unique to reproductive-age women.

PREGNANCY

Normally, pregnancy and childbirth are natural occurrences, but complications arise in 8% to 10% of pregnancies. The single most important factor in improving maternal and infant health is proper prenatal care, yet the United States remains one of only two industrialized nations that have yet to ensure universal health care for pregnant women (Bonifield, 1998). Early and continuing risk assessments, health promotion, and medical and psychosocial intervention with follow-up are the components of adequate prenatal care (Expert Panel on the Content of Prenatal Care, 1989). One of the goals of early prenatal care is identification of health problems and health-compromising behaviors that can be harmful to the fetus during initial stages of development.

Traditionally, obstetrical care has been delivered by a physician. With expanded roles in nursing, however, women may choose an advanced practice nurse as their primary care provider. Nurse practitioners and midwives deliver comprehensive prenatal care to women throughout their pregnancies in collaboration with other members of the health care team. Nurses play a significant role in the promotion of a healthy pregnancy.

Psychosocial Adaptations

Adapting to the maternal role is a complex social and cognitive process that is learned rather than intuitive. Reva Rubin (1984) wrote about certain tasks a woman must accomplish to prepare for the maternal role. These tasks include ensuring a safe passage for herself and child; ensuring social acceptance of the child by significant others; increasing ties in the construction of the identity and image of *I* and *you*; and exploring the meaning of the acts of giving and receiving. Gradually the woman must work through each of these tasks to adapt to the pregnancy. Each woman is unique in her manner of adaptation and is influenced by social and cultural factors.

Stressors influence the woman's ability to adapt and complete the tasks of her pregnancy. These stressors change as the pregnancy progresses, suggesting a need to tailor prenatal care to the different phases of childbearing. Typically, in the first trimester the woman deals with uncertainty and ambivalence with a focus on herself. The fetus becomes the primary focus during the second trimester with concerns of body image. During the third trimester, many women become dependent and vulnerable as preparations for the birth become the focus. Although the postpartum period seems focused on the newborn, developing an attachment to the baby begins early in the pregnancy and continues after the birth as bonding takes place.

Women also experience multiple worries during pregnancy, such as the baby's welfare, physical symptoms, emotional changes, body image changes, labor and birth, the relationship with the baby's father, and newborn behaviors (Affonso, Liu-Chiang, & Mayberry, 1999). The ability to cope with worry is influenced by personality, coping styles, spirituality, and cultural and social influences, (Johnson, 2002). Primary care nurses have an opportunity to provide support and education to expectant women as they progress through these developmental stages.

Cultural Concerns for Childbearing

Nurses are recognizing the importance of understanding the beliefs, values, and health practices of different cultures and how they influence health care. Interactions between persons of different cultures can be complicated by a lack of mutual understanding. Bringing new life into the world is part of every culture as a family adds a new member and generation. The birth strengthens cultural traditions and unifies families. This concept brings pregnancy and childbirth into the center of many cultural beliefs that may be less obvious in other settings (American College of Obstetricions and Gynecologists, 1998). Each culture has its own traditional beliefs and practices pertinent to childbearing. Key issues for industrial countries include impersonal medical care, marital instability, isolation of the nuclear family, economic pressure for mothers to work, deficiency of child care, and ambiguity in the definition of parental roles. Key issues for developing countries include poverty, malnutrition, family disruption, illiteracy, high rates of maternal and infant mortality, prostitution, and poor access to health care. These key issues affect the traditional beliefs and practices related to childbearing.

Achieving cultural competency involves an awareness and acceptance of cultural differences. Any approach to culturally sensitive care for women and their families must focus on the interaction between cultural meaning and biological function (Leininger, 1990). Beliefs about health, medical care, reproduction, and the role and status of women influence a society's view of childbirth and the formation of a family. At the same time, individual differences exist within cultures. How medical care is perceived and accessed, roles of the family members, pregnancy care, birth practices including recuperation, and infant feeding and care are issues to be discussed with pregnant women and their families. Every effort should be made to accommodate each person's beliefs and traditions.

Confirming Pregnancy and Assessment

Confirmation of pregnancy is based on signs and symptoms that can be divided into three categories: presumptive, probable, and positive evidence. Presumptive and probable evidence cannot confirm a pregnancy, whereas positive evidence can. The presumptive evidences of pregnancy are the subjective signs and symptoms women experience. Many of these symptoms can be caused by conditions other than pregnancy, making them the least reliable indicators of pregnancy. Probable evidence of pregnancy is objective data that can be obtained on examination. Most of these signs are related to the physical changes in the reproductive organs. Although these signs indicate a strong diagnosis of pregnancy, they can be false findings. Positive signs of pregnancy are present only with pregnancy. Table 16-4 lists signs and symptoms of pregnancy.

Normal gestation is 280 days (40 weeks) from the first day of the mother's last menstrual period or 266 days (38 weeks) from actual conception. Because actual ovulation is usually unknown, the delivery date is an approximation and is referred to as an estimated date of confinement. Normally the fundus enlarges at a predictable rate, which is approximately 1 cm per week of gestation. Measuring fundal height allows the provider to observe for normal growth and possible complications. Fundal height is measured from the symphysis pubis to the top of the fundus. The uterus should be palatable above the symphysis pubis between the twelfth and fourteenth weeks of gestation. By the twenty-second to the twenty-fourth weeks the uterus should be at the umbilicus. At term, the top of the fundus is close to the xiphoid process, until the fetus drops in the pelvis and becomes engaged. If a discrepancy occurs or the last menstrual period is unknown, an estimated gestational age can be determined by ultrasound. The earlier in a pregnancy, the more accurate are the dates, with the best results being in the first and second trimesters.

Risk Assessment

Initial and ongoing risk assessments are important components in prenatal care. Risk assessments include a comprehensive history, a thorough physical examination, and

Table **16-4**   **SIGNS AND SYMPTOMS OF PREGNANCY**

SIGNS	SYMPTOMS
Presumptive Evidence	
■ Amenorrhea	■ Nausea and vomiting
■ Abdominal enlargement and striae	■ Fatigue
■ Breast changes and tenderness	■ Weight gain
■ Vaginal mucosa discoloration (Chadwick sign)	■ Urinary frequency
■ Skin pigmentation	■ Constipation
	■ Quickening
Probable Evidence	
■ Cervical softening (Goodell sign)	Same as presumptive symptoms
■ Uterine changes:	
Softening of isthmus (Hegar sign)	
Ballottement	
Braxton-Hicks contractions	
■ Lab testing:	
Home pregnancy tests for human chorionic gonadotropin in maternal urine	
Serum human chorionic gonadotropin levels	
Radioimmunoassay	
Positive Evidence	
■ Auscultation of fetal heart sounds	—
■ Visualization of fetus by ultrasonography	
■ Fetal movement detected by examiner	

laboratory testing. The goal of these assessments is to identify women and fetuses at risk for developing complications. Results from laboratory tests can provide the primary care provider with information on chronic conditions such as diabetes, anemia, and hypertension; communicable diseases such as STDs, rubella, and hepatitis B; and genetic conditions such as spina bifida, Down syndrome, or other chromosomal abnormalities. This information provides the bases of assessment for possible risks of pregnancy complications. Besides ongoing assessments, genetic counseling may be appropriate. As the knowledge of genome mapping and its implication increases, more persons may have the need for genetic counseling. The purposes of counseling are (1) to advise couples before conception of the probability of an infant with a genetic disorder, (2) to advise couples after conception and fetal screening of whether a genetic disorder is found in the fetus(s), and (3) to inform couples of the options that are available to them (Chadwick, 1993).

Prenatal Care Schedule

In an uncomplicated pregnancy, approximately a dozen office visits will occur. Every visit is an opportunity for continued risk assessment, physical assessment, and education. After the initial visit, women should be examined approximately every 4 weeks until 28 weeks of gestation, every 2 to 3 weeks until 36 weeks of gestation, and weekly thereafter. Any medical or obstetric problems may require more frequent visits (American Academy of Pediatrics & American College of Obstetricians and Gynecologists, 1992). Box 16-2 provides a guide to the timing of screening procedures that may occur during each visit.

Prenatal records should contain all the data gathered during pregnancy in a systematic form. Most health care providers use some type of preprinted prenatal form to record all the information. These forms are available commercially or can be

---

Box 16-2 SCREENING PROCEDURES FOR HEALTH CARE VISITS DURING PREGNANCY

Initial Prenatal Visit
1. Complete medical and reproductive history.
2. Physical assessment including vital signs, weight, height, urine dipstick for albumin, glucose, and ketones. Abdominal exam with fetal heart rate, fetal movements, and fundal height. As fundus elevates out of the pelvis, it can be palpated just above the symphysis pubis at approximately 12 weeks. Eventually the fundus will rise to the level of the umbilicus at about 20 weeks and the xiphoid process near term. Pelvic exam with Pap smear, gonorrhea culture, and chlamydia testing.
   - ■ Nutritional assessment.
   - ■ Family history.
   - ■ History of current pregnancy, calculate estimated date of confinement.
   - ■ Psychosocial assessment.
3. Laboratory testing including pregnancy test, complete blood count, blood type and Rh, serology (RPR or VDRL), rubella, hepatitis B surface antigen, urinalysis, PPD (tuberculosis test). Offer HIV testing.

Ongoing Visits
Update history, including signs and symptoms of preterm labor.

Completed With Every Visit
Physical assessment, including vital signs, weight, urine dipstick for albumin, glucose, and ketones, fetal heart rate, fetal movements, fundal height, and Leopold maneuvers for fetal position.

First 12 Weeks
Perform chorionic villus sampling if a risk of inherited genetic disorders exists.

15-20 Weeks
1. Maternal serum alpha-fetoprotein.
2. Ultrasound screening.
3. Amniocentesis (may be done as early as 12 weeks).

24-28 Weeks
One-hour glucose tolerance test.

28-36 Weeks
1. Group beta strep culture at 36 weeks.
2. If woman is Rh negative, determine blood group antigen at 28 weeks.
3. Cervical exam at 36 weeks.

36-40 Weeks
1. Cervical exam.
2. Repeat laboratory testing as necessary.

developed by each institution or group. The forms should contain maternal health and obstetrical history, physical assessment, laboratory work done during the pregnancy, findings of each visit, and any other pertinent data. A copy of this record (as current as possible) needs to be available to the labor and delivery staff when the woman presents for delivery. This provides the staff with baseline knowledge of this woman and her pregnancy and allows them to deliver competent care.

Common Discomforts and Treatments

Pregnancy is a normal phenomenon; however, each woman adapts to pregnancy in her own way. Maternal physiological changes are caused by hormones and the physical changes arising from the growing uterus and other tissue. These changes have the potential to cause discomfort. Pregnancy education can provide women with knowledge of common discomforts and physical changes along with possible treatments. Table 16-5 lists common discomforts during pregnancy and possible treatments.

Fetal Assessment

One of the goals of prenatal care is to have as healthy a baby as possible. Fetal assessments are central to this goal. If changes in fetal conditions are noted, interventions can be implemented. The following are fetal assessment techniques.

Fetal Movement

Fetal movement is a reassuring sign. Normally a health fetus has 10 perceivable movements within 60 minutes (Lommel, 1990). Fetal assessment begins with the mother. The health care provider should instruct the mother to observe fetal movements throughout the day. If fetal activity seems less than usual, the women should be instructed to have something to drink or eat and then to rest in a quiet room while observing for fetal activity. The perception of four or more fetal movements in a 30-minute period is considered normal (Sadovsky, 1985). If fewer than four movements occur, observation should continue because movement is influenced by many factors, including fetal sleep cycles, maternal blood glucose levels, gestational age, maternal medications, maternal smoking, and maternal exercise. If fetal movement continues to be decreased or weak, the woman should notify her health care provider.

Nonstress Test

A nonstress test (NST) is a noninvasive, economical method of assessing fetal well-being and may be done in an outpatient setting or at home. Using electronic fetal monitoring (EFM), the fetal heart rate is observed for accelerations. In a healthy fetus with an intact central nervous system, fetal movements are associated with fetal heart accelerations. An NST is considered reactive when a minimum of two fetal heart rate accelerations of 15 beats per minute above baseline and lasting at least 15 seconds occur within a 20-minute time (American College of Obstetricians and Gynecologists, 1994a). A reactive NST provides current information on the fetus. If the NST is nonreactive, further testing is indicated.

Table 16-5	COMMON DISCOMFORTS OF PREGNANCY AND POSSIBLE TREATMENTS
PHYSIOLOGICAL CHANGE	**TREATMENT**
Nausea and vomiting (morning sickness)	Eat small, frequent meals. Eat dry toast or crackers before arising. Avoid foods with smells that bother. Avoid rich, fatty foods, spicy foods, and greasy foods. Drink fluids separately from meals.
Heartburn	Eat small, frequent meals. Sleep with extra pillow or elevate head of bed 6 inches. Avoid caffeine. Decrease or stop smoking. Use antacids as needed. Avoid those that are high in sodium or calcium.
Urinary frequency	Empty bladder regularly. Perform Kegel exercises to promote bladder control.
Backache	Maintain correct posture. Exercise regularly. Use exercises that will strengthen the back. Squat to pick up objects rather than bend over at the waist. Get back massages. Use heating pad on the lower back.
Constipation	Drink at least eight 8-ounce glasses of water daily. Avoid caffeine and carbonated beverages. Add food high in fiber to diet. Exercise daily. Use bulk laxatives or stool softeners as needed.
Hemorrhoids	Avoid straining for bowel movements. Drink plenty of water. Increase fiber in diet. Exercise regularly. Use sitz baths or warm soaks. Use witch hazel pads or anesthetic ointments. Call health care provider for bleeding or persistent pain.
Leg cramps	Extend affected leg and flex foot inward toward leg. Elevate legs during the day to improve circulation. Do calf stretches before bed. Increase intake of calcium or potassium if needed. Use aluminum hydroxide gel caps to help absorb phosphorus and raise calcium levels if prescribed by health care provider.
Swollen ankles	Avoid standing for long periods. Keep feet elevated. Drink plenty of water. Avoid foods high in sodium.
Varicosities	Avoid constricting clothing. Refrain from crossing legs at the knees. Elevate legs as much as possible. Wear support stockings. Avoid standing for long periods.
Nosebleeds	Use humidifiers. Use saline nose drops or spray.

Oxytocin Challenge Test or Contraction Stress Test

An oxytocin challenge test (OCT) indicates the response of the fetal heart rate to the stress of uterine contractions. If the woman is not having uterine contractions, nipple stimulation or intravenously administered oxytocin is used. The fetal heart rate and uterine contractions are observed via EFM until three contractions of at least 40 seconds duration occur within 10 minutes (American College of Obstetricians and Gynecologists, 1994a). The results of OCTs are categorized as follows:

- Negative OCT (normal): No late decelerations
- Positive OCT (abnormal): Late decelerations following 50% or more of contractions even if the contraction frequency is less than three in 1 minute
- Suspicious OCT (equivocal): Intermittent, late, or significant variable deceleration
- Unsatisfactory OCT: Fewer than three contractions per 10 minutes or quality of fetal heart rate monitor tracings inadequate for interpretation.

Since the introduction of the biophysical profile, use of OCTs has decreased greatly.

Biophysical Profile

In 1980 the biophysical profile (BPP) test was introduced as a form of intrauterine Apgar scoring (Manning, Platt, & Sipos, 1980). The BPP is a noninvasive procedure using ultrasound and electronic fetal monitoring (EFM). The five criteria that make up the BPP are shown in Table 16-6.

Interpretation of the BPP is similar to that of the Apgar score, with each criterion worth either zero or 2 points for a total possible score of 10. Normal is based on a score of 8 to 10. Equivocal is a score of 6, and a score of 4 or less is considered abnormal. Some practitioners have eliminated the nonstress test (NST) portion because movement, breathing, and fetal tone mimic the NST. This is known as a modified BPP and has a total possible score of 8.

Biochemical Testing

Couples whose fetuses are at risk for genetic abnormalities because of maternal age over 35 or a family history may consider further testing. The health care provider needs to explain the benefits and risks of the procedure.

Table 16-6   BIOPHYSICAL PROFILE

	POINTS	
CRITERIA	NONE	PRESENT
Reactive nonstress test	0	2
Fetal breathing movements (one or more episodes of 30 seconds or more in 30 minutes)	0	2
Fetal movement (three or more discrete body or limb movements in 30 minutes)	0	2
Fetal tone (one or more episodes of extension with return to flexion)	0	2
Quanitiation of amniotic fluid volume (one or more pockets of 2 cm or more in two perpendicular planes)	0	2

Amniocentesis is the collection of a small amount of amniotic fluid. A needle is inserted through the abdomen and into the uterus with the guidance of ultrasound. Amniocentesis may be done as early as 12 to 14 weeks but traditionally is done at 16 weeks of gestation. During the second trimester, amniocentesis is used to identify genetic diseases or birth defects. Later amniocentesis may be to assess fetal lung maturity, to test for infections, to remove fluid because of polyhydramnios, or to perform other evaluations of the pregnancy.

During chorionic villus sampling, a small amount of the chorionic (placental) tissue is removed for genetic testing via a catheter inserted through the cervix. Chorionic villus sampling can be done between 9 and 12 weeks of gestation. Some practitioners hesitate to use chorionic villus sampling because one of the complications is limb abnormalities in the fetus.

Management

Perinatal Education

Women seek safe passage for themselves and their babies during their pregnancies. This seeking may consist of a single approach or may combine several approaches (Patterson, Freese, & Goldenberg, 1990). Expectant parents need information about pregnancy and parenthood to be able to make informed decisions, take an active role in maintaining health during pregnancy and birth, and learn coping skills to deal with pregnancy, childbirth, and parenthood. These goals are realized through the provision of specific information about the components of a healthy pregnancy, the process of childbirth, the skills and tools available to deal with the process, and initial infant care and parenting.

Childbirth classes prepare the woman for all aspects of childbirth, including complications. The woman and her coach learn coping skills to approach childbirth in a positive manner. Increased confidence gained in childbirth classes is associated with a decreased perception and increase tolerance of pain during labor and lowers the use of drugs to manage labor pain (Lowe, 1996).

Classes usually occur in a series, with information broken down into subjects. A typical childbirth schedule includes the following subjects:

1. Pregnancy, focusing on physical and psychological changes, common concerns and discomforts, possible complications, nutrition, exercise, and sexuality
2. Common antepartum testing
3. Labor and birth, concentrating on anatomy and physiology of labor, the birth process, birth plans, signs of labor, when to go to the hospital, hospital admission and procedures, recovery, and a tour of the birthing facility
4. Coping techniques for labor, centering on relaxation, breathing techniques, comfort measures, and pain relief (nonpharmacological and pharmacological)
5. Complications of pregnancy and birth, including high-risk pregnancy and cesarean section
6. Support person, including the role of the coach and coaching techniques

7. Infant care, reviewing normal characteristics, general care and safety, and feeding (bottle and breast). Separate classes may be offered on infant care and breast-feeding as well as concerns of postpartum, teaching physiological and psychological changes, postpartum blues, role adaptation, family planning, and discharge plans.

All of these subjects in one course provide a comprehensive education. Some classes may exclude a portion of this information and cover it in another setting.

The Association of Women's Health, Obstetric, and Neonatal Nurses (1993) has published guidelines for class curricula and educator competencies. Other organizations such as the American Society for Psychoprophylaxis in Obstetrics and the International Childbirth Education Association offer certification for their instructors. Certification ensures that the instructors are prepared and knowledgeable about perinatal education. Some instructors may subscribe to a certain philosophy of birth and teach their methods. Examples of birthing methods may include the Bradley method, Lamaze, or water births.

Women, as consumers of health information, have demanded expanded childbirth education. Classes are no longer limited to just labor and delivery. Education is available in all areas of pregnancy, childbirth, and parenting. Some of the types of classes being taught are preconceptional classes, early pregnancy classes, exercise classes, childbirth classes, refresher classes, cesarean birth classes, vaginal birth after cesarean classes, breast-feeding classes, parenting classes, infant care classes, and postpartum classes. Classes for siblings and grandparents help other family members prepare for the birth. Usually classes are offered at a variety of times that are convenient for the expectant mother. Through education and discussion, women and their families can begin to adapt to their new roles (Humenick, 1998).

As the couple learns about birth, they are forming ideas of their own impending experience. Some couples have specific desires for their birth. Many couples have found that writing down their goals and expectations affords them open communication with their health care professionals and provides them with a unique experience. This tool is known as a birth plan. In collaboration with health care providers, couples can develop birth plans with realistic and achievable goals. Some of the topics that may be on a birth plan are the type of birth, support persons for the mother, birth setting, birth positions, labor management, immediate care after delivery, newborn care, and postpartum care.

Nutrition During Pregnancy

Adequate nutrition throughout pregnancy supports fetal growth and maternal health. Even with adequate nutrition, repeat pregnancies less than a year apart deplete maternal nutritional reserves. Although fetal growth may be protected, maternal health may decline. Weight gain and loss before and during pregnancy are related directly to the birth weight of the infant. An ideal weight gain of 25 to 35 pounds is recommended for pregnant women in developed countries. Weight gain should not be sudden or excessive, but steady (Nichols & Zwelling, 1997). Also refer to Chapter 11 on Nutrition.

Caloric intake. The RDA for women of childbearing age is approximately 2200 calories per day. Every pregnant woman hears the phrase "eating for two"; although this may be true to an extent, caloric intake during pregnancy needs to increase only 300 calories per day. A greater increase causes a greater weight increase (Centers for Disease Control and Prevention, 1997).

Folic acid. Folic acid can reduce the occurrence of neural tube defects such as spina bifida and anencephaly by at least 50% when consumed daily before conception and during early pregnancy (Centers for Disease Control and Prevention, 1998). It is recommended that all women of childbearing age who are capable of becoming pregnant consume 400 µg of folic acid daily.

Iron. Iron deficiency is one of the most common nutritional deficiencies. An estimated 11% of nonpregnant women of childbearing age have some level of iron deficiency (Hally, 1998). Inadequate amounts of iron intake or iron stores cause women of childbearing age to be at risk for anemia. The current RDA for iron is 30 mg/day. Adequate amounts of iron are difficult to obtain from food sources, so iron supplements are given.

Zinc. Zinc is required for synthesis of deoxyribonucleic acid and ribonucleic acid and thus for protein synthesis and cell differentiation, making it essential for normal fetal growth and development. Zinc is also necessary to synthesize breast milk during lactation. The RDA for zinc in the pregnant woman is 15 mg/day.

Calcium. During pregnancy women need to protect their own bone stores and support fetal bone mineralization. One group of women particularly at high risk for bone loss and osteoporosis are those women on long-term bed rest or who are taking steroids for high-risk pregnancies. The current RDA is 1200 mg/day for calcium.

Choosing an Infant Health Care Provider

During the pregnancy, the mother should choose a health care provider for her baby's health care. Just as the woman has options in health care, so too options exist for infant care. Advanced practice nurses such as family nurse practitioners, pediatric nurse practitioners, neonatal nurse practitioners, and certified nurse-midwives may care for infants, along with pediatricians and family medicine physicians. Recommendations for a health care provider may come from the woman's provider or other resources such as friends and family. The choices of some women may be limited by their insurance to a certain list of health care providers. The woman may want to contact several choices to interview before deciding who will be delivering care to her infant. Usually this occurs in the third trimester. When she is admitted to the hospital for the birth, a provider for the infant should have been chosen.

CHILDBIRTH

Women have a variety of choices for a health care professional during pregnancy. They may choose a certified nurse midwife, nurse practitioner, obstetrician, or a family practice physician. The role that each of these providers plays is slightly different, and women need to know what to expect from each. All four groups follow women during pregnancy and the postpartum period, but nurse practitioners usually do not deliver babies. Family practice physicians, nurse practitioners, and certified nurse-midwives can care for the baby as well. The certified nurse-midwife cares for low-risk women with a physician available for referral. The certified nurse-midwife is often present through most of the labor and birth, whereas a physician usually arrives for the birth. Additional labor support may come from a doula. A doula is trained professionally to provide labor support to women and their partners during labor and birth. The doula does not get involved with clinical tasks but provides physical, emotional, and informational support.

Besides choosing a health care provider, a woman can choose where she will deliver. To make the birth an intimate experience, institutions are moving from traditional labor rooms, delivery suites, and postpartum units to labor/deliver/recovery and labor/delivery/recovery/postpartum combination rooms within hospitals and freestanding birthing centers. Home delivery continues to be an option for some women.

Support During Labor

During labor, the woman needs to have support to help her through the process. Support can come from many sources. The support person may actively participate in labor or only be present. Most often the father of the baby fills this role. However, some women desire support from other relatives or friends. Also professional labor support persons (such as a doula) are becoming available (Doulas of North America, 1999). An experienced labor support person can reduce the length of labor, minimize the need for pain medications, and decrease the need for cesarean births (Klaus, Kennell, & Klaus, 1993). Having a support person increases a woman's satisfaction with childbirth. As birth has moved from the traditional delivery rooms to homelike rooms, health care has incorporated the woman's wishes for support. Many birthing suites follow a philosophy of family-centered care.

Health care personnel are striving to encourage women to participate in their care and adapting services to meet the needs of the family. Nursing care during childbirth includes physical and emotional care as well as education on the labor process. The Coalition for Improving Maternity Services published guidelines concerning services that meet the philosophical principles of mother-friendly childbirth (Box 16-3).

Development of a birth plan can help a woman identify options and choices in her health care. The birth plan is a tool that communicates to others the wishes of the woman and her support system. By writing her desires, a woman can consider what issues are important during her childbirth and those situations she would like to avoid. Topics that may be covered in a birth plan are labor management, family and partner participation, birth choices, care immediately after delivery, infant care and feeding options, postpartum care, and discharge planning. Active participation of the childbearing family allows them to make their birthing experience meaningful and unique.

Influences on Labor

Childbirth is a natural process, and health care providers are facilitators of the birth process. At times clinical interventions are necessary. During pregnancy the mother and

Box 16-3 TEN STEPS OF THE MOTHER-FRIENDLY CHILDBIRTH INITIATIVE FOR MOTHER-FRIENDLY HOSPITALS, BIRTH CENTERS, AND HOME BIRTH SERVICES

A mother-friendly hospital, birth center, or home birth service:

1. Offers all birthing mothers:
   - Unrestricted access to the birth companions of their choice, including fathers, partners, children, family members, and friends
   - Unrestricted access to continuous emotional and physical support from a skilled woman; for example, a doula or labor-support professional
   - Access to professional midwifery care
2. Provides accurate descriptive and statistical information to the public about its practices and procedures for birth care, including measures of intervention and outcomes.
3. Provides culturally competent care, that is, care that is sensitive and responsive to the specific beliefs, values, and customs of the mother's ethnicity and religion.
4. Provides the birthing mother with the freedom to walk, move about, and assume the positions of her choice during labor and birth (unless restriction is required specifically to correct a complication) and discourages the use of the lithotomy (flat on back with legs elevated) position.
5. Has clearly defined policies and procedures for the following:
   - Collaborating and consulting throughout the perinatal period with other maternity services, including communicating with the original caregiver when transfer from one birth site to another is necessary.
   - Linking the mother and baby to appropriate community resources, including prenatal and postdischarge follow-up and breast-feeding support.
6. Does not use practices and procedures routinely that are unsupported by scientific evidence, including but not limited to the following:
   - Shaving
   - Enemas
   - Intravenous drip
   - Withholding nourishment
   - Early rupture of membranes
   - Electronic fetal monitoring
7. Limits other interventions as follows:
   - Has an oxytocin use rate of 10% or less for induction and augmentation
   - Has an episiotomy rate of 20% or less, with a goal of 5% or less
   - Has a total cesarean rate of 10% or less in community hospitals and 15% or less in tertiary care (high-risk) hospitals
   - Has a vaginal birth after cesarean section rate of 60% or more with a goal of 75% or more
8. Educates staff in nondrug methods of pain relief and does not promote the use of analgesia or anesthetic drugs not specifically required to correct a complication.
9. Encourages all mothers and families, including those with sick or premature newborns or infants with congenital problems, to touch, hold, breast-feed, and care for their babies to the extent compatible with their conditions.
10. Discourages nonreligious circumcision of the newborn.
11. Strives to achieve the WHO-UNICEF "Ten Steps of the Baby-Friendly Hospital Initiative" to promote successful breast-feeding:
    - Has a written breast-feeding policy communicated to all health care staff
    - Trains all health care staff in skills necessary to implement this policy
    - Informs all pregnant women about the benefits and management of breast-feeding

Continued

Box 16-3 TEN STEPS OF THE MOTHER-FRIENDLY CHILDBIRTH INITIATIVE FOR MOTHER-FRIENDLY HOSPITALS, BIRTH CENTERS, AND HOME BIRTH SERVICES—CONT'D

- Helps mothers initiate breast-feeding within a half-hour of birth
- Shows mothers how to breast-feed and how to maintain lactation even if they should be separated from their infants
- Gives newborn infants no food or drink other than breast milk unless medically indicated
- Practices rooming in, allowing mothers and infants to remain together 24 hours a day
- Encourages breast-feeding on demanded
- Gives no artificial teats or pacifiers (also called *dummies* or *soothers*) to breast-feeding infants
- Fosters the establishment of breast-feeding support groups and refer mothers to them on discharge from hospitals or clinics

Copyright 1996 by the Coalition for Improving Maternity Services (CIMS).

---

fetus are preparing for the labor process. The success of that process is determined by many factors. Five essential factors known as the five *P*s are *p*assenger (the baby), *p*assageway (pelvis and reproductive structures), *p*ower (contractions), *p*osition (of mother and baby), and *p*sychological response (maternal sense of well-being).

Passenger

In 96% of pregnancies the fetus presents in the cephalic position. The bones of the head are not fused and have the ability to overlap and mold, allowing for passage through the pelvis. Although most fetuses enter the pelvis in the cephalic position, several variations can occur.

Fetal lie refers to the orientation of the long axis of the fetus in relation to the long axis of the woman. Longitudinal lie occurs when the fetus lies parallel to the long axis of the women. A transverse lie is when the fetus is at right angles to the long axis of the woman. An oblique lie is at an angle that is neither a right angle nor parallel.

Presentation is the fetal structure that enters the pelvis first and is closest to the cervix. Three types of presentation are cephalic, breech, and shoulder. Each of these presentations has its own variations. The cephalic can be vertex, face, brow, or military. Vertex is the normal position, with the neck flexed and the chin resting on the chest. This position is the most optimal position because the smallest diameter of the head is presenting. Breech presentations can be frank breech, complete breech, kneeling breech, and footling breech. Other presentations can be a shoulder or transverse lie. These presentations usually require delivery by cesarean birth.

Passageway

The bones and soft tissues of the pelvis influence the passageway. Although the bones of the pelvis are hard and do not give way to the passenger, the cartilage holding the pelvic bones together softens, allowing a small amount of stretching. The classification of the pelvis is based on the shape of the pelvic inlet and includes the gynecoid, android, anthropoid, and platypelloid.

Power

Involuntary and voluntary powers influence labor. The primary power of labor is uterine contractions, which are involuntary. Labor contractions of the uterus cause the cervix to efface and dilate, eventually forcing the fetus through the passageway. During the second stage of labor (complete dilatation until delivery), maternal pushing can assist in forcing the fetus through the passageway. Laboring women experience an involuntary urge to push when the presenting fetal part reaches the pelvic floor. Their bearing-down efforts are voluntary and known as secondary powers.

Position

Maternal position can influence pelvic size and contours. Changing position and walking affects the pelvis joints and facilitates fetal descent and rotation. Squatting enlarges the pelvic outlet by approximately 25%. A lying lateral position relaxes the pelvic muscles and promotes maternal circulation to the pelvic area and also facilitates fetal descent and rotation. Kneeling removes pressure on the maternal vena cava and helps rotate the fetus in the posterior position. Allowing the mother to move during labor encourages labor progression.

Psychological Response

A woman's ability to cope with labor is influenced by her psychological state. Anxiety and tension can cause release of catecholamines, which inhibit placental blood flow and uterine contractions. Relaxation promotes the labor process. Many factors influence how a woman is going to cope. Her previous experiences are the foundation of her current feeling. Her expectations of this birthing experience also influence her feelings. An exploration of these feelings can help to plan delivery care that is appropriate.

Assessment

Labor occurs as the fetus moves through the pelvis and birth canal to be expelled. Labor may occur at any time during a pregnancy; however, a term pregnancy is considered between 37 and 42 weeks. As a woman's body prepares for birth, she may experience one or more premonitory signs. These signs may begin as much as 2 weeks before delivery.

■ Fetal descent into the pelvic inlet is known as lightening or dropping and usually occurs approximately 2 weeks before the onset of labor. Breathing improves because of the expanded lung capacity; however, the woman experiences more pressure on the bladder, and frequency of urination increases. Lightening is more noticeable in primigravidas (first pregnancy).

■ Low back pain may increase because of the softening of the pelvic joints.

■ Braxton-Hicks contractions may increase and become painful on occasion.

- Vaginal mucus increases because of pelvic congestion. As the cervix becomes soft and dilates, the mucous plug may be passed through the vagina. Mucus mixed with pink or brown blood, which is known as bloody show, may occur.
- Some women have a slight weight loss of 1 to 3 pounds because of a shift in electrolytes caused by a change in estrogen and progesterone levels. The shift causes a fluid loss.
- Many women describe a burst of energy that is used to prepare their home. This is known as nesting.

The onset of true labor is often difficult to pinpoint. Many women experience a gradual onset of labor. True labor is defined as contractions with cervical change and progression in descent of the presenting part. The cervix must dilate and thin (efface). Dilatation goes from closed to approximately 10 cm. A term cervix is approximately 3 cm in length; this is called *thick* or *zero percent effacement*. As the cervix thins, the percentage increases until 100% is completely thinned. Also as labor progresses, the presenting fetal part descends through the pelvis. The degree of descent is measured by the station of the presenting part in comparison to the ischeal spines of the pelvis. A fetus that is not engaged in the pelvis is ballottable. Above the ischeal spines is -3 to -1. Even with the spines is 0 station, and below is +1 to +3.

Prodromal labor or false labor involves contractions without cervical change. Women who experience prodromal labor tend to become discouraged. Table 16-7 gives a comparison of true and false labor.

True labor follows a normal progression through four stages. Each stage is defined and has its own characteristics. The total length of labor should be less than 24 hours, with primigravidas tending to have longer labors than multigravidas.

First Stage of Labor: Dilatation

The first stage of labor is known as dilatation; it begins with the onset of true labor contractions and ends with complete dilatation of the cervix. Dilatation is usually the

Table 16-7	TRUE VS. FALSE LABOR
FALSE LABOR	**TRUE LABOR**
Discomfort is usually more in lower abdomen and groin.	Discomfort is usually felt in the back and works to the front.
Uterus is relaxed or mild to palpate.	Uterus is hard to palpate.
Contractions are irregular.	Contractions increase in frequency, duration, and intensity.
No cervical changes in effacement or dilatation.	Cervical change in effacement and dilatation.
No bloody show.	Bloody show.
A change in activity does not alter contractions or decreases them.	Contraction intensity increases when walking.

longest stage of labor and is subdivided in three phases. Each phase has its own characteristics based on maternal responses.

The early or latent phase is from the beginning of labor until 3 cm of dilatation. Contractions are usually every 5 to 10 minutes, lasting 30 to 45 seconds, and mild to palpable. Effacement is from none to 40%. Most women are able to talk during this phase. They may be excited, but anxiety is low. During this time they should contact their health care provider and prepare to go to the place they have chosen for the birth.

The second phase is known as the active phase. The cervix dilates from 4 to 7 cm, with 40% to 80% effacement. The presenting fetal part begins to descend further, -2 to 0 station. Contractions become stronger and the pain may increase. Relaxation techniques help to keep the woman focused on the task of labor. Many women become quiet and introspective, and they may depend on others for support as their self-confidence waivers.

Transition is the third phase, beginning at 8 cm and ending at 10 cm and complete effacement. The fetus descends to -1 to +1 station. Contractions continue to be strong and arrive approximately every 2 to 3 minutes, lasting 60 to 90 seconds. Nausea and vomiting, tremors, and an increased bloody show are common. Many women have an unbearable urge to push as the fetus descends to the pelvic floor. Women tend to become irritable and fatigued. Their coping ability decreases, and relaxation is difficult. When they speak, they are often speaking to their own bodies and their baby.

Nursing research has demonstrated that placing the woman in an upright position during second stage labor is more effective in giving birth (Mayberry & Strange, 1997; Shermer & Raines, 1997).

Second Stage of Labor: Infant Expulsion

The second stage of labor is the time from full cervical dilatation to birth of the newborn. As the fetus descends into the vagina, the urge to push may be uncontrollable. Traditionally, women have been taught to push holding their breath and bearing down for a count of 10. This method can cause hemodynamic changes in the mother and may produce abnormalities in the fetal heart rate. Alternative methods can be open-glottis or only pushing when the woman has the urge to push. Even women with epidural anesthesia may feel pressure or experience an urge to push, depending on the strength and level of the anesthetic.

An episiotomy may be performed during the delivery of the fetus. The decision to perform an episiotomy is made by the health care provider during the delivery. Episiotomies should not be routine but are used to prevent tearing, reduce time and stress, or allow room for an assisted delivery.

Indications for the use of forceps or vacuum may be maternal or fetal. Maternal indications include if the progression of second stage stops, maternal exhaustion, or a maternal medical condition such as cardiac disease that may become worse with pushing. Fetal indications are fetal distress or a preterm infant to prevent cranial damage during pushing. The following are types of assisted deliveries:

- Low or outlet forceps, where the head is visible at the perineum
- Midforceps, where the fetal head is at the ischial spines and the head may be in the anteroposterior position
- Vacuum, when a suction cup is applied to the presenting part and traction is exerted

After any assisted delivery the baby should be examined for possible injuries, including cephalhematoma, nerve damage, lacerations, or bruising. The use of forceps or vacuum also may increase the risk to the woman for lacerations of the vagina or perineum.

Third Stage of Labor: Placental Expulsion

The third stage is the time between the birth of the baby and delivery of the placenta. This stage is usually the shortest and may last only a few minutes. The mother may be excited and relieved that her baby is finally here. If possible, the baby should be placed on the mother's chest to be kept warm through the skin-to-skin method. This allows the mother to see and touch her baby immediately.

Most often the placenta delivers spontaneously; however, the placenta may need to be removed manually. Signs of spontaneous separation of the placenta include a gush of blood and lengthening of the umbilical cord. The fundus may rise in the abdomen, and the uterus becomes firm and global in shape. After delivery, the placenta should be inspected for any abnormalities or missing fragments that still may be in the uterus.

Fourth Stage of Labor: Immediate Postpartum

The fourth stage begins with the delivery of the placenta and lasts for the first several hours postpartum. Immediate postpartum recovery is an important maternal physiological transition time. The family is now in the beginning stages of adaptation to a family unit. The role of nurses is to facilitate early family attachment.

The physical assessment includes vital signs every 15 minutes, fundal checks, estimation of lochia, perineal inspection, and bladder inspection. For the women with epidural anesthesia, neuromuscular status with return of sensation should be assessed. The woman may have pain related to uterine involution or from the perineal area. Ice placed on the perineum decreases swelling and pain. Analgesics may be necessary. Hemorrhage is the most common complication of this stage of labor.

Admission Assessment

Admission to the birthing unit usually occurs during the first stage of labor. Obtaining a complete initial assessment depends on which phase of labor the woman is in and her ability to cope. Institutional policies and the primary health care provider determine laboratory testing, the starting of intravenous fluids, fetal monitoring, and other procedures. A patient's birth plan should be reviewed with the health care team and the patient during this time to provide individualized care. During admission, prenatal records should be obtained and reviewed. The history and assessment focuses on the status of the mother and infant. Essential information includes the following:

- Mother's and support person's names
- Health care provider's name

- Number of pregnancies and prior births, including types of birth
- History of prenatal care
- Status of membranes
- Estimated date of delivery
- Any problems with this pregnancy
- Allergies to medications or latex
- Time and type of last oral intake
- Maternal vital signs and fetal heart rate
- Cervical status and fetal position

Intrapartum Fetal Assessment

Monitoring the well-being of the fetus has been part of society for centuries. Fetal heart rates were first heard during the seventeenth century. Since that time many researchers have attempted to improve pregnancy outcomes through technology (Schmidt & McCartney, 2000). As advances are made in computers and biotechnology, the ability to monitor fetal well-being will increase. Currently, two approaches are used for intrapartum fetal assessment: intermittent auscultation and electronic fetal monitoring (EFM). The purpose of intrapartum fetal assessment is to evaluate fetal response to labor, looking for assurance of fetal well-being and identifying possible insults. Although either method of monitoring provides similar neonatal outcomes, EFM is the more widely used method of fetal surveillance in the United States and Canada (Feinstein, 2000).

Intermittent auscultation is done by listening to the fetal heart sounds with a fetoscope or a stethoscope. The fetal heart rate also can be assessed with Doppler ultrasound, which identifies movement of the fetal heart valve and converts feedback into an auditory sound or digital reading. Current recommendations state that intermittent auscultation should be done for 30 to 60 seconds after a contraction with varying intervals depending on risk factors and the stage of labor (Table 16-8) (Feinstein, 2000).

The decision to use intermittent auscultation usually is made by the health care provider; however, the woman should have input into that decision.

Originally, EFM was developed because of questions about the ability to assess fetal heart status accurately with auscultation (Schmidt & McCartney, 2000). Eventually the suggestion was made that changes in the fetal heart rate may be related to fetal hypoxia. As EFM was developed and technology improved, the ability to evaluate fetal oxygenation improved. Today, fetal monitoring may be accomplished through external and internal methods. Externally, Doppler ultrasound records fetal heart rate, and a tocodynamometer monitors uterine contractions. Any pregnant woman can use this method because it is noninvasive. Internal monitoring can only occur after the membranes have ruptured. Internal spiral electrodes directly measure the electrical activity of the fetal heart. Internal uterine pressure catheters accurately record the frequency, duration, and strength of uterine contractions. Both methods provide a permanent record via paper, electronic disks, or microfilm.

Table 16-8	RECOMMENDATIONS FOR INTERMITTENT AUSCULTATION		
AGENCY	LATENT PHASE	ACTIVE PHASE	SECOND STAGE
American College of Obstetricians and Gynecologists			
Low Risk		Every 30 minutes	Every 15 minutes
High Risk		Every 15 minutes	Every 5 minutes
Association of Women's Health, Obstetric and Neonatal Nurses			
Low Risk	Every hour	Every 30 minutes	Every 15 minutes
High Risk	Every 30 minutes	Every 15 minutes	Every 5 minutes
Society of Obstetricians and Gynecologists of Canada			
Low Risk	Every 30 minutes	Every 15 minutes	Every 5 minutes
High Risk	Every 30 minutes	Every 15 minutes	Every 5 minutes

ASSESS FETAL HEART RATE BEFORE	ASSESS FETAL HEART RATE AFTER
Ambulation	Admission of patient
Administration of medications	Artificial or spontaneous rupture of membranes
Administration of analgesia or anesthesia	Vaginal exam
Initiation of labor-enhancing procedures (e.g., amniotomy)	Ambulation
Transfer or discharge of patient	Recognition of abnormal uterine activity patterns Evaluation of oxytocin (maintenance; increase or decrease of dosage) Evaluation of analgesia or anesthesia (maintenance; increase or decrease of dosage)

Modified from Feinstein, N. F., Sprague, A., & Trepanier, M. J. (1999). *Fetal heart rate auscultation* (p. 27). Washington, DC: Association of Women's Health, Obstetric and Neonatal Nurses.

Pain Relief

Pain relief during the first stage of labor depends on the woman. Many factors influence pain response and may include previous experiences with pain, fatigue, anxiety and fear, culture, and preparation and support for this childbirth. Raines and Morgan (2000) found that differences exist between African-American and white women regarding descriptions and expectations about comfort and support during the labor and birth experience. White women were more fearful of loss of control and requested pain relief earlier than African-American women.

Labor support has long been considered the cornerstone of nursing care for women in labor. Nursing research has demonstrated that, although nurses perceive labor support as very important, the actual amount of time that nurses performed labor support was relatively small.

Nursing care of the laboring woman is both an art and science and is very individual in its implementation and interpretation. Therefore it is difficult to quantify. Additionally, labor nurses also have many barriers that may prevent them from spending as much time providing labor support as they would desire. Some of these barriers are the time-consuming tasks of documentation, electronic surveillance, medication administration, and assistance with medical interventions (Bowers, 2002; Raines & Morgan, 2000; Tumblin & Simkin, 2001). Nonpharmacological and pharmacological interventions should be made available.

Nonpharmacological Interventions

Nonpharmacological interventions focus on relaxation through a specific method such as biofeedback, breathing, self-hypnotism, acupressure, aromatherapy, water therapy, and music therapy. Position changes, ambulating, rocking, and using the birthing ball (large plastic ball women can position themselves against to provide counter-pressure) also may assist the woman in coping with pain and facilitating the labor process (Doulas of North America, 1999). These therapies may be used alone or in combination and with pharmacological agents. Through childbirth classes women can learn about many of these methods. Women may also have a labor doula who is a person specially trained to support the woman during labor and childbirth. Research has demonstrated that women require less pharmacological intervention when they have a doula (Doulas of North America, 1999).

Pharmacological Interventions

The goal of pharmacological management of labor discomfort is to provide adequate pain relief with as few side effects as possible to the mother and baby. The goal of analgesia is to change the perception of pain by raising the pain threshold or causing relaxation to decrease tension, whereas anesthesia eliminates pain by blocking nerve impulses to the brain.

Analgesia is systemic and crosses the blood-brain barrier and the placental barrier, thus affecting the fetus. The effect on the fetus depends on the amount the mother receives, the type of drug, and when she receives it. Barbiturates, tranquilizers, and narcotics usually are used for labor discomfort. The barbiturates phenobarbital (Nembutal) and secobarbital (Seconal) reduce tension and fear and provide sedation and sleep. Some health care providers use these drugs during prodromal labor to provide rest. They do not take away pain, however. Hydroxyzine (Vistaril) and promethazine (Phenergan) are tranquilizers that provide muscle relaxation and reduce anxiety. They also have antiemetic effects and may potentiate narcotics. Narcotics such as meperidine (Demerol), morphine, butorphanol (Stadol), nalbuphine (Nubain), fentanyl (Sublimaze), and sufentanil increase pain threshold and allow the woman to tolerate the pain. Drowsiness may occur, and uterine activity can be increased or decreased. These drugs may cause a decreased respiratory effort in the baby, so a narcotic antagonist should be available at delivery.

Regional Anesthesia

Regional anesthesia provides some pain relief and motor block and allows the mother to participate in the birth and have pain control without loss of consciousness. Disadvantages of regional pain control depend on the type used.

During a **paracervical block,** local anesthesia is injected transvaginally into the cervix that is dilated 4 to 6 cm. The lower uterine segment, cervix, and upper vagina are affected. Side effects may be fetal bradycardia. Use of this method of pain relief is declining because it is not always effective.

For a **pudendal block,** local anesthesia is injected into the pudendal nerves near each ischial spine. This provides pain relief to the lower vagina and part of the perineum. If an episotomy or perineal repair is needed, additional local anesthesia may be necessary for the perineum. A pudendal block does not provide relief of pain from uterine contractions. Complications to the woman may include a reaction to the drug, hematoma, or nerve block. Adverse reactions usually are not seen in the fetus.

Epidural anesthesia has become popular because it provides pain relief from contractions and the fetus moving through the vagina. The labor nurse is a major support to the laboring patient as well as the expectant father, regarding pain management in labor. Nurses' explanation of the normal responses to pain in labor, pain management options, and assistance with epidural insertion, all help to reduce the woman's and expectant father's levels of anxiety, fear, frustration, helplessness (Chapman, 2000).

In epidermal anesthesia, the epidural space is usually entered through the third and fourth lumbar vertebrae with a needle, and a catheter is threaded into the epidural space. The needle is removed and the catheter is left for continuous infusion or intermittent injections of medicine. The level of motor function and sensation depends on the type of medicine used. Epidural anesthesia can be used for vaginal and cesarean births. An epidural may be contraindicated for some women who have had previous spinal surgery or spinal abnormalities, coagulation defects or anticoagulation therapy, infections, and hypovolemia. Complications to the woman may include nausea, vomiting, pruritus, and respiratory depression, which can be a reaction to the drugs. During the insertion of the catheter, the dura may be punctured, causing spinal fluid to leak, which may result in a spinal headache. After injection of the medicine, a sympathetic reaction of vasodilation and hypotension may occur. This reaction can cause a decrease in blood flow to the uterus, leading to potential fetal distress. An intravenous fluid bolus of 500 to 1000 mL before the epidural may decrease the effects of systemic vasodilatation. If hypotension occurs, ephedrine administered intravenously can cause vasoconstriction to increase blood pressure. Bladder distention may occur with the decrease in sensation. Bladder distention may cause pain or physically impede the descent of the fetus.

Lastly, epidural anesthesia has been associated with lengthened labor and operative deliveries (Howell, 2000). However, the type and amount of drugs used can be factored into these possible complications. These factors may be decreased by waiting until the woman feels the urge to push instead of the traditional method of pushing when the cervix is dilated completely. This permits the fetus to descend into the birth canal and allows the woman to participate actively. The term *laboring down* has been applied to this method.

Spinal anesthesia is used commonly for cesarean births. A single injection provides sensory and motor function loss below the level of the block. In a spinal block, local anesthetic is injected through the third, fourth, and fifth lumbar vertebral spaces into the subarachnoid space and mixes with cerebrospinal fluid. The contraindications are similar to those for the epidural. Adverse reactions for the woman can be hypotension, bladder distention, and spinal headache. The use of a small-gauge needle (25 or 27 gauge) may decrease the incidence of spinal headache.

The use of **intrathecal narcotics** for labor is increasing. A narcotic is injected into the subarachnoid space, providing rapid pain relief yet maintaining motor function and sensation. An intrathecal narcotic usually is given during the active phase of labor. Although this is effective for pain, an intrathecal injection is limited by the duration of action of the drug used, so additional measures for pain may be necessary.

Complications of Labor and Birth

Malpresentation

The most common presenting fetal part is vertex. When other parts are presenting, they can influence the labor process. Breech presentations are associated with prematurity, multiparity, pelvic abnormalities, placenta previa, and some congenital anomalies. Increased fetal mortality and morbidity also are associated with a breech presentation, possibly because of trauma during the birth. Descent of the fetus into the pelvis may be slow; however, labor is not usually longer.

Transverse lies are associated with multigravidas possibly because of relaxed uterine and abdominal muscles. A compound presentation occurs when the fetus is in a unique position and presents a hand or arm alongside the presenting part. This compound presentation may interfere with the labor process.

Cesarean birth is not required for a breech presentation but commonly is performed, especially for nulliparous women. Vaginal birth may be attempted for a woman with a normal size and shape of pelvis and an estimated fetal mass of less than 3800 g. Cesarean birth is necessary for a transverse lie unless the fetus can be rotated by external version.

External version is an attempt to turn the fetus from a breech or a transverse lie to vertex. Usually a version is done after 37 weeks gestation and before the beginning of labor. An ultrasound is performed to confirm fetal position, assess amniotic fluid, locate the umbilical cord, and rule out any abnormalities. A tocolytic agent may be given to relax the uterus before the version. External version is accomplished by applying constant, gentle pressure on the maternal abdomen. Complications may include fetal bradycardia and placental abruption.

Fetal Size

Macrosomia involves an infant that weighs more than 4000 g (8.8 pounds) at birth. The greatest concern for large babies is they may not be able to adapt their heads and shoulders to the maternal pelvis. Shoulder dystocia occurs when the shoulders become impacted above the maternal symphysis pubis. Quick intervention is necessary because the umbilical cord is being compressed. Some of the methods of intervention may include McRobert's maneuver, where the woman flexes her thighs sharply against her abdomen to straighten the pelvic curve, a maternal squatting position, or applying pressure to the suprapubic area to displace the shoulder. Fundal pressure should not be used because this pushes the anterior shoulder against the woman's symphysis.

Cervical Ripening

Most women do not require intervention for labor to begin. However, some women may need clinical interventions to facilitate delivery. The type of intervention depends on maternal and fetal conditions. The cervix must be ripe, or favorable, to dilate. An assessment of the cervix can be done using a Bishop score. A score of 8 or more indicates the cervix is ready for birth and will respond to induction. The Bishop score is based on dilatation, effacement, station, consistency, and position of the cervix (Table 16-9).

When the cervix is not favorable, the health care provider may choose to use mechanical or pharmacological methods of cervical ripening. The most common mechanical method is stripping of the amniotic membranes or separating the membranes from the lower uterine segment. Although this can be done easily in the office, bleeding, spontaneous rupture of membranes, or infection can be complications. *Laminaria* or synthetic hygroscopic dilators extract water from the cervix, producing slow changes. Within 4 to 12 hours, they can be removed and the cervix reevaluated. Serial applications may be necessary.

Pharmacological methods for cervical ripening include prostaglandin gels such as misoprostol or low-dose oxytocin. The most common method is application of a prostaglandin E_2 gel (Prepidil) to the surface of the cervix or on a small, commercially prepared tampon (Cervidil). Additional doses of gel may be applied every 6 hours. Cervidil may be changed every 12 hours. Prostaglandin E_1 is given in the form of misoprostol, orally or intravaginally. Oral misoprostol has been associated with trends toward a vaginal birth and uterine tachysystole (Wing, Park, & Paul, 2000). Low-doses of oxytocin have not been shown to be effective for cervical ripening.

Table 16-9	BISHOP SCORE			
SCORING FACTORS	ASSIGNED NUMERICAL VALUE			
	0	1	2	3
Dilation	0	1-2	3-4	5-6
Effacement	1%-30%	40%-50%	60%-70%	80%
Station	-3	-2	-1/0	+1/+2
Consistency	Firm	Medium	Soft	—
Position	Posterior	Midposition	Anterior	—

Induction of Labor

The induction of labor may be necessary for maternal or fetal reasons. Because of the potential risks, induction of labor without medical indication is considered elective and should be avoided.

Maternal indications for induction include the following:

- Premature rupture of membranes
- Infection (chorioamnionitis)
- Pregnancy-induced hypertension/preeclampsia
- Medical illness (diabetic, pulmonary, or cardiac)
- History of rapid labor

Fetal indications for induction include the following:

- Fetal demise
- Postdate pregnancy (more than 41 weeks)
- Intrauterine growth restriction
- Nonreassuring fetal testing (NST or BPP)
- Fetal anomaly
- Macrosomia
- Fetal hydrops

Labor is induced by the administration of a synthetic version of the pituitary hormone oxytocin, which initiates contractions in a uterus. Oxytocin is given intravenously in low concentrations to avoid hyperstimulation of the uterus. The half-life of oxytocin is approximately 3 minutes, thus with intravenous use, the serum level and effects end quickly. Oxytocin should be delivered by a controlled infusion device not affected by needle size. A secondary line containing the oxytocin admixture should be piggybacked at the port closest to the patient. Oxytocin should not be administered without a physician at hand who is able to perform a cesarean birth (American College of Obstetricians and Gynecologists and American Academy of Pediatrics, 1997; American College of Obstetricians and Gynecologists 1999b).

Dosing protocols vary with the starting doses, dosing intervals and increments, and the maximum dose. Starting doses of 0.5 milliunits (mu) /minute to 1 milliunits (mu) /minute with increases of 1 to 2 mu /minute every 15 to 30 minutes is recommended by the American College of Obstetricians and Gynecologists (1999b). Individualized care is the goal of managing a patient on oxytocin, with a focus on assessing uterine activity, cervical dilatation, and maternal-fetal response. Auscultation can be used to assess fetal status using the guidelines prescribed for high-risk patients; however, most perinatal centers use EFM as the method of determining fetal response during oxytocin administration.

Oxytocin has an antidiuretic effect, resulting in decreased urine flow that may lead to water intoxication. The first symptoms of water intoxication are headache and vomiting. The most common adverse effect is uterine hyperstimulation, leading to fetal compromise and impaired oxygenation (Association of Women's Health, Obstetric and Neonatal Nurses, 1997).

Augmentation

When labor contractions begin spontaneously and then become weak, irregular, or ineffective, assistance is necessary to strengthen them. Amniotomy frequently is used but has not been shown to be effective. Nipple and breast stimulation releases endogenous pitocin, which can enhance labor. Oxytocin is the most common form of augmentation. The uterus tends to respond quickly to augmentation, and dosing intervals should be increased slowly (Simpson & Poole, 1998).

Vaginal Birth after Cesarean Section

The unwritten rule has been "once a c-section always a c-section." This rule is no longer true. Vaginal birth after cesarean section has become an option for some women. Ridley and others (2002) found that numerous internal and external factors influenced women's decisions to choose a vaginal birth after cesarean (VBAC). The dominant themes found were the woman's sense of control in the decision making process, physician encouragement for VBAC, and delivery-type outcome advantages that incorporate physical and emotional factors.

If the indication for the primary cesarean birth no longer exists, such as fetal distress or breech presentation, a trial of labor can occur. Studies have shown that a vaginal birth after cesarean section is safe, with a rise of 0.5% risk of uterine rupture through a lower uterine segment scar (Lyndon-Rochelle, 2001). No evidence indicates that administration of oxytocin to induce or augment labor or the use of epidural anesthesia is contraindicated (Caughey et al., 1999).

Complications of Pregnancy

Description

Childbearing is considered a normal process; however, complications can arise that threaten the fetus, the mother, or both.

Women with complicated pregnancies perceive their risks for negative outcomes as higher than do women with uncomplicated pregnancies. The strongest predictors of self-perception of pregnancy risk are the biomedical risk score and state anxiety. There is no relationship between stress, self-esteem, or social support and perception of risk. Therefore women with complicated pregnancies need to be assessed for their perception of risk (Cheung, 2001).

Conditions that complicate pregnancy can be divided into two groups: those that can exist at any time but when present during pregnancy may alter the course of the disease or complicate the pregnancy and those that are related to the pregnancy but do not exist at any other time. Pregnancy affects all body systems, and all systems make adjustments to accommodate the pregnancy. When a system is compromised before a pregnancy, the stress of pregnancy may exacerbate the problem or the pregnancy may be rejected. Some of the diseases that can affect reproduction are diabetes, heart disease, anemia, renal diseases, infections, and human immunodeficiency virus infection or acquired immunodeficiency syndrome. As discussed before, preconception care focuses on identifying women's reproductive risks before pregnancy, whereas counseling provides the safest environment for discussing a developing fetus (Nasso, 1997).

Complications Unique to Pregnancy

Hyperemesis gravidarum. Hyperemesis gravidarum is intractable vomiting beginning before the twentieth week of gestation and resulting in nutritional disturbances. The condition is associated with a loss of 5% or more of prepregnancy weight, electrolyte imbalances, dehydration, acidosis from starvation, alkalosis from loss of hydrochloric acid, ketonuria, and hypokalemia (Cowan, 1996). At present, the cause is unknown, but several theories exist. One is that there is extreme maternal sensitivity to the elevated hormone levels in early pregnancy.

Hemorrhagic disorders. The three most common causes of hemorrhage during the first half of pregnancy are ectopic pregnancy, abortion, and hydatidiform mole. Loss of the fetus occurs with each condition.

Ectopic pregnancy. An ectopic pregnancy is defined as the implantation of a fertilized ovum outside of the uterine cavity. Implantation can occur in the abdomen or cervix; however, the fallopian tube is the most common site, occurring in 92% of cases (Jehle, Krause, & Braen, 1994). Normally the fertilized ovum travels through the fallopian tubes over 4 to 5 days and implants into the uterus. Tubal obstruction often is cited as the primary reason for ectopic pregnancies. Major causes of obstruction are a history of tubal surgery, endometriosis, use of intrauterine devices, and pelvic infections. The incidence of ectopic pregnancies has increased with an increase in pelvic inflammatory disease, induced abortions, and changes in sexual behavior (Dimitry & Morcos, 1990). Prevention may be accomplished through education on these topics and treatment of pelvic infections. Ectopic pregnancy has been described as a disaster of human reproduction. Complications can lead to decreased chance of future pregnancies because of damaged or destroyed fallopian tubes or maternal death caused by abdominal hemorrhage. The classic signs of ectopic pregnancy are amenorrhea, lower abdominal pain, and vaginal bleeding or spotting. As the ovum begins to grow, pain may occur as the tissue is pulled and stretched or the fallopian tube ruptures. Pain radiating to the shoulder (Kehr's sign) may indicate abdominal bleeding caused by phrenic nerve irritation (Jehle et al., 1994). Other symptoms may include hypotension, rigid abdomen, tachycardia, or hyperpnea. Diagnosis is made by ultrasound and beta-human chorionic gonadotropin (β-hCG) levels. In an abnormal pregnancy, β-hCG is present but at lower levels than expected. Treatment depends on the symptoms, the location of implantation, and whether the tube is intact or ruptured. Medical management can occur if the tubes are not ruptured. However, when ectopic pregnancy results in rupture of the tubes, the goal is to control the bleeding and prevent hypovolemic shock. Women with ectopic pregnancies display several emotions, including grief, guilt, anger, fear, and self-blame. These women are also fearful of infertility because of a possible loss of the fallopian tubes.

Abortion. Abortion is defined as a pregnancy that ends before 20 weeks of gestation, spontaneously or electively. *Miscarriage* is the lay term for a spontaneous abortion. The exact incidence of spontaneous abortions is unknown because of the difficulty in recognizing early conceptions and losses. One estimate is that 15% of all recognized pregnancies end in spontaneous abortion. Most spontaneous abortions occur in the first 12 weeks of pregnancy, with the rate declining rapidly thereafter. The causes of spontaneous abortions vary. Chromosomal abnormalities and cervical incompetence are major causes. Other causes may include maternal infections, maternal endocrine disorders, luteal phase defects, abnormalities of the reproductive organs, or immune factors. Spontaneous abortion is divided into six categories: threatened, incomplete, missed, inevitable, complete, and recurrent. During the first trimester, approximately 25% of all women have spotting, or vaginal bleeding. Such pregnancies are known as threatened abortions. Roughly half of the women that experience spotting progress to inevitable abortions. Women should be instructed to call their care providers whenever vaginal bleeding is present. Bed rest often is recommended for vaginal bleeding; however, no valid basis for the practice is apparent. When nothing can be done to stop a spontaneous abortion, the abortion is considered inevitable. Usually the membranes rupture or the cervix dilates. If complete expulsion of the product of conception does not occur, the abortion is called incomplete. A complete abortion occurs when all products of conception are expelled from the uterus. A missed abortion occurs when the fetus dies in utero during the first 20 weeks of gestation but remains in the uterus. As long as no infection is present, a woman and her care provider may allow the mother to continue to carry the fetus until spontaneous abortion occurs. This may take several weeks. Recurrent spontaneous abortions are also known as habitual abortions, such as in women who have had three or more consecutive spontaneous abortions. Several factors may contribute to frequent spontaneous abortions. A history of sexually transmitted diseases, maternal systemic diseases such as lupus or diabetes, an immunological response, genetic abnormalities, abnormalities of the women's reproductive organs, and hormonal irregularities can affect pregnancy. Bleeding alone does not confirm an abortion. If an abortion is suspected before 8 weeks of gestation, two serum β-hCG levels are drawn 48 hours apart. In a normal pregnancy, the β-hCG level doubles in this time frame. Ultrasound can confirm a viable pregnancy. Appropriate treatment for spontaneous abortion is evacuation of the uterine contents. Ultrasound can be used to help determine if a fetus is still present and alive and also may be able to indicate if the abortion is complete. In the absence of evidence to support that an abortion is complete, curettage is indicated. Women who are Rh-negative should be given immune anti-D globulin (RhoGAM) to prevent sensitization after complete removal of tissue from the uterus. Complications of a spontaneous abortion include blood loss, infection, and disseminated intravascular coagulation. The woman should notify her primary caregiver of a temperature elevation, vaginal discharge with a foul odor, or abdominal pain. Psychological support is important for the family experiencing a spontaneous abortion. Many families feel an acute loss and grief with a spontaneous abortion. Women need reassurance that spontaneous abortions usually result from an abnormality and that their actions did not cause the abortion. Anger, disappointment, and sadness are common emotions. Their grief may follow the same model of grief described by Kübler-Ross (1969). Although the focus of the loss tends to be on women, their male partners also have a sense of sadness and loss, coupled with a feeling of uncertainty as to how to handle the situation (Murphy, 1998). Nursing has the opportunity to be supportive of these families during this grieving. For the grief process to last 6 or more months before the loss is accepted is not uncommon. Planning future pregnancies depends on the cause and treatment of the abortion. Some women may have an increased risk to abort again, whereas others will have no problems conceiving and carrying the pregnancy to term. Hemorrhagic conditions of late pregnancy include placenta previa, abruptio placentae, and disseminated intravascular coagulation. All of these can be life threatening to the fetus and mother.

Rh incompatibility. Rh disease occurs when the blood of the fetus and the mother is incompatible, causing destruction of fetal blood cells. Although this condition does not affect the mother, the baby can have jaundice, anemia, brain damage, heart failure, and death. Most human beings produce Rh factor, an inherited protein found on the surface of red blood cells; however, approximately 10% of human beings do not have the Rh protein. These persons are said to be Rh-negative. If an Rh-negative mother and Rh positive father conceive a child that inherits the Rh factor from the father, these Rh-positive cells may be introduced into the maternal blood system during the birth process. Because these cells are foreign to the mother, she can produce antibodies against them. During future pregnancies, if the fetus has Rh-positive blood, maternal Rh antibodies can cross the placenta and destroy fetal red blood cells.

To prevent Rh disease, an Rh-negative woman should receive an injection of the blood product Rh immunoglobulin (RhoGAM) within 72 hours of birth of an Rh-positive baby. The injection prevents sensitization in approximately 95% of Rh-negative women. Occasionally, some Rh-negative women become sensitized before delivery. For this reason, RhoGAM is given at 28 weeks of gestation. RhoGAM also should be given to women who have had a miscarriage or abortion, a blood transfusion of Rh-positive blood, ectopic pregnancy, amniocentesis, or chorionic villus sampling. The RhoGAM lasts approximately 12 weeks and so must be administered with each pregnancy.

Hypertension. Hypertensive disorders of pregnancy can result in life-threatening complications to the mother and fetus. The American College of Obstetricians and Gynecologists (1996b) has divided hypertension into two categories: chronic hypertension and pregnancy-induced hypertension. Chronic hypertension is an elevation of blood pressure before 20 weeks of gestation. Pregnancy-induced hypertension includes four classifications:

1. Pregnancy-induced hypertension is the development of hypertension (blood pressure greater than 140/90) during the second half of pregnancy in a previously normotensive woman.
2. Preeclampsia includes the involvement of the renal system leading to proteinuria.
3. Eclampsia involves the central nervous system with the presence of seizures.
4. HELLP (hemolysis, elevated liver enzymes, and low platelet count) syndrome presents a clinical picture dominated by hematological and hepatic signs and symptoms.

Multifetal pregnancy. A phenomenal increase in multiple births has occurred in recent years. According to the National Vital Statistics Report (2000), the twin birth rate is 28.1 per 1000 births and the triplet rate is 193.5 per 10,000 births. Many of the multiple gestations are caused by use of ovulation-stimulating drugs and in vitro fertilization. Women with multiple gestations are at risk for many of the complications of a singleton pregnancy such as preterm labor, anemia, intrauterine growth retardation, pregnancy-induced hypertension, abruptio placentae, and postpartum hemorrhage. Every maternal system has an increase in workload to accommodate the multiple gestation. Early diagnosis is an important factor in improving the perinatal outcome. Twins are suspected whenever uterine size is greater than ordinary for the expected point of the pregnancy, multiple large parts can be palpated in the abdomen, or more than one heart beat is heard. No biological tests are available for diagnosis of multiple gestations; however, ultrasound can aid in the diagnosis. The management of multiple gestations includes an increase in prenatal visits to every other week in the second trimester and every week in the third trimester. Weekly NSTs should begin at 28 weeks of gestation for serial fetal surveillance. The health care provider should observe for fetal growth rates and amniotic fluid volumes. An increase of 300 kcal/day beyond the 2500 kcal total for a normal pregnancy is recommended. Rest and comfort are important to a woman with multiple fetuses. Teaching of preterm labor signs and symptoms are necessary because early delivery is common.

Preterm labor and birth. Preterm labor is defined as uterine contractions and cervical dilatation before the thirty-seventh week of gestation. Some risks associated with preterm labor are prior preterm birth, uterine anomalies, urinary tract infections, polyhydramnios, and multiple gestation. The uterine contractions may or may not be painful but can be palpated. Cervical changes can be softening, dilatation, or effacement.

Predicting who will go into preterm labor has been difficult. Although several risk scoring systems have been developed, the preterm birth rate has not been lowered (Centers for Disease Control and Prevention, 1998). Recently biochemical markers have been developed to predict who might have preterm labor. The two most common markers are salivary estriol and fetal fibronectin. Salivary estriol is a form of estrogen that is produced by the fetus and is present in plasma at 9 weeks of gestation. The concentration of estriol has been shown to increase before preterm birth. The woman collects a small sample of saliva every 2 weeks for 10 weeks. The test is most accurate in predicting who will not have preterm birth, rather than who will deliver early.

Fetal fibronectins are produced during fetal life and are found in the cervical canal early in pregnancy and again late in pregnancy. If found between 24 and 34 weeks of gestation, fetal fibronectins may predict preterm labor. A specimen must be collected during a vaginal examination with a speculum. This test also has a high negative predictive value. Predicting who will have preterm labor may be possible, rather than who will not have preterm labor (Moore, 1999).

The exact cause of preterm labor is unknown and may be multifactorial. Preterm labor may be mistaken for normal changes within the maternal body during pregnancy. Education of pregnant women concerning the signs of preterm labor may be the best defense. If the woman suspects she is in labor, she should be evaluated. The assessment should include fetal monitoring, assessment of cervical status with cervical and vaginal cultures, assessment of amniotic fluid, and assessment of maternal vital signs looking for possible infections.

Treatment may begin with oral or parenteral hydration as indicated. Decreased maternal activity or bed rest may be indicated; however, bed rest never has been shown to decrease preterm birth. Women on long-term bed rest may develop complications from the bed rest. If preterm labor does not stop with these measures, tocolytic therapy may be started, which uses pharmaceuticals to suppress uterine activity. The most commonly used drugs are terbutaline, magnesium sulfate, indomethacin, nifedipine, and ritodrine. Although ritodrine is the only drug approved by the Food and Drug Administration for preterm labor, it may be the least used. These drugs should be used with caution because of the potential side effects to the woman and fetus. Maternal side effects are jitteriness, headache, heart palpitations, pulmonary edema, hypotension, hyperglycemia, and cardiac arrhythmias. Fetal side effect can include hyperglycemia, tachycardia, heart failure, and hyperinsulinemia. Promotion of fetal lung maturity can be encouraged with the administration of antenatal glucocorticoids. Although antenatal glucocorticoids have been in use since the early 1970s, widespread use began after the National Institutes of Health Concensus Development Conference Group (1995) recommended their use in all women between 24 and 34 weeks of gestation that are threatened with preterm labor. Fetal home monitoring may be indicated for women experiencing preterm labor.

Premature rupture of membranes. A rupture or leaking of the amniotic sac beginning at least 1 hour before the onset of labor is premature rupture of membranes. If rupture occurs before 37 weeks gestation, the term is *preterm premature rupture of membranes*. Premature rupture of membranes is confirmed by visualization of amniotic fluid in the vaginal vault on speculum examination, ferning (when viewing a sample of vaginal secretions under the microscope, specimen will have the appearance of ferns), and a positive nitrozine tape. When preterm premature rupture of membranes is suspected, sterile technique should be used to avoid the introduction of infection. As long as no signs of infection or fetal distress are present, the pregnancy can continue. This is known as expectant management.

Gestational diabetes. Gestational diabetes mellitus (GDM) is a carbohydrate intolerance of variable severity with an onset or first recognition during pregnancy. GDM occurs in approximately 2% to 7% of all pregnancies, with African-Americans, Hispanics, Southeast Asians, and Native Americans at increased risk (Expert Committee of the Diagnosis and Classification of Diabetes Mellitus, 1997). Insulin may or may not be required, and the condition may persist after the pregnancy. Those women that are at risk for GDM may include those who previously gave birth to an infant greater than 9 pounds (4000 g), previously had unexplained fetal death, previously had an infant with congenital anomalies, have maternal obesity greater than 20% above ideal weight, have hypertension, had GDM in a previous pregnancy, or have family history of diabetes. All pregnant women should be screened for GDM, according to the American Diabetes Association (1997). A 1-hour glucose challenge test between 24 and 28 weeks of gestation is recommended. If the blood glucose is greater than 120 mg/dL, a 3-hour glucose tolerance test is recommended. If the blood glucose is greater than 200 mg/dL on the glucose challenge test, a diagnosis of GDM can be made. A definitive diagnosis requires that two or more of the venous plasma (or serum) glucose concentrations be met or exceeded on the 3-hour glucose tolerance test. Those levels are as follows:

1. Fasting: 105 mg/dL
2. 1 hour: 190 mg/dL
3. 2 hours: 165 mg/dL
4. 3 hours: 145 mg/dL

Because GDM develops after the first trimester, GDM usually is not associated with spontaneous abortions or an increased incidence of congenital abnormalities. However, the effects are similar to those associated with preexisting diabetes. Maternal hyperglycemia can affect the woman and fetus. The woman is at increased risk for pregnancy-induced hypertension, urinary tract infections, ketoacidosis, polyhydramnios, and difficult labors. The effects of GDM on the fetus and neonate may include macrosomia, hypoglycemia, hypocalcemia, polycythemia, respiratory distress syndrome, hyperbilirubinemia, and perinatal death.

Therapeutic management should encompass diet, exercise, glucose monitoring, and fetal surveillance. Insulin therapy may or may not be needed. The dietary goal is to provide weight gain as close to a normal pregnancy as possible while preventing ketoacidosis. Exercise helps to use glucose and decrease insulin need; however, an exercise plan should take into account risk factors for the woman and fetus. Blood glucose levels can be monitored several times a day; however, to avoid hyperglycemia, postprandial measurements often are taken. The goal for women with GDM is to maintain euglycemia, which is target blood glucose levels within the 65 to 130 mg/dL range. By assessing the fetus regularly, the chances for complications are decreased. Teaching the pregnant women to do kick counts daily during the last trimester is an excellent assessment tool. Other means of fetal surveillance may include a nonstress test (NST), biophysical profile, and amniotic fluid index. Teaching the woman about GDM and how to live with it and control it are essential when providing care.

Cesarean birth.   Cesarean births have risen to 20.7% of all births (Centers for Disease Control and Prevention, 1998). A national goal for the *Healthy People 2010* initiative is to reduce the rate of cesarean births to no more than 15%, with the rate of primary cesarean births being no more than 12% of total births. Although the United States has decreased the rate of cesarean births, the rate is not near this goal.

Indications for performing a cesarean birth occur when the mother or fetus would be compromised by a vaginal delivery (Porrecco & Thorp, 1996). The following are some of the indications for cesarean birth:

- Active genital herpes
- Fetal distress, disease, or anomaly
- Fetal malpresentation or malposition
- Fetal macrosomia
- Prolapsed umbilical cord
- Cephalopelvic disproportion
- Placental abnormality (placenta previa or abruptio placentae)

■ Some previous uterine surgeries (classical cesarean birth)
■ Maternal disease process

Some women who have cesarean births have feelings of failure and inadequacy leading to guilt. They may have planned their births and did not anticipate any complications (DiMattero, 1996). Communication and support are essential to help them achieve a positive view of their birth experience.

Cesarean birth is major surgery and does have an increased risk over vaginal birth. Maternal complications may include infection, hemorrhage, urinary tract trauma, thrombophlebitis, paralytic ileus, atelectasis, and complications related to anesthesia. Besides the risks to the mother, the fetus may be at additional risk. Fetal complications may include injury, such as laceration or bruising, prematurity because of incorrect calculation of gestational age, and transient tachypnea.

The postpartum recovery period is usually longer and hospitalization is longer with cesarean births. Physiological concerns of women after cesarean birth may include fatigue, activity intolerance, and incisional problems. Pain control may be their primary concern for the first several days. Nursing care should follow the guidelines of a surgical client. During the prenatal period, the woman's primary care provider should explain that cesarean birth is a possible complication.

Uterine rupture. Uterine rupture is rare, with an incidence less than 0.05% in all pregnancies. Uterine rupture is associated with previous cesarean birth, trauma, oxytocin use, abruptio placentae, breech version, midforceps delivery, grand multiparity, and epidural anesthesia. Uterine rupture is considered an obstetrical emergency, and the care provider should know the signs and symptoms. The symptoms may vary depending on the extent of the rupture. The woman may have increased abdominal tenderness, vomiting, faintness, hypotonic uterine contractions, and lack of progress if the rupture is small or incomplete. The fetus eventually shows signs of fetal distress from the loss of blood. If the rupture is complete, the woman may complain of sudden sharp pain in her abdomen. She may shows signs of shock from the blood loss. A loss of the fetal heart rate may occur if the placenta separates. An emergency cesarean birth is necessary.

This section covers complications of pregnancy that can exist at any time but when present during pregnancy can alter the course of the disease or complicate the pregnancy.

Domestic violence. Domestic violence against women cuts across all socioeconomic and ethnic lines. Pregnancy is often the trigger for the beginning or escalation of violence in a relationship. Abuse concerns power and control and when a woman becomes pregnant, the partner may be jealous of the fetus or unable to control the stresses of the pregnancy. Physical abuse during pregnancy tends to be directed to the abdomen, breasts, or genitalia. The incidence of domestic violence is estimated to be 16%, which is one in six pregnant women (McFarlane, Parker, & Soeken, 1996). Janssen (2002) documents how domestic violence assessment can be incorporated in the care of obstetrics patients.

Substance abuse. The use of alcohol, tobacco, and illicit drugs such as marijuana and cocaine increases risk of complications to the mother and fetus. Substance abuse is not new but is increasing within the general population and during pregnancy. Multiple drug use is a common problem that can have a devastating effect on fetal and neonatal outcomes. Many of these problems become long-term physical and developmental problems for the neonate. Inadequate nutrition, inadequate prenatal care, and a higher incidence of STDs are associated with the use of drugs (Lieberman, 1998). Providing care to these women may take an interdisciplinary team for interventions.

Trauma. The leading cause of maternal death during pregnancy is trauma. The most frequent causes of injury are motor vehicle accidents, physical abuse, and falls (Lavery & Staten-McCormick, 1995). Head injuries are the most common, with abdominal injuries the second most common. Other major trauma includes spinal trauma, shock, open-chest trauma, pelvic fractures, or burns. Minor injuries may include lacerations, soft tissue injury, and fractures of the face, hand, foot, or long bones.

The primary goal in trauma is stabilization, remembering that two patients are involved—the mother and fetus. Fetal survival depends on maternal survival. Initially, the basic rules of resuscitation should be applied to the mother: Airway, Breathing, and Circulation. Maternal positioning can be accomplished with a wedge along either side for lateral displacement of the uterus. This minimizes compression of large blood vessels by the uterus. Electronic fetal monitoring is begun as soon as the mother is stabilized. Delivery may be necessary depending on gestational age and the extent of the injuries.

Preexisting diseases or chronic conditions also can place a woman at risk for further complications. The conditions may affect the pregnancy or the disease process. Some of those diseases may include cardiac diseases, diabetes, hypertension, renal diseases, postcancer therapy, or neurological diseases. Treatment of any existing medical problem should be managed in collaboration with the primary care provider.

Fetal Complications

The normal gestation is 280 days. During that time the normal fetus grows to an average length of 19 to 21 inches (48 to 53 cm) and 6 pounds 10 ounces to 8 pounds (3000 to 3600 g). This weight is known as average for gestational age. Human intrauterine growth charts have been developed to assess adequate fetal growth. When a question exists concerning size-for-dates estimate, an ultrasound can be performed.

Infants that weigh below the 10th percentile at term are considered small for gestational age. Small for gestational age infants and infants with intrauterine growth retardation are at risk for perinatal mortality and morbidity. Complications to those infants may include hypoglycemia, heat loss, meconium aspiration, and perinatal asphyxia.

An infant of more than 4000 g is considered large for gestational age. Such infants may be preterm, term, or postterm. They are associated with diabetic mothers and late birth dates. Trauma of delivery is the most common complication to these infants. Shoulder dystocia and birth trauma may be problems.

Postpartum Period

Once the baby has arrived, each system in the mother's body takes 4 to 6 weeks to return to a nonpregnant state. This time is known as the postpartum period. Not only is the woman's body returning to its prepregnant state, but also she is making psychosocial changes as new roles emerge. The postpartum period is often a stressful time physically and emotionally for the new parents. Physical fatigue, anxiety, and discomfort often contribute to depression and difficulty in role transition. Prenatal couple interventions and support for the couple to enhance their marital satisfaction may contribute to better role transition and fewer problems in the postpartum period (Bryan, 2000; Elek, Hudson, & Fleck, 2002; Stark, 2001).

Change in the reproductive system begins with the involution of the uterus as it contracts to its nonpregnant size. This may produce after-birth pains and some discomfort. Vaginal discharge progresses from lochia rubra to lochia serosa and finally to lochia alba, lasting 3 to 6 weeks. The perineum and vaginal walls may be edematous immediately follow the birth; however, healing and involution occur within the 6-week postpartum period.

Milk production by the breasts occurs on the second or third postpartum day in response to the release of prolactin. Engorgement of the breasts subsides in 2 to 3 days for non–breast-feeding women. If a mother chooses not to breast-feed, suppression of lactation needs to be started. Binding the breasts or wearing a tight-fitting bra 24 hours a day until the breasts become soft is the safest method to prevent breast engorgement. Ice packs to the breasts and analgesics relieve discomfort and pain. Women need to be instructed to avoid breast stimulation, warm showers directly to breasts, and pumping, which may stimulate milk production.

The cardiovascular system has an immediate decrease in blood volume at delivery related to blood loss; however, returning to the normal prepregnant volume takes 3 to 4 weeks. As blood shifts from extracellular to central circulation, cardiac output increases, and the kidneys excrete the excess fluid.

The urinary system may develop problems because of trauma or edema of the bladder, urethra, or urinary meatus after delivery. Diuresis begins within 12 hours after birth and continues through the first week postpartum. Kidney function returns to normal by 4 weeks after delivery.

Although physical needs of the woman seem to be a priority immediately postpartum, psychosocial adaptations are beginning. The birth of a child changes the family structure and roles of family members. How each individual reacts depends on previous experiences, the availability of a support system, cultural factors, and family influences. Attachment and bonding describe the initial steps of adaptation to forming a family. Traditionally, both concepts deal with the formation of a relationship between a mother and her newborn; however, all members of a family unit will have bonding and attachment issues (Mercer, 1985).

Bonding and attachment are gradual processes that lead to feelings of love and devotion that last throughout life. Interaction between the parents and child is necessary for bonding to occur. By encouraging unlimited contact, a nurse can provide an arena for bonding to begin.

Achieving the role of a parent with the confidence to care for the infant and comfort with the parental role many take several months. The transition to the maternal or paternal role follows four stages (Mercer, 1985):

1. The anticipatory stage grants the parents time to seek other role models.
2. The formal stage allows the parent to become acquainted with the infant and begin to take cues from the infant.
3. The informal stage encourages parents to respond to the infant as a unique individual.
4. The personal stage is attained when the parents feel a sense of harmony in their roles.

This process usually takes 4 to 6 months.

Postpartum blues is a mild, transient mood disturbance that frequently begins 1 to 10 days after birth and usually last no more than 2 weeks (Ugarriza, 1992). A possible cause of this emotional change may be the normal physiological drop in estrogen and progesterone. The symptoms may include anxiety, weeping, mood swings, and fatigue. Even though the condition may be upsetting to the mother, postpartum blues does not usually interfere with the mother's ability to participate in her own care or the care of her newborn. Education and support assist the mother through this condition.

Naturally, regaining a prepregnancy weight and fitness is a concern of many women, but exercise and dieting need to be moderate to maintain health and nutritional status. Women should resume routine exercise gradually, based on the woman's physical capability (American College of Obstetricians and Gynecologists, 1994b). If pain or other symptoms occur, exercise should be stopped. For women during the reproductive years, health maintenance and promotion should follow the guidelines of preconceptual care because the possibility of future pregnancies exists.

Postpartum Complications

The most common types of postpartum complications are hemorrhage, infections, thrombophlebitis, and depression. The following is a discussion of each condition.

Hemorrhage

Postpartum hemorrhage is defined as a blood loss greater than 500 mL in the first 24 hours after delivery. Late hemorrhage may occur up to 7 to 14 days postpartum. Postpartum hemorrhage occurs in approximately 4% of all deliveries and is responsible for one third of maternal deaths. Hemorrhage may be caused by uterine atony, lacerations of the gential tract, hematomas, retained placental fragments, or blood coagulation disorders. Treatment depends on the extent of the hemorrhage and its cause.

Postpartum Infections

Postpartum infections can be divided into three categories involving the breasts, urinary tract, or reproductive tract. Infections occur in approximately 6% of births in the United States. The most common is endometritis secondary to chorioamnionitis before birth.

Many infections are signaled by an elevated temperature and a feeling of malaise. Each type of infection should be treated depending on the symptoms.

Thrombophlebitis

Thrombophlebitis is an infection of a vessel in which a clot attaches to the vessel wall. The condition may occur in the legs or pelvis. Onset is usually 10 to 29 days postpartum but can occur earlier. Thrombophlebitis places the woman at risk for a pulmonary embolism and death related to obstruction of the lungs. Fortunately, thrombophlebitis occurs in less than 1% of all postpartum women.

Postpartum Depression and Psychosis

Postpartum depression and psychosis are maladaptations to the stress of the postpartum period. The mildest form of postpartum depression is the baby blues. Depression may occur in as many as 400,000 U.S. women each year (Beck & Gable, 2000). This phase passes quickly and may last only a few hours or days. Symptoms include mood swings, weepiness, fatigue, discomfort, and anorexia. The baby blues may be associated with the physical and hormonal changes in the woman's body. Postpartum depression can occur anytime during the first postpartum year but usually appears by the fourth postpartum week. The woman is usually tearful and despondent, having feelings of inadequacy, and feels she is not able to cope. She may have a lack of interest in herself or the baby and may have difficulty sleeping or concentrating. Professional help is usually necessary to return to her former state. Postpartum psychosis may manifest itself in a full psychotic break, with hallucinations and delusions. This condition is very dangerous for the mother and baby and could result in physical harm to either or both. Psychiatric care is needed immediately.

Lactation

Description

Most women choose how they are going to feed their babies before they give birth. *Healthy People 2010: National Health Promotion and Disease Prevention Objectives* goal is for 75% of all women to breast-feed. Although breast-feeding is increasing, the goal has not been attained (Fairbank et al., 1999).

Assessment and Management

Physical preparation for breast-feeding is questionable. The best preparation may lie in breast-feeding classes and education for the woman. The woman needs to be taught the process of breast-feeding, along with signs of adequate intake for the infant.

Complications of breast-feeding may be cracked nipples, mastitis, or difficulty latching on for the infant. Mastitis is an infection of the breast and usually presents with a high temperature and a hard, red, tender mass in one or both breasts. Treatment includes administering an analgesic, providing adequate fluids, binding the breast, applying heat for the breast-feeding mother and cold for the bottle-feeding mother.

INFERTILITY

Description

Having children is a valued experience by most women and until recently an expected norm within society. When a couple is unable to conceive, they are faced with a sense of failure. Such infertility can lead to stress and tension in the family and often to marital and sexual problems. Allan (2001) identified the critical attributes of nurses caring for infertile patients and how their interventions can positively impact the emotional outcomes of these families.

Infertility is defined as the failure to conceive after 1 full year of normal, regular intercourse without the use of any contraception or the inability to continue a pregnancy to live birth. The American Society for Reproductive Medicine (1998) states that infertility affects 6.1 million American women and their partners. This is 10% of the population of reproductive age.

In the United States, although infertility is not a serious health threat, personal, economic, and social consequences still exist. Diagnosis and treatment can be expensive and often are not covered by medical insurance. Treatments can be invasive and time-consuming. The stress of trying to conceive can be draining to a relationship. Infertility affects more than just the couple experiencing the problem; it affects the family and community.

Although infertility rates have been relatively constant for the past 3 decades, public perception is that infertility is on the rise. Several demographic and social factors have contributed to this misconception:

- Delaying childbirth decreases the number of years in which to achieve conception.
- An increase in physicians trained specifically in infertility increases public awareness of infertility (American College of Obstetricians and Gynecolgists, 1989b).
- Legalized abortions have decreased the number of babies available for adoption (Levine, Staiger, Kane, & Zimmerman, 1999).
- Improvements in drug therapy and assistive reproductive therapies have been developed and publicized (Schoener & Krysa, 1996).

Primary infertility occurs when a woman has never conceived or a man has never impregnated a woman. Secondary infertility happens when a woman has been pregnant in the past but is unable to conceive again or carry a fetus to a live birth. Fertility decreases as couples age. Men's sperm count is highest at age 20 and slowly decreases, with conception still possible in their 60s and 70s. Women's fertility decreases greatly after age 30 and continues to decrease steadily until menopause (Meyers et al., 1995). Many couples are delaying conception until their mid-30s because of personal, social, or economic reasons.

For a couple unable to conceive, the myth is that the woman is solely responsible. In fact, the source of infertility is almost evenly divided between the two partners. In approximately 40% of infertile couples, the male is the sole cause or a contributing factor to infertility. Forty percent of the time the cause can be associated with the female, and 20% of infertility is unexplained. More than one factor contributes to infertility in

25% of couples experiencing the condition. A diagnosis of unexplained infertility is made by exclusion after testing reveals no abnormality. When infertility becomes an issue, both partners should be evaluated and involved in the process (Ross & Niederberger, 1995).

Causes

Health habits can influence the ability to conceive. Nutritional status, weigh gain or loss, excessive exercise, smoking, alcohol intake, caffeine, and drug use, including prescription, over-the-counter, and illicit drugs, can decrease fertility. Infections, especially sexually transmitted diseases left untreated, can decrease fertility. When infertility is caused by infection, *Chlamydia, Neisseria gonorrhoeae*, and *Ureaplasma urealyticum* are the most common agents (Shane, 1993). Even though these organisms can be eliminated, sometimes they leave residual damage in the form of scar tissue. The scar tissue can block the fallopian tube, which accounts for 35% of all female infertility problems (American Society for Reproductive Medicine, 1998).

Female Factor Infertility

Tubal blockage and peritoneal factors (endometriosis) are the greatest contributing factors to female infertility (American Society of Reproductive Medicine, 1998) and may result from scarring of the reproductive organs. Abnormal or irregular ovulation accounts for one quarter of a woman's inability to conceive. Other factors may be related to physical abnormalities or infections of the reproductive organs, incompetent cervix, medical conditions, or immunological factors.

Male Factor Infertility

Sperm dysfunction is the greatest contributing factor to male factor infertility (American College of Obstetricians and Gynecologists, 1990). Sperm dysfunction includes low sperm count, poor sperm motility, or poor sperm morphology. Other factors may include abnormalities of the reproductive system, varicocele, infections, or drug use and sexual dysfunction (Ross & Niederberger, 1995). Lifestyle habits and environmental exposures may lead to abnormal spermatogenesis.

Assessment

The holistic philosophy of nursing is an excellent basis for care and guidance through the stages of reproductive life. Advanced practice nurses can provide gynecological care through the infertility process. Their role is to provide an appropriate course of evaluation and treatment. The couple should be seen together for the initial interview, helping to reiterate that infertility is a joint problem. The meeting establishes an understanding of what each person will undergo during testing. A comprehensive history includes partners' ages, occupations, medical conditions, surgical histories, and duration of unprotected intercourse. Coital frequency and habits should be noted to determine whether intercourse is taking place properly for conception. A basic knowledge of reproduction and sexual function is necessary for each couple. Intercourse every 2 to 3 days is usually sufficient to permit conception. Other information includes any previous pregnancy with another partner, history of sexually transmitted diseases, and the women's menstrual cycle along with any symptoms such as pain.

Male Evaluation

Ideally in a fertility workup, male factors should be ruled out first because testing is less invasive and complicated. During the physical examination, abnormalities of the genital structures, varicocele, testicular size, and the prostate should be noted. Tenderness may be an indication of infection. Initial laboratory testing of the male includes semen analysis, which evaluates semen volume, pH, density (sperm per milliliter), motility, some measurement of forward progression of sperm, and sperm morphology (Ross & Niederberger, 1995). Table 16-10 gives normal values for sperm.

A sperm penetration assay may be done to show whether the sperm has the ability to penetrate an egg. In addition, subtle hormonal abnormalities may impair fertility; therefore serum screening of follicle-stimulating hormone, luteinizing hormone, testosterone, and prolactin are recommended (Ross & Niederberger, 1995). If a male has a normal physical examination and semen analysis, then attention should be turned to the female.

Female Evaluation

A complete physical examination is necessary to rule out an underlying disease process or physical abnormality. Physical abnormalities may include a second vagina, false pouch, abnormal configurations of the uterus, ovarian cyst, infection, or tenderness. Initial laboratory tests include complete blood count and Pap smear and tests for rubella or *Chlamydia* (Shane, 1993). After the physical examination, ovulation should be documented on a calendar or daily record. Basal body temperature of the woman should be taken each morning before rising. During the cycle, a slight rise of

Table 16-10	CRITERIA FOR NORMAL SEMEN ANALYSIS (ON AT LEAST TWO OCCASIONS)	
SEMEN PARAMETER	**VALUE**
Volume	1.5-5.0 mL
Density	>20 million/mL
Motility	0.60%
Forward progression	>2 (scale of 1-4)
Morphology	>60% normal forms
Leukocytes	<1 million/mL
Agglutination	None
Hyperviscosity	None

From American College of Obstetricians and Gynecologists (1993). *Male infertility. (American College of Obstetricians and Gynecologists Bulletin 142).* Washington, DC: Author.

approximately 0.5°F at midcycle until menstruation is an indication that ovulation has occurred. The basal body temperature chart should not be used to schedule intercourse, because when the temperature rises, ovulation already has occurred. Changes in cervical mucosa also occur during a cycle. Observation of this mucus can provide additional information on ovulation. When ovulatory dysfunction is suspected, hormonal laboratory evaluation is necessary. Follicle-stimulating hormone, luteinizing hormone, prolactin, and thyroid-stimulating hormone levels are measured, and thyroid function studies are performed, with progesterone levels being measured 1 week after ovulation occurs. Pelvic ultrasound may be performed to detect ovarian cysts, polyps, or fibroids.

If sperm appear to be normal and ovulation has been confirmed, a postcoital test may be completed. When the female is ovulating, a sample of mucus is taken from the cervix 2 to 4 hours after intercourse. A positive result means live sperm are still present. The usefulness of this test has been debated, however (Cohlen, te Velde, & Habberma, 1999). Timing of the test, antibodies to sperm, cervical infections, or inadequate production of cervical mucus may interfere with the results.

The next step in the process of determining female infertility involves examining the uterus, ovaries, and fallopian tubes. A hysterosalpingogram determines whether the fallopian tubes are patent. A laparoscopy permits visualization of the external organs of the reproductive system. This is the only way to determine if external lesions are present. Adhesions can be removed at the time of the laparoscopy. These tests complete the normal sequence of testing for fertility patients (Table 16-11).

Other types of specialized testing are also available. The average length of time for an infertility workup is 6 months. The timing of testing often depends on the couple's desires and monetary considerations. Continued investigations should be based on any positive findings and the patients' desire and willingness to continue.

Management

The goal of treatment is to produce a viable pregnancy and child. How this goal is achieved is based on the cause of infertility. Interventions vary from the simple to the complex using advanced technology.

Simple lifestyle habits may be changed to increase fertility. For example, having the woman remain in a supine position with her hips on a pillow for 20 minutes after intercourse increases pooling of semen near the cervix. Lubricants or postcoital douching can decrease fertility and should be avoided. Sperm are affected negatively by heat; therefore, boxer shorts instead of jockey underwear for men decrease the body temperature, providing a cooler environment for sperm. Abstinence from male ejaculation except during ovulation can be detrimental to sperm. By abstaining for a period of 7 days, the number of abnormal or dead sperm increases (Weinberg & Wilcox, 1995).

Ovulation disorders occur in 20% of infertility cases. Hormone therapy can produce ovulation in 80% of the women, leading to a pregnancy rate of 40% (American College of Obstetricians and Gynecologists, 1989b). Clomiphene citrate is the most commonly

Table 16-11 INFERTILITY: CAUSES, TESTS, AND TREATMENTS

COMMON CAUSE	DIAGNOSTIC TESTS	TREATMENT PROCEDURES
Male Factors		
Low sperm count	Semen analysis	Antibiotics
Poor sperm motility	Sperm penetration assay	Hormone treatment
Poor sperm morphology		Micromanipulation: introcytoplasmic sperm injection into the ovum
Varicocele	Physical exam Sonogram	Varicocelectomy
Female Factors		
Peritoneal factors (endometriosis)	Laparoscopy	Fertility medication Surgery
Ovulation factors	Basal body temperature chart Endometrial biopsy	Fertility medication Egg donor
Tubal factors	Hysterosalpingogram Laparoscopy	In vitro fertilization Gamete intrafallopian transfer Zygote intrafallopian transfer
Cervical factors	Postcoital test	Antibiotics Hormone treatment Intrauterine insemination
Uterine factors	Hysterosalpingogram Hysteroscopy	Surgery
Immunology factors	Antiphospholipid antibodies Alloimmune risk tests Lupuslike antibodies Antithyroid antibodies	Treatment specific for immune needs
Interactive factors	Postcoital test Chromosomal studies of couple and any fetal losses	Intrauterine insemination
Unexplained factors	All	Any or all

Modified from American Society for Reproductive Medicine. (1998). *Fact sheet: Infertility*. Birmingham, AL: Author.

employed drug used to induce ovulation, with bromocriptine mesylate, gonadotropins, and gonadotropin-releasing hormone also being used (American College of Obstetricians and Gynecologists, 1996a). The side effects of these drugs can include hot flashes, headaches, nausea, breast tenderness, nervousness, depression, fatigue, insomnia, and irritability. Additionally, the risk of multiple gestation is increased. A greater incidence of ovarian cancer has been reported with prolonged use of these drugs (Rossing, Daling, Weiss, Moore, & Self, 1994). Currently, 6 months is the suggested length of administration for these drugs. These drugs are costly and often not covered by insurance. Table 16-12 presents drug types, success rates, and side effects.

Table 16-12	SUCCESS RATES AND SIDE EFFECTS OF VARIOUS AGENTS FOR INDUCTION OF OVULATION

DRUGS	OVULATION RATES (%)	PREGNANCY RATES (%)	MULTIPLE PREGNANCY RATES (%)	COMMON SIDE EFFECTS
Clomiphene citrate Clomid Serophene	≤80	≤40	≤8	Hot flashes, visual symptoms, nausea, and breast tenderness
Bromocriptine Parlodel	≤98	≤85	<1	Gastrointestinal irritation, orthostatic hypotension, nasal congestion, and headache
Gonadotropins Pregnyl Pergonal Humegon Repronex	30-100	20-90	≤30	Local (injection-related) and hyperstimulation syndrome
Gonadotropin-releasing hormone	30-100	20-90	≤12	Local (injection-related)

Modified from American College of Obstetricians and Gynecologists. (1994). *Managing the anovulatory state: Medical induction of ovulation. (American College of Obstetricians and Gynecologists Technical Bulletin 197).* Washington, DC: Author.

Assisted Reproductive Technologies

If fertility has not been achieved by other interventions, the couple may be candidates for assisted reproductive technologies. During the last two decades, technology has improved the chances of conception. A landmark in fertility technology was reached in 1978 when the first "test tube baby" was born. Today, in vitro fertilization is a commonplace treatment for infertility. Through the use of different techniques outside of the uterus, pregnancy can be achieved. Table 16-13 outlines types of assisted reproductive technologies, Table 16-14 shows the usage of such technologies, and Table 16-15 defines success rates as reported by the Centers for Disease Control and Prevention (2000).

Assisted reproductive technology is helping to redefine cultural norms (Sandelowski, 1999). Technology is helping to create new human arrangements, norms, and values. The use of new technologies may expose cultural and ethical concerns. Advanced practice nurses are in a position to assist women and their partners in understanding the controversies and concerns of assisted reproductive technology.

Intrauterine insemination is the process of collecting semen and then gently spinning it in a centrifuge to separate serum from sperm. The sperm then are placed high into the uterus through a small catheter, permitting the sperm to be closer to the fallopian tube.

Table 16-13   TYPES OF ASSISTED REPRODUCTIVE TECHNOLOGIES

TYPES OF ART	DESCRIPTION
Intrauterine insemination	Collect semen and gently spin to separate serum from sperm. Place semen high into the uterus through a small catheter, permitting the sperm to be closer to the fallopian tubes.
In vitro fertilization	Retrieve ovum or ova, vaginally or through laparoscopy. In the laboratory, the egg(s) and sperm are combined in a petri dish. Fertilization should occur in 2 to 3 days. The fertilized egg(s) are placed in the uterus through the vagina.
Gamete intrafallopian transfer	Eggs are retrieved through a laparoscopy, combined with concentrated sperm and placed directly into the fallopian tube, where fertilization occurs naturally.
Zygote intrafallopian transfer	Similar to in vitro fertilization except the zygote is placed directly into the tube through laparoscopy rather than into the uterus.
Introcytoplasmic sperm injection	A microscopic needle is inserted just under the capsule of the egg and one sperm is injected directly into the egg. The fertilized ovum then is placed in the uterus or fallopian tube for implantation.

Table 16-14   NATIONAL SUMMARY OF ASSISTED REPRODUCTIVE TECHNOLOGIES: (ART) 1997 PROGRAM PROFILE

PROGRAM CHARACTERISTICS	TYPE OF ART	ART PATIENT DIAGNOSIS
Total clinics 335	In vitro fertilization 93%	Tubal factor 27%
SART* member 96%	Gamete intrafallopian transfer 4%	Endometriosis 14%
Single women 76%	Zygote intrafallopian transfer 2%	Uterine factor 2%
Gestational carriers 37%	Combination 1%	Male factor 23%
Donor egg programs 78%	With introcytoplasmic sperm	Ovulatory dysfunction, 16%
Sharing of donor eggs 23%	injection 35%	Male factor 23%
	Unstimulated <1%	Other factors 8%
		Unexplained 10%

*Society of Artificial Reproductive Technology.

When infertility is caused by the male and cannot be treated, a donor sperm specimen can be used. The process is known as artificial insemination. Donors should be screened medically and then matched to the physical characteristics of the male partner. Frozen donor sperm is the appropriate type of specimen instead of using fresh sperm, therefore avoiding the risk of human immunodeficiency virus (Shane, 1993). If a couple are considering more than one child with the same genetic base, additional vials of sperm can be frozen for future use.

Table 16-15	1997 ASSISTED REPRODUCTIVE TECHNOLOGIES PREGNANCY SUCCESS RATES			
TYPE OF CYCLE	**AGE OF WOMEN**			
Fresh Embryos From Nondonor Eggs	*<35*	*35-38*	*39-40*	*>40*
Number of cycles	24,581	12,733	10,997	6,691
Pregnancies per 100 cycles	35.7	31.2	22.8	13.2
Live births per 100 cycles	30.7	25.5	17.1	7.6
Live births per 100 retrievals	33.8	29.6	20.9	9.9
Live births per 100 cycles	35.9	31.4	22.5	10.9
Cancellations per 100 cycles	9.3	14.0	18.3	22.9
Average number of embryos transferred	3.7	3.8	3.9	4.0
Twin gestation per 100 pregnancies	30.7	26.4	21.8	15.3
Triplet or more gestations per 100 pregnancies	13.7	11.3	6.8	2.8
Multiple live births per 100 live births	43.0	36.8	28.4	19.0
Frozen Embryos From Nondonor Eggs				
Number of transfers	4,862	2,144	1,385	774
Live births per 100 transfers	21.3	18.6	14.5	10.0
Avgerage number of embryos transferred	3.5	3.4	3.5	3.6
Donor Eggs				
Number of fresh transfers	547	480	846	2,625
Live births per 100 fresh transfers	40.8	41.9	36.6	40.2
Number of frozen transfers	177	134	213	958
Live births per 100 frozen transfers	16.4	22.4	19.3	23.6
Average number embryos transferred (fresh and frozen)	3.5	3.6	3.7	3.7

From Centers for Disease Control and Prevention. (2000). *Women's health data by state and U.S. territory.* Hyattsville, MD: National Center for Health Statistics.

In vitro fertilization is indicated for those women who have blocked or damaged fallopian tubes or unexplained infertility. In vitro fertilization uses ova retrieved vaginally with ultrasonograpic guidance or through laparoscopy. In the laboratory the eggs and sperm are combined in a petri dish. Fertilization should occur in 2 to 3 days. When this happens, the fertilized eggs are placed in the uterus through the vagina. Different protocols can be used, depending on the couple and the institution. Drug stimulation of the ovaries increases the number of eggs available for retrieval. Several eggs can be removed and fertilized and then cryopreserved for future use so that the couple does not need to repeat the initial procedure. Most clinics limit the number of eggs implanted because of an increased risk for multiple gestation. Natural cycle in vitro fertilization does not stimulate the ovaries and uses only the woman's eggs produced that month, usually one or two.

The gamete intrafallopian transfer is appropriate for women with normal fallopian tubes. Eggs are retrieved via laparoscopy, combined with concentrated sperm, and placed directly into the fallopian tube, where fertilization occurs naturally. The gamete intrafallopian transfer is acceptable to some religious groups that otherwise oppose in vitro fertilization.

Zygote intrafallopian transfer is similar to in vitro fertilization except that the zygote is placed directly into the tube through laparoscopy rather than into the uterus. This technique is not performed as often because of its cost and the ease of other techniques.

Introcytoplasmic sperm injection is a new treatment for male factor infertility. When the sperm are incapable of penetrating the shell of the ovum, a microscopic needle is inserted just under the capsule of the egg and one sperm is injected directly into the egg. The fertilized ovum then is placed in the uterus or tube for implantation.

Researchers are studying the possibility of preimplantation genetic diagnosis, which examines cells before implantation. Cells would be examined for possible defects or chromosome abnormalities. This allows couples to choose only unaffected embryos before transfer.

Another option is a surrogate mother carrying the genetic baby of the infertile couple. Sharan and others (2001) found that hospitalization of the genetic mother alongside the surrogate mother helped facilitate early bonding of the genetic parents.

Ethical Considerations

Social and legal aspects of infertility constantly are being debated by the religious community, the medical community, and society at large. Donor sperm and oocytes, surrogacy, storage of sperm and fertilized eggs, posthumous use of sperm, multiple pregnancies, cloning, selective reduction for multiple gestation, and ownership of cryopreserved fertilized ova are a few of the concerns. As knowledge of human reproductive biology expands, questions arise concerning individual values and interests versus those of society. Reproduction and parenting are social acts that are valued in society, but private reproductive decisions may have harmful effects. Women may be exploited, sex-distribution may be altered, or changes in social patterns may occur (Baird, 1997).

Laws and statutes vary from state to state. The American Society for Reproductive Medicine is a volunteer organization that is committed to maintaining ethical and medical standards and guidelines for reproductive medicine. Legal consultation is now part of the screening process in some clinics. Informed consent is essential for all parties before assisted reproductive technologies are used.

The cost of treating infertility per cycle is high. Depending on the treatment required, estimates range from a few hundred dollars to as high as $25,000 (American Society for Reproductive Medicine, 1998). The ability to access infertility assistance is limited to person with money or health insurance that covers infertility. Reimbursements by medical insurance vary. A few states have legislated that infertility services be covered by insurance. How to pay for infertility services has become an issue. Many couples cannot afford the services and are unable to receive treatment. The perception that infertility affects only white professional couples is not true. The fact is that poor couples with little education are more likely to be infertile (Abma, Chandra, Mosher, Peterson, & Piccinino, 1997). Typically, the affluent couples have the resources to seek and pay for infertility care.

Success rates of fertilization vary depending on the therapy. Scientific advances have increased the chance of fertility, but the possibility of delivering a viable baby is less than 40% (American Society of Reproductive Medicine, 1998).

Infertility affects the psychological, physical, and spiritual well-being of a couple. The ability to bear children is a central theme in the identification of being a woman. Infertility can cause a sense of loss of power and control, thus diminishing self-esteem for the couple. Deciding when to stop therapy is often stressful. Many couples find a rest from attempting to conceive is necessary. Counseling can help a couple cope with these difficult decisions. This is a role the advanced practice nurse can fulfill.

Learning to live with infertility has been related to the stages of death and dying (Kübler-Ross, 1969). Denial, anger, grief, and acceptance are the stages of adaptation that define the psychospiritual steps. Couples work through each stage and revisit them many times during their process. Remaining childless or even having a child often does not bring closure; many couples continue to view themselves as infertile (Schoener & Krysa, 1996).

ADOPTION

Adoption is an option for infertile couples and for those individuals who have a personal or social desire to adopt a child. Just like the infertility process, the adoption process may take many years, especially when one limits the choice of a child to a newborn. Adoptions can be arranged through an agency or independently and are no longer limited to couples; single-parent adoption is increasing.

More than 100,000 children are adopted in the United States each year (Gemignani, 1997). These adoptions include 10,000 children with special emotional or physical needs and 8000 international children. Adoption can occur across borders but may be more difficult. Laws vary from state to state and country to country. Legal counsel is often necessary to ensure all requirements and laws have been met.

As adoption is considered, a person should examine the reasons for adoption and become educated on the process. Adoptive parents describe the process as full of fear and anxiety, even though they consider themselves risk takers. Feelings of uncertainty, unpreparedness, and isolation, along with competition, a commitment to an unguaranteed investment, judgment, and ostracism from a variety of sources plague prospective adoptive parents (Lobar & Phillips, 1996).

Because adoption can be done publicly, privately, or independently, a decision on which process of adoption to pursue is necessary. The type of child—including age, race, sex, and any special needs—is a required decision for the couple or individual seeking to adopt. One issue is the type of adoption. At one time, adoptions were confidential and kept secret. Today, open adoption, where the birth parents and adoptive parents exchange information and meet, is becoming acceptable.

Adoption costs vary; usually a public agency is less expensive but may take the longest. Adoption fees average $12,000. If a couple has spent large amounts of money on infertility treatments, paying another fee for a child is difficult. Approximately one quarter of large corporations offer adoption benefits to their employees. The Small Business Job Protection Act of 1996 gives employers a tax break for offering adoption assistance up to $5,000 per child. The Family Medical Leave Act of 1993 allows new adoptive parents leave from their jobs.

Advanced practice nurses in primary care are in a unique position to offer support and encouragement with adoptions issues and to suggest resources for further help (Peterson, 1997). Primary care providers see the adoptive parents throughout the entire life cycle and can assess their needs, providing information and assistance as they adapt to their parenting roles.

Relinquishment

Traditionally, the focus of attention has been on the needs of adoptive parents rather than those of the birth mother. Most adoptions in the past were confidential and did not permit access to the birth mother. With current practices changing, the birth mother is more involved. These women naturally have a sense of loss and grief and may need assistance in dealing with those feelings. The process of relinquishment follows four major themes (Lauderdale, 1994):

1. The woman's feelings of being alone and pregnant
2. The decision-making process on the outcome of the pregnancy
3. The birth of the child without the acknowledgment of becoming a mother from family, friends, and hospital staff
4. How the experience has changed the women's life

Mothers relinquishing their babies have the same need for information and preparation for childbirth as any other woman (Keen-Payne & Bond, 1997). After the birth they may have greater needs because of the loss of the child. Open adoption has helped many of these women cope by allowing them some knowledge of their children. Through the holistic approach of nursing, women's health care nurses may function in multiple roles for women relinquishing their children including those of educator, counselor, and care manager.

ELECTIVE OR INDUCED ABORTIONS

Elective or induced abortions are voluntary methods for terminating a pregnancy. An elective abortion may be performed to preserve the health of the mother, end a pregnancy caused by rape or incest, or prevent the birth of a child with severe abnormalities. A woman may elect to terminate her pregnancy for personal, social, or economic reasons. Legalization of abortion in the United States occurred in 1973 with the Supreme Court decision in *Roe v. Wade.* Since that decision, abortion policy has remained one of the most controversial issues. Abortion involves social and ethical issues. Those who deliver health care to women must examine their own views on abortion.

The Centers for Disease Control and Prevention monitors the trends in elective abortions. Since 1990, the year in which the number of abortions was highest, the United States has had a steady decline in the number of abortions. The decrease is approximately 5% per year (Koonin, Smith, Ramick, & Strauss, 1998).

COMMON REPRODUCTIVE SYSTEM PROBLEMS

This last section covers the more common aspects of reproductive issues needing attention by health care providers. These issues relate specifically to the reproductive cycle and function.

Dysfunctional Uterine Bleeding

Description and Causes

The most common gynecological problems are related to menstruation or abnormal vaginal bleeding. Typical menstrual cycles last 28 days but may be 19 to 35 days apart. Irregular cycles are also common and may not indicate a problem. Abnormally long, short, or irregular cycles may create practical problems for individual women. Many women can have painful or heavy periods that disrupt their everyday lives. Women are aware that the pain will resolve within a few days only to return with predictable regularity and learn to plan activities around their menses. Because the pain and discomfort of menstruation has been viewed as normal, some women may not seek or gain treatment. Table 16-16 summarizes common reproductive problems.

Assessment

Abnormal uterine bleeding may occur across the entire life span. Dysfunctional uterine bleeding is a diagnosis of exclusion. Evaluation of abnormal bleeding warrants further investigation. A complete history includes the type, frequency, and length of bleeding; pregnancy history and current status; medical conditions; and effects on the woman and her lifestyle (American College of Obstetricians and Gynecologists, 1996a). Yearly physicals, including a pelvic examination and Pap smear, can provide a basis for diagnosing and treating problems. Although bleeding may have an underlying medical cause, often no medical reason exists for the symptoms. Fibroids and endometriosis are the most common causes of abnormal bleeding and pain (Engstrom et al., 1999)

Management

Treatment depends on the cause of the dysfunction bleeding. If conservative management does not satisfy the woman, pharmacological or surgical interventions may be necessary.

Dysmenorrhea

Description and Causes

Dysmenorrhea is pain experienced during or immediately before menstruation. Menstrual pain is common, causing women to lose more time from work than any other condition (Bingham, 1998). Although the pain is benign and will resolve itself within a

Table 16-16	COMMON HEALTH PROBLEMS OF REPRODUCTIVE-AGE WOMEN			
PROBLEM	**INCIDENCE**	**CAUSE**	**DIAGNOSIS**	**TREATMENT**
Dysfunctional uterine bleeding	Report of incidences vary	Diagnosis of exclusion	Complete history and physical exam; Pap smear Laboratory testing depends on findings of history and physical	Treat underlying cause
Dysmenorrhea	50% of menstruating women	Primary: no pathological condition in pelvic region Secondary: pathological condition in pelvic region	Complete history and physical exam Laboratory testing depends on findings of history and physical	Self-help measures: massage, exercise, biofeedback, eliminate caffeine and smoking NSAIDs*; oral contraceptives
Menorrhagia	30% of women of reproductive age	Pregnancy-related conditions Reproductive tract disorders Systemic conditions Dysfunctional uterine bleeding	Complete history and physical exam Laboratory testing: pregnancy test, complete blood count, serum ferritin, and other tests as indicated Pelvic ultrasound Tissue sampling by dilatation and curettage or hysteroscopy	Drug therapy: NSAIDs, oral contraceptives, progestins, gonadotropin-releasing hormone analogues, antifibrinolytics, and danazol Surgical interventions: hysterectomy or endometrial ablation
Amenorrhea	Varies with cause	Pregnancy, lactation, menopause, anatomical defects of the female reproductive system, ovarian failure, and endocrine imbalances	Complete history and physical exam Laboratory testing: pregnancy test, serum prolactin, TSH, LH, FSH, and estradiol Pelvic ultrasound MRI	Depends on cause and the needs of the woman

Table 16-16	COMMON HEALTH PROBLEMS OF REPRODUCTIVE-AGE WOMEN —CONT'D			
PROBLEM	**INCIDENCE**	**CAUSE**	**DIAGNOSIS**	**TREATMENT**
Endometriosis	1 in 10 women during the reproductive years	Implantation of endometrium outside the uterus	Direct visualization or biopsy is necessary for confirmation of the diagnosis.	Depends on symptoms and women's needs NSAIDs Alternative therapies Oral contraceptives Hormone therapy Surgical intervention: laser during laparoscopy or hysterectomy
Uterine fibroids	30% of women of reproductive age with an incidence among African-American women greater than in white women	Benign neoplasmic tumors of the uterine muscle	Complete history and physical exam Pelvis ultrasound MRI	Depends on desire of woman to maintain uterus Expectant management Myomectomy Hysterectomy
Premenstrual syndrome	May be as high as 97% of women at some time during their lives	Unknown cause	Complete history and physical exam to rule out any other disease processes	Lifestyle changes to decrease stress, increase exercise, maintain a balanced diet, and provide emotional support Drug therapy: vitamin B_6, benzodiazepines, selective serotonin reuptake inhibitors, oral micronized progesterone, and oral contraceptives

*NSAIDs, nonsteroidal antiinflammatory drugs; *TSH*, thyroid-stimulating hormone; *LH*, luteinizing hormone; *FSH*, follicle-stimulating hormone; *MRI*, magnetic resonance imaging.

few days, women affected by dysmenorrhea soon realize the pain will return with the next cycle.

Dysmenorrhea is categorized as primary or secondary. Primary dysmenorrhea is the most common and usually occurs in nulliparous young women. Painful menstruation occurs without a pathological condition in the pelvic region. Dysmenorrhea affects approximately 50% of menstruating women (American College of Obstetricians and Gynecologists, 1983). Secondary dysmenorrhea is caused by pathological conditions of the pelvic region, which should resolve when the cause is treated (Zhang & Li Wan Po,

1998). Some of the causes could be infection, endometriosis, fibroids, or a foreign object such as a tampon or an intrauterine device. If pain persists, a complete evaluation to determine the cause may be necessary for some women.

Assessment

Physical symptoms of dysmenorrhea may include cramping in the pelvic region, back pain, and gastrointestinal upsets of nausea, vomiting, and diarrhea. Psychological symptoms may include nervousness, depression, irritability, and sleeplessness. To diagnose primary dysmenorrhea, it is necessary to rule out any underlying pathological condition. A complete health history and physical is the basis of discovery. If a pathological condition is present, appropriate treatment for the specific problem is necessary.

Management

For primary dysmenorrhea, relief may come from self-help measures such as exercise, massage, biofeedback, eliminating caffeine, smoking cessation, and other tension-relieving measures. Drug therapy with nonsteroidal antiinflammatory drugs (NSAIDs) or analgesics can be effective in treating the pain. If the pain does not respond to analgesics, oral contraceptives are an option. The benefits of oral contraceptives are credited to a decreased prostaglandin synthesis, which causes the endometrium to atrophy.

Menorrhagia

Description and Causes

Menorrhagia is a greater than normal amount of vaginal bleeding and may have clots present. Approximately 30% of women of reproductive age experience menorrhagia (Hurskainen et al., 1998). Common causes of menorrhagia during the reproductive years can be divided into pregnancy-related conditions, reproductive tract disorders, systemic conditions, and dysfunctional uterine bleeding (Engstrom et al., 1999). The underlying pathological condition may include infections, fibroids, an intrauterine device, systemic diseases such as leukemia or diabetes, cancer, abortion, and cervical or endometrial polyps.

Assessment

Normal blood loss during a single menstruation is approximately 75 mL, varying from woman to woman and during different stages of each individual's life. Traditionally, more than 80 mL has been considered a heavy period. Recent studies indicate the risk of developing anemia from heavy menstrual bleeding occurs at a blood loss of 120 mL, not 80 mL (Janssen, Scholten, & Heintz, 1998). Determining blood loss usually is based on the woman's assessment of menstrual blood loss; however, personal judgment is not reliable. Only 40% to 53% of women complaining of excessive bleeding have true menorrhagia (Hurskainen et al., 1998). Assessing actual blood loss can be supported with a complete menstrual history, including frequency, duration, pattern, and amount

(Engstrom et al., 1999). Asking the woman to describe the amount of flow, to count the number and type of sanitary products used during a specific period, and to assess the amount of staining on the product can assist in establishing a pattern. Weighing the sanitary products before and after use can provide an estimate of menstrual blood loss.

Assessment of the women with complaints of heavy bleeding begins with a complete health history and physical examination. Initial laboratory testing includes a pregnancy test and complete blood count. Because prolonged or heavy bleeding may decrease iron stores, a serum ferritin level may be recommended to assess the woman's iron reserves (Engstrom et al., 1999). Other laboratory testing should be based on the findings during the history and physical examination.

Standard evaluation and treatment has been a dilatation and curettage to remove tissue for evaluation. However, endocrine disorders often are associated with menorrhagia making a dilatation and curettage ineffective as a therapeutic procedure (American College of Obstetricians and Gynecologists, 1996). Today, tissue samples can be obtained through hysteroscopy in the office or in an outpatient setting, with transvaginal ultrasound allowing visualization of the pelvic region. Each of these procedures is less invasive and reduces costs for women and insurance companies. Detection of uterine abnormalities such as polyps and fibroids can be assessed with ultrasound, along with an evaluation of the uterine body.

Management

Treatment depends on the patient's diagnosis, age, and needs. Drug therapy may consist of NSAIDs for pain and inflammation, oral contraceptives, progestins, gonadotropin-releasing hormone analogues, antifibrinolytics, and danazol (Chen & Giudice, 1998).

Interventional radiology has been used to cut off the blood flow to fibroids, which destroys them. If bleeding continues and the woman has completed childbearing, a hysterectomy should be considered if medical therapies have failed. Another surgical modality developed in the last decade is endometrial ablation. The endometrium is permanently destroyed by thermal energy or removed through a hysteroscope. The thermal procedure can be done in the office under local anesthesia, thus reducing postoperative complications, pain, and cost (Chen & Giudice, 1998). Although advanced practice nurses can manage treatments and therapies, the surgical techniques of dilatation and curettage, hysteroscopy, hysterectomy, and endometrial ablation require a physician's skill.

Amenorrhea

Description and Causes

Amenorrhea is the complete cessation of menses for more than 6 months (Baird, 1997). Changes in menstruation may be caused by normal physiological causes such as pregnancy (the most common cause), lactation, and menopause. Amenorrhea is not a diagnosis in itself and should be regarded as pathological when present during the reproductive years. Treatment depends on the cause, which can be anatomical, ovarian failure, or endocrine imbalances. Anatomical causes include defects or absences of the uterus or vagina. Amenorrhea resulting from ovarian malfunction is associated with endocrine conditions. Any malfunction in the endocrine system can cause a disruption in the menstrual cycle. Endocrine imbalances are the most common form of amenorrhea and can include disorders of the ovaries, anterior pituitary, adrenal glands, thyroid, or the hypothalamus (American College of Obstetricians and Gynecologists, 1989a). Besides physiological problems with the endocrine system, weight loss, anorexia, excessive exercise, or stress can alter the function of the hypothalamus, thereby preventing ovulation (Baird, 1997).

Assessment

A female who has never menstruated is said to have primary amenorrhea. Secondary amenorrhea is the absence of menstruation in women with past menses.

Diagnosis begins with a complete history and physical examination. Pregnancy is the most common cause of amenorrhea and must be ruled out first. Other laboratory testing includes serum prolactin, thyroid-stimulating hormone, luteinizing hormone, follicle-stimulating hormone, and estradiol. Pelvic ultrasound or magnetic resonance imaging can rule out any pelvic abnormalities.

Management

Treatment depends on the results of the tests and the presenting problem. Amenorrhea has no debilitating effect on a woman's health but is always a symptom of some other process. Treatment depends on the cause and the needs of the woman.

Endometriosis

Description and Causes

Endometriosis occurs when endometrial tissue travels through the fallopian tubes and implants outside of the uterus on other pelvic structures. The implanted endometrial tissue responds to hormonal changes as it would inside the uterus. With each cycle the tissues multiply and enlarge—if conception does not occur—and then fragment and bleed, leading to inflammation and scarring (Corwin, 1997). Scarring from endometriosis can cause blockage of the fallopian tubes, preventing conception, which makes endometriosis the largest contributing factor to female infertility (American Society for Reproductive Medicine, 1998).

Determining the exact number of women affected by endometriosis has been difficult because many women may be asymptomatic or have unusual or vague symptoms. As many as 1 in 10 females may be affected by endometriosis during the reproductive years (Pepping, 1994). In the United States endometriosis is most common in white females during their early to middle reproductive years.

Assessment

Symptoms of endometriosis vary with each woman. The degree of endometriosis does not seem to correlate with the symptoms. Some women with advanced endometriosis may have few to no symptoms, whereas other women with minimal disease are affected with pain, bleeding, or sexual dysfunction (American College of Obstetricians and Gynecologists, 1999). Symptoms may include dysmenorrhea, dyspareunia (painful intercourse), pelvic pain, spotting or irregular uterine bleeding, and infertility. Advanced disease attached to the rectum or urinary tract may cause rectal or urinary bleeding and painful defecation.

A history and physical examination can suggest a diagnosis of endometriosis, but direct visualization or biopsy is necessary for confirmation of the diagnosis (American College of Obstetricians and Gynecologists, 1999a).

Management

Treatment depends on the severity of the symptoms and the woman's needs and can be accomplished by analgesics, hormones, surgery, or combined approaches. Mild to moderate pain can be managed with NSAIDs. For those women not trying to conceive, drug therapy with oral contraceptives or hormonal therapy (gonadotropin-realeasing hormone analogues) to suppress the growth of endometriosis lesions may be a choice. Either of these therapies can be initiated without confirmation of a diagnosis (American College of Obstetricians and Gynecologists, 1999a). For mild discomfort, relief may come from alternative therapies such as exercise, massage, biofeedback, and other tension-relieving measures. When conservative therapies are not effective in decreasing or controlling the symptoms, surgical intervention may be indicated, including laser treatment during laparoscopy or, for those women who have completed their families, hysterectomy.

A primary practitioner must have an understanding of the medical aspects of this disease along with the social and psychological costs. Endometriosis symptoms can influence self-esteem and interfere with women's daily lives. Nursing interventions should be designed to relieve pain.

Uterine Fibroids

Description and Causes

Fibroids (uterine leiomyomata) are the most common benign neoplasmic tumors of the uterine muscle. Fibroids occur in 30% of women of reproductive age with an incidence among African-American women greater than white women (Cramer, 1992). Usually appearing in the middle reproductive years and slow growing, fibroids are often asymptomatic and may be found during routine pelvic exams. Because fibroids are slow growing, symptoms more often are seen in the later reproductive years or around menopause.

Assessment

Heavy bleeding that may cause anemia, pelvic pain, and urinary frequency is common. Although seldom seen in pregnancy, large fibroids may interfere with conception and place the pregnant woman at increased risk for abortion, preterm labor, or postpartum hemorrhage.

Uterine fibroids can be detected in 95% of women on physical examination (American College of Obstetricians and Gynecologists, 1996a). Confirmation of the diagnosis can be accomplished with ultrasound, magnetic resonance imaging, or direct laparoscopy.

Management

Treatment depends on the symptoms and desire of the woman to maintain her uterus for future pregnancies. If symptoms are mild or absent, expectant management of physical assessments yearly are appropriate. Other symptoms can be treated with NSAIDs or oral contraceptives. Myomectomy for the removal of the symptomatic fibroids is appropriate for the woman wishing to retain her uterus, knowing reoccurrence is common. If childbearing is complete, hysterectomy is appropriate. Gonadotropin-releasing hormone analogues reduce uterine volume and fibroid size and pelvic symptoms and improve anemia by decreasing vaginal bleeding (Lethaby, Vollenhoven, & Sowter, 1999). Drug therapy should not be considered a cure because, as soon as therapy is discontinued, the fibroids will regrow and symptoms will return. However, gonadotropin-releasing hormone analogue therapy for 3 to 4 months before surgery may decrease the uterine size to allow for a vaginal, instead of an abdominal, hysterectomy. Interventional radiology may remove the fibroid without surgical intervention.

Nursing interventions depend on the patient's desire. The role of the advanced practice nurse as primary caregiver includes assessments, yearly physical examinations, and supporting the woman's decisions in the management of fibroids. Comanagement with a physician partner is necessary when surgery is indicated.

Premenstrual Syndrome

Description and Causes

Premenstrual syndrome (PMS) is a common condition with medical and psychiatric aspects affecting as many as 97% of women at some time during their lives (Kraemer & Kraemer, 1998). However, a uniform definition or diagnostic criteria in the literature and in practice is lacking. With no definition to guide research, a clear cause of the syndrome has not emerged, nor have effective treatments been developed (Cahill, 1998). Symptoms encompass physical and emotional changes during the luteal phase of the menstrual cycle and diminish during the remainder of the cycle. High levels of estradiol and progesterone are characteristic of the luteal secretory phase, causing edema in the endometrium. Withdrawal of estradiol and progesterone results in tissue sloughing (Abraham, 1983). Symptoms usually are present 7 to 12 days before menses and absent or mild during the week of menstruation.

Establishing the pathological course of PMS continues to be elusive because of the difference in symptoms and normal hormonal changes occurring during the premenstrual period. Many hypotheses have been cited as reasons for PMS. Some of the following are currently under investigation: nutritional deficits possibly related to vitamin B_6, ovarian hormonal imbalance, fluid retention produced by an increase in progesterone-estrogen levels, or dysfunction of neurotransmitter endorphins.

Assessment

Symptoms of PMS vary from woman to woman and may vary from cycle to cycle. Typically, behavioral symptoms are characterized by mood swings, irritability, depression, anxiety, fatigue, and forgetfulness. Physical symptoms may include swelling, breast tenderness, acne, abdominal bloating, gastrointestinal upset, headaches, and an increased appetite.

Most of the time, recognition of PMS comes from the woman or nonmedical associates of hers rather than a medical clinician (Kraemer & Kraemer, 1998). Self-diagnosis often leads to self-help; consequently, fewer than 40% of women seek medical help for PMS (Swann, 1995). If a woman seeks care for PMS, exact symptoms need to be identified and a comparison of her menstrual cycle needs to be established. The woman should keep a calendar with the dates of her menstrual periods, the dates of symptoms, the symptoms and their severity, and self-treatment that may or may not have improved the symptoms. Determining estradiol, progesterone, and prolactin levels during the most severe symptoms may help to determine a hormonal imbalance. The woman also needs a complete physical examination, including blood pressure, weight, heart and lung assessment, breast examination, and pelvic examination. Careful consideration should be given to signs of endometriosis or dysmenorrhea, which are often present in women with PMS.

Management

Just as symptoms vary, treatment for PMS varies, and a combination of treatment modalities may be necessary. Treatments can be divided into two categories: medical and natural. Natural approaches usually begin with education and lifestyle changes to decrease stress, increase exercise, maintain a balanced diet, avoid caffeine, and provide emotional support. The medical approach focuses on balancing hormone levels and providing comfort. Drug therapy with vitamin B_6, benzodiazepines, selective serotonin reuptake inhibitors, oral micronized progesterone, and suppression of ovulation with hormonal agents such as medroxyprogesterone acetate or oral contraceptives may offer relief from some symptoms (American College of Obstetricians and Gynecologists, 1995). NSAIDs, diuretics, and high-protein, low-salt, and low-sugar diets also may be prescribed.

Nursing management for a woman with PMS indicates a need for individual approaches. Objective data gathering with careful evaluation is necessary. Women need to know that their complaints are legitimate and their care provider is willing to assess their problem before advising treatment.

SUMMARY

Women's health care is no longer focused solely on pregnancy but is designed to meet the needs of women across the life span. Women's health care is being recognized as a legitimate specialty practice, with more health care providers practicing in this area, including advanced practice nurses. Nurse practitioners, nurse midwives, and clinical nurse specialists are all providing care within the field of women's health. Women of reproductive age have a conundrum of complex variables that affect their health. Nurses' holistic approach to health care provides women with an opportunity to access care that addresses their entire biopsychosocial needs.

REFERENCES

Abma, J., Chandra, A., Mosher, W., Peterson, L., & Piccinino, L. (1997). Fertility, family planning, and women's health: New data from the 1995 National Survey of Family Growth. *Vital Health Stat, 23*(19).

Abraham, G. (1983). Nutritional factors in the etiology of the premenstrual tension syndrome. *Journal of Reproductive Medicine, 28*(464).

Affonso, D., Liu-Chiang, C., & Mayberry, L. (1999). Worry: Conceptual dimensions and relevance to child-bearing woman. *Health Care for Women International, 20*(3), 227–236.

Allan, H. (2001). A "good enough" nurse: Supporting patients in a fertility unit. *Nursing Inquiry, 8* (1), 51–60.

American Academy of Pediatrics & American College of Obstetricians and Gynecologists. (1992). *Guidelines for perinatal care* (3rd ed.). Elk Grove Village, IL: Authors.

American College of Obstetricians and Gynecologists. (1983). *Dysmenorrhea (American College of Obstetricians and Gynecologists Technical Bulletin 68).* Washington, DC: Author.

American College of Obstetricians and Gynecologists. (1989a). *Amenorrhea (American College of Obstetricians and Gynecologists Technical Bulletin 128).* Washington, DC: Author.

American College of Obstetricians and Gynecologists. (1989b). *Infertility (American College of Obstetricians and Gynecologists Technical Bulletin 125).* Washington, DC: Author.

American College of Obstetricians and Gynecologists. (1993). *Male infertility (American College of Obstetricians and Gynecologists Technical Bulletin 142).* Washington, DC: Author.

American College of Obstetricians and Gynecologists. (1994). *Managing the anovulatory state: Medical induction of ovulation (American College of Obstetricians and Gynecologists Technical Bulletin 197).* Washington, DC: Author.

American College of Obstetricians and Gynecologists. (1994a). *Antepartum fetal surveillance (American College of Obstetricians and Gynecologists Technical Bulletin 188).* Washington, DC: Author.

American College of Obstetricians and Gynecologists. (1994b). *Exercise during pregnancy and the postpartum period (American College of Obstetricians and Gynecologists Technical Bulletin 189).* Washington, DC: Author.

American College of Obstetricians and Gynecologists (1995). *Premenstrual syndrome (American College of Obstetricians and Gynecologists Technical Bulletin 155).* Washington, DC: Author.

American College of Obstetricians and Gynecologists. (1996a). *Guidelines for women's health care.* Washington, DC: Author.

American College of Obstetricians and Gynecologists. (1996b). *Hypertension in pregnancy (American College of Obstetricians and Gynecologists Technical Bulletin 219).* Washington, DC: Author.

American College of Obstetricians and Gynecologists. (1998). *Cultural competency in health care (American College of Obstetricians and Gynecologists Committee Opinion 201).* Washington, DC: Author.

American College of Obstetricians and Gynecologists. (1999a). *Endometriosis (American College of Obstetricians and Gynecologists Technical Bulletin 11).* Washington, DC: Author.

American College of Obstetricians and Gynecologists. (1999b). *Induction of labor (American College of Obstetricians and Gynecologists Technical Bulletin 10).* Washington, DC: Author.

American College of Obstetricians and Gynecologists & American Academy of Pediatrics. (1997). *Guidelines for perinatal care* (4th Ed.). Elk Grove Village, IL, and Washington, DC: Author.

American Diabetes Association. (1997). Position statement: Gestational diabetes mellitus. *Diabetic Care, 20* (Suppl.), S44.

American Society for Reproductive Medicine. (1998). *Fact sheet: Infertility.* Birmingham, AL: Author.

Association of Women's Health, Obstetric and Neonatal Nurses. (1993). *Competencies and program guidelines for nurse providers of perinatal education.* Washington, DC: Author.

Association of Women's Health, Obstetric and Neonatal Nurses. (1997). *Standards and guidelines for professional nursing practice in the care of women and newborns* (5th Ed.). Washington, DC: Author.

Baird, D. (1997). Amenorrhoea. *Lancet, 350*(9073), 275–279.

Beck, C., & Gable, R. (2000). Postpartum Depression Screen Scale: Development and psychometric testing. *Nursing Research, 49*(5), 272–282.

Berry, R., Li, Z., Erickson, J., Li, S., Moore, C., Wang, H., et al. (1999). Prevention of neural-tube defect with folic acid in China. China–United States Collaborative Project for Neural Tube Defect Prevention. *New England Journal of Medicine, 341*(20), 1485–1490.

Bingham, K. (1998). Women's health. *Nursing Standard, 12*(40), 26–27.

Bonifield, S. (1998). A cost-saving analysis of prenatal interventions. *Journal of Healthcare Management, 43*(5), 443–451.

Bowers, B. (2002). Mothers' experiences of labor support: exploration of qualitative research. *Journal of Obstetric, Gynecologic, and Neonatal Nursing, 31* (6), 742–752.

Bryan, A. (2000). Enhancing parent-child interaction with a prenatal couple intervention. *MNC The American Journal of Maternal/Child Nursing, 25* (3), 139–145.

Cahill, C. (1998). Differences in cortisol, a stress hormone, in women with turmoil-type premenstrual symptoms. *Nursing Research, 47*(5), 278–283.

Caughey, A., Shipp, T., Repke, J., Zelop, C., Cohen, A., & Liberman, E. (1999). Rate of uterine rupture during a trial of labor in women with one or two prior cesarean deliveries. *American Journal of Obstetrics and Gynecology, 181*(4), 872–876.

Centers for Disease Control and Prevention. (1997). Update: Prevalence of overweight among children, adolescents, and adults—United States, 1988–1994. *Morbidity and Mortality Weekly Reports, 46*, 199–202, 721–723.

Centers for Disease Control and Prevention. (1998). *Behavioral Risk Factor Surveillance System (BRFSS) Summary of Prevalence Report.* Altanta, GA: Department of Health and Human Services, Centers for Disease Control and Prevention.

Chadwick, R. (1993). What counts as success in genetic counseling? *Journal of Medical Ethics, 19*, 43.

Chapman, L. (2000). Expectant fathers and labor epidurals. *MNC The American Journal of Maternal/Child Nursing, 25* (3), 133–138.

Chen, B., & Giudice, L. (1998). Dysfunctional uterine bleeding. *Western Journal of Medicine, 169*(5), 280–284.

Cheung, L. (2001). Complicated and uncomplicated pregnancies: Women's perception of risk. *Journal of Obstetric, Gynecologic, and Neonatal Nursing, 30* (20), 192–201.

Cohlen, B., te Velde, E., & Habberma, J. (1999). Postcoital testing. *British Medical Journal, 318*(7189), 1008–1009.

Corwin, E. (1997). Endometriosis: Pathology, diagnosis, and treatment. *Nurse Practitioner, 22*(10), 35–42.

Cowan, M. (1996). Hyperemesis gravidarum: Implications for home care and infusion therapies. *Journal of Intravenous Nursing, 19*, 46–58.

Craft, N. (1997). The childbearing years and after. *British Medical Journal, 7118*(315), 1301–1305.

Cramer, D. (1992). Epidemiology of myomas. *Seminars in Reproductive Endocrinology, 10*, 320–324.

DiMattero, R. (1996). Cesarean childbirth and psychosocial outcomes: A meta-analysis. *Health Psychology, 15*(4) 303–314.

Dimitry, E., & Morcos, M. (1990). The increasing incidence of ectopic pregnancy: 193 cases in ten years in the Medway towns. *British Journal of Obstetrics and Gynaecology, 10*(3), 181–185.

Doswell, W., & Erlen, J. (1998). Multicultural issues and ethical concerns in the delivery of nursing care interventions. *Nursing Clinics of North America, 33*(2), 353–361.

Doulas of North America. (1999). *Mission statement.* Retrieved from *www.dona.com.*

Doyle, W., Crawford, M., Srivastava, A., & Costeloe, K. (1999). Interpregnancy nutrition intervention with mothers of low-birth-weight babies living in an inner city area: A feasibility study. *Journal of Human Nutrition and Dietetics, 12*(6), 517–527.

Droste, T. (1998). It pays to immunize adults. *Business & Health (Special Report)*, pp. 8–11.

Elek, S., Hudson, D., & Fleck, M. (2002). Couples' experience with fatigue during the transition to parenthood. *Journal of Family Nursing, 8* (3), 221–240.

Engstrom, J., Rose, R., Brill, A., Polhill, K., Lukanich, C., & Fritz, L. (1999). Midwifery care of the woman with menorrhagia. *Journal of Nurse-Midwifery, 44*(2), 89–105.

Expert Committee of the Diagnosis and Classification of Diabetes Mellitus. (1997). Report of the Expert Committee of the Diagnosis and Classification of Diabetes Mellitus. *Diabetes Care, 20*(7), 1183–1187.

Expert Panel on the Content of Prenatal Care. (1989). *Caring for our future: The content of prenatal care.* Washington, DC: Public Health Service.

Fairbank, L., Lister-Sharpe, D., Renfrew, M., Woolridge, M., Sowdwn, A., & O'Meara, S. (1999). Interventions for promoting the initiation of breastfeeding. *Cochrane Library Database of Systematic Reviews,* p. 4.

Feinstein, N. F., (2000). Fetal heart rate auscultation: Current and future practice. *Journal of Obstetric, Gynecologic, and Neonatal Nursing, 29*(3), 306–315.

Gale, J., Fothergill-Bourbonnais, F., & Chamberlain, M. (2001). Measuring nursing support during childbirth. *MNC The American Journal of Maternal/Child Nursing, 26* (5), 264–271.

Gemignani, J. (1997). And baby makes three. *Business & Health, 15*(6), 55–59.

Glei, D. (1999). Measuring contraceptive use patterns among teenage and adult women. *Family Planning Perspectives, 31*(2), 73–81.

Gramling, I., Lambert, V., & Pursley-Crotteau, S., (1998). Coping in young women: Theoretical retroduction. *Journal of Advanced Nursing, 28*(5), 1082–1091.

Hackley, B., (1999). Immunizations in pregnancy: A public health perspective. *Journal of Nurse-Midwifery, 44*(2), 106–117.

Hally, S. (1998). Nutrition in reproductive health. *Journal of Nurse-Midwifery 43*(6), 459–470.

Harrington, C. (2002). Labor intensive: labor and delivery nursing in the 21st century. *Nursing Spectrum (New England Edition), 6* (8), 6–7.

Heaton, T., Jacobson, C., & Holland, K. (1999). Persistence and change in decisions to remain childless. *Journal of Marriage and the Family, 61*(2), 531–539.

Howell, C. J. (2000). Epidural vs. nonepidural for pain relief in labour. *Cochrane Library Database of Systematic Reviews,* Computer File(2) CD000 331.

Humenick, S. (1998). Poetry inspired by the Coalition to Improve Maternity Services (CIMS) and the Mother-Friendly Initiative. *Journal of Perinatal Education, 7*(2), 5–6.

Hurskainen, R., Teperi, J., Turpeinen, U., Grenman, S., Kivela, A., Kujansuu, E., et al. (1998). Combined laboratory and diary method for objective assessment of menstrual blood loss. *Acta Obstetricia et Gynecologica Scandinavica, 77*(2), 201–201.

Janssen, P. (2002). Introducing domestic violence in a postpartum clinical setting. *Maternal & Child Health Journal, 6* (3), 195–203.

Janssen, C., Scholten, P., & Heintz, A. (1998). Reconsidering menorrhagia in gynecological practice. Is a 30-year-old definition still valid? *European Journal of Obstetrics, Gynecology, & Reproductive Biology, 78*(1), 69–72.

Jehle, D., Krause, R., & Braen, G. (1994). Ectopic pregnancy. *Emergency Medicine Clinics of North America, 12*(1), 55–72.

Johnson, K. O. (2002). The lived experience of spirituality in pregnancy. *Communicating Nursing Research, 35* (10), 298.

Keen-Payne, R., & Bond, M. (1997). Voices of clients and caregivers in a maternity home: Pregnant women considering relinquishment. *Western Journal of Nursing Research, 19*(2), 190–204.

Klaus, M., Kennell, J., & Klaus, P. (1993). *Mothering the mother.* New York: Addison-Wesley.

Koonin, L., Smith, J., Ramick, M., & Strauss, L., (1998). Abortion surveillance: United States, 1995. *Morbidity & Mortality Weekly Report, 47*(2), 31–40.

Kraemer, G., & Kraemer, R. (1998). Premenstrual syndrome: Diagnosis and treatment experiences. *Journal of Women's Health, 7*(7), 893–904.

Kübler-Ross, E. (1969). *On death and dying.* New York: Macmillan.

Lauderdale, J. (1994). Infant relinquishment through adoption. *Image: The Journal of Nursing Scholarship, 26*(3), 213–217.

Lavery, J., & Staten-McCormick, M. (1995). Management of moderate to severe trauma in pregnancy. *Obstetrics and Gynecology Clinics of North America, 22*(1), 69–88.

Leininger, M. (1990). Issues, questions, and concerns related to the nursing diagnosis cultural movement from a transcultural nursing perspective. *Journal of Transcultural Nursing, 2*(1), 23–32.

Lethaby, A., Vollenhoven, B., & Sowter, M. (1999). Pre-operative GnRH analogue therapy before hysterectomy or myomectomy for uterine fibroids. *Cochrane Library, 1,* 18.

Levine, P., Staiger, D., Kane, T., & Zimmerman, D. (1999). *Roe vs. Wade* and American fertility. *American Journal of Public Health, 89*(2), 199–203.

Lewis, K., & Moon, S. (1997). Always single and single again women: A qualitative study. *Journal of Marital and Family Therapy, 23*(2), 115–134.

Lieberman, L. (1998). Overview of substance abuse prevention and treatment approaches in urban, multicultural settings: The Center of Substance Abuse Prevention programs for pregnant and postpartum women and their infants. *Women's Health, 8*(4), 208–217.

Lobar, S., & Phillips, S. (1996). Parents who utilize private infant adoption: An ethnographic analysis. *Issues in Comprehensive Pediatric Nursing, 19*(1), 65–76.

Lommel, L. (1990). Antepartal fetal surveillance. In W. L. Star, M. T. Shannon, L. N. Sammons, L. Lommel, & Y. Gutierrez (Eds.), *Ambulatory obstetrics: Protocols for nurse practitioners/nurse midwives* (2nd ed.). San Francisco: School of Nursing, University of California.

Lowe, N. (1996). The pain and discomfort of labor and birth. *Journal of Obstetric, Gynecologic, and Neonatal Nursing, 25*(1), 82–92.

Lucas, V. A. (1991). An investigation of the health care preferences of the lesbian population. *Health Care for Women International, 24*, 25–30.

Lyndon-Rochelle, M. (2001). Risk of uterine rupture during labor among women with a prior cesarean. *The New England Journal of Medicine, 1*, 345.

Manning, F., Pratt, L., & Sipos, L. (1980). Antepartum fetal evaluation: Development of a fetal biophysical profile. *American Journal of Obstetrics and Gynecology, 136*(6), 787–795.

Manogin, T., Bechtel, G., & Rami, J. (2000). Caring behavior by nurses: Women's perception during childbirth. *Journal of Obstetric, Gynecologic, and Neonatal Nursing, 29* (2), 153–157.

Mayberry, L., & Strange, L. (1997). Strategies for designing a research utilization project with labor and delivery nurses. *Journal of Obstetric, Gynecologic, and Neonatal Nursing, 26* (6), 701–708.

McFarlane, J., Parker, B., & Soeken, K. (1996). Abuse during pregnancy: Associations with maternal health and infant birth weight. *Nursing Research, 45*(1), 37–42.

Mercer, R. (1985). The process of maternal role attainment. *Nursing Research, 34*(4), 198–204.

Meyers, M., Diamond, R., Kezur, D., Scharf, C., Weinshel, M., & Rait, DS. (1995). An infertility primer for family therapists: I. Medical, social, and psychological dimensions. *Family Process, 34*(2) 219–229.

Miltner, R. (2002). More than support: nursing interventions provided to women in labor. *Journal of Obstetric, Gynecologic, and Neonatal Nursing, 31* (6), 753–761.

Moore, M. (1999). Biochemical markers for preterm birth. *MNC The American Journal of Maternal/Child Nursing, 24*, 66–74.

Morin, K. (1998a). Perinatal outcomes of obese women: A review of the literature. *Journal of Obstetric, Gynecologic, and Neonatal Nursing, 27*(4), 431–440.

Morin, K. (1998b). Promoting gynecologic health in young and middle-aged women. *Holistic Nursing Practice, 2*(12), 17–28.

Murphy, F. (1998). The experience of early miscarriage from a male perspective. *Journal of Clinical Nursing, 7*(4), 325–332.

Nasso, J. (1997). Planning for pregnancy: A preconceptual health program. *MNC The American Journal of Maternal/Child Nursing, 22*(3), 142–146.

National Institutes of Health Consensus Development Conference Group. (1995). Effects of corticosteriods for fetal maturation on perinatal outcomes. *American Journal of Obstetrics and Gynecology, 173*, 246–252.

National Vital Statistics Reports. (2000). *Births, marriages, divorces, and deaths: Provisional data for January-December 2000, 49*(6). Washington, DC: National Center for Health Statistics.

National Women's Law Center. (2000). *Making the grade on women's health*. Washington, DC: Author.

Nichols, F., & Zwelling, E. (1997). *Maternal-newborn nursing: Theory & practice*. Philadelphia: W. B. Saunders.

1996 American Academy of Nursing Expert Panel on Women's Health (1997). Women's health and women's health care: Recommendations of the 1996 AAN Expert Panel on Women's Health. *Nursing Outlook, 45*(1), 7–15.

Patterson, E., Freese, M., & Goldenberg, R., (1990). Seeking safe passage: Utilizing health care during pregnancy. *Image, 22*(1), 27.

Pepping, P. (1994). Endometriosis: A nursing perspective. *Innovations in Women's Health Nursing, 1*(1), 2.

Peters, K., Kochanek, K., & Murphy, S. (1998). Birth trends in the United States. *National Vital Statistics Reports, 47*(9), 22.

Peterson, E. (1997). Supporting the adoptive family: A developmental approach. *American Journal of Maternal Child Nursing, 22*(3), 147–152.

Porrecco, R., & Thorp, J. (1996). The cesarean birth epidemic: Trends, causes, and solutions. *American Journal of Obstetrics and Gynecology, 175*(2), 369–374.

Pouliot, M., Despres, J., Lemieux, S., Moorjani, S., Bouchard, C., Tremblay, A., et al. (1994). Waist circumference and abdominal sagittal diameter: Best simple anthropometric indexes of abdominal visceral adipose tissue accumulation and related cardiovascular risk in men and women. *American Journal of Cardiology, 73*(7), 460–468.

Quimby, C. (1994). Women and the family of the future. *Journal of Obstetric, Gynecologic, and Neonatal Nursing, 23*(2), 113–123.

Rafferty, M. (1998). Prevention services in primary care: Taking time, setting priorities. *Western Journal of Medicine, 169*(5), 269–275.

Raines, P., & Morgan, Z. (2000). Culturally sensitive care during childbirth. *Applied Nursing Research, 13*(4), 167–172.

Ridley, R., Davis, P., Bright, J., & Sinclair, D. (2002). What influences a woman to choose vaginal birth after cesarean? *Journal of Obstetric, Gynecologic, and Neonatal Nursing, 31* (6), 665–672.

Riemann, M., & Kanstrup Hansen, I. (2000). Effects on the foetus of exercise in pregnancy. *Scandinavian Journal of Medicine & Science in Sports, 10*(1), 12–19.

Ross, L., & Niederberger, C. (1995). Male infertility: Diagnosis and treatment. *Comprehensive Therapy, 21*(6), 276–282.

Rossing, W., Daling, J., Weiss, N., Moore, D., & Self, S. (1994). Ovarian tumors in a cohort of infertile women. *New England Journal of Medicine, 331*(12), 771–776.

Rubin, R. (1984). *Maternal identity and the maternal experience.* New York: Springer-Verlag.

Sadovsky, E. (1985). Monitoring fetal movements: A useful screening test. *Comtemporary Obstetrics and Gynecology, 25*, 123–127.

Sandelowski, M. (1999). Cultural, conceptive technology, and nursing. *International Journal of Nursing Studies, 36*(1), 13–20.

Schmidt, J., & McCartney, P. (2000). History and development of fetal heart assessment: A composite. *Journal of Obstetric, Gynecologic, and Neonatal Nursing, 29*(3), 295–305.

Schoener, C., & Krysa, L. (1996). The comfort and discomfort of infertility. *Journal of Obstetric, Gynecologic, and Neonatal Nursing, 25*(2), 167–172.

Shane, J. (1993). Evaluation and treatment of infertility. *Clinical Symposia, 45*(2), 3–32.

Sharan, H., Yahav, J., Peleg, D., Ben-Rafael, Z., & Merlob, P. (2001). Hospitalization for early bonding of the genetic mother after a surrogate pregnancy. *Birth, 28* (4), 270–273.

Shaw, R., Brickley, M., Evans, L., & Edwards, M. (1998). Perceptions of women on the impact of menorrhagia on their health using multi-attribute utility assessment. *British Journal of Obstetrics & Gynaecology, 105*(11), 1155–1159.

Shermer, R., & Raines, D. (1997). Positioning during second stage of labor: moving back to basics. *Journal of Obstetric, Gynecologic, and Neonatal Nursing, 26*(6), 727–734.

Simpson, K. R., & Poole, J. H. (1998). *Cervical ripening and induction and augmentation of labor.* Washington, DC: Association of Women's Health, Obstetric and Neonatal Nurses.

Spatz, D. (1996). The role of advanced practice nurses in the 21st century. *Nursing Clinics of North America, 31*(2), 269–277.

Stark, M. (2001). Relationship of psychosocial tasks of pregnancy and attentional functioning in the third trimester. *Research in Nursing & Health, 24* (3), 194–202.

Summers, L., & Price, R. (1993). Preconception care. *Journal of Nurse-Midwifery, 38*(4), 188–198.

Swann, C. (1995). A discourse analytic approach to women's experiences of premenstrual syndrome. *Journal of Mental Health, 4*(4), 359–367.

Tessaro, I., Campbell, M., Benedict, S., Kelsey, K., Heisler-MacKinnon, J., Belton, L., et al. (1998). Developing a worksite health promotion intervention: Health works for women. *American Journal of Health Behavior, 22*(6), 434–442.

Tumblin, A., & Simkin, P. (2001). Pregnant women's perception of their nurse's role during labor and delivery. *Birth, 28* (1), 52–56.

U.S. Census Bureau. (1999). *Population trends in women,* April 14, 2000, *www.census.gov.*

U.S. Department of Health and Human Services. (1996). *Physical activity and health: A report of the Surgeon General.* Atlanta, GA: U.S. Department of Health and Human Services, Centers for

Disease Control and Prevention, & National Center of Chronic Disease Prevention and Health Promotion.

U.S. Department of Health and Human Services. (1998). *Public health reports, May-June* (DHHS Publication 017-022-01405-5). Washington, DC: Author.

U.S. Department of Health and Human Services. (2000). *Healthy people 2010: Understanding and improving health* (2nd ed.) (DHHS Publication 017-001-00550-9). Washington, DC: Author.

Ugarriza, D. (1992). Postpartum affective disorders: Incidence and treatment. *Journal of Psychosocial Nursing, 30*(5), 29–32.

Weinberg, C., & Wilcox, A. (1995). A model for estimating the potency and survival of human gametes in vivo. *Biometrics, 51*(2), 405–412.

Weisman, C. (1997). Changing definitions of women's health: Implications for health care policy. *Maternal & Child Health Journal, 1*(3), 179–189.

Wilbur, J., Miller, A., Montgomery, A., & Chandler, P. (1998). Women's physical activity pattern: Nursing implications. *Journal of Obstetric, Gynecologic, and Neonatal Nursing, 27*(4), 383–392.

Wing, D., Park, M., & Paul, R. (2000). A randomized comparison of oral and intravaginal misoprostol for labor induction. *Obstetrics and Gynecology, 95*(6), 905–908.

Wright, L., & Leahey, M. (1994). *Nurses and families: A guide to family assessment and intervention.* Philadelphia: F. A. Davis.

Writing Group of the AAN Expert Panel on Women's Health. (1996). Women's health and women's health care. *Nursing Outlook, 45*(1), 7–15.

Zeidenstein, L. (1990). Gynecological and childbearing needs of lesbians. *Journal of Nurse-Midwifery, 35*(1), 10–18.

Zhang, W., & Li Wan Po, A. (1998). Efficacy of minor analgesics in primary dysmenorrhoea: A systematic review. *British Journal of Obstetrics & Gynaecology, 105*(7), 780–780.

Zucker, C., Wright, J., & Meyer, E. (1999). *Daily word for women* (p. 22). Emmaar, PA: Daybreak Books.

RESOURCES

Association of Women's Health, Obstetric and Neonatal Nurses: *www.awhonn.org*
American Society of Reproductive Medicine: *www.asrm.org*
Society for Artificial Reproductive Technology: *www.sart.org/home.html*
Doulas of North America: *www.dona.org*
La Leche League: *www.lalecheleague.org*
Childbirth Education: *www.childbirth.org; www.bradleybirth.com; www.lamaze=childbirth.com*
World Health Organization: *who.int/en*
Lactation: *www.nursingmother.com*
Centers for Disease Control and Prevention: *www.cdc.gov*
Department of Health and Human Services: *www.4woman.gov*
American College of Obstetricians and Gynecologists: *www.acog.org*

Chapter 17

Health Concerns of Women in Midlife

Carole Kanusky

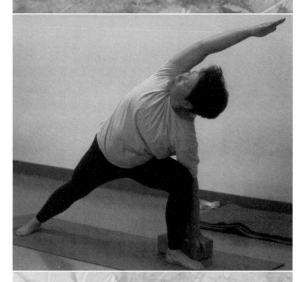

Defining moments or situations in life can be a positive catalyst as the turning point in your life.

Dave Pelzer

INTRODUCTION

During a woman's childbearing years, she is usually most diligent about meeting her health needs. But as years and outside pressures from family, work, and social contacts take hold of her time and energy, her own health is often neglected. In the past, she may have focused on her growing family but now, at midlife, she maybe faced with aging parents and their specific health needs. Today, many women find themselves "sandwiched" in a position of balancing care for two generations simultaneously. Responsibilities associated with the multiple roles that a woman fulfills leave little time for personal care and nurturing.

Midlife can present a golden opportunity for personal introspection, to assess one's health status, identify certain health risks, and acknowledge areas where there is need for health promotion and disease prevention. For health care providers, the midlife woman presents a unique challenge—to individualize her health care as she traverses a period of major life changes. The nursing care of these women should be designed to assess and support ongoing health needs necessary for optimal wellness. The clinician, once thought of as the knowledge expert, now assumes the role of assisting the woman to develop and enhance those actions that are identified as part of that woman's self-care system.

In the past, little attention was focused on midlife women's health issues other than menopause. Only within the past decade or so has research centered on health promotion for what is now the most rapidly growing age population in the United States—midlife women. More than 40 million American women are now postmenopausal and by the year 2010, that number will exceed 60 million (Lindsay, 1999). These women will often live at least 30 years past menopause with a life expectancy of 81 years of age (Blackwell & Blackwell, 1997; Rousseau. 1998). As contemporary midlife women age, their longevity is likely to strain the resources of health care as we know it today. How midlife women currently use health services to promote health and prevent disease becomes particularly important in anticipating future needs and availability of entitlement programs for the elderly.

The National Institutes of Health (NIH) launched a campaign in 1991 to expand the role of women in clinical trials and initiated clinical research specifically on midlife health concerns, including menopause, cardiovascular disease, osteoporosis, and hormone replacement therapy. Women are now being encouraged to make wise health decisions based on identification of health risks, preventive disease education, and personal psychosocial forces that define their health-seeking options, preferences, and behavior. Besides education and socioeconomic factors, cultural beliefs and practices also affect the health status of women by influencing their use of health care services and their confidence and acceptance of recommended prevention and treatment strategies.

Many issues confront women as they journey through the midlife transition. The biologic changes may trigger a sense of loss: the end of fertility and childbearing ability. For some, it may mean the end of their femininity. For women who are mothers, this time coincides with major developmental changes in the lives of their children (adolescence, leaving home, college, marriage). The significance, irreversibility, and unpredictability of menopause may create a feeling of personal distress and loss of control. On a more positive note, many women welcome menopause with open arms as they no longer have to contend with the possibility of a midlife pregnancy and having to deal with monthly periods. It is not surprising that many psychosocial issues related to a woman's multiple roles surface at this time and need to be addressed as part of the health assessment of the midlife woman.

DEFINITION OF MIDLIFE

Early concepts of midlife were defined by a change in a woman's role that occurred when the children finished school, left home, and the woman often sought employment outside the home. Now adult children stay at home much longer and many women have remained in the work force while raising a family. Today such a definition of midlife can present a problem when women in their late 30s and 40s become pregnant and think of college expenses rather than retirement.

Some have used menopause as a historical marker for midlife, linking this part of life to the end of reproductive years. Others more appropriately use age boundaries such as 45 to 65 years to signal midlife (Callahan & Paris, 1997). For women, such limits tend to differentiate between reproductive and non-reproductive years. Regardless of the definition used to delineate midlife, it is important to appreciate the biosociocultural perspective in which an age cohort of women arrive at this unique time of their lives.

Menopause is often considered a turning point in a woman's life, amidst an array of biologic, psychological, social, and spiritual changes. It should mark the beginning of new experiences, filled with adventure and good health. It is during this time that women often search for a new role or purpose in life and may be willing to focus on their own health and wellness.

Unfortunately, in the United States much emphasis is placed on youth, fertility, and vitality. Midlife women experiencing the normal aging process are often made to feel less feminine and less valued as members of society. Long used by health care providers, the biomedical model has supported the negativism associated with midlife and the concept of menopause as a disease process. Women are seen as victims of a deficiency disease (Blackwell & Blackwell, 1997; Winterich & Umberson, 1999).

Today, women are seeking answers, sharing their own experiences and wanting to be heard. "By adopting a biosociocultural perspective, practitioners can provide information about the biological and social factors associated with menopause, thus enabling women to adapt to midlife changes and have confidence in their self-care abilities" (Ellis & Kanusky, 1996, p.45). The emphasis is on the education and empowerment of midlife women and the acceptance of menopause, not as a disease, but as a natural stage of life. A dilemma faced by midlife women and their practitioners is striking the proper balance between accepting the medicalization of menopause or viewing menopause as a normal physiologic life event that allows women to take advantage of health care interventions aimed at preventing chronic disease in later years.

A more holistic approach to menopause and midlife allows for an appreciation of how cultural and social factors affect health promotion behavior, thus enabling women to adapt more easily to change. Participants in the Massachusetts Women's Health Study (the largest and most comprehensive study of midlife women) support the argument that menopause is not, and should not be, viewed as a negative experience. The majority of women interviewed in this study found the physical changes associated with menopause to be unproblematic, but most agree with the cultural perception that women become depressed during menopause for any number of reasons (Winterich & Umbertson, 1999).

HEALTH FOCUS

The greatest disease burden, because of increasing incidence with age, is borne by women 50 years and older. Midlife is often the period of life when women have their first experience with a chronic disease such as high blood pressure, arthritis, heart disease, or diabetes. Hospitalization for this age cohort is most frequently for heart disease, cancer, gallbladder disease, diabetes, and depression. The most common surgical procedures are hysterectomy and cholecystectomy. Cardiovascular disease is the leading cause of death in women in the United States. Before menopause, women rarely develop heart disease, but, by age 50, they have a 50% chance of developing heart disease (Mosca, 2000; Rousseau, 1998). Some risk factors such as gender and age cannot be changed but modifying one's lifestyle and focusing on disease prevention can alter many factors.

The design of care for midlife women is the identification of risk factors through assessment and screening, reduction of health risks through education and behavior modification, and the development of a prevention program designed to support optimum health. The aim is to raise women's awareness of what they can do to prevent disease and protect their quality of life in later years. Chronic medical conditions seen in this age group do not negate the ability of a woman to achieve an optimal state of well-being through ongoing education and health care.

PHYSIOLOGIC AGE-RELATED CHANGES

Menopause is the major physiologic change for midlife women. Many women in the United States view menopause as a turning point in their lives. Some have very positive feelings such as freedom from the need for contraception while others sense a great loss in the change from the reproductive to non-reproductive state. Much of what menopause means to a woman lies within her culture and self-image. Besides the physical changes affecting women 45 to 65 years of age, the cultural, occupational, personal, and family factors must be examined when providing care.

Jones (1997) states that discussion about declining estrogen and symptoms can reinforce a medical representation of menopause. However, the movement in women's health has described menopause as a natural change in a woman's body that may or may not require lifestyle adjustments. For some women, their response to health-related body changes associated with menopause depends on their anticipation of how severe these changes will be and how their lifestyle will be affected. Although many women do experience some degree of body change, they tend to view menopause as a transitional stage of life rather than strictly as a medical condition. It is interesting to note that Japanese women do not have a word for "hot flash" and Canadian women report fewer problems with menopause than American women (Winterich & Umberson, 1999). The complexity of meanings that women give to this phase of their life makes a social definition of menopause difficult. For each woman, her concept of menopause will be based on interrelated social and cultural contexts (Andrist & MacPherson, 2001).

By definition, menopause is the cessation of ovarian function resulting from depletion of ovarian follicles, diagnosed by 1 complete year without any vaginal bleeding. In the United States, the median age for menopause is approximately 51 years. Before age 40, it is considered premature menopause and after age 55, as late menopause. The age of menopause is thought to be genetically related and, contrary to myths, not related to age at menarche, number of pregnancies, or use of oral contraceptives. The one factor that may affect menopausal age is smoking. Smokers tend to reach menopause up to 2 years earlier than nonsmokers, placing smokers at increased risk for diseases associated with low estrogen levels (North American Menopause Society, 2000b). The diagnosis of menopause is supported by a history of symptoms and laboratory values. Perimenopause is the transitional phase before actual menopause when there are observed changes in normal menstrual flow and interval, with or without the onset of vasomotor symptoms (i.e. hot flashes). The word climacteric may also be used to characterize the 5 to 10 years before complete cessation of estrogen production, identified by noncyclic uterine bleeding caused by anovulation or sporadic ovulation. Box 17-1 lists selected menopause terms and definitions.

During midlife, the ovaries are becoming more resistant to the action of FSH, producing decreasing amounts of estrogen, progesterone, androgen, and inhibin. The result is loss of the negative feedback from ovarian estrogen production that increases secretion of FSH and LH. Eventually there is a sustained elevation of FSH, indicating onset on menopause (Kendig & Sanford, 1998). In a woman who has had a hysterectomy, it is difficult to distinguish between perimenopause and menopause. Both may have similar symptoms and elevated FSH levels. However, a menopausal woman will no longer experience cyclic breast tenderness.

BODY RESPONSE TO ESTROGEN DEFICIENCY

The most common physiological symptoms seen during the perimenopause period leading up to menopause involve the central nervous system. These may include hot flashes, night sweats, fatigue, depression, headache, palpitations, and anxiety. The "hot flash" (also called "hot flush") is the sensation of extreme heat often accompanied by sweating, flushing, and anxiety, which starts on the chest or neck area and spreads up to the face. Hot flashes usually last from 2 to 5 minutes, occurring at any time and as irregularly as once a week or several times a day. The hot flash is the second most frequent perimenopausal symptom (after irregular bleeding) and is considered the hallmark sign of the perimenopause. Night sweats occur when a hot flash awakens a woman from a sound sleep, drenched in perspiration and unable to return to sleep. During the climacteric, sleep is less efficient with decreased periods of REM sleep.

BOX 17-1 MENOPAUSE TERMS

Perimenopause
The period surrounding menopause. It usually starts in the mid-to-late 40s with the onset of characteristic physical and emotional changes. It ends 1 year after the cessation of menses.

Menopause
The very last menses, typically in the early 50s, resulting from depletion of ovarian follicles and declining estrogen.

Postmenopause
The time after 12 consecutive months without any menstrual bleeding.

Premature menopause
Occurs before the age of 40.

Late menopause
Occurs after the age of 55.

Modified from AWHONN (1998). *Standards and guidelines for professional nursing practice in the care of women and newborns,* Washington, DC: AWHONN.

These sleep disturbances often lead to fatigue, irritability, and poor concentration during the day. The incidence of hot flashes reported in literature varies. According to Rousseau (1998) approximately 70% of women experience daily hot flashes for some period of time. These vasomotor symptoms reflect instability between the hypothalamus and autonomic nervous system and may continue for many years or just a few months. Hot flashes typically stop on their own but there is no way of predicting when that will occur. Women who do seek medical care for hot flashes often present with multiple symptoms such as insomnia, mood swings, and depression.

The etiology of the hot flash leaves room for some speculation, but most research indicates it results from a decrease in estrogen and inhibin levels that affect the temperature-regulating center in the hypothalamus. This often happens while women are still experiencing regular menstrual cycles. Potential triggers for hot flashes include stressful situations, alcohol, caffeine, spicy foods, extreme heat, and enclosed spaces.

There are other physical responses to estrogen deficiency that a woman may notice (Table 17-1). For example, epidermal skin has a significant number of estrogen receptors. As levels of estrogen drop, skin loses its tensile strength, turgor, and skin collagen, causing dryness and wrinkles. Sebaceous and sweat glands have reduced function related to the loss of estrogen-binding receptors, primarily located in the face, hands, and breast tissue, followed by thighs and adipose tissue. Breast tissue may lose form and firmness as a woman ages. Irregular body hair distribution and hirsutism may develop as a reflection of androgen secretion by the ovaries instead of estrogen.

Table **17-1**   PHYSIOLOGIC AND PSYCHOLOGIC MANIFESTATIONS OF MENOPAUSE

ORGAN/BODY SYSTEM	EFFECT FROM DECLINING ESTROGEN	MANIFESTATION
Vasomotor	Instability between hypothalamus and autonomic nervous system	Hot flashes, night sweats, palpitations
Ovary	Number of ovarian follicles producing estrogen decreases	Irregular menstrual cycles
Vagina/vulva	Vagina becomes shorter and narrower; loss of rugae, paleness of epithelia, brittle pubic hair	Easily traumatized; prone to infection, vaginal dryness, dyspareunia, pruritus
Epidermis	Loss of elasticity and collagen; sebaceous and sweat glands have decreased function	Wrinkling and dryness of skin
Breast	Atrophy of glandular tissue	Change in shape
Urinary system	Atrophy of bladder and urethral structure	Frequency, urgency, increase in urinary incontinence, prone to infection
Mental status	Possibly endocrine hormone-related	Mood swings, loss of memory, anxiety, irritability, loss of libido

From Neinstein, L. S., Juliani, M. A., & Shapiro, J. (1996a). Psychosocial development in normal adolescents. In L. S. Neinstein (Ed.), *Adolescent health care: A practical guide* (3rd ed., pp. 40–45). Baltimore: Williams & Wilkins.

The vagina and urethra are also estrogen-sensitive tissue and within 2 to 3 years of estrogen deficiency, some degree of atrophy occurs. The vaginal epithelium tends to become thin and dry, frequently causing vaginitis and affecting sexual function/pleasure. A menstrual history will disclose symptoms of these vaginal changes. Physical examination will reveal thinning and paleness of vaginal epithelia, disappearance of vaginal rugae, brittle pubic hair, and possible chronic infection. Symptoms such as dyspareunia, pain on penetration, burning, and pruritus respond well to estrogen treatment. Urethral changes coincide with vaginal changes, and urinary symptoms may appear but generally respond well to appropriate treatment. Symptoms of urinary incontinence occur in 31% of perimenopausal women at least once a month, possibly related to decreased bladder and urethral tissue (Sampselle et al., 1997).

Midlife women and health care providers are now focusing on the metabolic responses to decreasing estrogen levels, often referred to as the "silent killers," osteoporosis and cardiovascular heart disease. Bone loss actually begins long before menopause, affecting some 25 million women aged 45 and older. As women enter menopause and lose the protective properties of estrogen, bone resorption outpaces bone remodeling, resulting in bone loss (Kendig & Sanford, 1998). Before vertebral or hip fracture, there are no symptoms associated with osteoporosis, making it a "silent killer." The value of drug therapy in slowing osteoclastic resorption is discussed later in this chapter. Mentioned also will be the optimal approach to any osteoporosis program aimed at educating young people about the value of good nutrition and exercise.

Today, coronary heart disease (CHD) is the leading cause of death as well as significant cause of disability in American women (King & Mosca, 2000). Although coronary heart disease generally develops 6 to 10 years later in women than men, by the time women reach their 70s, their death rate is equivalent to that of men. The toll of CHD on African-American women is particularly alarming compared to white women of the same age. Premenopausal cardiovascular protection from estrogen is lost after menopause and adverse lipid changes are noted in many women past 45 years of age. CHD risk substantially increases in postmenopausal women and in women who have surgically induced menopause (via hysterectomy) at an early age. Discussion of risk factors and modification of these risks through education will be developed further in this chapter.

COMPREHENSIVE MIDLIFE ASSESSMENT

The standard health care encounter includes a health and psychosocial history, physical examination, laboratory evaluation, assessment of risk factors, and a program of preventive services. There are standardized health assessment tools that address issues such as health risk and functional status. The woman before the office visit can fill out these screening tools. Once scored, they indicate risk factors and areas needing health education.

Effective interviewing and interpersonal skills are required in order to conduct a meaningful history and physical examination. Language and terminology must be matched to the woman's level of understanding, culture, and background. Questions pertinent to women 45 to 65 years include menstrual history or hormone therapy; related vaginal bleeding; signs of menopause, specifically vasomotor flushes; bowel or urinary complaints; weight gain; sexual function and satisfaction; and personal health habits and lifestyle practices, such as smoking, alcohol use, and nutrition. Clinicians should be aware of nonverbal cues such as body movements, facial expressions, and signs of anxiety. Such cues may indicate an unspoken fear or concern on the woman's part and a hesitancy to raise questions.

After obtaining a thorough history, a complete review of systems is indicated. In preparation for the physical examination, explain all procedures beforehand. Blood pressure, height, and weight screening should be conducted initially. Blood pressure should be screened at every visit. It is known that the incidence of hypertension rises steadily with age and hypertension has been identified as the leading risk factor for heart disease (Maldon-Kay, 1997; Mosca, 2000). Confirmation of hypertension should be made after a series of elevated readings on three separate occasions with the woman at rest. Early recognition and treatment of hypertension has been shown to significantly reduce morbidity and mortality from heart disease (Callahan & Paris, 1997; Denke, 1999).

Measurement of a woman's height and weight should be part of every visit. An annual review of one's height can identify loss of inches possibly related to osteoporosis. Weight should also be monitored since recent studies indicate that an estimated 55% of women 55 to 75 years of age are overweight (King & Mosca, 2000). Careful measurement of height and weight ratio is the initial step in the clinical assessment of overweight. Overweight has been defined in relation to tables of desirable weight, generally designed by insurance companies. The degree of overweight can be best expressed by use of body mass index (BMI). This index is the body weight in kilograms divided by the square of the height in meters. Obesity refers to an abnormally high proportion of body fat. An ideal weight is a body mass index (BMI) between 18.5 to 24.9 kg/m^2 for women over 35 years, based on height, and is associated with low health risk. A BMI of 27 to 30 may be considered overweight, while a BMI greater than 30 is synonymous with obesity (King & Mosca, 2000). Excessive body weight is associated with certain lifestyle practices such as smoking, alcohol consumption, lack of regular exercise, and a diet high in fat. Studies have shown that there is increased risk for diabetes, hypertension, heart disease, and certain cancers associated with being overweight.

Early diagnosis of breast disease should be a priority in caring for the midlife woman. Breast cancer screening should consist of a professional breast examination, education on breast self-exam, and mammography. Several large studies have shown that breast cancer mortality is decreased by 30% in women ages 50 to 74 by use of comprehensive breast screening (Callahan & Paris, 1997).

Papanicolaou (Pap) smears are recommended for all women who have been or are sexually active, regardless of age. Done yearly as a screening for precancerous and cancerous conditions of the cervix and vagina, Pap smears have accounted for a significant decrease in mortality. During the pelvic examination, inspection of the vaginal mucosa should be noted for evidence of declining estrogen. At this time, a digital rectal exam with fecal occult blood test should be performed as a screening for colorectal cancer.

Laboratory tests that may be considered for this age cohort include:

1. Serum follicle-stimulating hormone (FSH)
2. Serum luteinizing hormone (LH)
3. Baseline thyroid-stimulating hormone
4. If at risk, human immunodeficiency virus (HIV) testing.
5. If not previously assessed, a lipid profile before hormone replacement therapy (HRT)

During the years before menopause, many women have rising FSH levels, reflecting a declining follicular pool. Hormonal testing, although controversial, can confirm the decline of the production of ovarian estrogen, resulting in elevated FSH levels (greater than 40m IU/ml) and to a lesser degree raised LH levels (McNagny, 1999; Rousseau, 1998). The ovaries do not produce enough estrogen to inhibit hypothalamic release of gonadotropin-releasing hormone (GnRH). Continued release of GnRH results in elevated FSH/LH levels as ovulation ceases. Both FSH and LH decline slowly over time with advancing age.

Thyroid testing is suggested because thyroid disorders are among the more common endocrine abnormalities in women and can affect many aspects of a woman's life. Thyroid disease can alter menstruation and fertility, mimic depression or other psychiatric disorders, and complicate pregnancy. Left untreated, thyroid disease can also impact the cardiovascular, skeletal, and central nervous system. Screening for thyroid function in women 45 to 65 is best performed with a panel that includes T_4, T_3 RU, and TSH. This provides thyroid values within the context of the woman's individual hormonal status (Sakornbut, 1997).

Infectious disease prevention focuses on a review of the woman's immunization record. All adults should be immune to diphtheria and tetanus if they received the complete series as a child. An adult tetanus booster is then indicated every 10 years. Any adult born after 1957 should have received the measles, mumps, and rubella (MMR) vaccine. If there is no documentation or proof of vaccination, the vaccine should be administered, especially to high-risk groups such as health care workers and international travelers (Stevenson, 1999). Several other vaccinations such as influenza, pneumococcal, and hepatitis B may be indicated based on the woman's occupation, contact with chronically ill or immune-compromised patients, or if the woman herself has a chronic health condition. Screening for tuberculosis should also be done for women under similar circumstances (Sakornbut, 1997). Travelers planning a trip out of the country should contact their local health department for advice on required immunizations for that travel destination.

All current medications, both prescription and over-the-counter (OTC) drugs, should be reviewed during the health history. Determine the reason for taking any reported medications, validate accurate dosage, question if there have been any adverse reactions or side effects, and discuss possible drug interactions.

HEALTH PROMOTION/DISEASE PREVENTION

Health promotion and disease prevention in midlife women is focused on preventing the short-term and long-term effects from decreasing ovarian function. In addition to hormone replacement therapy or its alternatives, which will be presented next, midlife women need specific guidance on nutrition, exercise, and cancer screening.

Nutrition

Calcium is a critical mineral for midlife women in order to prevent osteoporosis. Optimal calcium intake for the nonpregnant female should be approximately 1000 mg/day. In postmenopausal women not on estrogen replacement therapy, the recommendation is 1200 to 1500 mg/day and for those on estrogen 1000 mg/day. A glass of milk provides 300 mg of calcium and many products such as orange juice, bread, and cereals are now fortified with calcium. Soybeans, leafy green vegetables, tofu and other dairy products (including non-fat cheeses and milk) contain calcium. Up to 1500 mg of calcium daily does not increase the risk of developing kidney stones. Adequate vitamin D is necessary as it facilitates intestinal absorption of calcium and stimulation of osteoblast synthesis of osteocalcin. Just 15 minutes of sunshine daily will provide what the body needs of natural vitamin D. The elderly and housebound may need to take a multivitamin containing the recommended dose of 400 IU vitamin D. The practice of vitamin D and calcium supplementation in the elderly has been suggested to reduce hip fractures. Andrews (1998) reports that there is a high prevalence of vitamin D deficiency in the elderly and argues the case for supplementation, especially for those bedridden. Midlife women should also have a diet low in fat and cholesterol because of their increased risk for heart disease. A diet that is rich in calcium and low in fat will help them achieve and maintain their ideal weight.

Exercise

Prevention of osteoporosis should be a health priority for all women and their clinicians. Although some risk factors cannot be controlled, there are many that can. One's lifestyle definitely has an effect on bone density and the risk of osteoporosis. Physical activity (weight bearing) for 30 minutes for at least 3 days a week will strengthen bone. The relationship between aerobic fitness and bone loss in healthy midlife women has been well documented. The findings show a positive effect of regular exercise on bone change as well as an improvement in cardiovascular health. Adverse habits such as smoking or excessive alcohol consumption, which impair bone remodeling, are associated with a risk of osteoporosis and are to be avoided. As always, counseling on these issues should be part of the well woman examination, leading toward a healthy lifestyle. Screening for osteoporosis should include identification of the woman's risk factors, physical assessment, education on healthy lifestyle behavior, measurement of height, and discussion on the choice of treatment to prevent or treat osteoporosis.

Cancer Screening and Detection

Midlife women are at higher risk for all cancers merely because of the aging process. Cancer in midlife women will be presented in depth later in this chapter. For the purposes of health promotion and disease prevention, midlife women need to be screened annually for the following cancers: breast, cervical, uterine, ovarian, skin, and colon. All midlife women should receive an annual mammogram, pap smear, pelvic examination, rectal examination, breast examination, skin assessment, and testing of stool for occult blood. The goal of cancer screening is early detection. The earlier the detection, the more successful the outcome, which will promote health and prevent recurrences or metastasis. Box 17-2 summarizes the health promotion and disease prevention activities for midlife women.

Hormone Replacement Therapy

Menopause is a natural event in a woman's life. Although not a disease, menopause is associated with short-term and long-term effects resulting from decreasing ovarian function. Most women will spend one third of their lives postmenopausal. To combat adverse conditions that may be brought about by menopause, many clinicians previously advised women to consider hormone replacement therapy (HRT). Although the treatment of menopausal symptoms was previously the most widely recognized reason for estrogen replacement therapy (ERT), a secondary purpose just as important was the hypothetical prevention of the long-term effects of decreased estrogen (Graziottin, 1999).

Although estrogen was first approved in the 1940s for postmenopausal women, it was not readily used until the 1960s when it was prescribed for menopausal hot flashes and urogenital symptoms. Early descriptions of menopause called it a state of failure or deficiency of ovarian function; a disease defined by specific symptomatology and only treated by estrogen replacement. During the 1970s there was evidence of an increased incidence of endometrial cancer that led to a decrease in usage. By mid-1980, progestin was added to estrogen therapy to reduce the risk of endometrial cancer. When the U.S. Food and Drug Administration acknowledged the correlation between estrogen and the prevention of osteoporosis, use of hormone therapy greatly increased. Medications prescribed for postmenopausal hormone therapy became some of the most widely distributed drugs in the history of the pharamaceutical industry. The National Institutes of Health Women's Health Initiative (WHI) focused on a long-term study of the effects of menopause on women and the impact of HRT, ERT, exercise, and nutrition on postmenopausal women. The WHI made an unprecedented decision in 2002 to stop a portion of the study early as a result of findings that indicated an increased risk to women in the estrogen-progestin combination group. Findings demonstrated a slightly increased risk for intact women (with a uterus) in the combination group for cardiovascular disease and breast cancer (Writing Group for the Women's Health Initiative Investigations, 2002).

The WHI reported their findings as hazardous ratios (HR). The ratio of hazards is essentially a relative risk, not an absolute risk. For example, an HR of 0.63 indicates that the risk of a condition was decreased by 37% and an HR of 1.41 indicates the risk of developing a condition increased by 41% (Brucker & Youngkin, 2002). The WHI reported the following HR values for the combination group: coronary heart disease—HR 1.29; stroke—HR 1.41; pulmonary embolism—HR 2.13; total cardiovascular disease—HR 1.22, and breast cancer—HR 1.26.

Box 17-2 HEALTH PROMOTION/DISEASE PREVENTION FOR WOMEN IN MIDLIFE

History	Physical Exam	Laboratory Tests	Risk Assessment	Immunizations
Medical history: Review of systems, signs/ symptoms of cancer, heart disease	Blood pressure, height, weight	Pap smear as indicated	Tobacco/alcohol/ drug use	Tetanus/diphtheria booster every 10 years
Ob-gyn history: Age of menarche, menstrual history, hormonal therapy related to vaginal bleeding, age of first coitus, consensual/ nonconsensual sexual practices, safe sex practices, signs/symptoms of menopause, bowel and urinary complaints, STDs*, contraception, number of partners, sexual orientation, function, and satisfaction	Visual acuity Oral cavity exam Palpation of thyroid Breast exam Cardiovascular assessment Skin exam Lymph node exam Pelvic exam Rectal exam	Mammogram annually Fecal blood testing annually Dipstick urinalysis Sigmoidoscopy every 3 to 5 years after age 50, earlier as indicated Nonfasting total blood cholesterol every 5 years, more frequently as indicated Fasting blood glucose as indicated Tuberculosis skin test in high-risk patients Thyroid function tests as indicated STD screening for gonorrhea, chlamydia, VDRL; HIV counseling, and testing Glaucoma testing as indicated	Symptoms of physical/ emotional abuse Symptoms of depression, suicide, and abnormal bereavement Evidence of social isolation Symptoms of emotional abuse or physical abuse Symptoms of increased stress Risk factors for STDs, unintended pregnancy, high-risk pregnancy Driving motor vehicle Lack of regular exercise Body mass index calculation Excessive dietary intake or lack of dietary intake Sun/ultraviolet light exposure/reduction Prevention strategies	Measles/mumps/ rubella if given before 1957 Hepatitis B Influenza annually if high risk Pneumococcal vaccine if high risk
Surgical history Family history of breast/ovarian cancer, cardiovascular disease, diabetes Current medications, prescriptions, and over-the- counter drugs Self-care, dietary		Vision screening Pregnancy test as indicated Serum FSH Serum LH Baseline thyroid- stimulating hormone Lipid profile prior to HRT	Use of smoke detector in homes Use of seat belts in motor vehicles, use of helmets in skateboarding, rollerblading Cessation of tobacco, alcohol/drugs Limiting alcohol intake Avoidance of driving, being a passenger in a car driven by someone under the	

Continued

Box 17-2 HEALTH PROMOTION/DISEASE PREVENTION FOR WOMEN IN MIDLIFE—CONT'D

History	Physical Exam	Laboratory Tests	Risk Assessment	Immunizations
intake, weight gain, regular exercise, tobacco/alcohol/ drug use Functional status and psychosocial history: History of child, abuse/neglect, domestic violence, emotional/ physical abuse by parents Worklife exposure to environmental hazards			influence of alcohol Modifiable factors: Health promotion activities, exercise and physical activity, nutrition, stress management Smoking cessation Dietary plan: restriction of fat, cholesterol; adequate intake of iron, calcium, maintaining balanced diet Avoidance of bingeing and purging for weight control Teaching breast self-exam Teaching signs/ symptoms of cancer, Pap smears for cervical cancer, cardiovascular disease Discussion of osteoporosis prevention Discussion of hormone therapy: estrogen/ androgen Discussion of domestic violence and resources Contraception and STD risk reduction Violent behavior, ways to reduce risk Available resources like family support, finances, etc. Discussion of stress reduction in employment settings	

Box 17-2 HEALTH PROMOTION/DISEASE PREVENTION FOR WOMEN IN MIDLIFE—
CONT'D

History	Physical Exam	Laboratory Tests	Risk Assessment	Immunizations
			Assessment of workplace environment safety	
			Diet intake—decreased calories, calcium, fiber and fluid, fat	
			Secondary prevention of further problems (complications) from existing health problems	
			Clinical breast exam and mammography for breast cancer	
			Blood pressure screening for hypertension	

*STDs, sexually transmitted diseases.

On a positive note, the WHI also found the following HR values for the combination group: colorectal cancer—HR 0.63 and hip fracture—HR 0.66. The reason the study was stopped was that the relative risks to the study group were greater than the potential benefits (Writing Group for the Women's Health Initiative Investigations, 2002). These findings were limited to the intact group (women with a uterus) receiving combination estrogen and progestin therapy. The other study groups within the WHI are continuing the study as planned, and the results will not be released until after the completion of the study.

Numerous other research studies have investigated the impact of HRT on various menopausal symptoms and diseases. Brucker and Youngkin (2002) summarized the findings of these studies. They stated that HRT has had mixed outcomes regarding its impact on Alzheimer's disease although HRT has demonstrated a positive impact on depression, mood swings, hot flashes, insomnia, vaginal dryness, and skin changes. Choosing what to do for these short-term and potentially long-term effects of estrogen decline can be confusing to many women. Evaluation of personal risk factors in making a decision about hormone therapy will be discussed later in the chapter.

Women in the United States begin the transition to menopause at about age 47, possibly going through a period of several years with irregular menstrual cycles, hot flashes and night sweats, until about age 51 when they experience menopause. In healthy, non-smoking women, low-dose estrogen oral contraceptives may be prescribed to improve perimenopausal menstrual changes such as irregular bleeding and for menopausal symptoms such as hot flashes. The peak use of hormone therapy is found

BOX 17-3 INDICATIONS FOR HORMONE REPLACEMENT THERAPY (HRT)

Candidates for HRT include:
- All menopausal or perimenopausal women with symptoms of estrogen deficiency: vasomotor, genitourinary, changes in mood or mentation.
- Women with or at risk for osteoporosis, particularly women with premature ovarian failure or those who experienced oophorectomy at an early age.

among women 50 to 59 years of age. Current research indicates that the use of hormones varies with ethnicity; access to health care mediated by education, income, and insurance; and women's own health awareness. White women are more likely to use hormone therapy than African-Americans, suggesting that women who use hormones are possibly better educated, more affluent, and have fewer coronary risk factors (Massey, Hupp, Kreisberg, Alpert, & Hoff, 2000). This hormonal use may reflect a greater perceived risk for osteoporosis rather than heart disease among white women. Limited access to health care for many African-American and Hispanic women may account for minimal use of hormones along with a cultural belief system that relies more on natural therapies. Women who have experienced early surgical or induced menopause are often prescribed hormone treatment for long-term benefits and are more compliant with their medication. The need for continued use should be evaluated annually, especially after 50 years of age (North American Menopause Society, 2000b).

Meanwhile, the decision to take hormones and which hormone regimen to follow should be thoroughly discussed by the woman and her practitioner. The role of the health care provider is to facilitate decision-making. Clearly it is not to make a decision for the patient. Women want the opportunity to choose whether or not to start HRT but need guidance and information to make that informed decision. Symptoms should be reviewed and advice given as to which ones are directly related to estrogen deficiency. The risks and benefits of hormone therapy need to be summarized in light of each woman's individual disease risk factors (Box 17-3). Graziottin (1999) reports that women are more willing to accept HRT and be compliant if their physician has made them feel like an active partner in the decision process.

Wilhelm (2002) found that self-efficacy was a greater predictor of a woman's intent to adopt HRT than support or knowledge. However, all three factors combined affected the intent to adopt HRT to a greater degree than any of the variables independently.

Benefits

The decision to initiate HRT is rarely based on one symptom or risk factor. An overall risk/benefit assessment should be conducted for each woman. Historically, unopposed estrogen replacement therapy (ERT) has been widely used for over 50 years to treat menopause-related symptoms (McNagny, 1999). HRT has now been approved by the Food and Drug Administration (FDA) for the prevention and management of osteoporosis (Writing Group of the PEPI Trial, 1996) by preserving bone mineral density. The choice of hormone regimen may include unopposed estrogen or estrogen plus a progestogen (if the uterus is intact), available in many forms to individualize treatment. There are several routes of administration for hormones, including oral, transdermal patch, intramuscular injection, and subdermal implants. Estrogen taken orally, by patch, or injection has been found to be beneficial in reducing or stopping short-term changes such as hot flashes, mood swings, sleep disturbance, and vaginal dryness. These forms of estrogen may reduce a woman's risk for cardiovascular disease and osteoporosis. Estrogen vaginal cream, used for vaginal dryness and bladder symptoms, is thought to have only a localized effect. This preparation of estrogen offers no relief from hot flashes and other short-term effects, nor does it provide protection from long-term effects such as osteoporosis and heart disease. There is an estrogen vaginal ring for localized therapy that, if administered in high doses with significant absorption from the vagina, may have some systemic estrogenic benefits (Czarpata, 1999), Ruggiero and Likis (2002) summarize the physiology and pharmacology of ERT and HRT, and Rousseau (2001) documents evidence-based practice guidelines for ERT and HRT.

A primary benefit of estrogen is thought to be its effect on the cardiovascular system to inhibit arteriosclerosis and to help maintain normal cardiac and arterial functions (Yoder, 1997). Because cardiovascular disease is the leading cause of death in women, this desirable benefit of estrogen should be weighed against any other personal risks from hormone therapy (North American Menopause Society, 2000a). Recent research shows that a postmenopausal woman on hormone therapy has a 50% less chance of developing heart disease than a woman not on therapy. Yoder (1997) cites that the protective cardiac benefits of estrogen are lost within 3 years of discontinuing hormone therapy. Studies have also shown that in postmenopausal women, oral estrogen reduces low-density lipoproteins (LDL) associated with cardiovascular disease by 10% to 15% while increasing levels of desirable high-density lipoproteins (HDL) 20% to 30% (Mosca, 2000). There are also beneficial effects on vascular endothelial function and reduction of platelet adhesiveness that may contribute to a lowered risk for stroke and myocardial infarction in women receiving estrogen. A trend toward an increase in triglycerides with oral estrogen has been noted. For this reason, transdermal estrogen, which has very little influence on lipids, may be better suited for a woman with long-standing elevated triglyceride levels (North American Menopause Society, 2000a). A disadvantage of combined oral estrogen and progestin therapy may be a lowering of HDL because of the action of progestin reducing estrogen's protective effects on the heart. In 2002, the WHI demonstrated a negative impact of combination therapy on cardiovascular disease.

There is now abundant evidence that exogenous estrogen reduces the risk of osteoporosis in postmenopausal women. Despite the recognized value of estrogen therapy, however, there is reported under use of estrogen among older, postmenopausal women, particularly African-American women (DeMasters, 2000). It is thought that when these women experienced menopause, the risk for osteoporosis was not recognized and hormone replacement therapy was not commonly prescribed. Studies now show that osteoporosis is closely associated with estrogen deficiency. After menopause, bone mineral density loss averages 1% to 2% annually for the first 5 years. Estrogen inhibits bone resorption and increases intestinal absorption of calcium, preventing bone loss and minimally increasing bone density. All estrogens, regardless of route of administration or in combination with progestin, reduce bone loss.

Approximately 20% of white women over 50 years of age have osteoporosis of the hip and spine. The benefit for women on hormone therapy is a 35% to 40% reduction in risk for osteoporosis (Yoder, 1997). The greatest impact of estrogen on bone occurs when therapy is started within the first few years after menopause. Protection against bone loss lasts until hormone replacement is discontinued, and then bone loss returns to the former postmenopausal rate (DeMasters, 2000). However, Keating, Cleary, Rossi, Zaslovsky, and Ayanian (1999) suggest that starting long-term estrogen replacement in a woman aged 60 or older has bone-conserving benefit equal to approximately that of early postmenopausal therapy.

Hormone therapy and calcium supplementations are being considered for older women, especially those who experienced early menopause (before age 40). Further loss of bone can be slowed and the risk of fractures reduced. The positive impact of hormone therapy has been documented in women 65 and older (North American Menopause Society, 2000a). Whether estrogen's cardiovascular protection has any significance in the very old has yet to be determined.

If postmenopausal hormone therapy were demonstrated to have a definite beneficial effect on the risk for Alzheimer's disease, this would be a forceful reason to recommend treatment for the elderly. However, there is not conclusive evidence at this time; in fact, many of the findings are contradictory. Paganini-Hill and Henderson (1996) cite a study of 8877 women that indicates that hormone therapy reduces the risk for Alzheimer's and related dementia by 33%, possibly delaying the onset of these diseases by 5 years. It is thought that estrogen has a protective effect on nerve cells in the brain and may somehow prevent nerve cell death. Although there are plausible biological actions as to how estrogen can improve cognitive function, most reviews emphasize that current research information is incomplete (DeMasters, 2000; McNagny, 1999). Perhaps the ongoing Women's Health Initiative Memory Study (2002), measuring the rate of Alzheimer's disease in postmenopausal women randomly assigned to either HRT/ERT or placebo, will provide more definitive answers.

There is a common perception that urinary incontinence and decreased sexual desire are inevitable aspects of aging in a woman. Systemic or local estrogen can be effective in preventing or reducing urogenital atrophy, which leads to some forms of incontinence. The vaginal dryness that accounts for painful intercourse and lack of interest in sexual intimacy can be improved with estrogen and possibly the use of a lubricant. Midlife sexuality is discussed later in this chapter.

Risks

Unopposed estrogen (ERT) has been identified as creating a higher risk for endometrial cancer in women with an intact uterus. This risk has been effectively nullified by the addition of progestin to estrogen. Like progesterone production in ovulatory women, exogenous progesterone will prevent hyperplasia in postmenopausal women, thus reducing risk for endometrial cancer.

Even after the benefit-to-risk ratio has been explained, many women will take their estrogen sporadically or not at all. A primary reason may be the fear of cancer or the resumption of menstrual bleeding as a most unfavorable aspect of hormonal therapy. Conflicting studies have been reported regarding a possible link between ERT/HRT and breast cancer and duration of therapy. Graziottin (1999) reports several studies that show no increase in the risk of developing breast cancer if a woman is on HRT less than 5 years. The risk does appear to increase 30% to 40% with long-term therapy of 5 to 15 years (North American Menopause Society, 2000a), and the WHI (2002) has documented a HR of 1.26. Treatment-induced withdrawal bleeding or breakthrough bleeding in women taking cyclic HRT with progestin may be bothersome enough to cause some women to stop taking their medication. Education about what to expect for the first 6 months or longer is a vital link in how compliant a patient will be.

An abundance of indirect evidence indicates estrogen plays a role in breast cancer. Breast tissue has estrogen and progesterone receptors that have a proliferative effect when stimulated. Across the lifespan, women are exposed to sex hormones longer than ever before, from earlier menarche, low parity, to late menopause. Clinical observations indicate prolonged exposure to estrogen increases the risk for breast cancer, but a definitive cause/effect relationship has yet to be announced. Women with a strong risk for breast cancer (i.e., mother or sister with a history of breast cancer) are advised to carefully consider estrogen therapy. Nonetheless, recent research reports that low-dose, short-term estrogen may not increase risk as originally thought nor does the possible risk remain once hormone therapy is discontinued (Graziottin, 1999). It may be the case that a past history of breast cancer may not automatically disqualify women from HRT. Although caution is advised in prescribing estrogen to women with known genetic breast cancer mutations, estrogen might be considered for the relief of menopausal symptoms in breast cancer survivors without genetic susceptibility (Willis, 1997).

Fibrocystic breast changes do respond variably to postmenopausal HRT. The presence of existing fibrocystic changes or cyclic mastalgia does not always eliminate women from using hormone therapy. In either case, an informed decision should be mutually made between provider and woman after all individual risks and benefits have been weighed. Contraindications for long-term therapy are uncommon but include undiagnosed vaginal bleeding, active breast or endometrial cancer, active liver or gallbladder disease, and active thrombophlebitis. Low-dose temporary treatment with estrogen cream may be a solution for atrophic symptoms in these women.

Migraine headaches, very common in women, are not an absolute contraindication to hormone therapy but the route and regimen are important factors. Counseling should include an explanation that any interruption of a woman's regimen for more than a few days may exacerbate her headaches. If exacerbation or frequent recurrence occurs with fluctuating hormone levels during transition, the following strategies may be tried: lowering the dose of estrogen, changing from a cyclic to a continuous regimen, and using transdermal administration (McNagny, 1999).

Use of Androgens

Androgen (testosterone) deprivation after menopause is an important factor contributing to the decline of sexuality seen in postmenopausal women. Androgens are metabolically active in skin, muscle, and bone and are thought to play a role in one's libido. Because of a gradual decline, androgen levels are only noticeably decreased after 10 years (Scharbo-DeHaan, 1996). There is little if any effect on the peripheral physiologic response associated with menopause. The potential benefits of androgen treatment combined with estrogen include improvement in psychologic well-being and an increase in sexual behavior. Androgens do not protect the endometrium, and a progestin must be administered. There is concern that with androgen supplementation, the mitigating effect of this drug lowers estrogen's beneficial effects on lipids (DeMasters, 2000). Women with a low HDL cholesterol level, cardiovascular disease, or a strong family history of heart disease should avoid estrogen-androgen therapy. Limiting use of androgen to an as-needed form of therapy may be the most effective approach, considering the boost in libido may decline if used daily over a long period of time (DeMasters, 2000).

The only FDA-approved androgen product for women is a combination of esterified estrogens and methyltestosterone (MT), a synthetic oral compound that is more potent than testosterone. Marketed as Estratest, it is indicated for the treatment of moderate to severe vasomotor symptoms unresponsive to ERT but not for sexual dysfunction. However, many women do report increased sexual desire while on the medication. Monitoring of a woman's free testosterone levels as well as lipid profile should be performed if on therapy more than 6 months. There is a custom-compounded preparation of testosterone, which anecdotal evidence indicates, improves libido. However, data is limited and caution is indicated.

Available Regimens

The usual regimen of hormone therapy consists of estrogen (unopposed), which is usually only for women without a uterus, or an estrogen-progestin combination for women with an intact uterus. Concurrent estrogen/progestogen therapy decreases the risk of endometrial hyperplasia and possible endometrial cancer by reducing estrogen receptor activity (North American Menopause Society, 2000a). Progestin can be added to estrogen either cyclically or continually every month. Continuous unopposed estrogen therapy is 0.625 mg of conjugated estrogen, esterified estrogen, or estradiol pipate. The dose for micronized estradiol is 1 mg and 0.05 mg for transdermal estradiol. Administration of estrogen alone may produce less withdrawal bleeding, possibly more benefit on bone and the heart, but does increase the risk of endometrial hyperplasia.

A cyclic regimen of estrogen/progestin follows the normal reproductive cycle. During the estrogen only phase, the endometrium exhibits some proliferative effect. When progestin is added, the endometrium is suppressed, and, when withdrawn, bleeding will occur. Combined regimens use the same dose of estrogen and add 2.5 to 10 mg of medroxyprogesterone acetate (MPA). A common regimen calls for 25 days of estrogen, adding progestin (10 mg medroxyprogesterone acetate) the first 14 days of the month or the last 10 days of estrogen, respectively. Women will experience vaginal bleeding on an anticipated day of the month. Complaints with this sequential regimen include breast tenderness, bloating, fluid retention, and depression. These problems are related to the dose of progestin.

The continuous combined regimen allows for lower-dose progestin that may increase patient compliance. Daily estrogen is combined with 2.5 mg medroxyprogesterone, and both are taken every day. The biggest concern women have with continuous regimen is breakthrough bleeding during the first 4 to 6 months. This breakthrough bleeding affects 50% to 80% of women, particularly during the first year and is similar to that seen with oral contraceptives (DeMasters, 2000). The WHI (2002) findings indicate an increased risk for cardiovascular disease and breast cancer with combined therapy.

A modification of the cyclic regimen is now being used with favorable response. Estrogen is taken daily and a progestin added every 3 months for 14 days. Withdrawal bleeding occurs predictably just every 3 months, increasing adherence to therapy. There is some speculation that this approach may result in heavier bleeding initially and a slight increase of hyperplasia (DeMasters, 2000). Women on hormone therapy will need constant support and educational preparation to allay anxiety and encourage

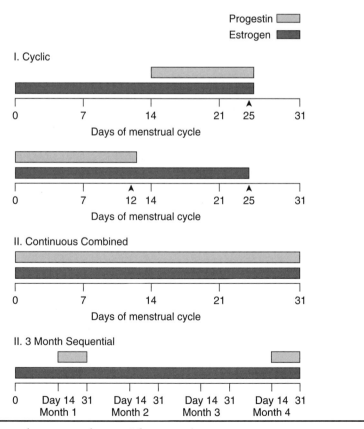

Figure **17-1** Common hormone replacement therapy regimens.

Table **17-2** **ALTERNATIVES TO ESTROGEN FOR PERIMENOPAUSAL SYMPTOMS**

HERB	ACTION	CAUTION
Vitamin E	Reduces hot flashes by decreasing FSH and LH; source: wheat germ, whole grains, soybeans	Ingest with meals; supplementation 400 to 800 IU
Vitamin B$_6$	Possibly reduces hot flashes but mostly used for irritability; source: Brewer's yeast, bran, wheat germ	5 to 25 mg/day not to exceed 100 mg
Chamomile	Reduces cramps; relieves insomnia	Anyone with hay fever should use caution
Garlic	Inhibits breast cancer; helps lower blood pressure and lipids; acts as an antioxidant	Avoid large amounts if on regular aspirin therapy
Ginseng	Improves memory; increases longevity; improves sex drive; decreases fatigue	Not to be taken with vitamin C nor by persons with diabetes
St. John's wort	Reduces depression	Large doses or long-term use may cause sensitivity to sun
Lubricants (water soluble)	Relieves vaginal dryness; improves sexual enjoyment	
Black cohosh	Binds to estrogen receptors and reduces hot flashes	
Dong quai	Relieves symptoms of menopause, especially hot flashes	
Primrose oil	Contains gamma-linolenic, which is a precursor to prostaglandins; reduces hot flashes and PMS symptoms	

Source: Lindsay, S. (1999). Menopause, naturally exploring alternatives to traditional hormone replacement therapy, *AWHONN Lifelines* 3(5), 35.

compliance. They need to be part of the decision process and fully understand the risks and benefits to improve compliance. Figure 17-1 illustrates common HRT regimens.

Duration of Therapy

The decision to start hormone therapy can be very confusing. There are risks and benefits for each individual to weigh and discuss with her health care provider. Knowing when to stop, if at all, presents more concern. The decision to continue therapy rests on the indications and reasons for beginning hormone replacement therapy initially. If relief of short-term vasomotor symptoms was the goal, then 2 to 5 years is appropriate. If symptoms reoccur, HRT may be resumed for an additional 2 to 5 years. If long-term prevention or treatment of osteoporosis was the intent, then ideally therapy should be continued as long as the prophylactic benefit is obtained. For some women this may be a lifelong therapy because studies are still inconclusive regarding hormone therapy in the very old.

Alternatives to Estrogen

Alternative medicine includes herbal therapies, nutritional supplements, homeopathy, biofeedback, osteopathy, massage, aromatherapy, naturopathy, and traditional Chinese therapies such as acupuncture. These alternative therapies recognize the mind, body, emotional, and environmental connection. There still remains some disbelief regarding alternative therapies, despite the hundreds of years they have been practiced. If used wisely, health care providers and their patients can benefit from the wide range of therapeutic options now available for women as they transition through menopause (Table 17-2).

For those women who cannot take hormones or who choose not to, alternatives to estrogen may help to alleviate symptoms and enhance quality of life. A growing body of research supports the use of phytoestrogens in treating menopausal symptoms, focusing on a "natural" approach to health care. Phytoestrogens are natural compounds in certain plants, herbs, and seeds that are similar in chemical structure to steroidal estrogen produced by the body. In cultures where plant foods make up a large part of the diet, women seem to have fewer, if any, menopausal symptoms. Compared to approximately 85% of women in Western cultures, less than 25% of Asian women experience hot flashes (Ramsey, Ross, & Fischer, 1999). Their daily diet is extremely high in soy, a plant rich in estrogen. Western women who wish to try soy products should understand that hot flashes might decrease by only 45%, compared to the 80% to 90% reduction claimed by estrogen replacement (McNagny, 1999). Ongoing studies indicate soy protein may have cardiovascular benefits, inhibit cancer tumor growth in animals, and protect against bone loss (Lindsay, 1999). Natural food sources of phytoestrogens include soybeans, lentils, whole-grain cereals, flaxseed, and dried seaweed.

Botanicals (herbs) are the fastest growing choice of alternative care therapies on the market. Approximately one in three Americans use herbal products to manage symptoms or to maintain a state of well-being (Learn & Higgins, 1999). Women should be cautious when considering these alternatives because ideal dosage and major "active ingredients" have not been determined. The U.S. Food and Drug Administration has been unsuccessful at regulating herbs and other supplements. It is not known yet what effect these natural compounds will have on long-term postmenopausal diseases. It is important that a woman understands the mechanism of action of a substance or product and discusses potential side effects with her health care provider. For instance, dong quai, which is an estrogen precursor, is often recommended for menopausal symptoms, especially hot flashes. Not many people know dong quai is a coumarin and affects blood clotting. Therefore this herb should be not be used in women who have absolute contraindications to estrogen therapy, who experience heavy menstrual periods, nor for those on blood-thinning medications (Learn & Higgins, 1999). Herbs can have medicinal properties and potential life-threatening side effects. Health care providers should initiate open discussion with patients concerning the risks of taking herbs and the potential for drug interaction with other prescriptions or over-the-counter medications.

Certain vitamins have been reported to help some women with menopausal problems, but this evidence is anecdotal and may take weeks before there are signs of any benefit. Vitamins such as vitamin E (400 to 800 IU daily) and vitamin D (400 to 1000 IU daily) are thought to have some beneficial properties in lowering the risk of cardiovascular disease, osteoporosis, and in decreasing menopausal symptoms (Lindsay, 1999).

Nonprescription medications are available to treat vulvovaginal changes, such as vaginal dryness and atrophic vaginitis that result from declining estrogen levels. These symptoms usually do not become troublesome until several years past menopause. Vaginal lubricants, such as Astroglide, K-Y Jelly, Lubrin, and Moist Again, are available without prescription and help maintain vaginal moisture in women with mild vaginal atrophy. Replens is a vaginal moisturizer, which helps keep the vagina acidic to guard against infection. It is not a lubricant, but its effects make sexual activity more pleasant. For moderate to severe vaginal problems, a low-dose estrogen cream may be considered for short-term use to help restore vaginal blood flow and improve the elasticity of tissue.

A physical problem that often responds well to alternative therapy is incontinence. A large percentage of women with new-onset incontinence have a reversible cause such as urinary tract infection or weakened muscle tone because of decreased estrogen. Pelvic floor strengthening exercises and the use of biofeedback have been shown to improve stress incontinence. Kegel exercises, which consist of repeated contraction and relaxation of the urethral and vaginal muscles, help restore muscle tone. Some women have even reported an improvement in their sex life after learning to perform Kegel exercises.

Graziottin (1999) reports that clonidine, an alpha-adrenergic agonist, is useful for hot flashes, but its efficacy is limited because of possible hypotension. Veralipride also reduces peripheral vascular resistance and may be used for hot flashes. Both treatments are less effective than HRT and have serious side effects. Tibolone is a synthetic steroid with estrogenic, progestogenic, and androgenic properties. In postmenopausal women, it can be used to treat vasomotor, urogenital, and psychological symptoms. Although it does not cause endometrial hyperplasia, it does cause vaginal bleeding. For this reason, it is not prescripted until 1 year after menopause has been confirmed by 12 months of no vaginal bleeding.

For some women, alternative chemical compounds now available help reduce the risk of breast cancer, heart disease, and osteoporosis. Selective estrogen receptor modulators (SERMs) are nonhormonal agents that show great promise for the preventive health of midlife women. These compounds bind with estrogen receptors and activate them, eliciting mixed agonist/antagonist reaction, depending on the specific tissue involved. The two most clinically tested SERMs in postmenopausal women are tamoxifen and raloxifene. The FDA has approved the use of tamoxifen for primary prevention of breast cancer in high-risk women; it also displays beneficial estrogen-like effects on bone and serum cholesterol. Raloxifene has been approved for the prevention of osteoporosis, and it acts as an antagonist to both uterine and breast tissue (DeMasters, 2000; Kendig & Sanford, 1998). Neither drug should be used to treat the common complaints women have from loss of estrogen, but they certainly have a bright future in preserving the health of postmenopausal women.

Lifestyle modification in many cases can be just as potent as a prescriptive drug. Regular aerobic exercise, heart-healthy eating, no smoking, and limiting alcohol and caffeine have been shown to minimize the risk for cardiovascular disease and osteoporosis. Once diagnosed, symptoms associated with osteoporosis may be decreased by the use of the drugs, calcitonin, bisphosphonates, and tibolone, although long-term effects of these drugs are not known.

Compliance with hormone therapy begins with patient education during the decision-making process. Follow-up care also increases compliance. A return visit 3 months after starting HRT as well as communication via telephone calls should alleviate any concerns the woman may have. If all is going well, an annual examination for age-appropriate screening can be scheduled.

The next section will cover some of the more common health concerns of midlife women. These health concerns were chosen as focus areas because research shows that risk identification and lifestyle modification can impact outcome. Education and preventive health care are major subjects that the clinician must emphasize to women as they age.

Osteoporosis

Osteoporosis is a global disease affecting up to 25 million Americans, 80% of them women (Darovic, 1997; Lindsay, 1999). This condition is especially devastating to a woman's quality of life as well as being responsible for more than 1.5 million osteoporosis-related fractures annually (NIH, 2000). Often the patient is asymptomatic until fractures occur. The associated costs of osteoporosis far exceed $13.8 billion annually in the United States alone (NIH, 2000). Cooney (1997) refers to osteoporosis as a pediatric disease with a geriatric outcome. A young person's patterns of diet, exercise, and use of alcohol and tobacco have a long-lasting effect on bone.

Causes

Osteoporosis is defined as a degenerative disease characterized by progressive loss of bone mass with resulting fractures. The reduction of bone strength or bone mineral content causes the bone to become fragile and brittle, allowing bone to break with minimal stress. Healthy bone is continuously undergoing a process called *remodeling*, whereby bone resorption (removal of bone tissue) equals bone formation (Figure 17-2). Bone loss occurs when the amount resorbed is not fully replaced. A major contributor to accelerated bone loss at midlife is the loss of intrinsic estrogen. In addition to estrogen depletion, ethnicity, age, ovarian function, lifestyle choices related to smoking, diet, and exercise, are contributing factors to the disease. Pregnancy, lactation, and immobilization also influence bone mass.

Osteoporosis can strike at any age, but symptoms are more common in older people (Box 17-4). The higher percentage of women affected, one in four, is thought to be related to hormonal changes at midlife and that men typically have larger, stronger bones during the first half of their life.

The risk factors listed in Box 17-4 affect the calcium content of bone and increase the likelihood of bone fractures later in life. Diseases such as hyperthyroidism and rheumatoid arthritis may also predispose a woman to osteoporosis. Osteoporosis is less

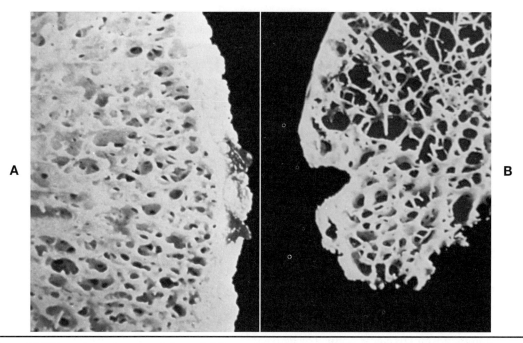

Figure 17-2 Normal vs. osteooporotic bone. **A,** Microscopic view of normal bone. **B,** Typical osteoporotic bone. (From Maher, A. B., Salmond, S. W., & Pellino, T. A. [2002]. *Orthopedic nursing* [3rd ed., p. 426]. Philadelphia: W. B. Saunders.)

BOX 17-4 MAJOR RISK FACTORS FOR OSTEOPOROSIS

Advancing age
Small frame
Caucasian or Asian race
Female gender
Family history
Poor nutrition
Smoking
Excessive alcohol use
Sedentary lifestyle
Steroid use

common in African-Americans, because of denser initial bone mass, and in obese women who have higher circulating levels of estrogen. However, Bailey, Combs, Rogers, and Stanley (2000) state that 10% of African-American women past age 50 have osteoporosis and an additional 30% have bone density low enough to put them at great risk for developing osteoporosis. Ninety-seven percent of bone mass is reached before a young woman reaches 19 years of age. The onset of spinal bone loss may begin even before a woman reaches 30 but is rather slow until menopause (Cooney, 1997). Bone density in the femur starts to decrease between 30 to 35, and, by age 40, resorption begins to exceed formation. The highest rate of bone loss will occur within the first 5 to 6 years after menopause (Andrews, 1998). Seventy-five percent of bone loss that occurs in women after menopause is related to estrogen deficiency rather than the aging process. The bone loss associated with postmenopause and declining estrogen initially starts at a site enriched in trabecular bone, namely the vertebral spine and pelvis (Kendig & Sanford, 1998). Such bone fragility places women at increased risk of fractures in those areas.

There are no early warning signs of osteoporosis and bone damage. Half of a woman's bone mass may be lost before a fracture occurs or a diagnosis of osteoporosis is confirmed. Vertebral bone is especially vulnerable, accounting for 50% of all fractures, and leading to the characteristic dorsal kyphosis or "dowager's hump." As bone loss occurs, there is a gradual loss of height. The average woman not on estrogen therapy may expect to lose an 1 to 1.5 inches in height as part of the normal aging process. Height loss greater than 1.5 inches may be associated with vertebral compression fractures indicative of osteoporosis.

Hip fractures occur in about 250,000 women per year with a mortality rate of 12% to 20% within 1 year of the event with more than 50% being unable to return to independent living, costing billions of dollars in medical care (Kendig & Sanford, 1998). The risk of hip fracture equals the risk of breast, uterine, and ovarian cancer combined. In fact, hip fractures and their complications kill more postmenopausal women than breast cancer (DeMasters, 2000).

Assessment

The good news is that osteoporosis is a preventable disease. Elimination of all but genetic risk factors at an early age will play a significant role in preventing this crippling disease from happening later in life. Currently, there is no cure for osteoporosis, but early diagnosis and treatment can help slow down the disease process. Perhaps the most important defense against osteoporosis is a healthy lifestyle, starting at a young age, aimed at building and maintaining strong bones. For older women, a simple nursing intervention and screening tool is to measure the height of all females older than age 25 with each office visit and to educate women as to the importance of this intervention (Cooney, 1997).

Traditional x-rays cannot reveal demineralization of bone until approximately 30% of bone mineral has been lost. A bone mineral density test has the ability to determine bone loss and detect osteoporosis when bone loss is less than 3% and long before a fracture happens (Cooney, 1997). DEXA (dual energy x-ray absorptiometry) provides reliable measurements and uses a minimal level of radiation when scanning for osteoporosis. Studies conducted by Weinstein and Ullery (2000) using bone densitometry confirm that estrogen increases bone mineral density, with age being directly related to bone loss and weight being inversely related.

Biochemical markers are used to track both formation and resorption. Two serum proteins, alkaline phosphatase and serum osteocalcin, are bone formation markers that might be considered for future screening to predict rate of bone loss and to monitor therapeutic response. Bone resorption markers that appear in urine are hydroxyproline and hydroxy lysine. Because these markers vary from day to day by 25% to 30%, it is necessary to take baseline measurements as well as serial testing. Certain diseases can greatly affect bone turnover markers, such as Paget's disease, renal insufficiency, rheumatoid arthritis, malignancy, alcohol or tobacco use, or long-term steroid use (Eastell, 1998). Identification of a variant of the vitamin D receptor gene, which is involved with bone formation, indicates the potential for future development of genetic screening for osteoporosis.

Management

Drug therapy for osteoporosis may include calcium supplement, vitamin D metabolites, estrogen, and a category of drugs known as bisphosphonates that claim to slow down resorption and help increase bone mass. Bisphosphonates are oral medications that do not provide relief from short-term menopause symptoms (hot flashes, insomnia) nor do they reduce the risk of cardiovascular disease in women. Alendronate (Fosamax) is the only bisphosphonate that the FDA has approved for the prevention and treatment of osteoporosis in postmenopausal women. Treatment has been shown to increase bone mineral density in areas prone to fracture, such as the vertebrae and femur. Alendronate and other bisphosphonates are poorly absorbed and, if not taken as directed, can cause difficulty swallowing, esophagitis, and gastric ulcers. Fosamax must be taken on an empty stomach followed by 30 minutes without any food or drink. The patient should not lie down during this time. Etidronate, another bisphosphonate, was once approved for use only in Paget's disease but is now being studied as a treatment for postmenopausal osteoporosis (Andrews, 1998).

Calcitonin, a hormone produced by the thyroid, has been used for its effects in aiding calcium absorption and inhibiting resorption. There is some documentation it increases vertebral bone mineral density. Calcitonin has been poorly accepted by patients when administered via a subcutaneous or intramuscular route. A nasal form of calcitonin (Calcimar, Miacalcin) made from salmon has been approved in conjunction with a calcium supplement for the treatment of osteoporosis but not the prevention of the disease. A nasal spray has been found to be more acceptable to some patients than injections. One study using nasal spray calcitonin in older postmenopausal women with low bone mass showed promising results arresting bone loss, particularly in osteoporotic women 5 years postmenopause (Andrews, 1998).

A method of preventing osteoporosis in women in the reproductive years is the use of oral contraceptives. Once women are postmenopausal, research has shown that a daily regimen of 0.625 mg of conjugated estrogen or 0.5 mg estradiol will reduce the risk of osteoporosis up to 60%. Progestin, when added to estrogen, leads to an increase in bone formation by aiding in calcium absorption. There has been a positive impact of hormone therapy on the bones of women over age 65, which presents a strong argument in favor of treating older women with estrogen.

Selective estrogen receptor modulators (SERMs) provide the benefit of estrogen on bone without the adverse effect on the endometrium or breasts. The first SERM used in the United States was tamoxifen for breast cancer therapy, and it is now being used in some women at high risk for osteoporosis. Raloxifene (Evista), another SERM, was recently approved for both the prevention and treatment of osteoporosis. It has been reported to lower low-density cholesterol (LDL) and does not increase high-density cholesterol (HDL) or triglyceride levels. Side effects are an increase in hot flashes and deep vein thrombosis (Andrews, 1998).

New treatments now under study are sodium fluoride and parathyroid hormone. Both drugs stimulate bone formation rather than inhibit bone loss (Andrews, 1998). Sodium fluoride has been around for a number of years but has potential toxicity problems. For that reason, until approved by the FDA, it should not be prescribed. The parathyroid hormone is currently being reviewed as an oral preparation to prevent and treat osteoporosis. Some women are using phytoestrogens because of their weak estrogen-like properties, but scientific studies are not available to document a proven effect on fracture reduction.

In a review of 18 randomized controlled clinical trials, Bonaiuti and others (2002) found that aerobic, weight-bearing resistance and walking exercise were all effective in increasing bone mineral density of the spine in postmenopausal women. Walking was also effective on the hip and aerobics on the wrist.

Existing data on children and adolescent girls suggest that current levels of dietary calcium may not be sufficient to achieve optimal bone mass density at maturity, leading to increased risk for osteoporosis. On a national average daily basis, only 12.7% of teenage girls ages 12 to 19 get the recommended dietary allowance of calcium for strong bones (Cooney, 1997). Young women with eating disorders such as anorexia and bulimia increase their risk for osteoporosis in later years because of insufficient absorption of calcium.

Heart Disease

Cardiovascular disease is the leading cause of death and disability in American women over 50, and every year approximately one half million women will die from this disease (Mosca, 2000). The predominant clinical manifestation is coronary heart disease (CHD). Approximately 233,000 women die of myocardial infarction and over 87,000 from strokes (Kendig & Sanford, 1998). Many women do not believe that they are at risk. A common misconception is that heart disease kills only men. Women may fear dying from breast cancer more than they do from heart disease.

Causes

Men experience more heart attacks at an earlier age than women, but women have less chance of surviving. More women will die (42%) from a myocardial infarction within the first year after an incident than men (24%) (King & Mosca, 2000). For women, signs of heart disease generally do not appear until about 10 years later than for their male counterparts or when they are postmenopausal (Kuhn, McMahon, & Creekmore, 1999; Mosca, 2000). Gender contrast based on anatomic differences in the heart and coronary arteries of men and women and ovarian hormonal factors may be responsible for delaying the development of CHD in women. During the reproductive years, women seem protected from CHD by high levels of high-density lipoproteins, attributed to high estrogen levels. Mosca (2000) cites the Framingham Study that total cholesterol levels are increased after menopause primarily because of a decrease in low-density lipoproteins (LDL) and a slight decrease in high-density lipoproteins (HDL). The risk of mortality from CHD is proportionate to a net reduction in total cholesterol levels.

Assessment

The most common presenting symptom of coronary heart disease in women is chest pain. Women presenting with chest pain, particularly premenopausal women, are often diagnosed as "anxious" or "reacting to stress" and denied a full cardiac workup. Often women have vague symptoms not associated with heart disease such as nausea, sweating, shortness of breath, and dizziness, especially during physical activity and lasting only a few minutes. Frequently these symptoms go unreported for some time. King and Mosca (2000) report that women not only fail to see the dangers of CHD but are less likely than men to be counseled during a routine health exam regarding blood pressure, nutrition, physical activity, smoking, and weight reduction.

Risk factors for CHD are classified as nonmodifiable and modifiable (Box 17-5). When looking at nonmodifiable factors, family history of early CHD is a very strong predictor of disease. A family history of heart disease may reflect a function of a learned family lifestyle that promotes years of unhealthy lifestyle choices. Race is a factor, especially for women of African-American ancestry who are at greater risk for CHD with a higher incidence and earlier mortality (King & Mosca, 2000). Women are all particularly vulnerable to the effects diabetes has on coronary vessel tone, hypertension, and lipid levels. Women with diabetes exhibit an incidence of CHD similar to that of men who do not have diabetes and even greater than men with diabetes (Kendig & Sanford, 1998). King and Mosca (2000) cite a three- to seven-fold increase of CHD in diabetic women. The onset of gestational

---

BOX 17-5 RISK FACTORS FOR CORONARY HEART DISEASE

Nonmodifiable Factors
Advancing age
Family history
Gender
Race
Diabetes

Modifiable Factors
Hypertension
Smoking
Hyperlipidemia
Obesity
Sedentary lifestyle
Menopause

diabetes during pregnancy has been found to be an indicator of higher CHD risk in 30% of those women later in life (Kuhn, McMahon, & Creekmore, 1999).

Hypertension, a modifiable risk, is defined as systolic pressure equal to or greater than 140 mm Hg and diastolic pressure equal to or greater than 90 mm Hg. High blood pressure is thought to be the strongest predictor of CHD. It has been suggested that a 10 mm Hg increase in systolic blood pressure in women may result in a 20% to 30% increase in CHD risk (Kendig & Sanford, 1998). Hypertension causes changes in the vascular system that promote the atherosclerotic process. Factors that can modify blood pressure include weight, exercise, smoking, alcohol abuse, and high sodium intake. A nontraditional risk factor reported in the Framingham Health Study identifies a relationship between Type A behavior and CHD in women. Women with Type A behavior who were followed for 8 years showed twice as much CHD as women with Type B behavior.

Kuhn, McMahon, and Creekmore (1999) see smoking as the most controllable risk factor for CHD. Women are smoking more than men, increasing their risk for cardiovascular disease with each and every cigarette smoked. For every pack smoked, they increase their risk two to four times more than nonsmoking women. Even if a woman smokes only one to four cigarettes a day, she has doubled her risk of heart disease (Kuhn, McMahon, & Creekmore, 1999). Nicotine, the active ingredient in tobacco smoke, causes spasm in small arteries, affects clotting factors, accelerates atherosclerosis, and increases LDL while decreasing HDL. Smoking also decreases estrogen levels, possibly leading to early menopause. Benefit from smoking cessation is realized almost immediately, and, within 3 to 5 years, the risk approximates that of a nonsmoker (Kuhn, McMahon, & Creekmore, 1999). Smoking cessation definitely reduces stroke risk, regardless of the woman's age when she started smoking, the number of cigarettes smoked, and her age when she stopped smoking.

It is now recognized that hormones can account for some variation between men's and women's lipid profile. Current recommendations are that total serum cholesterol should be less than 200 mg/dL. A level greater than 265 is associated with twice the risk of CHD than a level of 205 or lower (Kuhn, McMahon, & Creekmore, 1999). More than one third of American women have cholesterol levels that put them at increased risk for heart disease. A 25% reduction in total blood cholesterol can significantly reduce cardiovascular disease. Modifiable factors to keep cholesterol levels within normal levels include eating a heart-healthy diet, controlling weight, performing aerobic exercise, and not smoking. Women also tend to have high blood triglycerides, which can be controlled by reducing dietary fat intake.

More than 17 million American women are defined as being at least 20% above ideal body weight or having a body mass index greater than 30 (Kuhn, McMahon, & Creekmore, 1999). Epidemiological evidence supports the theory that a diet high in vegetable and low in animal protein reduces the risk for CHD (Ramsey, Ross, & Fischer, 1999). Obesity is directly associated with CHD by predisposing women to hypertension and unfavorable LDL/HDL cholesterol ratios. Of significance is excessive abdominal fat (a waist to hip ratio > 0.8), creating an apple-shaped appearance, which is an indicator of increased risk (King & Mosca, 1999).

Another controllable factor for developing CHD is physical inactivity. Women now in midlife or older were generally discouraged from participating in active exercise or vigorous sports in their youth, based largely on gender constraints. Low levels of physical activity as a child may have placed these women at increased risk for disease commonly associated with aging. Today, some form of physical exercise for 30 minutes daily or as much as possible is recommended to reduce CHD risk from a sedentary lifestyle. The benefit of exercise is evident by an increase in HDL levels, a decrease in blood sugar levels, and a decrease in triglycerides (Kendig & Sanford, 1998).

Hormonal status plays an important role in identifying risk factors for women, especially those postmenopausal. Women who experienced early menopause or who had an oophorectomy before age 35 have a seven-fold increase in CHD risk attributed to more years without the protective effects of estrogen (Massey, Hupp, Kreisberg, Alpert, & Hoff, 2000).

It has been well documented that estrogen is associated with a protective effect against CHD. Estrogen therapy can reduce heart disease risk up to 50% in women by decreasing LDL levels, increasing HDL levels, and lowering lipoproteins (DeMasters, 2000). The impact of estrogen therapy on the lipid profile is maintained as long as the woman remains on estrogen. The WHI (2002) findings indicate that the effect of progestin, when combined with estrogen replacement, reduces the protective effect of the estrogen and increases the risk of cardiovascular disease. Some studies, such as the Postmenopausal Estrogen/Progestin Interventions trial (PEPI), indicate a decrease in HDL levels but results are influenced by dose and duration of administration of progestin (De Masters, 2000). For women with an intact uterus, the PEPI results support the use of estrogen/progestin for the best effect on high-density levels without any increased risk of endometrial hyperplasia. Women approaching menopause should undergo a careful evaluation of individual risk factors for heart disease before making a decision regarding HRT. It should be noted that women with existing heart disease and on combined hormone therapy may not receive the same degree of cardiovascular protection and will require closer evaluation (De Masters, 2000).

The most effective strategy for reducing coronary heart disease in women is primary prevention through education and risk factor modification. Unless women realize the threat CHD presents to their well-being, they are unlikely to accept recommendations or change lifestyle behavior.

Cancers

This discussion of cancer will focus on the information that advanced practice nurses use in ambulatory settings. Emphasis will be placed on assessment and patient education. Management will be discussed briefly, but an indepth discussion of surgical radiation and chemotherapeutic interventions are beyond the scope of this text.

Breast Cancer

Menopause is not associated with increased cancer risk. However, cancer rates tend to increase with age so at midlife women are more aware of disease occurrence. The fear of breast cancer in this age cohort is quite prevalent, potentially underestimating the risk of heart disease and osteoporosis. Such fear, combined with an awareness of the association between estrogen and breast cancer, may influence a woman not to try HRT. Midlife women, already observing the effects of aging on their bodies, may perceive the loss of a breast from cancer as a final insult to their once youthful image. The horror of cancer and its treatment causes fear and anxiety for women who have any type of breast symptoms. For some, this fear motivates them to seek medical attention, while for others, it paralyzes them. Concern over breast cancer is indeed warranted: breast cancer now occurs in one in every eight women over a lifetime with more than 183,000 women diagnosed each year. Excluding skin cancer, it is the most common malignancy in women, and second only to lung cancer as a cause of cancer mortality in women (American Cancer Society, 2000; Nogueira & Appling, 2000). Breast cancer is rare in women under 30, rises among women in their early 40s, levels off about age 45, and then spirals again after 55 until approximately 75 years of age. The incidence increases with age, with a median age at diagnosis of 64 years. Although risk factors exist for breast cancer, age is the only factor in 70% of women diagnosed (Kendig & Sanford, 1998). Over 75% of women diagnosed are age 50 and older (Abraham & Seremetis, 1997). The sharp rise in incidence rates across the lifespan has been largely attributed to use of mammography as a screening tool. However, the higher mortality in a specific race, such as African-Americans, may be attributed to limited access to early breast health screening and adequate treatment.

Causes. The precise etiology of breast cancer is unclear but several factors are associated with an increased risk: advancing age, positive family history, previous breast cancer, high fat diet, alcohol use, early menarche, late menopause, hormonal factors, and nulliparity. Breast cancer is 1.5 to 3 times more likely to occur in women whose mother or sister had a history of breast cancer. Six percent of all women with breast cancer have a positive family history. If two first-degree relatives are affected, the risk jumps to 4 to 6 times when compared to that of a woman with a negative history for breast cancer (Couzi & Davidson, 1997). When assessing a woman's risk for breast cancer based on family history, genetic susceptibility for mutations in BRCA 1 and BRCA 2 (the first two genes to be implicated in hereditary breast and breast-ovarian cancer syndromes) accounts for 30% to 70% of all familial breast cancer. Research has also shown that these two genetic mutations are linked to 5% to 10% of all cervical cancers (Nogueira & Appling, 2000). However, it is important to recognize that there is enormous variation in risk, depending on the characteristics of the cancer of the affected relative. Certain cultures, such as Ashkenazi Jewish women specifically from Eastern European descent, have three known mutations within the BRCA1 and BRCA2 genes that increases their risk of breast cancer (Nogueira & Appling, 2000). Genetic testing for breast cancer has opened a new area of exploration for women and health care professionals regarding cancer screening, prophylactic treatment options, and ethical issues surrounding the reporting of test results.

Early menarche (before 12), late menopause (after 55), nulliparity, and delayed childbearing (after 30) have been associated with an increased risk of breast cancer but to what extent is unclear. The hypothesis is that there is a longer lifetime exposure to the proliferative effects of estrogen on breast tissue as a result of large numbers of ovulatory cycles during the reproductive years. Bear in mind, however, that 70% of all breast cancers occur without any significant risk factor (Nogueira & Appling, 2000). A woman whose menarche occurred at age 12 has a 30% increase in risk of breast cancer as compared to a woman who started menstruating at 15 years or older. Natural menopause after age 55 doubles the risk factor for breast cancer. In comparison, women who have had bilateral oophorectomies before age 40 have a 50% decrease in risk over a lifetime. An early age, full-term pregnancy may offer substantial protection against breast cancer while a woman who delays childbearing until 35 or later increases her risk factor twofold. Nulliparous women are at increased risk for breast cancer as compared to parous women. The protective effect of multiparity has been noted mostly in women aged 40 to 50 years (Couzi & Davidson, 1997). Breastfeeding appears to decrease risk up to 30%, but the protective effect is seen only in the premenopausal years and not after menopause and only if the woman lactated for at least 1 full year. Studies have focused on women of certain cultures, such as Asian, who tend to have a lower incidence of breast cancer, possibly related to a diet lower in fat and higher in soybeans, along with leaner bodies. The hypothesis that a high-fat diet increases risk of breast cancer, based on a study correlating worldwide incidence of breast cancer with per capita fat intake, continues to be researched through the WHI (Furniss, 2000).

The role of oral contraceptives and HRT in the development of breast cancer remains under discussion. Results from the 16-year cohort analysis of women in the Nurses Health Study, indicate the relative risk for breast cancer was slightly higher in women who have been on hormone replacement longer than 5 years (Abraham & Seremetis, 1997). Willis (1997) reports that "out of every 100 women on estrogen replacement therapy, 13 will develop breast cancer between the ages of 50 and 80 years, but only three of those 13 cases will be related to hormonal use." Some research reports a slight decrease in risk of fatal breast cancer associated with HRT simply because these women are healthier, less likely to smoke, and tend to participate in regular breast cancer screening. The WHI (2002) found a slightly increased risk of breast cancer in intact women taking combination HRT. It is possible that women on constant, low levels of estrogen replacement therapy have less risk because of the different chemical composition and estrogenic effect on breast tissue than with endogenous hormones (Willis, 1997). When counseling patients about hormone replacement, the proven benefits of HRT need to be weighed against the woman's personal risk for breast cancer before making a decision. By virtue of the magnitude of the postmenopausal population, more research concerning long-term use of hormones is essential to provide the answers women are seeking.

Assessment. Risk assessment provides the opportunity to identify and appropriately counsel women at moderate or high risk for breast cancer. One tool used to assess risk factors for breast cancer is the GAIL Model Risk Assessment Tool, developed by the National Cancer Institute. Information is obtained pertaining to the woman's age, number of first-degree relatives with breast cancer, age of first delivery, age at menarche, number of breast biopsies, and presence of endometrial atypical hyperplasia.

Women can actually take this assessment on the Internet (see Resources) and figure their 5-year risk and lifetime risk (Furniss, 2000).

The aim of breast cancer screening is to detect disease at the earliest possible stage. The three accepted methods of breast cancer detection include breast self-examination (BSE), professional breast examination, and mammography. According to the American Cancer Society (ACS), breast self-examination accounts for detection of approximately 80% of all breast masses, yet many women fail to carry out this simple monthly procedure. Contributing factors may be fear and anxiety of discovering a lump, lack of knowledge on how to perform BSE, cultural beliefs regarding body manipulation, lack of perceived risk of breast cancer, and apathy. The American Cancer Society and the American College of Obstetricians and Gynecologists recommend the following schedule for all asymptomatic women (Couzi & Davidson, 1997):

1. Breast self-examination every month for women older than 20
2. Clinical breast examination annually
3. Mammography starting with a baseline at 40, then a mammogram every 1 to 2 years between 40 and 50, then a yearly mammogram after age 50

Controversy exists as to the usefulness of a baseline mammogram at a younger age, unless the woman is in a high-risk category. A 30% reduction in mortality has been proven in women ages 50 to 69 who undergo mammogram screening (Abraham & Seremetis, 1997). Both the ACS and ACOG recommend annual mammography for women over 50 but no upper age has been identified at which screening should be stopped. The National Institutes of Health Breast Cancer Screening Forum and the American Geriatric Society recommend annual clinical breast examination and mammography every 2 years for women ages 65 to 75 years.

Management. There has been increasing interest in the development of "chemoprevention" or "chemosuppression" directed at inhibiting neoplastic development through pharmacologic measures. Clinical trials are investigating the prophylactic use of the drugs tamoxifen and raloxifene in women who are at increased risk for breast cancer, especially postmenopause (Nogueria & Appling, 2000). In the past, tamoxifen has been used to promote tumor regression and to delay recurrence of a tumor sensitive to estrogen and progesterone. Several large studies have shown that tamoxifen decreases the risk of invasive breast cancer by blocking the effects of estrogen on breast tissue. However, side effects have been noted, including an increased risk of endometrial cancer, pulmonary embolism, stroke, deep vein thrombosis, and cataracts (Nogueria & Appling, 2000). The newer drug raloxifene appears to decrease the risk of breast cancer without increasing the risk of endometrial cancer (Furniss, 2000). Another option some women at high risk consider is prophylactic mastectomy. Even with the removal of the breast, cancer cells can still be present in surrounding tissue. A breast cancer specialist should counsel these women when considering this option.

Concerns about breast symptoms are among the most common complaints clinicians hear. The fear of breast cancer causes great anxiety and stress for women who have breast symptoms. Educating women about breast health is paramount so that possible cancer can be diagnosed early and receive immediate referral, thus reducing mortality associated with breast cancer. The good news is that 97% of women diagnosed with breast cancer at an early stage survive for longer than 5 years (American Cancer Society, 2000).

Lung Cancer

The fact that lung cancer has surpassed breast cancer as the number one cancer death among women indicates the need for aggressive action aimed at this preventable disease (Williams & Sandler, 2001).

Causes. Over 90% of all cancers of the lung, trachea, and bronchus are attributable to tobacco. Although the rate of lung cancer is decreasing among Caucasian men, it is increasing among African-American men and among women of both races. The age that women start smoking is getting younger as well. According to the American Cancer Society, there is a 30% increased risk of a nonsmoker who lives with a smoker dying of lung cancer than that of a nonsmoker living with a nonsmoker (Williams, 1997). Other risk factors for lung cancer beside second-hand smoke include occupational exposure to asbestos and radon gas. Lung cancer has no early symptoms making early detection almost impossible. Because of this, lung cancer has the lowest 5-year survival rate of any cancer. Over the last 25 years, survival rates have not increased significantly at all (Williams & Sandler, 2001). Over 90% of patients die of the disease. Once symptoms appear, they include persistent cough, chest pain, wheezing breath sounds, coughing up blood, shortness of breath, and recurring pneumonia. Chest x-ray, sputum analysis, and fiberoptic examination of the bronchial passages assist diagnosis. Research is pointing the way to screen for lung cancer using specific biomarkers, which may indicate a predisposition to smoking-related carcinogenesis (Williams & Sandler, 2001).

Management. Smoking cessation remains the best strategy to decreasing mortality from lung cancer. For individuals who have smoked less than 20 years and then stop, their lung cancer risk steadily declines until after 15 years of abstinence, their risk is almost that of a nonsmoker (Williams, 1997). The tobacco industry has marketed cigarette smoking to women, with over half of female smokers starting before the age of 13, as a way to be provocative, seductive, and thin. Smoking cessation programs must address the concerns of women of all ages and include education on the life-long effects of smoking to their bodies.

Gynecological Cancers

Gynecological malignancies still remain an important cause of morbidity and mortality in women. The traditional focus for cervical, endometrial, and ovarian cancers has been early detection and prompt treatment. Each of these cancers will be reviewed with a proposed shift toward prevention.

Cervical cancer. The greatest risk factor for developing cervical cancer is not having, or rarely having a Papanicolaou (Pap) smear. Half of the cervical cancers in the United States occur in women who have never been screened, and over 60% occur in women who have not had a Pap smear in the 5 years preceding their diagnosis. Cervical cancer is the third most common reproductive cancer in women in the United States (Furniss, 2000). In countries where there are inadequate Pap smear screening programs, cervical cancer is the leading cause of cancer death among women. Even with the Pap test as a part of the annual examination, 4600 American women were expected to die of cervical cancer in 2000 out of 12,800 newly diagnosed cases (Furniss, 2000; Greenlee, Murray, & Bolden, 2000).

Causes. Cervical carcinoma in situ (CIS) is associated with women ages 25 to 35, whereas invasive cervical cancer tends to occur more in older women (Williams, 1997). Wilmoth and Spinelli (2000), in discussing sexuality in cancer patients, state that by the end of 2001, two thirds of newly diagnosed cases of invasive cervical cancer will occur in women younger than 50. Be aware that even women in their 80s have been diagnosed with invasive cervical cancer. This older segment of women often gets overlooked in screening programs. Fortunately, the incidence of invasive cervical cancer has decreased for most American women because of annual screening, and survival rates have increased. However, the incidence of in situ cancers is increasing, possibly because of early detection.

Assessment. All women who are sexually active or 18 years and older should have an annual Pap and pelvic examination. Some physicians feel that if a woman has three or more consecutive normal annual examinations, the Pap may be performed less frequently, possibly every 3 to 5 years. A high-risk woman should continue having annual Pap smear screening. There is no upper age limit on screening. Unfortunately, there is almost a 50% failure rate in diagnosing invasive cervical cancer, depending on the reliability of the collection technique used and the reviewing cytologist (Huff, 2000).

A complete sexual history provides the woman and her clinician an opportunity to discuss risk factors and to make an informed decision about the frequency of testing. Bear in mind that any abnormality on screening immediately creates fear in the woman's mind, and results should be discussed immediately. In an attempt to improve on the Pap test, the FDA in 1996 approved the use of a new technique for collection called the Thin Prep Pap test. Early studies found Thin Prep to be significantly more effective as a mass screening tool for cervical cancer. However, in 1998, the American College of Obstetricians and Gynecologists called for a large, population-based study before they would claim any advantage over the traditional method of collection (Huff, 2000).

Identified risk factors for cervical cancer include early age at first intercourse, multiple sex partners, "high-risk" male consort, low socioeconomic status, and early age at childbearing. Viral agents, such as herpes simplex, human papilloma virus (HPV) and human immunodeficiency virus (HIV) are likely cofactors in the development of cervical cancer. Strong evidence has emerged linking HPV 16 and HPV 18 infection with 93% of cervical cancer and is considered the primary cause of cervical neoplasia (Furniss, 2000; Williams, 1997). The presence of other cofactors, including exposure to carcinogens in cigarette smoking and in utero exposure to diethylstilbestrol (DES), have also been associated with cervical cancer.

Management. Lifestyle changes and better patient education regarding the impact of sexual behavior on one's health could decrease many of the cancer risk factors found in a sexually active population. Because cervical cancer behaves like a sexually transmitted disease, barrier contraception and spermicidal foam act as antiviral agents, reducing exposure to infectious agents. The Hybrid Capture II, a human papilloma virus DNA test, is available to help identify women who have underlying lesions related to HPV and potentially greater risk for cervical cancer. Furniss (2000) states the best prevention for cervical cancer is abstinence or a monogamous relationship. Because that may not be a choice for every woman, the development of new drugs such as Imiquimod hold promise for the prevention of cervical cancer. As an antiviral agent, it stimulates the body's immune system to recognize and destroy viral cells such as HPV that lead to cervical dysplasia. Other preventive strategies include a high dietary intake of vitamin C, which has an antioxidant effect and enhances the immune system, and the addition of folate and beta cartotene supplementation (Furniss, 2000).

There are no symptoms with the pre-invasive stage of cervical cancer. The most common symptoms of invasive cancer are abnormal bleeding and vaginal discharge (Huff, 2000). Pain and systemic manifestations occur late in the disease. A characteristic aching pain in the lower abdominal quadrant or low back region may indicate that the tumor has reached the pelvic side wall and is pressing on the nerve trunks (Williams, 1997). Most women with an abnormal Pap smear have a treatable precancerous condition called *cervical dysplasia* (CIN). The use of colposcopy has allowed for a more conservative treatment approach to this disease. Treatment for invasive cervical cancer is surgery, radiation, or both, depending on the stage of disease, the patient's age and general health, and the surgeon's clinical judgement. The importance of annual screening cannot be stressed enough as half of the women diagnosed with advanced invasive cervical cancer never had a routine Pap test (Furniss, 2000).

Uterine cancer. Uterine or endometrial cancer is the most common gynecological cancer affecting the female reproductive organs (Furniss, 2000). The uterus is composed of two layers, the endometrium or inner layer and a muscular outer layer known as the myometrium. Uterine cancer most often develops in the endometrium. It affects predominantly postmenopausal women, with an average age of 61 at the time of diagnosis, and has a higher incidence among white women than African-American women (Wilmoth & Spinelli, 2000). According to the American Cancer Society (2000) over 36,000 new cases of uterine cancer and 6500 deaths were predicted for the year 2000.

Causes. Williams (1997) attributes the rise in incidence of endometrial tumors to an aging population; a high-fat diet, which may influence metabolism of circulating hormones; and estrogen replacement therapy without the protective benefit of progestin. In a woman with a uterus, the use of unopposed estrogen increases the risk of endometrial cancer 2 to 3 times after 3 years of exposure. Thus unopposed estrogen therapy is no longer recommended for a woman with an intact uterus. Hormonal therapy with progestin may be used both adjunctively to prevent recurrence and as a treatment for advanced disease (Wilmoth & Spinelli, 2000).

Assessment. Predisposition to endometrial cancer follows years of unopposed estrogen related to early menarche, late menopause, infertility, low parity, and obesity. Women with diabetes are 2 to 3 times more likely to have endometrial cancer compared to women who do not have the disease. Hypertension is also a risk factor found in over half of the women with diagnosed endometrial cancer (Kendig & Sanford, 1998). Endometrial hyperplasia is a known precursor to the development of endometrial cancer and requires prompt treatment. There is a familial tendency, although there is no genetic marker for endometrial cancer at this time. In addition, women who have had breast or ovarian cancer are at higher risk for endometrial cancer (American Cancer Society, 2000; Williams, 1997).

The one significant sign of endometrial cancer is abnormal or dysfunctional uterine bleeding (DUB), specifically in postmenopausal women. One in ten women postmenopause will complain of uterine bleeding. Often postmenopausal women will exhibit premalignant changes of atypical endometrial hyperplasia before actually developing an overt carcinoma and the accompanying pain that occurs late in the disease process. Bleeding in pre- and perimenopausal women is usually not associated with endometrial cancer but is more related to anovulatory cycles. Although the Pap test is not a screening tool for endometrial cancer, any reported atypical endometrial cells found should warrant further investigation whether bleeding is present or not and regardless of the woman's age.

Routine screening by biopsy for the asymptomatic woman is neither practical nor cost effective. The criteria for performing endometrial sampling (biopsy) include the following:

■ Any postmenopausal bleeding
■ Postmenopausal women on long-term unopposed exogenous estrogen
■ Premenopausal women with polycystic ovary disease
■ Women on tamoxifen therapy
■ Obese, nulliparous women with a history of diabetes or hypertension

Management. Treatment for endometrial cancer depends on the stage of the tumor, the size of the uterus, the degree of cancer cell differentiation, and the woman's general medical condition (Williams, 1997). The procedure commonly performed is hysterectomy, with or without radiation therapy. The cure rate is very high if diagnosed early, as these tumors tend to be well differentiated and localized. When detected in an invasive stage, the survival rate drops dramatically.

Preventive strategies for endometrial cancer include use of combination oral contraceptives or combined hormone therapy. The progestin offsets the effect of endogenous estrogen production and causes a decidual change in the endometrium.

Ovarian cancer. Ovarian cancer deaths in the United States exceed those of cervical and endometrial cancer combined. It is estimated 2 out of 70 women will be diagnosed with ovarian cancer. The onset is insidious, and it is usually not diagnosed in an early stage. The lack of early symptoms conceals ovarian cancer until it frequently spreads beyond the ovaries to the upper abdomen or further sites. Almost 15,000 American women die each year from ovarian cancer, largely because the disease could not be detected early enough for effective treatment. The 5-year survival rate with ovarian cancer is approximately 93% when the cancer is localized but drops dramatically to below 40% when advanced disease is diagnosed, despite extensive surgery and chemotherapy (Wilmoth & Spinelli, 2000). Tumors of the ovary are most common in the 40 to 70 age group, with a higher incidence among Western industrialized nations than elsewhere in the world. Women with a strong family history may develop the disease and be diagnosed at a much younger age. A first-degree relative with ovarian cancer raises a woman's risk three times (Furniss, 2000).

Causes. The causes of ovarian cancer are still unclear but there is evidence that altered endocrine function may be a contributing factor. Unfortunately, some women with breast, colon, or endometrial cancer have developed ovarian cancer at the same time, supporting the theory of a common etiology among cancers. Reduction in the number of ovulations through pregnancy before age 25, early menopause, and long-term oral contraceptive use appears to provide some protection against this disease. Risk factors include aging, especially for women 45 to 60; postmenopause; mother or sister with ovarian, colon, or breast cancer; and environmental exposure to certain agents such as asbestos and talc.

Furniss (2000) describes several biologic tumor markers associated with ovarian cancer. Although CA 125 is found elevated in many women with ovarian cancer, it is not specific for this cancer and may be elevated with other malignancies. For now it is not sensitive enough to serve as a screening tool. The discovery of two breast cancer susceptibility genes, BRCA-1 and BRCA-2, has opened a new genetic field for women at high risk of ovarian cancer based on familial history.

Assessment. Diagnosis of ovarian cancer is difficult compared to other gynecologic cancers where vaginal bleeding is an early clue. The most common sign of ovarian cancer is ascites or an increase in abdominal girth accompanied by vague gastrointestinal complaints. No effective means of mass screening has been developed. Any postmenopausal woman who has a palpable ovary or mass should have a laparoscopic examination.

Management. Treatment is dictated by the stage of disease at the time of diagnosis and often includes a total abdominal hysterectomy and bilateral salpingo-oophorectomy plus lymph node sampling. Adjuvant chemotherapy has been proven effective in improving the survival rate in ovarian cancer and is often started immediately after surgery. Some women, having completed their childbearing and having a first-degree relative with ovarian cancer, may elect to have a prophylactic oophorectomy performed. Preventive strategies include use of combined oral contraceptives, which if taken for 10 years, can reduce a woman's risk of ovarian cancer by almost 80%. The irony of using long-term oral contraceptives to reduce endometrial and ovarian cancers is that there is an associated increased risk for cervical cancer. There is, however, an effective screening for early detection of cervical cancer with the annual Pap test. Hence, the beneficial effects on endometrial and ovarian cancer might outweigh the adverse effect of oral contraceptives on cervical cancer.

Gynecologic cancer summary. Gynecologic cancers, such as breast, cervical, uterine, or ovarian, have a profound physical and emotional impact on a woman's sense of identity and her sexuality. Her decisions about various treatments, particularly in younger years, have lasting consequences. Women who lose a part of their body to cancer feel a significant loss, not only of the organ removed but also of the pleasure associated with sexual functioning. Williams (1997) reports that because breast cancer is the most common female cancer and breast removal the most common treatment, sexual problems arise more often than with any other cancer. With any cancer, discussion of a woman's sexuality should be addressed in the very beginning.

Skin Cancer

The three most common skin cancers in the United States are basal cell carcinoma, squamous cell carcinoma, and malignant melanoma.

Causes. Basal cell and squamous cell cancers are the most typical and are easily treated, but malignant melanomas account for almost all the deaths. The incidence of malignant melanoma is increasing because of the popularity of outdoor recreation and suntans.

Assessment. Areas of the body that are exposed repeatedly to the sun such as the face, chest, back, shoulders, and legs are sites of most skin cancers. Women who frequently sunbathe, those with fair skin, and outdoor workers are particularly at risk.

Management. Skin cancer can be avoided by protecting oneself from continued exposure to ultraviolet rays of the sun (Duey, Smith, & Johnson, 1997) (Box 17-6).

Because women tend to discover skin cancer at an earlier stage than men, the overall cure rate is higher in women. Skin cancer screening should be incorporated into the annual physical examination. Women should be instructed on examining their skin regularly for signs of new growths or changes in existing ones, particularly a change in size, shape, or color of a mole; a sore that never heals; and painless scaly or crusted patches of skin.

Colon Cancer

Colorectal cancer in women is an underappreciated but preventable cancer. Colon cancer is the third most common cause of cancer deaths in women after lung and breast cancer. Although 40% of the 65,000 women diagnosed each year eventually die, it is highly curable if diagnosed at an early stage (Donovan & Syngal, 1998). The risk of colon cancer increases after age 40 with 90% of women diagnosed being 50 years or older. The incidence is slightly higher in African-American women. The exact cause of colon cancer is unknown, but acknowledged risk factors include advancing age; familial history or personal history of other colon disease, specifically ulcerative colitis; alcohol and cigarette smoking of long duration; and possibly a diet high in fat and low in fiber.

BOX 17-6 COMMON SKIN CANCER PRECAUTIONS

- Avoid sun exposure, especially if fair skinned
- Protect infants and children (an increased risk may be associated with exposure in the first decade)
- Avoid the sun if on certain medications (such as tetracycline, tricyclics, antihistamines, antipsychotics, hypoglycemics, diuretics, antineoplastics, and retin A)
- Use sunscreen with an appropriate sun protective factor (SPF) and as directed by the manufacturer
- Avoid peak time for ultraviolet rays: 10 AM to 2 PM
- Wear light-colored clothing and a hat
- Beware of reflective surfaces such as water, cement, snow that enhance the rays of the sun

Women with a history of breast, endometrial, or ovarian cancer may be at a greater risk for colon cancer. Occupational exposure to asbestos and mineral oil may increase the risk as well. Having a first-degree relative with colon cancer greatly increases a woman's risk of disease over her lifetime.

Assessment. Most colon cancers start as benign colonic polyps and simple removal reduces the risk of cancer tremendously. The woman with colon cancer may be asymptomatic for long time, making annual screening very important. A change in bowel habits, rectal bleeding, abdominal pain or bloating, unexplained weight loss, and fatigue are possible symptoms. The United States Preventive Task Force has recommended universal screening for colon cancer starting at age 50 with an annual digital rectal exam and a non-invasive fecal occult blood test. Thereafter, every 5 to 7 years a flexible sigmoidoscopy is advised (Donovan & Syngal, 1998). A positive fecal occult test may lead to a diagnosis long before symptoms appear.

Management. Colon cancer is curable surgically if found before metastasis spreads into the peritoneum, surrounding tissue, and lymph nodes. The most important factor in reducing one's risk of colon cancer is primary prevention (i.e., change in diet) and secondary prevention (i.e., adequate screening for all women over 50). Donovan and Syngal (1998) report that annual screening and subsequent surveillance can reduce colon deaths by 75%. Table 17-3 summarizes the signs and symptoms and diagnostic tests related to cancers in women.

Midlife Sexuality

Sexuality is an important part of the total woman, integral to her health, quality of life, and general well-being. Continued sexual activity as one grows older contributes to an active social life and general physical and mental health. However, contraceptive practices should be assessed for all women entering midlife who are at risk for pregnancy. Many perimenopausal women are still potentially fertile despite irregular menstrual cycles. If a midlife woman has unprotected intercourse without becoming pregnant, she may falsely assume she has become infertile. Because the average age of menopause is about 51 years, sexually active women need contraception until they have completely gone through menopause.

All forms of contraception are available. Some women may choose to use low-dose estrogen/progestin oral contraceptives until menopause and then consider HRT. Low-dose birth control pills during midlife re-establish a regular menstrual pattern, minimize perimenopausal symptoms, and postpone bone loss associated with osteoporosis. The absolute contraindication for oral contraceptives in this age group is smoking, which has been known to increase the risk of stroke, myocardial infarction, and blood clots. The use of an intrauterine device (IUD) may be appropriate for midlife women as long as there is no history of menorrhagia, fibroids, or positive cultures for *Gonorrhea* and *Chlamydia.* Contraceptive jelly or foam with a diaphragm may be advantageous to the perimenopausal woman for alleviating vaginal dryness. The condom may present a problem for midlife couples as penile sensitivity and degree of erection decreases.

Table 17-3	CANCERS IN WOMEN		
TYPE	**HISTORY**	**SIGNS/SYMPTOMS**	**DIAGNOSTIC TEST**
Breast	Family history is significant	Painless mass, nipple discharge, dimpling	BSE, mammogram, clinical exam
Lung	Closely correlates with long-term smoking	No early symptoms; later persistent cough	Chest x-ray, sputum analysis, fiberoptic exam
Cervical	History of STDs, especially HPV	Abnormal bleeding and vaginal discharge	Pap smear
Uterine	Years of unopposed estrogen	Abnormal bleeding, especially in menopausal women	Endometrial biopsy
Ovarian	Seen in women with other cancers	Non-specific; abdominal bloating, pain, intestinal complaints	Bimanual exam
Skin	Repeated exposure to the sun	New growths or changes in existing ones; a sore that never heals	Visual inspection
Colon	History of ulcerative colitis; possibly high-fat diet	Change in bowel habits, rectal bleeding, bloating, weight loss	Digital rectal exam, fecal occult blood test

Assessment

It is important during a screening examination, to routinely inquire about sexual functioning. In a quiet, private area the clinician should introduce the subject of sexuality and satisfaction in an open and forthright manner. As part of a woman's sexual history, the clinician inquires about the woman's current sex life, including sexual orientation and number of partners; sexual difficulties such as pain with intercourse, lack of sexual desire, or a decrease in vaginal lubrication with sexual arousal; and any concerns the woman may have about her sexual functioning (Katz, 2000). Asking such questions sends the message that the clinician recognizes the subject is important to the woman and is a legitimate topic of concern. It also allows for assessment of domestic violence and sexual abuse. There is the opportunity to educate the woman regarding normal changes that may occur with age in sexual functioning. It is important that the clinician be comfortable initiating such discussions and remain neutral to comments and descriptions she may hear (Katz, 2000).

With age, men experience slower arousal, lack of sustained erection, decreased penile sensitivity, and a decrease in libido as testosterone levels drop. It is important that the woman understand that changes brought about by age affect her partner as well as herself. Major sexual changes that occur in the aging woman because of decreasing estrogen involve a reduction in vaginal lubrication, loss of vaginal elasticity, and a slower response cycle with decreased intensity of orgasm (Box 17-7). Decreased libido and clitoral response seem to be related to levels of free testosterone. Postmenopausal urogenital atrophy causes a feeling of dryness, vaginal irritation and burning with coitus, and possible vaginal spotting after intercourse.

Management

Sexually active women tend to have less complaints of vaginal atrophy, possibly related to a maintained vaginal vasculature and circulation. Most women after age 55 do experience some vascular changes that decrease their arousal and intensity of muscular contractions during orgasm (Alexander, 1997). Use of estrogen, either topically or systemically, helps restore vaginal circulation and improves vaginal tone and reduces dryness. The decline in sexual activity associated with perimenopause is often influenced by culture and attitudes rather than by hormones. Two important factors to a satisfactory sex life are the strength of the couple's relationship and the physical condition of each partner. A consideration would include any medications that either partner may be taking that could affect sexual performance. Agents such as antihypertensives, sedatives, antidepressants, antihistamines, alcohol, and nicotine can adversely affect sexual performance.

The inability to communicate with a partner about one's needs and desires very often affects sexual fulfillment. Sexual behaviors that may need to be modified include taking more time for arousal, alternative positions, and use of water-soluble lubricants. For long-term partners, boredom and old habits can stand in the way. Women can learn to be more open with their partners about what they enjoy in the way of stimulation, touch, and position. Important determinants of sexual activity in the aging woman are the unavailability of a partner because of divorce or death or a nonfunctional male partner. Midlife women who are divorced or widowed and rejoining the dating scene may have concerns about sexually transmitted diseases and "safe sex." Any behavior identified as high-risk will place a woman in danger regardless of her age. This includes having unprotected sex, multiple partners, and vaginal intercourse or oral sex with someone who uses illicit, intravenous drugs. Sexual issues with lesbian patients are similar to those of heterosexual women and should be openly discussed (Woodson, 1997).

Urinary Incontinence

Urinary incontinence is defined as involuntary loss of urine and is often considered a "female" problem although it does affect men in significant numbers. Most women who

---

BOX 17-7 SEXUAL MODIFICATIONS

- Increased time for foreplay
- Use of water-soluble lubricant
- Variations in positioning
- Increased communication between partners
- Perineal exercises to increase muscle tone
- Estrogen therapy

develop urinary incontinence never discuss this problem with their health care provider. They believe problems with urinary control are a consequence of "normal aging" and childbirth and that incontinence is not treatable. Store shelves are packed with adult absorbent products, conveying the message that incontinence is "normal." On the contrary, this condition is not normal and is a symptom of an underlying problem. Some 13 million Americans suffer with urinary incontinence, more than half women. Nearly one in every two women will experience episodes of incontinence between the ages of 45 (the most common age of onset) and 64 years (Czarapata & McKillips, 1997), often resulting in profound embarrassment and modifications in lifestyle. Incontinence has a profound effect on a woman's life. It can cause loss of independence and privacy, considerable embarrassment and loss of self-esteem, and possibly even loss of her job. Yet it is treatable in most cases. Even partial improvement in symptoms may restore quality of life. Women will suffer in silence with urinary incontinence, typically waiting 3 to 4 years before they visit a health care provider for help. It appears that urinary incontinence drastically lowers the quality of life of peri- and postmenopausal women yet they wait to seek medical treatment (Ushiroyama, Ikeda, & Ueki, 1999). This hesitancy may be attributed to a clinician's lack of evaluating and assessing this condition as well as the patient's embarrassment. It is the clinician's responsibility to approach the subject of bladder control and voiding habits in a caring manner with every midlife woman (Gallo, Fallon, & Staskins, 1997). Assessing the onset and severity will aid in diagnosis and treatment. Although most people associate incontinence with old age, it knows no age limit. Gallo, Fallon, and Staskins cite the prevalence of incontinence for women ages 45 to 64 to range from 8% to 15%, increasing to 25% after age 65. Incontinence will be addressed in greater depth in Chapter 18.

Mental Health Issues

Historically, women's mental health care has focused on women's responses to reproduction and hormonal changes. There is a growing need to center on more global issues such as domestic violence, depression, and substance abuse. Addressing women's health concerns involves recognizing and responding to their mental as well as physical health needs.

Domestic Violence

There is no single definition of domestic violence that satisfies medical, social, and criminal justice purposes. Typically the term refers to violence in any form perpetrated against females within the context of family or intimate relationships. Violence toward women is definitely a significant health issue that crosses all age, racial, ethnic, educational, or socioeconomic lines. Historically, domestic violence had been accepted as a private matter between two people in the confines of their bedroom. Most of the sexual violence against a woman is committed by someone she knows. The term "intimate" violence has been recently coined to describe such violence at the hands of partners, husbands, dates, friends, and close acquaintances (Draucker & Madsen, 1999). Every year 8% to 12% of American women in a relationship experience at least one episode of severe violence that includes physical injury, being threatened with a weapon, or being verbally abused (ACOG, 1999).

It is now acknowledged that without intervention, the violence continues in the home and escalates, often ending in death. Since 1985, the United States Surgeon General's Office has viewed domestic violence as a major health problem that carries with it many health-related implications (Ryan & King, 1998). From a global perspective, domestic violence is so prevalent it is considered an epidemic. The issue of domestic violence is costing our society thousands of human lives lost, millions of dollars in health care, and substantial psychological harm to the family unit, including depression, substance abuse, sexual dysfunction, anxiety disorders, and symptoms of posttraumatic shock (Drucker & Madsen, 1999).

There is a mind set about violence against women that often precludes effective intervention. Certain myths often perpetuate more violence. Ryan and King (1998) cite the following myths that cloud society's understanding of the depth of domestic violence in America today:

- Violence occurs only in problem families or certain ethnic groups
- Only a small percentage of women are really abused
- The abuse cannot be so bad if the woman doesn't leave
- Family violence rarely escalates to homicide

Domestic violence—be it called *battering, spouse abuse,* or *intimate violence*—is the most common form of family violence and the most common cause of injuries to women that require medical attention. The National Health Objective for *Healthy People 2000* addressed domestic violence and specified that at least 90% of our country's hospital emergency departments should have protocols in place to identify, treat, and refer patients who experience assault or other form of violence (Coker, Smith, Bethea, King, & McKeown, 2000). The Surgeon General's Task Force on Violence further called for the development of both prevention and intervention programs for use by health care providers in all settings (Ryan & King, 1998).

More than half the women murdered in this country are killed by husbands or boyfriends or by men they had a relationship with in the past such as ex-husbands (Poirier, 1997). Injuries resulting from domestic violence outnumber automobile accidents, muggings, and rapes combined. Gantt and Bickford (1999) report 7% or some 3.9 million American women are physically abused and 37% (20.7 million) were either verbally or emotionally abused by their spouse or partner. The act of abuse is repetitive in nature and many women report being assaulted repeatedly within a short span of time. It has been speculated that as high as 43% of abuse cases are not even reported to the police because of the secretive nature surrounding domestic violence (Poirier, 1997). Nationally, 30% of women seen in emergency rooms were identified as having injuries or complaints consistent with some form of abuse (Gantt & Bickford, 1999). The most common physical complaints of these women are chronic pain and insomnia. Irritable bowel syndrome, arthritis, pelvic inflammatory disease, urinary tract infections, depression, migraine headaches, and neurologic damage are also associated with years of physical abuse (Coker, Smith, Bethea, King, & McKeown, 2000). Domestic

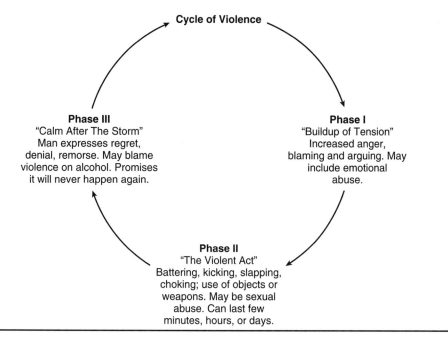

Cycle of Violence

Phase III
"Calm After The Storm"
Man expresses regret,
denial, remorse. May blame
violence on alcohol. Promises
it will never happen again.

Phase I
"Buildup of Tension"
Increased anger,
blaming and arguing. May
include emotional
abuse.

Phase II
"The Violent Act"
Battering, kicking, slapping,
choking; use of objects or
weapons. May be sexual
abuse. Can last few
minutes, hours, or days.

Figure **17-3** The cycle of violence.

violence also accounts for one in four suicide attempts by women; half of those attempts are by African-American women. But violence does not stop with younger women. Elder abuse has also become a serious problem for older women, with estimates of 1% to 4% being abused either in a health care facility or in their own home by a caregiver.

Domestic violence can include physical abuse, sexual abuse, verbal and emotional abuse, and destruction of personal property. Clever abusers may never have to resort to physical harm if they can gain control over the other person through tactics such as fear, isolation, and destruction of self-esteem. The cycle of violence occurs in three phases-the tension building phase; the acute, violent period; and the honeymoon phase or period of loving contrition (ACOG, 1999) (Figure 17-3).

Causes. During the tension-building phase of the cycle of violence, the woman attempts to avoid angering her partner. Often, the male will start with abusive remarks, progress to minor physical abuse, such as slapping or pushing, followed by intimidation and shouting. There can be emotional abuse whereby phone calls are monitored, outside social contact is limited, medical care denied, and money withheld. At some point the man's anger boils over and he brutally attacks the woman. The acute battering phase may involve kicking, choking, hitting, or threats with a weapon. Sexual abuse, forcing the woman to perform sexual activities against her will, or preventing her from using birth control or protection against sexually transmitted diseases, may occur. The battering may go on for hours or days. After the violence ends, the man tries to justify his actions by recounting events that led to his anger or blaming substances (alcohol or drugs) for his behavior. The honeymoon phase is the calm after the storm. The man asks forgiveness and assures the woman that it will never happen again. Many battered women have a unique relationship with their abuser, often including feelings of dependency, love, affection, and fear. Eighty-five percent of abused women will attempt to leave at least once, if not more often, before finally being able to end the relationship because of a misplaced concept of love, fear, and self-worth (Coker et al., 2000).

Assessment. In addition to the physical pain, battered women feel frightened, ashamed, isolated, guilty, and will not admit to the abuse unless directly asked. Providing quality health care involves integrating knowledge of domestic violence into clinical practice. This means asking *every* woman about abuse and violence in her life. The American Nurses' Association in their position statement *Physical Violence Against Women* (1991) supported routine assessment and documentation for physical abuse in every health care institution and community setting, specifically targeting women at high risk, including pregnant women and women presenting in the emergency room in crisis.

All interviews should be conducted in a private place without children or family members in the room. Confidentiality must be ensured. Direct questions, asked in a nonjudgmental manner and aimed at specific behavior, are most effective in allowing the woman to talk about her abuse. Empathetic listening is important to establishing rapport.

Management. Should the abused woman decide to return home, it is important to discuss the development of a safety plan that can be implemented in an emergency. Clinicians need to be supportive of the woman's decision if she is fearful of leaving. By inquiring and expressing concern, clinicians can provide a safe and caring environment for women to reflect and consider their options. Information on the cycle of violence and resources should be discussed so the woman understands that she is not at fault and does not desire this punishment. Even if the woman is reluctant to end the relationship now, she knows that the health care provider is a source of support and information when she is ready to leave the situation. Health care providers and community domestic violence programs should work closely together to ensure a prompt response to the needs of battered women and to change the perspective of violence from a medical problem to societal issue. Often not only is the woman in danger but her children may be. Abuse may be considered a learned behavior, and it is recognized that many abusers came from families where this behavior was practiced. Children who are abused or who witness violence eventually come to imitate such behavior as a "learned phenomenon" and often become controlling and abusive as adults (Poirier, 1997). Clearly, violence against women is a significant health problem that affects women of all ages in all areas of health and well-being.

Depression

In the late 1800s, it was thought that depression in women was related to changes in their reproductive function but it was never scientifically proven. It was known that a sudden change in hormonal activity, such as surgical menopause, often led to severe depression (Schmidt, Roca, Bloch, & Rubinow, 1997). The unresolved question of the relationship between depression and perimenopause has resurfaced as more is known about the impact gonadal steriods have on the central nervous system. Schmidt and others (1997) cite epidemiological studies that report no increase in the prevalence of major depression in women at midlife (ages 45 to 55), yet that same article cites other studies that show the increase in episodes of major depression in midlife women is twice that of men. What is known is that depression limits daily living, affects one's state of physical and mental well-being, and impinges on the person's ability to earn a living or care for her family.

Clinically, depression is defined as a transient or persistent mood change, with sufficient physical or mental symptoms (such as impaired cognitive or motor function) that are severe enough to warrant diagnosis as an illness (Moore, 2000). One in four women can expect to experience at least one episode of clinical depression during their lifetime, which is twice that of men (Moore, 2000).

Causes. Gender differences in the function of neurotransmitters and neurostructures may be involved in maintaining mood, and these differences may increase the vulnerability of women to depression (Schmidt et al., 1997). Desai and Jann (2000) cite a change in estrogen levels, leading to modulation of serotonergic function, that may increase the risk of depression. Stressful life events over a long period may also modulate neurotransmitter activity, contributing to a biological basis for depression. Szewczyk and Chennault (1997) refer to the prevalence of depression as a "reflection of biologic factors that may interact with social, psychological, and psychosocial influences."

Assessment. Risk factors for depression include a history of prior episode, family history of depression, chronic illness or pain, and sexual dysfunction (Box 17-8). Prior incident of depression is the strongest predictor of subsequent events. Having a first-degree biological relative with major depression puts a woman at 1.5 to 3 times greater risk (Desai & Jann, 2000). Certain psychosocial factors may place a woman at risk, including loss of a parent while a young child, an unhappy or abusive marriage, sexual abuse, level of education, financial problems, single parenthood, and the stress of multiple roles within society (Hall, 1997). Single mothers are almost three times more likely than married mothers to experience a major episode of depression (Desai & Jann, 2000).

Besides affecting mood, depression influences other brain functions as well. It may be physiological symptoms that bring a woman to her clinician rather than psychological complaints. Depressed women may complain of chronic fatigue, inability to perform at work, headaches, weight loss or gain, sleep disturbance, and constipation. On further questioning, feelings of extreme sadness and worthlessness or guilt surface, along with difficulty concentrating, disinterest in daily activities, and suicidal ideation. Because the symptoms of depression are vague and overlap other medical illnesses, a complete history is essential. An accurate diagnosis requires differentiation between depression and underlying medical conditions such as thyroid disorders, vitamin deficiency (specifically vitamin B_{12}), Cushing syndrome, diabetes, stroke, and certain degenerative neurologic disorders such as Parkinson's disease, Alzheimer's disease, and multiple sclerosis. Substance abuse, especially cocaine and alcohol, may precipitate depressive symptoms. Medications such as digoxin, beta-blockers, and corticosteriods may also trigger depressive manifestations. Abstinence from these substances can

BOX 17-8 RISK FACTORS FOR DEPRESSION

History
Prior episode of depression
Family history of depression
Chronic or severe medical illness
Early childhood loss of a parent
Sexual abuse as a child or adult

Psychosocial Factors
Unhappy or abusive marriage
Single parenthood
Financial problems

effectively reduce the symptoms. Affective changes at perimenopause may be secondary to occurrence of vasomotor changes or other physical symptoms of midlife. Desai and Jann (2000) report an increased risk of depression at menopause in the woman who has a history of premenstrual syndrome, prior depressive episodes, is caring for aging parents, or has a chronic condition herself.

Management. Almost 90% of depression is treatable. Treatment includes cognitive behavioral therapy and interpersonal psychotherapy as the first choice for mild to moderate depression. Antidepressants commonly prescribed include tricyclics (Elavil), heterocyclics (Wellbutrin), selective serotin reuptake inhibitors (Prozac), and monoamine oxidase inhibitors (Nardil). Unfortunately, only one-third of women with depression are identified and adequately treated (Moore, 2000). The difficulty lies with diagnosing depression in face of overshadowing somatic complaints and lack of provider expertise and knowledge about depression. Other obstacles, such as social stigma, misunderstanding about the disease, and lack of mental health insurance benefits often prevent women from seeking treatment. Ongoing evaluation of the status of depression is important because there is a 50% incidence of recurrence at least once (Moore, 2000). Advancement of patient education focused on healthy coping skills and stress management programs can forestall some of the mental and physical reactions that lead to mental illness. As part of patient education, it should be emphasized that depression is a medical illness and not a personal weakness, and in most cases can be effectively treated.

Alcohol and Drug Dependency

For clarity, alcohol and drug abuse is defined as the illegal or non-medical use of a psychoactive substance. Alcohol and drug dependency is further defined as the need for repeated doses of the substance to "feel good." Chemical dependency has both physical and psychological elements. Psychological dependence refers to impaired control over drinking or use of drugs, whereas physiological or physical dependence refers to tolerance and withdrawal symptoms.

Causes. Substance abuse/dependency is multifaceted with many interacting factors that predispose the person to addictive behavior. Gender, age, race, physiology, and genetics all contribute to addiction. Family history of addiction is a strong predictor. Female physiology and hormonal fluctuations may influence the metabolism of alcohol and the dose-related effects of other drugs. Women and men experience substance abuse at differing rates, but men, ages 15 to 54, tend to have twice as many alcohol and drug-related problems as women (Naegle, 1997). Women exhibit effects of long-term drinking sooner than men and die earlier from alcohol-related complications.

Historically, alcohol was the drug most often used by women during the 18th and 19th centuries. Alcohol-based elixirs containing opiates were consumed for dental problems, painful menstruation, any female organ problem, gastrointestinal disorders, and infectious diseases. These elixirs could be mail ordered from a mail order catalog or purchased at a local store. Today, because alcohol is so widely available and socially acceptable, one can easily forget it is a drug with many harmful effects. Alcohol is the most commonly used drug in the United States (McGann & Spangler, 1997). Excessive consumption of alcohol and other drugs can cause serious health problems and moderate to severe psychiatric symptoms resulting from central nervous system damage (Naegle, 1997). Research has shown that women progress more rapidly through the disease process of alcoholism than men but have drinking problems at a later age. Physical effects may include permanent brain impairment or stroke; hypertension or heart failure; possible increased risk of breast cancer, hepatitis, and cirrhosis; increased risk of osteoporosis; irregular menstrual cycles, infertility, and birth defects; and permanent peripheral nerve impairment. There have been a few documented benefits from alcohol consumption, but the amount of ingested alcohol is very modest, one drink per day or less (McGann & Spangler, 1997).

Six out of ten women identify themselves as drinkers, with the percentage of women over men increasing. In Caucasian women, alcohol abuse peaks in their 20s. African-American women have the highest incidence of alcohol abuse in their 40s. Hispanic women have a fairly low rate of alcohol abuse across the lifespan. Alcoholism in elderly women reflects either long-term drinking habits or late onset as a response to life changes or stresses. Either way, alcoholism often goes undiagnosed because of inappropriate screening and numerous somatic complaints that cover up the underlying problem.

Assessment. The use of a brief screening questionnaire can help clinicians identify women in need of further evaluation for alcohol abuse. The four-item CAGE questionnaire has good sensitivity and specificity to allow for use as a screening tool (McGann & Spangler, 1997) (Box 17-9). One "YES" response should raise the clinician's suspicions.

Management. Early recognition of alcohol abuse is essential if effective interventions are to be implemented and long-term health problems minimized. Treatment issues particular to women include missed diagnosis of alcohol and drug abuse, child care concerns, fear of losing the children, and the social stigma of alcohol abuse, which appears more intense for women. Vocational training, marital counseling, financial counseling, parenting skills, coexistent psychiatric disorders, and coexistent addictions are areas of special focus for women in treatment centers.

Illicit Drug Use

Psychological or emotional issues are antecedents to alcohol and drug use among women. More women than men turn to self-medication with prescription or over-the-counter drugs to help them cope with stress and anxiety. The Public Health Task Force on Women's Health Issues in 1985 reported older women will take sedatives, tranquilizers, hypnotics, and other drugs (both over-the-counter and prescription) twice as often as older men. Some women will use any drug that is available—legal or illegal. Twenty-five percent of cocaine, marijuana, and heroin users are women dependent on drugs to handle an affective disorder (Naegle, 1997). Cocaine usage is increasing, particularly in low-income, inner-city areas.

Causes. Cocaine acts as both a stimulant and local anesthetic. It produces a rush of euphoria and energy, but the effect wears off rather quickly, leaving the person desiring another dose. The medical complications from cocaine do not vary between the sexes. Cocaine is absorbed from all mucous membranes, metabolized by the liver, and excreted in urine. Cocaine possesses direct cardiotoxic effects that can cause seizures, dysrhythmias, myocardial infarction, left ventricular failure, and sudden death (Beebe, 1997). Abstinence from cocaine in an addicted person will produce anxiety, fatigue, depression, irritability, and sleep disturbances.

Heroin and marijuana are used to dull the senses, provide a sense of detachment from the real world, and induce sleep. Abuse of either drug has serious medical complications, especially heroin, which is injected under the skin, into a vein, or snorted through the nose. There is some controversy regarding the smoking of marijuana for pain relief in chronically ill patients. In a healthy individual, even occasional use has been shown to place additional stress on the heart. Chronic use of marijuana can cause an amotivational syndrome and, as with other inhaled substances, severe damage to the lungs (McGann & Spangler, 1997).

Management. Treatment for drug abuse is similar to that offered in alcohol treatment programs. Most programs involve intensive counseling, education, and support groups over a long period of time. Screening for illicit drug use during a clinical interview can be done but expect a high false-negative rate. When asked, women will more readily admit to alcohol abuse and cigarettes than to the use of illicit drugs (McGann & Spangler, 1997).

Smoking

Tobacco is the most widely abused drug in the United States although many smokers would never admit to being addicted. The fact that lung cancer has surpassed breast

---

BOX 17-9 SCREENING QUESTIONS FOR ALCOHOL ABUSE

C. Have you ever felt the need to *c*ut down on your drinking?
A. Have people ever *a*nnoyed you by criticizing your drinking?
G. Have you ever felt bad or *g*uilty about drinking?
E. Have you ever had a drink first thing in the morning to steady your nerves or get rid of a hangover (*e*ye-opener)?

cancer as the leading cause of cancer death in women indicates the extent of this epidemic. According to the American Cancer Society (2000), lung cancer mortality rates are 13 times higher for female smokers as compared to women who never smoked.

Traditionally, smoking was seen as "unladylike," but newer marketing campaigns have made smoking popular and sexy and promote it as a way to reduce weight (Ernster, Kaufman, Nichter, Samet, & Yoon, 2000). This may explain why smoking among female teenagers is increasing so rapidly. For adolescents, smoking serves as a way to appear mature, particularly desirous for teenage girls who are developmentally more advanced than boys their own age. Not surprisingly, girls are more likely to report that cigarette smoking helps with their weight control. Unforutnately, marketing aimed at women has resulted in the increase seen in female smokers. The World Health Organization International Conference in 1999 stated over 200 million women smoke, and, by the year 2025, the number will almost triple. In developing countries, smoking has become a symbol of women's liberation and freedom from traditional gender roles (Ernster et al., 2000).

Causes. Smoking has been shown to be associated with several types of cancer, such as mouth, esophagus, uterine, cervical, kidney, and bladder (Ernster et al., 2000). Smoking is a major risk factor for cardiovascular disease in all women who smoke more than a pack a day. Women on oral contraceptives who smoke have a greater risk for heart disease than nonsmokers and are warned not to take birth control pills if they smoke. Earlier studies found that the risk for cardiovascular disease was 20- to 40-fold higher in smoking women on oral contraceptives than in non-smoking women. Recent studies show a decrease in risk based on newer formulations of oral contraceptives; however, the relative risk remains (Ernster et al., 2000). Smoking in midlife women is often associated with an increased consumption of alcohol, increased stroke risk, increased risk for osteoporosis, earlier menopause by 1 to 2 years, and premature skin wrinkling. Although the effect of smoking on bone density in premenopausal women has not been conclusively proven, many studies indicate postmenopausal women who smoke have a lower bone density than non-smokers and an increased risk for osteoporosis (Ernster et al., 2000).

Management. To stop smoking is the single most important step a person can take to improve their health and reduce risk. Like illegal drugs, users develop a tolerance to nicotine and crave more and more. Treatment is aimed at gradually eliminating the addiction and includes use of nicotine substitutes to reduce the craving for nicotine, smoking cessation programs, female support groups, and stress management skills. The best health advice remains never to smoke. However, women who are current smokers can achieve substantial reduction in their risk for many diseases, notably stroke, if they quit. Ernster and others (2000) propose a multi-prong strategy against tobacco use that includes changes in legislation, taxation, and benefits to the tobacco industry; a ban on advertising and promotion of tobacco products, increased consumer education about health risks, and increased access to smoking cessation programs.

SUMMARY

The nursing management of midlife women consists of supportive counseling, careful assessment, and education. The goal of health care is the identification of risk factors through comprehensive assessment and screening and the development of a prevention-based program designed to support optimum health across the lifespan. By adopting a biosociocultural perspective to midlife transitions, clinicians can better educate women about the physical, mental, social, and cultural factors associated with this transition, thus enabling women to adapt to midlife changes with ease and confidence in their self-care abilities. For as long as menopause is represented primarily as a medical condition rather than a natural physiological process within a woman's lifetime, it will only serve to reinforce negative stereotypes about women's bodies (Jones, 1997). Through preventive health care and education, women can be empowered to use midlife transition as a positive catalyst for the remainder of their golden years.

REFERENCES

Abraham, C., & Seremetis, S. (1997). Breast health at midlife: Guidelines for screening and patient evaluation. *Geriatrics, 52*(6), 58–65.

ACOG Educational Bulletin on Domestic Violence Number 257 (1999). *International Journal of Gynecology & Obstetrics, 71*(2000), 79–87.

Alexander, B. (1997). Women's sexuality—A paradigm shift. In J. Rosenfeld (Ed.), *Women's health in primary care* (pp. 277–288). Baltimore: Williams & Wilkins.

American Cancer Society (2000). *Cancer facts and figures 2000.* New York: Author. *www.cancer.org.*

Andrews, W. (1998). What's new in preventing and treating osteoporosis? *Postgraduate Medicine, 104*(4), 89–97.

Andrist, L. C., & MacPherson, K. I. (2001). Conceptual models for women's health research: Reclaiming menopause, exemplar of nursing's contribution to feminist scholarship. *Annual Review of Nursing Research, 19*, 29–60.

Association of Women's Health, Obstetric and Neonatal Nurses. (1998). *Standards and guidelines for professional nursing practice of women and newborns* (5th ed.). Washington, DC: Author.

Bailey, K., Combs, M., Rogers, L. & Stanley, K. (2000). Measuring up: Could this simple nursing intervention help prevent osteoporosis? *AWHONN Lifelines, 4*(2), 41–44.

Beebe, D. (1997). Addictive behaviors. In J. Rosenfeld (Ed.), *Women's health in primary care* (pp. 227–240). Baltimore: Williams & Wilkins.

Blackwell, J., & Blackwell, D. (1997). Menopause: Life event or medical disease. *Clinical Nurse Specialist, 11*(1), 7–9.

Bonaiuti, D., Shea, B., Iovine, R., Negrini, S., Robinson, V., et al. (2002). Exercise for preventing and treating osteoporosis in postmenopausal women (Cochrane Review). In *The Cochrane Library*, Issue 3, Update Software.

Brucker, M., & Youngkin, E. (2002). What's a women to do? Exploring HRT questions raised by the Women's Health Initiative. *AWHONN Lifelines, 6*(5), 408–467.

Callahan, E., & Paris, B. (1997). Midlife periodic health exam in the primary care practice. *Geriatrics, 52*(10), 60–76.

Coker, A., Smith, P., Bethea, L., King, M., & McKeown, R. (2000). Physical health consequences of physical and psychological intimate partner violence. *Archives of Family Medicine, 2*(5), 451–457.

Cooney, B. (1997). Preventing osteoporosis. *AWHONN Lifelines, 1*(5), 25–26.

Couzi, R., & Davidson, N. (1997). Breast cancer. In J. Rosenfeld (Ed.), *Women's health in primary care* (pp. 683–702). Baltimore: Williams & Wilkins.

Czarpata, B. (1999). Managing urinary incontinence. *Patient Care for Nurse Practitioners, 2*(4), 37–48.

Czarpata, B., & McKillips, K. (1997). Silent suffering—Helping women find the path to continence. *AWHONN Lifelines, 1*(2), 29–34.

Darovic, G. (1997). Caring for patients with osteoporosis. *Nursing 97,* May, 50–51.

DeMasters, J. (2000). A clinician's guide to understanding the dilemma. *AWHONN Lifelines, 4*(2), 27–35.

Denke, M. (1999). Primary prevention of coronary heart disease in postmenopausal women. *The American Journal of Medicine, 107*(2A), 48S–50S.

Desai, H., & Jann, M. (2000) Major depression in women: A review of the literature. *Journal of the American Pharmaceutical Association, 40*(4), 525–537.

Donovan J., & Syngal, S. (1998). Colorectal cancer in women: An underappreciated but preventable risk. *Journal Women's Health, 7*(1), 45–48.

Draucker, C., & Madsen, C. (1999). Women dwelling with violence. *Image: Journal of Nursing Scholarship, 31*(4), 327–332.

Duey, C., Smith, W., & Johnson, T. (1997). Patients must receive education on universal sun safety precautions. *Oncology Nursing Forum, 24*(3), 457–458.

Eastell, R. (1998). Treatment of postmenopausal osteoporosis. *New England Journal of Medicine, 333*, 736–746.

Ellis, J., & Kanusky, C. (1996). Addressing women's midlife concerns—Profile of an issues forum. *Advance for Nurse Practitioners, 4*(5), 45–50.

Ernster, V., Kaufman, N., Nichter, M., Samet, J. & Yoon, S. (2000). Women and tobacco: Moving from policy to action. *Bulletin of the World Health Organization, 78*(7), 891–897.

Furniss, K. (2000). Tomatoes, Pap smears, and tea? Adopting behaviors thay may prevent reproductive cancers and improve health. *Journal of Obstetric, Gynecologic, and Neonatal Nursing, 29*(6), 641–652.

Gallo, M., Fallon, P., & Staskin, D. (1997). Urinary incontinence: Steps to evaluation, diagnosis, and treatment. *The Nurse Practitioner, 22*(2), 21–44.

Gantt, L., & Bickford, A. (1999). Screening for domestic violence. *AWHONN Lifelines, 3*(2), 36–42.

Graziottin, A. (1999). Strategies for effectively addressing women's concerns about menopouse and HRT. *Maturitas, 33,* S15–S23.

Greenlee, R., Murray, T. & Bolden, S. (2000). Cancer statistics 2000. *Cancer Journal for Clinicians, 50*(1), 7–33.

Hall, K. (1997). Depression and anxiety. In J. Rosenfeld (Ed.), *Women's health in primary care* (pp. 183–203). Baltimore: Williams & Wilkins.

Huff, B. (2000). Screening for cervical cancer. *AWHONN Lifelines, 4*(3), 53–55.

Jones, J, (1997). Representations of menopause and their health care implications: A qualitative study. *American Journal of Preventive Medicine, 13*(1), 58–65.

Katz, A. (2000). Birds do it, bees do it, let's talk about it: The nurse's role in sexuality counseling. *AWHONN Lifelines, 4*(5), 40–41.

Keating, N., Cleary, P., Rossi, A., Zaslovsky, A., & Ayanian, J. (1999). Use of hormone replacement therapy by postmenopausal women in the United States. *Annals of Internal Medicine, 130*(7), 545–553.

Kendig, S., & Sanford, D. (1998). *Midlife and menopause: Celebrating women's health.* AWHONN Symposia Series. Washington, DC: AWHONN.

King, K., & Mosca, L. (2000). Prevention of heart disease in women: Recommendations for management of risk factors. *Progress in Cardiovascular Nursing, Spring*, 36–42.

Kuhn, J., McMahon, P., & Creekmore, S. (1999). Stopping a silent killer: Preventing heart disease in women. *AWHONN Lifelines, 3*(2), 31–35.

Learn, C., & Higgins, P. (1999). Harmonizing herbs: Managing menopause with help from Mother Earth. *AWHONN Lifelines, 3*(5), 39–43.

Lindsay, S. (1999). Menopause, naturally exploring alternatives to traditional hormone replacement therapy. *AWHONN Lifelines, 3*(5), 32–38.

Madlon-Kay, D. (1997). Preventive health care—Adulthood. In J. Rosenfeld (Ed.), *Women's health in primary care* (pp. 75–92). Baltimore: Williams & Wilkins.

Massey, C., Hupp, C., Kreisberg, M., Alpert, M. & Hoff, C. (2000). Estrogen replacement therapy is underutilized among postmenopausal women at high risk for coronary heart disease. *The American Journal of Medical Sciences, 320*(2), 124–127.

McGann, K., & Spangler, J. (1997). Alcohol, tobacco, and illicit drug use among women. *Primary Care, 24*(1), 113–123.

McNagny, S. E. (1999). Prescribing hormone replacement therapy for menopausal symptoms. *Annals of Internal Medicine, 131*(8), 605–616.

Moore, D. (2000). An expression of depression: Help end the suffering by recognizing the signs. *AWHONN Lifelines, 4*(4), 11–13.

Mosca, L. (2000). The role of hormone replacement therapy in the prevention of postmenopausal heart disease. *Archives of Internal Medicine, 160*, August, 2263–2272.

Murabito, J. (1995). Women and cardiovascular disease: Contributions from the Pramingham Heart Study. *Journal of the American Medical Women's Association, 50*(2), 35–39, 55.

Naegle, M. (1997). Understanding women with dual diagnosis. *Journal of Obstetric, Gynecologic, and Neonatal Nursing, 26*(5), 567–575.

National Institutes of Health, Osteoporosis and Related Bone Diseases, National Resource Center (2000). *Fast facts on osteoporosis. http://www.osteo.org/osteofastfact.html.*

Nogueira, S., & Appling, S. (2000). Breast cancer: Genetics, risks, and strategies. *Nursing Clinics of North America, 35*(3), 663–669.

North American Menopause Society (2000a). A decision tree for the use of estrogen replacement therapy or hormone replacement therapy in postmenopausal women: Consensus opinion of the North American Menopause Society. *The Journal of the North American Menopause Society, 7*(2), 76–86.

Paganini-Hill, A., & Henderson, V, (1996). Estrogen replacement therapy and risk of Alzheimer disease. *Archives of Internal Medicine, 28:156*(19), 2213–2217.

Poirier, L. (1997). The importance of screening for domestic violence in all women. *The Nurse Practitioner, 22*(5), 105–122.

Ramsey, L., Ross, B., & Fischer, R. (1999). Phytoestrogens and the management of menopause. *Advance for Nurse Practitioners, 7*(5), 27–30.

Rosenfeld, J. (1997). Urinary incontinence. In J. Rosenfeld (Ed.), *Women's health in primary care* (pp. 727–735). Baltimore: Williams & Wilkins.

Rousseau, M. (2001). Evidence-based practice in women's health: hormone therapy for women in menopause. *Journal of Midwifery Women's Health, 96*(13), 167–180.

Rousseau, M. (1998). Women's midlife health—reframing menopause. *Journal of Nurse-Midwifery, 43*(3), 208–223.

Ruggiero, R. J., & Likis, F. E. (2002). Estrogen: Physiology, pharmacology and formulations for replacement hormone. *Journal of Midwifery Women's Health, 47*(13), 130–138.

Ryan, J., & King, M. (1998). Scanning for violence. *AWHONN Lifelines, 2*(3), 36–41.

Sakornbut, E. (1997). Preventive health care—Perimenopausal years. In J. Rosenfeld (Ed.), *Women's health in primary care* (pp. 739–761). Baltimore: Williams & Wilkins.

Sampselle, C., Burns, P., Dougherty, M., Newman, D., Thomas, K., & Wyman, J. (1997). Continence for women: Evidence-based practice. *Journal of Obstetric, Gynecologic, and Neonatal Nursing, 26*(4), 375–385.

Scharbo-DeHaan, M. (1996). Hormone replacement therapy. *Nurse Practitioner, 21*(12pt 2), 1–13.

Schmidt, P., Roca, C., Bloch, M., & Rubinow, D. (1997). The perimenopause and affective disorders. *Seminars in Reproductive Endocrinology, 15*(1), 91–98.

Stevenson, A. (1999). Immunizations for women and children. *Journal of Obstetric, Gynecologic, and Neonatal Nursing, 28*(5), 534–544.

Szewczyk, M., & Chennault, S. (1997). Depression and related disorders. *Primary Care, 24*(1), 83–99.

Ushiroyama, T., Ikeda, A., & Ueki, M. (1999). Prevalence, incidence, and awareness in the treatment of menopausal urinary incontinence. *Maturitas, 33*, 127–132.

Vesser, P., Fost, S., Evans, S., & Sreed, A. (2002). Today's HRT chaos. A compendium for prescribers. *Advanced Nurse Practitioner, 10*(6), 57–60, 62, 102.

Weinstein, L., & Ullery, B. (2000). Identification of at-risk women for osteoporosis screening. *American Journal of Obstetrics and Gynecology, 183*(3), 547–549.

Wilhelm, S. (2002). Factors affecting a woman's intent to adopt hormone replacement therapy for menopause. *Journal of Obstetric, Gynecologic, and Neonatal Nursing, 31*(6), 698–707.

Williams, R. (1997). Cancer. In K. Allen & J. Phillips (Eds.), *Women's health across the lifespan* (pp. 193–219). Philadelphia: J. B. Lippincott.

Williams, M., & Sandler, A. (2001). The epidemiology of lung cancer. *Cancer Treatment, 105*, 31–52.

Willis, D. (1997). Does estrogen replacement therapy reduce the risk of fatal breast cancer in postmenopausal women? *Maturitas, 27*, 105–108.

Wilmoth, M., & Spinelli, A. (2000). Sexual implications of gynecologic cancer treatments. *Journal of Obstetric, Gynecologic, and Neonatal Nursing, 29*(4), 413–421.

Winterich, J., & Umberson, D. (1999). How women experience menopause: The importance of social context. *Journal of Women & Aging, 11*(4), 57–73.

Woodson, S. (1997). Sexual health across the lifespan. *AWHONN Lifelines, 1*(4), 34–39.

Writing Group of the PEPI Trial. (1996). Effects of hormonal therapy on bone mineral density: Results from the postmenopausal estrogen/progestin interventions (PEPI). *Journal of the American Medical Association, 276*, 1389–1396.

Writing Group for the Women's Health Initiative Investigations. (2002). Risks and benefits of estrogen plus progestin in healthy postmenopausal women. *Journal of the American Medical Association, 288*(3), 321–333.

Yoder, M. (1997, March/April). Hormone replacement therapy: A question of benefits and risks. *Women's Health Research Update (*Supplement to the *Ireland Report)*, 1–4.

RESOURCES

National Women's Health Network
514 10th Street NW, Suite 400
Washington, DC 20004
202-347-1140
www.womenshealthnetwork.org

Older Women's League
666 11th Street NW, Suite 700
Washington, DC 20001
202-783-6686
www.owl-national.org

The American College of Obstetricians and Gynecologists
409 12th Street SW
P.O. Box 96920
Washington, DC 20090
202-638-5577
www.acog.org

The North American Menopause Society
P.O. Box 94527
Cleveland, OH 44101
440-442-7550
www.menopause.org

National Osteoporosis Foundation
1232 22nd Street NW
Washington, DC 20037
202-223-2226
www.nof.org

American Heart Association
National Center
7272 Greenville Avenue
Dallas, TX 75231
1-800-242-8721
www.americanheart.org

American Association of Retired Persons (AARP)
601 E Street NW
Washington, DC 20049
1-800-424-3410
www.aarp.org

American Cancer Society: *www.cancer.org or* **1-800-ACS-2345**
Breast Cancer GAIL Model Risk Assessment Tool: *www.cancernet.nci.gov/clinpdq/risk/*
    EstimatingBreastCancer Risks.html or **1-800-898-9702**
Midlife Women's Network: 1-800-886-4354
National Women's Health Resource Center: *www.info.health/women.org*
Women's Health Initiative: *www.whi.org* or *www.nhibi.nihgov/whi/index.html*
Association of Women's Health, Obstetric and Neonatal Nurses: *www.awhonn.org*

Chapter 18

Health Care for Older Women

Judith Bunnell Sellers

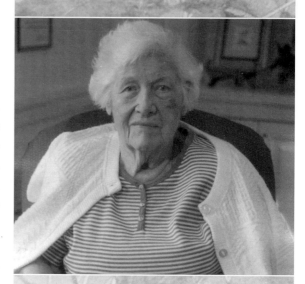

Not enjoyment, and not sorrow,

Is our destined end or way;

But to act, that each tomorrow

Find us farther than today.

Let us then be up and doing,

With a heart for any fate;

Still achieving, still pursuing,

Learn to labor and to wait.

Henry Wadsworth Longfellow

INTRODUCTION

Gerontology and geriatric nursing are changing continually as research on aging provides new information. Most authors consider the elderly to be anyone more than 65 years of age. Older women, particularly women more than 85 years of age, are being viewed as the survivors. As this population of women ages further, a new interest is growing in discovering the secrets of successful aging from them. In the near future, older women, especially women 85 and older, will make up a larger percentage of the population. With the increase in life expectancy, more women will be living into their 90s, which means that the term *elderly* will cover a 30-year life span.

Women in this 30-year span will be diverse. Social and health-related issues will become increasingly complex. For most women, with increased age comes an increase in chronic disease and a decrease in function. The elderly woman of the future may present a different picture because she may benefit from new findings regarding prevention and treatment.

Gender differences exist for life expectancy, mortality, and chronic illness, although the reasons for the differences are not always clear. On average, women live longer and are less likely to have conditions that are life threatening than men. Women are more likely than men to have disabling conditions such as arthritis, as well as having a variety of conditions that limit activity (Federal Interagency Forum on Aging-Related Statistics, 2000; Kramarow, Lentzner, Rooks, Weeks, & Saydah, 1999; Manton, 1997; Markides, 1990). Beginning at age 65 and continuing past 75, arthritis and hypertension are the two most common chronic conditions in women (Federal Interagency Forum, 2000; Taeuber, 1996). Apart from hypertension, no other cardiovascular conditions are among the top five chronic diseases in women (Manton, 1997; Markides, 1990).

Self-rated health, one measure frequently used to determine the health of a population that corresponds with provider ratings of health among the elderly, can help the women's health care nurse understand the perception the older woman has about her health. Using self-rated health, the majority of women 65 to 74 rate their health as excellent, very good, or good (71.7%).

Another 20% rate their health as fair. Thus only a small percentage of elderly women rate their health as poor. Of those 75 to 84, almost 66% rate their health between excellent and good, 23% rate their health as fair, and around 11% rate their health as poor. A majority of women ages 65 to 74 and 75 to 84 rate their health excellent to good (74% and 68%, respectively). Thus apparently most women do not relate chronic conditions that they may be experiencing with poor health (Federal Interagency Forum, 2000; Kramarow et al., 1999; Taeuber, 1996).

This chapter attempts to equip the women's health care nurse with some information needed to provide holistic care for older women. Although a great deal of information is presented, the information is not intended to be all-inclusive. Research, and particularly studies on older women, is continually identifying new aspects of aging and new strategies to improve women's health care. The nurse will find caring for the older woman an exciting and fulfilling challenge. The practitioner who provides primary care for an older woman is positioned truly to affect her patient's quality of life.

The first area to be addressed is the dramatic shift in the aging population. Population statistics and changes in family structure and the implications of the changes in family structure are summarized. This will assist the reader in understanding the extent of health care need by the year 2030. Health care of the growing elderly population is complex because of the many changes that occur with aging. For this reason, the second section presents normal physiological changes associated with aging, with emphasis on specific changes related to women. The nurse will be able to relate normal age-related changes to the comprehensive geriatric assessment information presented in the third major section. The fourth section deals with the usual health promotion and disease prevention activities of screening, nutrition, and exercise programs, with an emphasis on older women. Finally, in the fifth section, eleven issues that have a direct effect on the quality of life of the older woman are presented in some detail, including a focus on each issue and the particular assessment and management of each. These issues are poverty, grandparents as parents, elder abuse, polypharmacy, falls, sexuality, incontinence, depression, bereavement, alcoholism, and suicide.

DEMOGRAPHICS

Population Growth and Life Expectancy

Major changes in the population age distribution will occur in the near future. These changes are being called the rectangularization of the population. Instead of a pyramid, where large numbers of persons are in lower age groups and fewer in older age groups, the population is becoming more evenly distributed across all age groups (Byyny & Speroff, 1996; Nusselder & Mackenbach, 1997).

In 1776 the total population in the United States was 2.5 million. Of those, 1 in 50 were 65 or older, whereas 50% were under the age of 16. A dramatic shift has occurred in the 1990s and the shift continues into the twenty-first century. In 1990, only 25% of the population was under 16 and one in seven was 65 or older. Between 1980 and 1990 the elderly population grew 22%, whereas the total population only grew 9%. When the baby boom generation (those born between 1946 and 1964) become 65, the elderly population will have grown exponentially. Instead of one in seven, one in five will be 65 or older. Those 85 and older will grow from 3 million in 1990 to 17 million by the year 2050 (Administration on Aging, 1998; Federal Interagency Forum, 2000; Schick & Schick, 1994; Taeuber, 1996; U.S. Bureau of the Census 1997). We now need to divide the elderly population into specific age groups because of the different health-related issues for the aging population. Classification may be the young-old (65 to 74), the old (75 to 84), and the old-old (85 and older).

African Americans, Hispanics, and others such as Asian Americans who are 65 and older will represent 32% of the population by the year 2050, an increase of 18% between 1990 and 2050. Life expectancy will increase for persons of all races. However, white elders will continue to have a longer life expectancy than members of other racial and ethnic groups. An African-American female at 65 in 1990 can expect to live another 17.6 years, whereas her white counterpart can expect to live 19 more years. An African-American male at 65 in 1990 can expect to live 14.2 more years; a white male, 15.3 more years. Overall, for white persons, by the year 2040, the life expectancy of females at age 65 will be 22.3 more years and of males at age 65, 17.3 more years (Administration on Aging, 1998; Federal Interagency Forum, 2000; Schick & Schick, 1994; Taeuber, 1996; U.S. Bureau of the Census 1997).

Interestingly, for those 85 and older the ratio of men to women will be 39 to 100 by 2050. Elderly women usually are widowed, whereas elderly men tend to be married. If men are widowed, they are 7 times more likely to remarry than are women. Table 18-1 provides statistics on the marital status of men and women, comparing 1990 with 2040. Although not shown on the table, the numbers of never married, widowed, and divorced elderly women will increase with age (Administration on Aging, 1998; Schick & Schick 1994; Taeuber, 1996; U.S. Bureau of the Census, 1997). Therefore the nurse is anticipated to be providing primary care for a large number of single elderly women (Johnson, 1992).

The increase in life expectancy has many implications. Of major importance to the elderly woman is the availability of caregivers. An increased number of women will be

Table 18-1	PERCENT OF MARRIED AND WIDOWED BY AGE AND GENDER FOR 1990 AND 2040

	1990		2040	
AGE	FEMALE	MALE	FEMALE	MALE
Married				
65-74	53.2	80.2	58	73
75 and older	25.4	70	30.8	65
Widowed				
65-74	36.1	8.5	21.5	6.4
75 and older	65.6	23.7	48.7	19.6

Sources: Schick, F., & Schick, R. (Eds.). (1994). *Statistical handbook on aging in Americans.* Phoenix, AZ: Oryx Press. Taeuber, C. (Ed). (1996). *Statistical handbook on women in America* (2nd ed.). Phoenix, AZ: Oryx Press. U.S. Bureau of the Census. (1997). *Sixty-five plus in the United States.* Washington, D.C.: Economics and Statistics Administration, U.S. Department of Commerce.

old-old, and more generations will be living at one time. More frequently, older persons live with a spouse, plus have living children, grandchildren, and great-grandchildren. In addition, older adults will spend a greater number of years with chronic illness. With more chronic illness and a longer life expectancy come an increased need to have a caregiver, and more responsibility will fall on the family to provide care for a longer period of time (Himes, 1992b; Taeuber, 1996; U.S. Bureau of the Census, 1997).

In addition to the predicted increased life expectancy and the large increase in the number of women 85 and older, changes in family structure are related to a decrease in fertility and patterns of marriage that influence the availability of caregivers for the older woman. With increasing age comes an increase in chronic illnesses that in turn may decrease the functional status of the older person and increase the need for nonspousal caregivers. Although most caregivers are spouses, women live longer than men and therefore will be in need of caregivers. A daughter usually becomes the primary caregiver. In a large longitudinal epidemiological study (Freedman, 1996), the elderly who had a spouse as a caregiver were less likely to enter a nursing home. Elderly without a spouse to care for them were 50% more likely to enter a nursing home than women with a spouse. In addition, women who had neither a spouse nor a daughter were at high risk for nursing home admission. Thus the availability of caregivers is a major issue for the older woman and therefore the nurse.

Fertility

Unfortunately, although the need for a family caregiver will increase, the availability of a family caregiver may decrease. Those who are now old are the first population to analyze. In the 1930s these persons were in their childbearing years during the Great Depression. During the 1930s the birth rate was low, creating a childless older population. Of those women now 85 to 89, 20% of the white population and 28% of the African-American population did not have children. Many old-old, therefore, have no family to provide care.

The women who were born between 1945 and 1965 are the second group to analyze. This group, now middle aged, often has children as well as older parents who may be frail or disabled. This is the "sandwich" generation that will experience the stress of providing care for children and aged, chronically ill parents.

As this large cohort ages, they too will be subject to increased disability because of chronic illness, and they may also need care. Also, a decline in fertility among the baby boomer generation will leave fewer caregivers for the elderly in that cohort when they reach 85. The outcome will be fewer family members available to assume the caregiver role, and the need for creative, affordable living and caregiving facilities.

Finally, the baby boomer's children are the third group to analyze. Fertility patterns of these women have two characteristics. The first is early childbearing, creating young parents and grandparents. Frequently, the young parent is single and in need of financial and emotional support from parents. The second trend is that of late childbearing. During the 1980s, the birthrate for women over 30 increased more than for any age group. This means that grandparents are older and, again, the parent is responsible for care of the older parent and a child (Himes, 1992a). Therefore among the increasing elderly population will be families with children and grandchildren who also will have to take on the caregiving role.

Marriage

Adding complexity to the structure of the older person's family are present trends to marry later, to have single-parent families, and not to marry. In the year 2000, the prediction was that among the white population age 65 and older 11.5% of women and 7.3% of men would be unmarried and childless. Among the African-American population in the same age group, 20% of the females and 18% of the males would be unmarried and childless (Federal Interagency Forum, 2000; Himes, 1992b).

Controversy exists about the family available to be caregivers. Himes (1992a) found that in the population as a whole, a high rate of marriage and a high fertility continues. Johnson (1992), however, points out that the divorce rate continues to rise, women are having children later in life, and the fertility rate is dropping. Although Himes (1992a) maintains that the older person will have a spouse and children available for caregiving, Johnson (1992) believes that older women will need to rely on fewer children or long-term care organizations for caregiving. In a recent publication by the American Association of Retired Persons Public Policy Institute (1997) the ratio of potential family caregivers decreases from 11:1 in 1990 to 6:1 and 4:1 in 2030 and 2050, respectively. Therefore fewer family members are expected to be available for assuming the caregiving role of the elderly woman.

Conclusion

Demographic predictions indicate that the nurse will be providing care to a hardy group of women ages 85 and older. This population of women will be single, living alone, in poverty, and possibly without caregivers. The family structure will be complex with multigenerational families, often living together. Older women will be a challenge for the health care team. Old-old women are considered the survivors who may provide answers to aging well. Advanced practice nurses, in addition to providing primary care, have the opportunity to develop research programs aimed at identifying characteristics of the old-old and the influence of health promotion through the life span, as well as important health promotion measures to improve the quality of life of older women. The nurse will be providing primary care to the older woman in many settings. A comprehensive health assessment is crucial to appropriate management of care. However, before beginning a geriatric assessment, the nurse must know the implications normal physiological changes will have on the assessment findings.

PHYSIOLOGICAL AGE-RELATED CHANGES

Normal age-related physiological changes must be included in the analysis of findings from a geriatric assessment before an appropriate management plan is developed. Aging often is associated with declining function and chronic disease. When the field of gerontology began, aging and disease were synonymous. With longitudinal research, what was once thought to be inevitable with age was determined to be more likely to be caused by environmental, social, and genetic influences. Many changes that occur with aging result from poor nutrition, poverty, smoking, use of alcohol and medications, and lack of physical activity rather than from aging alone (Metter, Conwit, Tobin, & Fozard, 1997).

Biological aging, as discussed in this section, examines normal physiological changes. To be considered normal aging, these changes must be universal, nonreversible, inevitable alterations in function. This means that no matter what health measures the person takes, the changes continue to occur. Although the changes are progressive, the functional level of the person is strongly influenced by preventive health measures such as exercise, smoking cessation, improved diet, and appropriate use of medications. Additionally, although the physiological changes are universal, the rate of functional decline varies between individuals.

Most changes happen gradually. The peak efficiency of the body is between ages 30 and 40, after which a slow decline in function of organ systems occurs. Because the organs have a great deal of reserve capacity, the decline does not become clinically observable until the loss is significant. The significance of the loss of function of an organ depends on the rate of deterioration and the needed level of performance. The important factor in function is the ability of the organ to respond to demand. Table 18-2 provides detailed information about physiological changes and the clinical significance of the changes from the perspective of the history, physical, and diagnostic tests. The clinical significance (findings) is what relates to all physiological changes. Changes in laboratory findings that are consistent for the elderly are included, although no reference values exist for the elderly and changes in laboratory values associated with aging are not clear.

In the field of gerontology, researchers try to explain age-related changes. In addition to the many changes itemized in Table 18-2 is a need to discuss possible reasons for the physiological changes. Many interrelated changes are noted for the older woman, along with the relationship of estrogen to aging.

Table 18-2

AGE-RELATED PHYSIOLOGICAL CHANGES AND CLINICAL SIGNIFICANCE

ORGAN/SYSTEM	PHYSIOLOGICAL CHANGE	CLINICAL SIGNIFICANCE
Cardiovascular	Arteries elongate and intimate thicken Sclerosis of heart valves; valvular stiffness Decreased number of pacemaker cells and Purkinje fibers Increased fibrous tissue Decreased automaticity Left ventricular hypertrophy Decreased resting heart rate Decreased receptor activity	Systolic ejection murmur Arrhythmias Atrial and ventricular ectopic beats Decreased heart rate in response to stress Decreased cardiac output with stress Diastolic dysfunction S3 heart sound common, especially with hypertension
Respiratory	Decreased ciliary activity Decreased elasticity Decreased chest wall compliance Loss of elastic recoil Decreased respiratory muscle strength	Forced expiratory volume in first second decreases Decrease in oxygen uptake Decreased vital capacity Decreased cough reflex; susceptibility to infection
Musculoskeletal	Loss of trabecular bone Loss of cartilage Decreased lean body mass Decreased total water Increased total fat	Osteoporosis and fractures Loss of height Stooped posture Arthritis Pain Decreased strength and endurance Decreased drug volume distribution of water-soluble drugs or lean body mass (LBM) Increased drug volume distribution of highly lipid-soluble drugs
Immune	Decreased thymic activity Decreased lymphocyte response Decreased production of interleukin-2 Decreased T cell activity	Increased susceptibility to infection Increased autoimmune disorders and neoplasms
Endocrine	Decreased triiodothyronine Decreased hormone receptors Decreased sensitivity of target organs Increased norepinephrine Decreased adrenergic response Increased vasopressin Endocrine gland failure	Hypothyroidism Menopause Diabetes mellitus
Renal	Decreased glomerular filtration Increased abnormal glomeruli Decreased renal blood flow Decreased ability to concentrate urine	Drug toxicity Poor response to changes in fluid volume Poor response to sodium increases or decreases Increased plasma half-life of drugs excreted by the kidney

Table 18-2	AGE-RELATED PHYSIOLOGICAL CHANGES AND CLINICAL SIGNIFICANCE—CONT'D	
ORGAN/SYSTEM	**PHYSIOLOGICAL CHANGE**	**CLINICAL SIGNIFICANCE**
Gastrointestinal	Decreased saliva Decreased hydrochloric acid production Decreased calcium absorption Increased pH in proximal small intestine Decreased intrinsic factor Decreased thirst Reduced hepatic enzyme activity Decreased hepatic blood flow	Dehydration Decreased gastric emptying Altered drug absorption Risk for pernicious anemia and bacterial growth Reduced hepatic metabolism of drugs with high lipid extraction ratios
Neurological	Decreased cholinergic neurons Decreased number of neurons Decreased number of cortical cells Decreased brain weight Decreased rapid eye movement and stage 4 sleep Decreased cerebral blood flow Decreased oxygenation Impaired baroreceptor function Orthostatic hypotension Decreased neurotransmitter synthesis, especially acetylcholine, dopamine, and serotonin	Slower motor response Slower reaction time Slower motor skills Increased learning time Increased processing time Decreased hours of sleep Increased light sleep Increased sensitivity to anticholinergic drugs Decrease in responsiveness to adrenergic drugs
Skin	Atrophy of sweat glands Altered fat–lean mass ratio Decreased collagen Decreased subcutaneous fat	Hypo- and hyperthermia Fragile skin and pressure sores Wrinkles
Sensory	Eyes: Lens stiffening Opacity of lens Pupil size reduction Lens growth Macular changes Ears: Ossicles degenerate Eustachian tube obstruction Atrophy of external auditory meatus Atrophy of hair cells Loss of auditory neurons Taste: Loss of taste buds and altered taste sensation	Eyes: Decreased accommodation Hyperopia Decreased acuity Decreased color sensitivity Decreased depth perception Night glare Intolerance to glare Ears: Decreased perception of high frequencies Decreased ability to differentiate pitch Taste: Malnutrition

Continued

Table 18-2	AGE-RELATED PHYSIOLOGICAL CHANGES AND CLINICAL SIGNIFICANCE—CONT'D	
ORGAN/SYSTEM	**PHYSIOLOGICAL CHANGE**	**CLINICAL SIGNIFICANCE**

Laboratory values	Increased: Alkaline phosphatase
	  Uric acid (equivocal)
	  Blood urea nitrogen
	  Erythrocyte sedimentation rate
	  Two-hour postprandial blood glucose
	Decreased: Albumin
	  Creatinine clearance
	  White blood cells
	  Magnesium
	  Hemoglobin
	  Specific gravity of urine
		Chance of missing a diagnosis or diagnosing inappropriately

Sources: Byyny, R., & Speroff, L. (1996). *A clinical guide for the care of older women* (2nd ed.). Baltimore: Williams & Wilkins. Calkins, E., Ford, A., & Katz, R. (1992). *Practice of geriatrics*. Philadelphia: W. B. Saunders. Kane, R., Ouslander, J., & Abrass, I. (1999). *Essentials of clinical geriatrics* (4th ed.). New York: McGraw-Hill. Semla, T., Beizer, J., & Higbee, M. (1997). *Geriatric dosage handbook* (3rd ed.). Cleveland, OH: Lexi-Comp.

Cardiovascular System

Decreased rate of calcium release and removal may explain the decreased speed of contraction and relaxation of the heart muscle. The adrenergic receptors necessary for the response to beta-adrenergic stimulation decrease. With a decrease in adrenergic receptors, the heart is less able to respond to stress. A decrease in digitalis receptors also may occur. The decline in adrenergic and digitalis receptors results in decreased effectiveness of catecholamines and increased sensitivity to beta-blockers and calcium channel blockers (Calkins, Ford, & Katz, 1992; Kane, Ouslander, & Abrass, 1999).

Resting heart rate declines about 4 beats per minute per decade after age 30. The maximum heart rate also declines with age although it is higher in women than in men. Although the mechanisms for this decline are unclear, a decrease in adrenergic receptors or sinus node pacemaker cells is probably the cause (Calkins et al., 1992).

Most sources report a decrease in cardiac output with age, but findings of the Baltimore Longitudinal Study suggest that resting cardiac output remains the same. Cardiac output does, however, decrease when the heart is under stress, such as during exercise. In addition to a decreased cardiac output, stroke volume, oxygen uptake, and maximum heart rate decrease with exercise (Calkins et al., 1992; Byyny & Speroff, 1996).

A significant difference occurs between the heart weight in women compared with that in men between the ages of 40 and 70. A significant correlation also exists between age and percentage of fat in the heart among women but not men. Higher heart weight and more fat accumulation may be caused by the loss of estrogen at menopause (Kitzman & Edwards, 1990).

Women have a higher mean heart rate for 24 hours than men, even during sleep. An electrocardiogram reveals an elongated Q-T interval, making women more at risk for sudden death than males. Women are more at risk for death during antiarrhythmic therapy than men, and antiarrhythmic medications cause 70% of drug-related torsades de pointes, significantly more in women than men. Finally, peripheral vascular disease in the absence of diabetes is less severe in women than in men possibly because of the effect of estrogen on arterial walls (Legato, 1997).

Coronary heart disease occurs about 10 years later in women than in men. However, women are more likely to die in the first few weeks following the first myocardial infarction (MI). In addition, women are more likely to have a second MI within the first year. Estrogen is implicated in many findings related to coronary artery disease. Box 18-1 outlines findings related to the function of estrogen on the cardiovascular system.

Respiratory System

With age the chest wall is unable to expand and the lungs lose the capacity to recoil, resulting in increased residual volume and a decreased vital capacity. The total lung capacity also probably decreases in women, the result of loss of height and narrowing of intervertebral disk space (Saltzman, 1992). The forced expiratory volume is altered and varies extremely among individuals and probably is influenced by smoking, exposure to

---

Box 18-1 FUNCTION OF ESTROGEN ON THE CARDIOVASCULAR SYSTEM

Myocardium
■ Protects the myocardium, providing relative immunity to coronary artery disease.

Arterial Walls
■ Inhibits the production of adhesive molecules that promote platelet aggregation by endothelial cells.
■ Inhibits calcium entry into and release from the vascular smooth muscle cells by promoting the manufacture and release of an endothelial-produced relaxing factor.
■ Promotes coronary vasodilation and restores vasodilating quality of acetylcholine in women with atherosclerosis.
■ Stabilizes arterial flow and eliminates vasomotor instability that causes hot flashes by restoring and modulating the response of the vasculature to catecholamines.
■ Estrogen receptors in the atrium and ventricular walls create protection from atherosclerotic plaque formation.

Lipid Profile
■ Maintains optimal serum lipid profile.
■ Promotes production of high-density lipoproteins.
■ Promotes catabolism of low-density lipoproteins in hepatic cells.
■ Production of high-density lipoproteins and catabolism of low-density lipoproteins inhibits cholesterol oxidation and entry into arterial walls.

Source: Legato, M. (1997). Gender-specific physiology: How real is it? How important is it? *International Journal of Fertility 4*, 19–29.

environmental pollutants, and the presence of disease states. Also, although the partial pressure of carbon dioxide values remain the same as in a younger adult, arterial partial pressure of oxygen (PaO_2) declines steadily. Arterial oxygen value can be estimated using the formula: $PaO_2 = 100 - (0.34 \times age)$ (Byyny & Speroff, 1996).

Response of the respiratory system to exercise is limited by age alterations, pathological conditions, and environmental factors. The response to hypercapnia and hypoxia declines. A decrease in exercise tolerance is likely caused by the diminished cardiac response and changes in the function of the respiratory system. Exercise training tends to improve respiratory muscle endurance (Saltzman, 1992).

Musculoskeletal System

Changes in bone density and muscle mass continue to be areas of intense interest and investigation in gerontology. Although age-related changes are reported, questions and research continue to identify the multiple factors involved.

Although loss of bone is common, especially in postmenopausal women, osteoporosis may not result. Women with dense bone structure in youth, those with adequate calcium intake, those who perform weight-bearing exercise, and those who are dark skinned are at less risk than those without these characteristics. A recent study (Krall et al., 1997) of bone mineral density (BMD) found that men and women had a decline in BMD at the femoral neck at about 0.03% to 0.05% per year after age 65. Women, however, had a 0.03% decline per year after age 65 in BMD at the trochanter and whole body, whereas men had no significant related change.

Although loss of skeletal muscle mass is part of aging, the rate of loss can be slowed by strength training (Lexell, 1995; Tseng, Marsh, Hamilton, & Booth, 1995). Skeletal muscle begins to atrophy around age 30 but with only a slight decline until age 50. From age 50 to 80 a 30% decrease in muscle mass may occur. However, the role of inactivity, altered mitochondrial concentration, and activity in the muscle and the changes in the neuromuscular system remain unclear.

Muscular strength peaks between the ages of 20 and 30 and then begins to decline between ages 40 and 50. Women reach their peak strength earlier than men and start to have loss sooner, but total loss appears to be less than in men (Hurley, 1995). Much of the loss of strength is thought to be caused by the loss of skeletal muscle. Phillips, Rook, Siddle, Bruce, and Woledge (1993) suggest that loss of strength in women after menopause could be prevented by hormone replacement and strength training. However, no longitudinal studies lend support to this idea. The decrease in the ability of lymphocytes to proliferate may be caused by a decrease in lymphokines and a decreased ability to respond to signals outside the cell (Kane et al., 1999). With aging, cell-mediated immunity, antibody responses, and loss of activating factors, including interleukin-2, decrease.

In women, a relationship between gonadal steroids, particularly estrogen, and immune response is believed to influence the development of autoimmune diseases, although the mechanism is unknown. Women have more diagnoses of systemic lupus erythematosis, Sjögren syndrome, rheumatoid arthritis, multiple sclerosis, scleroderma, and mixed connective tissue disease than men. Women also respond more aggressively than men to *Escherichia coli*, viral illness, and parasitic infections, probably because of a higher immunoglobulin level. Cell-mediated immune responses are not as aggressive in women as in men.

With an understanding of the physiological changes and possible mechanisms of change that occur with aging, as well as the clinical implications, findings from a comprehensive geriatric assessment can be placed in context. Assessment is the key to geriatric care, and the interdisciplinary team is the key to management of a plan of care. Plans must use assessment data to focus on helping the woman reach an optimal level of function. The review of systems, physical findings, and disease orientation may provide the practitioner with treatable conditions, but they do not suffice for planning comprehensive care of the elderly. A complete assessment that focuses on functional level plus traditional system-based assessments gives a picture of overall well-being and quality of life and guides the efforts of the interdisciplinary team (Siegler, Hyer, Fulmer, & Mezey, 1998).

Renal System

Renal mass and size begin to decrease at about age 40. The major consideration for the aging kidney is the decrease in glomerular filtration rate, which occurs because of the decreased number of normal and functioning nephrons and a decrease in renal blood flow. Glomerular filtration decreases about 0.75 mL/minute/year after age 40. Although serum creatinine does not decline, creatinine clearance may decline significantly.

In addition to a decline in glomerular filtration rate, the ability of the kidney to concentrate urine and conserve fluid also declines with age. The kidney is less efficient in reacting to water increases and decreases and to changes in sodium intake. Diuretics and hypotonic intravenous fluids often lead to hyponatremia, volume depletion, and orthostatic hypotension. A sudden increase in sodium may result in pulmonary edema.

Immune System

The thymus gland involutes after puberty, with an accompanying decrease in thymic hormone. The result may be an increase in autoantibodies and alterations in the functions of T cell and B cell interaction. These changes result in an inability to activate the sequence needed to fight disease. The host is unable to discriminate between self and nonself (Blass, Cherniak, & Weksler, 1992).

COMPREHENSIVE GERIATRIC ASSESSMENT
Interview Challenges

Because of the complexity of the older woman, the history is crucial. Obtaining the history can sometimes be frustrating. Frequently responses to questions are in the form of stories, and these may seem to be on unrelated tangents. In addition, the woman has a desire to answer correctly, a fear of being diagnosed as cognitively impaired, and a dislike of being rushed. The skilled practitioner will be able to discern important points in the stories and guide the interview without appearing judgmental or hurried.

Kane and others (1999) outline problems frequently encountered during interviews with elderly patients:

1. **Atypical presentation:** The older person seldom is a textbook picture of disease. Symptoms of acute conditions may be vague and nonspecific, which is associated with the normal physiological changes of aging plus possible cognitive impairment that alters the response to disease states.

2. **Underreporting of symptoms:** Not only does the older person have an atypical presentation that alters how she reports symptoms, but also the person may minimize symptoms. This reluctance often is caused by several levels of fear relating to diagnosis, hospitalization or nursing home placement, loss of independence, and loss of cognitive abilities. The older person also may have an underlying depression that influences responses to questions.

3. **Multiple complaints:** Given the multiple problems, many complaints are often vague. The practitioner may see the client for one problem, then another, and another. Frequently, this situation is caused by an underlying depression that presents as somatization. Also, the older person usually has multiple chronic illnesses that make identification of specific problems difficult.

4. **Communication:** Difficulty hearing and seeing and slower psychomotor response time may add to the challenges of atypical presentation, multiple complaints, and underreported symptoms.

5. **Agenda:** Although not identified in Kane and others (1999), the older person usually has an agenda and goal for visiting the health care provider. The practitioner must identify the patient's priorities rather than her own. If the concerns that brought the older person to the provider are not addressed, successful outcomes are not possible. Box 18-2 offers some ideas for overcoming some of the difficulties encountered during assessment of the older woman.

History

The history includes health patterns, past and present medical care, and social, psychological, and financial aspects. If the client has an acute illness or exacerbation of an existing illness, the assessment data may not reflect true abilities. Assessing functional health patterns before the current episode and during and after illness is important. Functional assessment of conditions before the current problem assists the practitioner and client in setting mutually acceptable goals for treatment and identifying appropriate members of the interdisciplinary team needed for additional evaluation and treatment plans.

Specific concerns of the nurse on completing the history of an older woman are adequate nutrition, risk of falls, poverty, incontinence, polypharmacy, abuse/neglect, caregiving, and depression. Each of these topics is discussed in later sections. Box 18-3 outlines key points to cover when taking a history.

Box 18-2 SUGGESTIONS FOR OVERCOMING DIFFICULTIES IN ASSESSING THE OLDER PERSON

Lighting
Make sure the room is well lighted with as little glare as possible.

Noise
Try to eliminate outside noises and decrease distractions.

Interview
Speak slowly, deepen the voice, face the person, and ask one question at a time. Use other informants for accuracy and completeness of assessment data or to validate information.

Time
Because of the level of detail and extent of information needed for a comprehensive assessment, scheduling multiple short visits may be necessary. Being on time allows for a complete assessment. Do not rush for answers to questions, and avoid assuming the answer to questions.

Questions
Make questions specific for important symptoms.

Differential Diagnosis
Consider all possibilities and do not automatically rule out diseases based on atypical presentation.

Primary Provider
Try to be the provider the older woman sees at each visit. Know the typical presentation and be aware of new or changing complaints.

Source: Kane, R., Ouslander, J., & Abrass, I. (1999). *Essentials of clinical geriatrics* (4th ed.). New York: McGraw-Hill.

Instruments

The functional level encompasses multiple domains. Changes in one domain create a domino effect because, with increasing age, the woman has less reserve capacity to cope and adapt to change. The functional level refers to the ability of the older woman to perform activities needed in everyday life. A functional assessment, covering multiple domains, helps focus on abilities rather than disabilities.

Measures of functional level help the clinician to identify changes and begin the process of identifying causative factors and developing a treatment plan. The ideal instrument is one that is easy to administer, is short, is able to detect even small changes over time, and measures the domain of interest. In addition, many instruments have cutoff scores that assist in the identifying increased frailty, the woman at risk, and the need for additional support.

This section identifies only a few of the many assessment instruments and includes those most frequently used for assessment of the elderly and those that meet the criteria of being easy to use, short, and sensitive to change (Gallo, Reichel, & Anderson, 1995). The instruments are not discussed in detail or reproduced in this text. Most geriatric

---

Box 18-3 GERIATRIC ASSESSMENT HISTORY

Medical
- Surgical
- Illnesses and hospitalizations
- Health practices such as immunization, mammogram, Pap smear, and tuberculosis history and testing
- Medication use: Request a brown bag to be brought with all medications including over-the-counter and herbal
- Complementary health practices

Health Patterns
- Exercise/activity: Include daily routine, functional status, activities of daily living, and instrumental activities of daily living
- Nutrition
- Sleep
- Cognition: baseline and changes
- Elimination: Include incontinence and use of laxatives
- Value/belief: Include advance directive, religion, and religious practices
- Self-concept and coping: Include support systems, family, abuse, and depression

Sexuality
- Health promotion: Include personal perception of health and goals for treatment

Social
- Location of family members and frequency of contact, friendships and frequency of contact, and social activities
- Problems maintaining social contacts such as transportation or disability

Psychological
- Depression, dementia, and cognition

Financial
- Ask questions such as: Do you have enough money to pay your bills and buy food? Do you have enough money to buy medicines and food? These questions often help identify real or potential problems.

Source: Kane, R., Ouslander, J., & Abrass, I. (1999). *Essentials of clinical geriatrics* (4th ed.). New York: McGraw-Hill.

---

texts (Gallo et al., 1995; Kane et al., 1999; Leuckenotte, 1996) include the actual scales and also many other assessment instruments for other domains (social, values, economic, and dementia).

One important reason for the older woman to have a consistent provider is to assess her at different points along the continuum of care. With information about a variety of levels of function, the nurse will be able to assess changes. Box 18-4 lists commonly used assessments.

The self-care scales include activities of daily living (ADL) and instrumental activities of daily living (IADL). The IADL scales are particularly useful for the older woman because the items focus on tasks usually identified with women (housekeeping, laundry, shopping, cooking, and telephoning). The psychological scales concentrate on

Box 18-4 INSTRUMENTS COMMONLY USED FOR GERIATRIC FUNCTIONAL ASSESSMENT

Self-Care
■ Katz Index of Activities of Daily Living (Katz, Ford, Moskowitz, Jackson, & Jaffee, 1963): Easy to use and quick to administer. Measures activities of daily living. Can be used to identify areas for intervention and the ability to live independently.

■ Barthel Index (Mahoney & Barthel, 1965): Numerical scoring. Measures activities of daily living.

■ The Five Item Instrumental Activities of Daily Living Screening Questionnaire (Fillenbaum, 1985): Identifies changes in function and is easy to administer.

Psychological
■ Geriatric Depression Scale (Yesavage, Brink, & Rose, 1983; Sheikh & Yesavage, 1986): Only depression scale developed specifically for the elderly. Easy to administer (30 or 15 items) and has threshold scores for level of depression. Used for screening purposes only. Validity decreases with increased cognitive impairment.

■ Beck Depression Inventory (Beck, Ward, Mendelson, Mock, & Ergaugh, 1961): Began with 21 symptom categories with four choices for each. Shorter version is now available (Beck & Beck, 1972): Thirteen items identify levels of depression. Inventory is short and less complex than original.

Cognitive
■ Short Portable Mental Status Questionnaire (Pfeiffer, 1975): Ten-item questionnaire is easy to administer and does not require vision; adjusts for race and educational status.

■ Folstein Mini-Mental State Examination (Folstein, Folstein, & McHugh, 1975): Most frequently used screening instrument; short and easy to administer but eyesight is required; not adjusted for educational level. Differentiates between normal vs. dementia or delirium but not depression.

Comprehensive
■ OARS (Older Americans Resources and Services) Multidimensional Functional Assessment Questionnaire (Duke University, Center for the Study of Aging and Human Development, 1974): Excellent instrument that measures five domains of function. Good for use in all aspects of geriatric assessment and management. Long and difficult to complete; interviewer instructions are required. Possible to choose certain parts for use in assessment.

depression, whereas the cognitive scales focus on mental status and confusion. For scales that look at dementia, see Gallo and others (1995). One final comprehensive assessment instrument that measures multiple domains is the Older Americans Resources and Services Multidimensional Assessment; however, the assessment rarely is used in its entirety.

Physical Examination

The physical examination of the older woman is essentially the same as any complete physical. As issues of concern for the older woman are discussed in this chapter, specific areas of focus for the physical examination and diagnostic testing will be addressed within the context of the health promotion and disease prevention model.

HEALTH PROMOTION AND DISEASE PREVENTION

Basic Principles

The importance of health promotion and disease prevention programs for older women cannot be stressed enough. Prevention, nutrition, and exercise not only have an impact on quality of life but also affect the issues of women and aging to be discussed later in the chapter. However, research in the area of health promotion for elderly populations has been inadequate. Most health promotion programs focus on health behaviors and changing those behaviors most likely to be successful using the most efficient methods. Hickey and Stilwell (1991) maintain that research has not adequately identified the behaviors or methods to change behaviors. Epidemiological data about older populations is lacking, research is poorly designed and not randomized, and clinical trials are usually not included. If clinical trials are done, the elderly often are excluded because of assumptions about the health benefit to older persons.

Preventive and health promotion programs for the older adult must be interdisciplinary. To promote successful aging as defined by Rowe and Kahn (1997) and to meet the goals of health promotion and disease prevention, all professionals need to be included in the health plan. The interdisciplinary team working with the elderly person should include a primary provider, physical therapist, occupational therapist, nutritionist, pharmacist, medical social worker, counselor, psychopharmacologist, and a case manager (Siegler et al., 1998).

With population projections for the next 20 years and the increase in chronic disease in the past 20 years and continued increase in the next 20 to 30 years, the interest concerning health promotion and disease prevention is heightened. The realization is that with the projected increases in the elderly population, health care costs will skyrocket, as will rates of disability. Strategies for health promotion and disease prevention are taking on more importance. Research is pointing to a relationship between health behaviors and disease. By decreasing risk factors, disease may also decrease (Rowe & Kahn, 1997). In the discipline of geriatrics, the goal is to maximize the functional level of the older person. To reach the goal, strategies need to be aimed at identifying and modifying risk factors that decrease function and developing mechanisms to increase function (Schmidt, 1994).

If one uses the definition of prevention as "enhancing autonomy and functional independence," as proposed by Schmidt (1994), using the traditional definitions of prevention with elderly clients becomes difficult. Traditionally, primary prevention prevents disease from occurring through removal of risk factors. Secondary prevention aims at early detection (preferably before symptoms occur), early treatment, and prevention of complications. Tertiary prevention focuses on prevention of progress of disease and disability. These definitions are too narrow for the elderly population.

Prevention now needs to be aimed at a "low probability of disease and disease-related disability, high cognitive and physical functional capacity, and active engagement with life" (Rowe & Kahn, 1997, p. 433). Primary, secondary, and tertiary prevention are incorporated into this definition, which provides a framework for the nurse to design health promotion and disease prevention interventions for elderly populations.

When using the expanded definition, the nurse is able to involve the older woman in health promotion and disease prevention activities. For instance, using the first part of the definition, creating a "low probability of disease and disease-related disability," primary prevention now includes prevention of injury, prevention of osteoporosis and removal of risks for iatrogenic illness, immunization, and improving health habits in the areas of smoking, exercise, nutrition, and alcohol. Secondary prevention is accomplished through early diagnosis of new diseases or the exacerbation of current illnesses; tertiary prevention is accomplished by minimizing disease-related disability with rehabilitation.

The second and third parts of the definition proposed by Rowe and Kahn (1997), reaching a high cognitive and physical functional level and having an active engagement with life, imply that the older woman is involved actively in health promotion activities, activity, and social interaction. The definition indicates the value an older woman places on independence. The nurse is able to use this value to facilitate cognitive, physical, and social activities.

Health promotion and disease prevention are not strictly separable for the elderly population. Currently, outcome measures related to health promotion and disease prevention strategies, such as the relationship between changes in health behaviors and functional level or other health indicators, are poorly defined (Schmidt, 1994). Outcome studies could, in addition to functional level, include the relationship of interventions to the number of acute episodes and hospitalizations and a decrease in mortality rates.

To date, secondary and particularly tertiary prevention have been the basis of health care for the elderly. Tertiary prevention is expensive and does not address early prevention. Tertiary prevention also assumes that once disease occurs, primary prevention is of little use.

Using the broad definition of health promotion, the primary care provider is in a position to assist elderly women in activities that decrease disability, retard the progression of illness, and improve functional status. Elderly women are placed at risk for multiple reasons. The reasons that will be discussed are culture, early detection and treatment, exercise, and nutrition.

Cultural Considerations

Most women approach health and health care differently from the way men do. As reported by Franks, Gold, and Clancy (1996), women are more likely to have regular physical examinations and preventive care than men. Regular checkups and preventive health care are associated with longevity in women but not in men. In addition, women have a more positive attitude about health. Women live longer and have less cardiovascular disease until about the age of 80. However, women experience more chronic illness, especially diabetes and hypertension. Women get sick, but men die.

Unfortunately, this simplistic view of women and health does not address the problems underlying health promotion. A great deal of economic inequality exists in health, health care, and mortality. Looking at self-rated health, about 29% of white women 65 and older rate their health as fair or poor, whereas 47% of African-American women in the same age group rate their health as fair to poor (Schick & Schick, 1994). The privileged tend to have better access to health care, are in better health, and have less disability in later life (Mutcheler & Burr, 1994; Stoller & Gibson, 1994). The less privileged—those who have had fewer educational opportunities, are poor, and have a lower occupational status—die earlier. Disadvantaged women tend to seek health care later in the progression of illness and are therefore sicker when presenting to the provider.

Within gerontological literature, a continued hypothesis is that age, racial group, and female gender place an older person in double and triple jeopardy. The belief is that the process of aging, normal and pathological, places the older person at risk for illness and disability. As factors associated with being non-white (particularly African-American) and female are added into the equation, the risk doubles and triples, respectively. Ferraro and Farmer (1996) questioned the double jeopardy hypothesis as related to aging alone. They found that a lifelong risk exists for African-American elderly. The longitudinal data showed that African-Americans had more chronic illness and disability that began early in life. Thus African-American women over 65 are at greater risk of chronic illness, disability, and early mortality becauses of lifelong risk exposure. This risk is not genetic but social and economic.

Multiple barriers to health care are experienced more by elderly women, particularly the disadvantaged, than by elderly men. Financial barriers include the amount of deductible and copay from health insurance, the cost of services that are needed but not covered, and the premiums for coverage. As has been noted, older women are not as likely to have been in the labor force for long periods of time and may or may not have access to health care benefits. Barriers to actual health care and treatment include the convenience of health care, a decrease in mobility and the ability to drive, fewer providers in poor and rural areas, and discrimination in health care (Mutcheler & Burr, 1994; Stoller & Gibson, 1994).

Discrimination in health care has many faces. Giacomini (1996) examined the association between race and gender in receiving hospital-based procedures. In California, African-American, Hispanic, and Asian women had fewer high-technology medical procedures than white women, and all females had fewer procedures than men. Although age was not identified specifically, of nine procedures examined by the researcher, at least three are performed frequently on elderly clients (hip replacement, angioplasty, and pacemaker implants).

More specific discrimination related to age and gender was found by McLaughlin, Soumerai, and Willison (1996), who examined the use of standard lifesaving drugs after myocardial infarction (MI). The standard of care after MI includes thrombolytics, beta-blockers, and aspirin. Patients 75 and older, compared with those 64 and younger, were significantly less likely to receive the standard medication, especially the thrombolytic agents. Additionally, elderly women were significantly less likely to receive aspirin or thrombolytics. Thus elderly women appear to be undertreated with potentially lifesaving drugs.

Discrimination also was found in treatment of elderly women with breast cancer (Hillner, Penberthy, & Desch, 1996). The researchers used a sample of 3361 women who had surgery for breast cancer. Controlling for coexisting conditions, findings showed a decrease of 67% per decade in the use of chemotherapy. The differences in use of radiation therapy also were striking. Sixty-six percent of the women age 65 to 69 received radiation therapy, whereas only 7% of those 85 and older received radiation therapy. Finally, the assessment of axillary nodes was less likely to occur with increasing age. As in the study of the women after MI, the standard of care was not followed as the age of the patient increased. Indeed, older women are less likely to have chemotherapy or radiation therapy after surgery for breast cancer. The study, however, did not discuss the informed consent given the patient or report patient wishes concerning chemotherapy or radiation therapy.

Early Detection and Treatment: Screening

Screening is designed to be a cost-effective approach for a large segment of the population. Hickey and Stilwell (1991) discuss a variety of pros and cons for screening the elderly population, pointing out that research is limited as to the benefits, risks, and feasibility, particularly for cancer. In addition to the cost and invasive quality of screening programs, the problem of underreporting of symptoms in the older population occurs. The lack of reporting, whether because of fear of diagnosis or belief that cancer cannot be prevented or treated, limits the efficacy of widespread screening.

Screening for cancer is an example of problems with early detection and treatment among older women. Breast cancer is one of the leading causes of death among women, with more than 50% of the incidence occurring in women over 60. Mammograms help identify breast cancer early in the course of the disease, yet health care providers do not always recommend mammograms for older women. Possibly because of poor screening or late reporting of symptoms, breast cancer in elderly women often is detected late in the disease process. Screening for cervical cancer is equally discouraging among older women, although abnormal results may be 2 to 3 times more likely after 65, and debate continues about the need for Papanicolaou (Pap) smear screening after age 65 (Byyny & Speroff, 1996; Hickey & Stilwell, 1991).

At a different level of argument, however, treatment of cancer is often invasive, disabling or disfiguring, painful, and uncomfortable. Quality of life issues need to be explored with the patient and family by taking into consideration patient wishes and considering that life expectancy may not be longer with or without treatment for cancer with comorbid conditions. Hickey and Stilwell (1991) believe the goal of cancer detection and treatment should be directed at those with early stages of disease.

Numerous guides for screening of older women exist. Box 18-5 represents general guidelines for screening.

Box 18-5 SCREENING GUIDELINES FOR THE OLDER WOMAN

Recommendations for Screening
Every Visit
Generally, every visit should include information on smoking, alcohol use, weight and height, and blood pressure.
Annually from age 60
Breast examination
Mammogram
Pelvic examination
Rectal examination
Occult blood
Hearing
Vision
Immunizations
Pneumovaccine (once)
Influenza: every year after 65
Tetanus-diphtheria: every 10 years after age 60
Laboratory
Lipid profile: every 5 years if not at risk
Thyroid: every 2 years
Pap smear: 3 years consecutive normal and then every 3 years
Tuberculosis
Two-stage purified protein derivative: If first test is negative, repeat 2 to 4 weeks later.

Sources: Byyny, R., & Speroff, L. (1996). *A clinical guide for the care of older women* (2nd ed.). Baltimore: Williams & Wilkins. Kane, R., Ouslander, J., & Abrass, I. (1999). *Essentials of clinical geriatrics* (4th ed.). New York: McGraw-Hill.

Exercise

Biological changes in the cardiovascular, respiratory, and musculoskeletal systems plus inactivity, role stress, poverty, loss, and depression predispose women to chronic illness and place them at risk for disability. The stresses of poverty, declining health, and widowhood, common among elderly women, contribute to feelings of depression. Chronic disorders such as bunions, spinal degeneration, bladder infections, and stress disorders decrease the motivation to exercise, which in turn results in inactivity, decreased muscle strength, decreased endurance, and poor balance. Depression, stress, chronic illness, alcohol, and medications such as tranquilizers and sleeping medications may alter movement patterns and cognition. Changes in musculoskeletal, neurological, and cognitive function predispose the older woman to falls (O'Brien & Vertinsky, 1991; Woollacott, 2000).

Findings from the Baltimore Longitudinal Study (Metter et al., 1997) indicate a decline in strength and power in men and women beginning at age 40. A growing belief, verified in part by research focusing on exercise, is that much of the loss of skeletal muscle can be attributed to lack of exercise. O'Brien and Vertinsky (1991) report that 30% to 60% of the general population does not do any physical activity, and, of those 65 and older, 42% or more acknowledge that they lead sedentary lives.

Although the percentage of women over 65 who participate in exercise activities has increased since 1985 (44%), 39% continue to report a sedentary life style (Federal Interagency Forum, 2000). O'Brien and Vertinsky (1991) would agree with Hickey and Stilwell (1991) that research related to exercise and women over 70 is lacking. Data on walking, the most often suggested form of exercise for women, are lacking and absent for those 80 and older.

The benefits of participating in regular exercise are many. In the short term, women report that they immediately feel better. Improvements noted include a positive mood, decreased stress, better sleep, and improved self-concept and self-esteem. In addition, exercise programs often place women in social groups with peers, thereby enlarging the social network. Long-term benefits include improvement in chronic conditions, increased longevity with increased quality of life, and improvements in cardiovascular, respiratory, and musculoskeletal functioning.

Although women can verbalize the benefits of an exercise program, a recent study of 114 community-dwelling women age 70 and older found that the perception of the risks of exercise prevented participation in an exercise program (Cousins, 2000). The researcher, using open-ended questions, found that the perceived risks included joint damage, heart attack, breathlessness, overexertion, and fatigue. Although this study sample was small, the results indicate the importance of discussing concerns about exercise.

Developing an Exercise Program

Any exercise program needs to focus on more than one type of exercise. In discussions of cardiovascular risk, aerobic exercise is most often mentioned as a means to decrease blood pressure, improve the lipid profile, and aid in weight reduction. Dallas (1997) developed a 10-week walking program for women. Women walked 45 minutes 3 times a week at 60% to 70% of the maximum heart rate. Significant improvement was found in four of the seven indicators. A significant change in cardiovascular fitness occurred as measured by an increase of almost 12 steps per minute. Weight loss, decreased waist-to-hip ratio, and a decrease in the body mass index indicated that walking was beneficial for overweight women. Unfortunately, the sample was small ($n = 22$), white, and of a higher socioeconomic status.

Although aerobic exercise must be included in a health promotion program for women, a need also exists for women to participate in resistance exercises to improve flexibility, strength, and balance. Within the goals of health promotion, decreasing risk of falling and fear of falling are important for prevention and for maintaining an optimal functional level. Progressive resistance training in 87-year-old women increased muscle strength by 90%, velocity in gait 12%, and ability to climb stairs 28% in 10 weeks (Metter et al., 1997). Resistance training started slowly, with gradual increments. The researchers noted that results might not be apparent for 12 weeks or more. Motivating the woman to continue and showing even small changes are important. Improved mood may occur early in the exercise program, and this may be the motivation to continue.

Exercise in older women improves strength in lower limb muscles, leading to increased walking speed, cadence, balance, and stride length. These improvements were associated with improved ankle strength and strength of hip extension (Lord et al., 1996). Weight-bearing exercises also are being found to maintain or even increase bone mineral density (BMD).

McCartney, Hicks, Martin, and Webber (1996) conducted a randomized control trial of weight training and aerobic exercise in 142 females and males age 60 to 80. Women and men improved significantly in measures of strength and endurance. After completing the 2-year study, women participants in the exercise program had increased strength with muscle hypertrophy and increased endurance in stair climbing, walking, and cycling. In addition, although bone density measurements did not change significantly in exercisers, a 1% *decrease* in whole body bone mineral content occurred in the control group of nonexercisers.

Snow, Shaw, Winters, and Witzke (2000) used weighted vests to study the benefit of exercise on BMD in the hip. One group of elderly women used weighted vests, and the control group did not. The researchers found that BMD significantly increased for the women using vests, whereas those without the weighted vests had a decline in BMD. In addition to increases in BMD, women who used the vests had continued the exercise program at the 5-year follow-up.

As youngsters, many older women frequently were socialized not to exercise, and thus they have never participated in an exercise program. Given the importance of aerobic exercise, starting with a walking program is ideal. In addition to decreasing cardiovascular risk, walking may help prevent loss of bone mass through placing stress on long bones and improving strength, endurance, and balance. Aerobic training also decreases the risk of back pain, breast and female reproductive cancers, diabetes, obesity, and stroke (Fentem, 1994).

When beginning a new exercise program, women should begin with small goals such as walking a short distance. Increases in distance and speed can be gradual. Studies show that the elderly need at least 12 weeks of an exercise program to feel results. Changes may not be apparent quickly, so consistent support and encouragement are needed to maintain motivation and participation in the program. The ultimate goal of aerobic activity is 20 to 30 minutes 3 times a week at 65% to 75% maximal heart rate. However, evauation and exercise program development need to be individualized.

Nutrition

Older women frequently have problems related to poor nutrition and over- and undernutrition (Byyny & Speroff, 1996). Nutritional status has an affect on multiple functional and cognitive aspects of aging. Causative factors involve physiological changes, chronic illness, medications, and psychosocial issues. Changes in the gastrointestinal system, as well as changes in taste, may contribute to malnutrition in the elderly. However, many chronic conditions and accompanying dietary restrictions, multiple medications that decrease appetite, physical and financial changes, loneliness, and alcohol intake are more important factors in poor nutrition among the elderly. Food preparation may be a problem because of arthritic pain and deformity; eating may be a problem because of chronic obstructive pulmonary disease and congestive heart failure and the accompanying shortness of breath when eating; appetite may be poor because of loss of companionship at mealtime, medications that cause nausea, or a decrease in basal metabolic rate; and obtaining food may be a problem because of inadequate finances, poor transportation, or physical inability to shop.

Widowhood often is mentioned as an event that places a woman at risk for nutritional inadequacy; however, the reasons for this are not clear. In a 3-year ethnographic study of 64 widows in two rural communities (Quandt, McDonald, Arcury, Bell, & Vitoling, 2000), certain themes were identified relating to nutritional inadequacies. The themes were changes in obtaining food, preparing food, types of food eaten, frequency of eating, and having a supply of food on hand. Preparation and meal times often were related to the husband's nutritional needs during a terminal illness, which often created changes in nutritional practices that continued into widowhood. After the death of the husband, preparation of food was a problem because of the lack of structure for meal preparation. Women reported a decreased interest in food and a lack of scheduled meal times as problems. In addition, many rural women stopped vegetable gardening, avoided asking others for rides to the store, skipped meals, ate take-out food, had poorly balanced meals, and did not stock a freezer or preserve foods.

Although many changes, as mentioned previously, can lead to undernutrition, obesity is a more common problem (Byyny & Speroff, 1996; Kramarow et al., 1999). Frequently, the elderly eat foods high in fat because they taste good, are readily available, and require little preparation. In addition, elders often relate food to being healthy.

Obesity and being overweight are not synonymous. Obesity is excess body fat caused by excess storage of triglycerides in adipose tissue. A person may be overweight but not obese. However, unless the practitioner has an accurate means to determine body fat, body weight is an indicator. Weight that is 20% or more than ideal weight (indicative of excess adipose tissue) is high enough to alter physiological functioning. Women then are placed at risk for a decrease in life expectancy, hypercholesterolemia, hypertriglyceridemia, hypertension, and diabetes. In addition to multiple genetic, psychological, cultural, and physical factors, women have a lower metabolic rate, especially after menopause. Women therefore are at risk for obesity and its sequelae.

In addition to trying to help elderly women maintain appropriate nutrition, the provider is faced with the potential for dehydration among elderly clients. Although salivation decreases, the older person does not feel thirsty. Compounding the problem is often the fear of incontinence. Older persons may avoid drinking fluids because they believe that they will "have an accident." The result is not only dehydration but also confusion and isolation.

Nutritional Assessment and Management

The nurse must be able to identify persons at risk for malnutrition. Factors associated with obtaining and preparing foods, meal schedules, and the type of food must be included in the assessment. A complete 24-hour intake is not necessary for screening.

Two measures that have been developed are quick and easy to use. The first is the Nutritional Risk Index published and distributed by the Nutrition Screening Initiative (1991). The Nutrition Screening Initiative is a multidisciplinary effort led by the American Academy of Family Physicians, American Dietetic Association, the National Council on Aging, and 25 other organizations committed to incorporating nutrition screening and intervention into the health care delivery system. The risk index identifies factors, other than physical, that place the older person at risk. The second is the Food Guide Pyramid, which identifies foods the client is eating and the adequacy of her diet. Before using the pyramid, the provider asks what the person ate the day before or what is typically eaten during the day. The answer does not have to be absolutely accurate. If some foods are not mentioned, the nurse should ask if they are ever eaten. Identifying approximate amounts is useful, but questions have to be in terms the person understands. The person's usual intake then may be compared with the requirements identified by the Food Guide Pyramid. Table 18-3 gives one way to use the pyramid for screening (intake amounts and adequacy are examples only, as if provided by a client).

Table 18-3 indicates the client does not have adequate nutrition. When using the Nutritional Risk Index and the Pyramid, the provider is able to begin a differential diagnosis, consider needs for education and counseling, identify financial barriers, and consider collaboration with a nutritionist, psychologist, physical therapist, or social worker. The provider also is able to identify areas in need of additional in-depth assessment.

All clients need a detailed history and physical examination. Laboratory data are useful, especially the following indicators of nutritional adequacy: hemoglobin, hematocrit, complete blood count, albumin, and folate (vitamin B_{12}). In counseling and teaching dietary adjustments, remember that although caloric intake may be decreased, nutrient intake is not necessarily decreased. Making sure the diet is supplemented also is important. In addition, dietary instruction falls on deaf ears if culture, ability to obtain food, ability to cook, ability to taste foods (decline in taste buds and decline in ability to taste sweet and salty), and likes and dislikes are not taken into account. In addition, meal time is a social event. Eating alone may decrease the appetite, motivation to cook and eat, and enjoyment of meals.

Table **18-3**   **EXAMPLE CLIENT ASSESSMENT USING THE FOOD GUIDE PYRAMID**

FOOD	REQUIRED AMOUNT	TYPICAL INTAKE (24 HOURS)	ADEQUACY
Bread, cereal, rice, and pasta	6-11 servings	4 servings	(–) at least 2
Vegetable group	3-5 servings	6 servings	(+) 1
Fruit group	2-4 servings	0 servings	(–) at least 2
Milk, yogurt, and cheese	2-3 servings	2 servings	Adequate
Meat, poultry, fish, beans, eggs, and nuts	2-3 servings	5 servings	(+) 2 servings
Fats, oils, and sweets	Sparingly	(+) 3 servings	3 servings

Collaboration with the geriatric team is important for successful management because of the multiple causes of malnutrition. Because of the need to involve many members of the team, a case manager is necessary. The following list identifies team members and their contributions to the management of malnutrition:

- *Physical therapist:* Assists with exercise program and follow-up.
- *Social worker:* Addresses financial support, identifies possible social dining opportunities, and assists with problems of transportation to obtain needed foods.
- *Psychosocial counseler:* Assesses psychosocial needs and counsels as needed.
- *Nutritionist:* Assesses, teaches, and counsels concerning diet and nutrition.
- *Occupational therapist:* Teaches those whose physical limitations make cooking impossible or difficult new ways to cook and organize kitchen.
- *Home health nurse:* Is a consistent visitor, offers support to the woman, and reports to the team.

Box 18-6 summarizes the health promotion and disease prevention activities for the older woman.

WOMEN'S ISSUES IN AGING

The following section discusses issues that are of particular concern to older women. Not only do women have specific needs in the area of health promotion as described previously, but also they have problems that can lead to disease, disability, poor cognition, and overall decreases in quality of life. The 11 issues presented in detail are poverty, grandparents as parents, elder abuse, polypharmacy, falls, sexuality, incontinence, depression, bereavement, alcoholism, and suicide.

Poverty

More elderly women than men live at or below the national poverty level, and African-American and Hispanic women are almost 2 times more likely to live in poverty than white women (Kramarow et al., 1999). In 1992 only 13% of the elderly were poor; however, of the 13%, 71% were women. Close to 75% of the elderly poor in the United States are women, even though a majority of the elderly have incomes of $25,000 per year. The poverty threshold is an amount set by the federal government. The poor have an income below the set threshold. The near poor have an income of 25% higher than the poverty threshold. The poverty threshold for a single person living alone age 65 and older in 1992 was $6729, and the near poor threshold was $8411 (U.S. Bureau of the Census, 1993). Box 18-7 provides a profile of women in poverty.

Poverty among elderly women results from multiple, complex factors. Many women have a transition into poverty in old age. Most retirement income is based on a work history that covers many years, salary increases, and retirement benefits. Generally, those in professional and management positions have higher incomes in retirement. For elderly women, work history is often a negative factor because many women did not pay into Social Security, did not have employment out of the home, and did not have any retirement income. Therefore for the married elderly woman, the spouse's work

Box 18-6 SUMMARY OF HEALTH PROMOTION AND DISEASE PREVENTION ACTIVITIES IN OLDER WOMEN

History	*Physical Exam*	*Laboratory Tests*	*Risk Assessment*	*Immunization*
Complete medical history: Review of systems for signs and symptoms of cancer, heart disease, autoimmune disease, or respiratory disease	Height, weight, blood pressure, and hearing	Pap smear as indicated	Changes in cognitive function, health promotion avtivities, support systems; signs and symptoms of depression, alcoholism, poverty, or polypharmacy	Tetanus/diphtheria booster every 10 years after age 60
Obstetric/ gynecological history: Gastrointestinal and genitourinary systems, menopause, sexual patterns, and polypharmacy	Visual acuity Oral cavity exam Palpation of thyroid Cardiovascular assessment Respiratory Musculoskeletal Skin exam Lymph node Pelvic exam Rectal exam Gastrointestinal exam Genitourinary	Mammogram annually from age 60 Rubella titer as indicated Fecal blood testing annually after age 50 Sigmoidoscopy every 3-5 years after age 50; earlier as indicated Nonfasting total blood lipid profile every 5 years; more frequently as indicated Fasting blood glucose as indicated Tuberculosis skin test in high-risk women Sexually transmitted disease screening: Gonorrhea, if needed, chlamydia, VDRL* test, human immunodeficiency virus counseling and testing Glaucoma testing as indicated Vision screening Thyroid test every 2 years	Tobacco, alcohol, or drug use Symptoms of physical or emotional abuse Symptoms of depression, suicide, or abnormal bereavement behavior Evidence of social isolation Symptoms of increased stress Lack of regular exercise Excessive dietary intake or lack of dietary intake Sun and ultraviolet light exposure Evidence of social isolation, increased stress, and limited financial resources Prevention strategies Prevention of falls Hot water heater temperature reduction to less than 130°F (54°C)	Rubella vaccine as indicated Hepatitis B Influenza annually after age 65 if high risk Pneumococcal vaccine if high risk
Mental health history: Depression, dementia, cognition, sleep, elimination, values, and advance directives				
Surgical history: Hysterectomy				
Family history: Breast or ovarian cancer, cardiovascular disease, and diabetes				
Current medications: Prescription and over-the-counter				
Self-care: Functional status, dietary intake, regular exercise, tobacco, alcohol, and drug use				

*VDRL, Venereal Disease Research Laboratory.

Box 18-6 SUMMARY OF HEALTH PROMOTION AND DISEASE PREVENTION ACTIVITIES IN OLDER WOMEN

History	Physical Exam	Laboratory Tests	Risk Assessment	Immunization
Psychosocial history: History of child abuse or neglect, domestic violence, location of family members, and frequency of family contact, ability to maintain social activities, parenting of grandchildren			Use of smoke detector in home Use of seat belts in motor vehicles, Use of helmets on rollerblades Cessation of tobacco, alcohol, or drug use Limiting alcohol intake Avoiding being a passenger in a car driven by someone under the influence of alcohol Regular exercise program Dietary plan: Restriction of fat and cholesterol, adequate intake of iron and calcium, maintaining balanced diet Teach breast self-exam Teach signs and symptoms of cancer and cardiovascular disease Discuss osteoporosis prevention Discuss the following: Sexually transmitted disease risk reduction, violent behavior and ways to reduce risk, available resources, sunlight and ultraviolet light exposure Discuss stress reduction in employment settings Assess workplace environmental safety	

Box 18-7 WOMEN AND POVERTY: FACTS AND FIGURES

Poverty: Age and Ethnicity
White women
Ages 65-69: 28% poor or near poor
Ages 75 and older: 20% poor
Ages 85 and older: 58% poor or near poor
African-American women
Ages 65-74: 35% poor
Ages 75 and older: 43% poor
Hispanic women
Ages 65-74: 22% poor
Ages 75 and older: 32% poor

Poverty: Living Alone
White: 23% poor or near poor
African American: 50% poor or near poor
Hispanic: 58% poor or near poor

Poverty: Age 62 and Older by Marital Status
Widowed: 22%
Divorced: 27%
Separated: 37%
Married: 6%

Source: U.S. Bureau of the Census. (1993). *Poverty in the United States* (Current Population Reports, Series P60). Washington DC: Government Printing Office.

history, salary, and retirement plan are important. When the marital status changes, women often transition into poverty (McLaughlin & Jensen, 2000).

Census data indicate that older women living alone face the greatest risk for poverty. Many females suddenly find themselves poor after the death of their husbands. Women reaching old age now were socialized to believe that income security came with marriage. Women are less likely to receive a pension than men, and, if they receive a pension, it is likely to be 50% less than that for men of the same age. Only 22% of women over 65 report receiving a pension, whereas 49% of the men over 65 report receiving a pension. Women received an average income from pensions of $5432 per year; men received $10,031 per year.

Older women are financially underprotected and are among the most vulnerable segment of our population. Many women must rely on Social Security benefits for income. As Burkhauser (1994) points out, the policies of the Social Security system are made by married men using a traditional model of income and work. The greatest level of protection in the Social Security trust fund is for the traditional married male.

Even though never intended to be a major source of income on retirement, Social Security for many elderly is a primary source of income. Social Security benefits are determined by payroll deductions and the number of credits (usually four credits per year) accrued. Benefits are based on an average of earnings over the years worked. The number of earnings years used is 35. Therefore, for years of nonemployment (not paying into the system), zeros are placed into the equation. The more money earned and the longer the individual was employed, the higher the benefit.

With the death of a spouse, Social Security benefits drop dramatically. The woman may choose to receive her husband's Social Security benefit or the benefit from her work history. Because of the sporadic nature of work and low-paying employment, 61% of widows receive more income using the survivor benefit than their own (Social Security Administration, 1993).

Poverty and Health Care

Medicare Part A. Medicare was designed to provide affordable health care for everyone over the age of 65. The information provided in this chapter is not extensive for two main reasons. First, the relationship between Medicare and managed care is in a state of change. Second, given the population projections for women eligible for Medicare, the known information about the increase in chronic disease with aging, and the stress on the Medicare system, changes in coverage must be expected (Moon & Gage, 1997). For detailed, regularly updated information on Medicare and other federally funded plans, refer to *http://www.medicare.gov/whatis.html.*

Women or their spouses over 65 who have paid into Social Security for at least 10 years are entitled to receive Medicare Part A. This is a hospital insurance plan and is available without cost if the woman or her spouse is receiving or is eligible to receive retirement benefits from Social Security or the Railroad Pension Fund.

Medicare Part A helps pay for hospitalization, home care, hospice care, and benefits for skilled nursing facilities. The coverage, however, has limitations. Medicare Part A is not a comprehensive health care plan and does not pay for health needs most frequently encountered among elderly women. Medicare Part A does not cover dentures, eyeglasses, hearing aids, appointments to prescribe and fit eyeglasses or hearing aides, prescription medications, and routine physical checkups.

Medicare Part B. Medicare Part B is considered medical insurance and is available to elderly who are able to pay a monthly premium. As of 1995, the monthly premium was $46.10 or $553.20 per year. This is an increase from $36.60 per month in 1994. In 1998 the premium was $43.80 per month. By the year 2002 the premium will have reached $67 and by the year 2007 will increase to $105.50 per month. These increases place a burden on women who are already in poverty (Moon & Gage, 1997).

Having Medicare Part B has many advantages, even though the insurance has a deductible. Medicare Part B pays about 80% of approved charges. Medicare Part B *helps* pay for services of health care providers; outpatient hospital services; home health visits not covered in part A; diagnostic x-ray, laboratory, and other tests; ambulance services; and medical services and supplies. Part B also covers some preventive care such as mammography, Pap smears, and outpatient therapies.

Medicaid. Medicaid is a program that provides financial help to states and counties so that they can then pay for medical care for the aged poor, blind, disabled, and families with dependent children. Medicaid requires that the older person have few assets. If eligibility requirements are met, Medicaid covers the cost of the Medicare deductibles and pays for preventive health care, as well as acute care and long-term stays in nursing facilities. Medicare covers the first 100 days of a nursing facility stay. After that, if the older person has assets, these must be spent until such assets are almost gone. Older women with few assets and low income rely on Medicaid for health care. More than 75% of the residents of nursing facilities are women whose stays are paid for by Medicaid (Moon & Gage, 1997).

Older women, even those covered by Medicare, must use out-of-pocket resources to cover health care costs. Analysis of out-of-pocket spending indicates that major disparities exist between older women and older men and those with chronic illnesses. On the average, women must spend a higher percentage of their annual income on health care than men, and this gap widens with increasing age (Crystal, Johnson, Harman, Sambamoorthi, & Kumar, 2000; Foley & Gibson, 2000). Costs include payments to providers, insurance premiums, and medications. Insurance premiums account for an average of 28.5% of the older woman's annual income. Women also tend to have a higher burden of prescription drug costs than men. Given the limited income and greater number of chronic illnesses among older women, health care costs impose an extra financial burden. Finally, even with adequate insurance coverage, older women may not have adequate health care because of financial burdens of caregiving, living arrangements, or provider attitudes.

Assessment

The practitioner is not always called on to complete a financial assessment. However, as part of a comprehensive geriatric assessment, knowledge about financial status assists the nurse in assessing and managing care. If finances are a major problem for the older woman and the cost of care is viewed as impossible, health care management will fail. Frequently, the older person gives the impression that enough money is available, but, with direct questions, the practitioner discovers a different story. The older person prioritizes expenses. Food is one of the first areas to save on when money is tight, so many questions relate to money available to buy food.

The following are some suggested interview questions:

- Do you have enough money to meet your monthly bills?
- Do you have enough money to buy food?
- Do you have enough money to buy medicines?
- What do you eat every day?
- How do you cook your food?
- How do you get to the store?
- When did you last go to the doctor?
- How do you get to the doctor?
- When did you last go to the dentist?
- When was your last Pap smear or mammogram?
- Do you have Medicare Part A or Part B?

Management

The geriatric interdisciplinary team is needed to manage the financial needs of the older person. The social service team member will be able to identify potential resources and assist the person and family to access the services. Again, the advanced practitioner case manager provides continuity and helps prevent losing the patient in the complex system.

Grandparent as Parent

Grandparenting is not usually considered a problem. An exploration of all the issues in aging, however, indicates that grandparents raising grandchildren may contribute to poverty and depression. If one examines transition timelines through life, grandparents have no place for raising grandchildren. Family transitions at age 50 begin looking at retirement, children leaving home, empty nest, and widowhood. Traditionally, for the middle class, grandparenting is a time of playing with grandchildren, having fun, and sending them home. Today, 3.7 million adults in mid-life or older are caring for 3.9 million grandchildren with neither parent present, a 53% increase since 1990. Fifty-one percent of these grandparents are married couples. The number of households with a grandchild in residence is about 353,000. In addition, about 260,000 mid-life or older adults in nontraditional households have a grandchild as part of the home without a parent present (American Association of Retired Persons [AARP], 1997; Beltran, 2000; Chalfie, 1994).

Now known as the skip generation, these grandparents are torn between loyalty to their own child and the grandchild. They must make difficult choices. The most common reason for the grandparent to be raising the grandchild is because of substance abuse by the parent (Beltran, 2000; Chalfie, 1994; Kelley, 1993). Child abuse and neglect or abandonment, teenage mothers unable to care for the child, death of the parent, parental unemployment or divorce, incarceration, and human immunodeficiency virus and acquired immunodeficiency syndrome are other reasons grandparents must assume the second-time-around role of parent.

The demographic information to date indicates that most of the grandparents raising grandchildren are women from age 45 to over 75. The median age is 57 with 75% between 45 and 64, 23% between 65 and 74, and 7% age 75 and older. The median age for women (45 to 64) raising grandchildren is 54 but the median age for women 65 to 74 is 70. Among those surveyed, grandparent ethnicity was overwhelmingly white (AARP, 1997; Beltran, 2000; Kelley, 1993). However, a suspicion is that many women do not report the expanded grandparenting role. The 2000 U.S. Census was the first one to have questions about grandparents raising grandchildren. In the urban areas of California, and in Detroit and New York City, the majority of grandparents raising grandchildren were African-American (Wagner, 1995). The educational level of most grandparents raising grandchildren tends to be less than high school or high school (AARP, 1997; Kelley, 1993).

Forty-one percent of the women who are grandparents and are raising children are below the poverty level or near poor, and 56% earn less than $20,000, compared with 26% of the traditional family (families not raising grandchildren) with children. The median income of the grandparent-as-parent family is half that of the traditional family with children. In addition to assuming the role of parent for grandchildren, younger grandparents often are raising children, working, and possibly coping with their own aging parents. With increased age, many of the women are on fixed income. Among the grandparents raising grandchildren surveyed (AARP, 1997), 42% were working, 46% were on fixed incomes, and 12% were on a fixed income and working.

In the study by Kelley (1993) the ages of the grandchildren ranged from 2 or fewer years (11%) to 19 years (4%). About 18% of the grandchildren were age 3 to 4 and 18% were 12 to 16 years of age. Many grandchildren were in elementary school (46%). Most grandparents believed their role as parents a second time around was permanent. Usually only one grandchild is being raised by a grandmother; however, many women had two or three grandchildren to raise (AARP, 1997; Kelley, 1993)

Grandparenting by African-Americans and Hispanics

Little information is available about African-American and Hispanic grandparents. However, a recent report (AARP, 1997) on African-American and Hispanic grandparents raising grandchildren showed some startling differences between whites and other racial groups. African-American and Hispanic grandparents lived alone in urban areas, caring for two or more children on an income under $20,000, and had 12 or fewer years of education. White grandparents were usually married, caring for less than two grandchildren, often working and earning more than $40,000 per year and had more than 12 years of education. The problems of the two groups studied centered around physical and psychological limitations and finances.

The AARP (1997) report identified differences between African-American and Hispanic grandparents in the types of support (including the use of agencies, importance of legal problems, medical costs, help with daily responsibilities, and support groups) and types of outreach communication available. African-American grandparents seek support from agencies that offer education and an opportunity to talk about frustrations about their new role. Hispanic grandparents look for assistance in dealing with all the problems encountered. Both groups mistrust social service agencies.

Further, in this study, African-American grandparents reported that legal issues were problematic, but Hispanics felt that legal issues were not particularly important. African-American women found medical costs burdensome because they paid most medical costs. Medicaid, however, covered the medical costs of the grandchildren of the Hispanic population. Generally, the Hispanic population identified a need for respite care, whereas the African-American group identified the need for day care and homework assistance for the children.

Support group involvement was different between the two populations. African-American grandparents found that support groups were helpful in providing emotional support, a way to have friends and a peer group having similar problems, and an educational opportunity to relearn parenting skills. Hispanics were not as enthusiastic about support groups. Although willing to attend support groups if talks were given on specific topics or were a means for referral, they were uncomfortable talking about problems with the group.

Outreach was problematic for both groups. Most effective in identifying grandparents serving as parents and providing assistance was communication from one grandparent to another about possible support services and flyers placed in churches or grocery stores. Once in a support group, the best way of communicating was on a personal level through telephone calls or one-on-one conversations. Once in a support group, African-Americans and Hispanics seemed to be more aware of information provided through television and newspapers. Hispanics stressed the need for using Spanish to provide information.

Specific Issues Facing Grandparents Raising Grandchildren

The problems experienced by grandparents raising grandchildren include the traditional task of managing developmental issues. More important, however, are totally new problems and concerns that include legal, financial, health and health care, including psychological and emotional concerns, social isolation, and housing problems (AARP, 1997, Wagner, 1995).

Legal. Legal status is one of the first concerns to be faced. Many grandparents assume informal responsibility. In most states today, to obtain public assistance the grandparent must have some legally recognized status. What seems simple, such as registration of the child in school and making health care decisions, can become major problems if no legal relationship exists between the grandparent and child. This means that the grandparent must adopt, obtain guardianship, or become a recognized foster parent for the grandchild (AARP, 1997; Beltran, 2000; Chalfie, 1994; Wagner, 1995).

Economic. Financial responsibilities are another concern. As noted previously, the majority of women raising grandchildren have a low, often fixed income. If the grandparent is still working, taking on the responsibility of a parent again may mean leaving a job or decreasing hours on the job. This often means increased poverty, loss of any financial cushion, and loss of health benefits. Retired women already on a low Social Security income must add costs of caring for the grandchildren. Planning for retirement and retirement savings does not usually include costs associated with raising young children (AARP, 1997; Beltran, 2000; Chalfie, 1994; Minkler & Roe, 1996).

One form of economic support that was available to the grandparent (Aid to Families with Dependent Children, part of the Social Security Act) was repealed in 1996 and was replaced by Temporary Assistance for Needy Families, also a welfare program. States rely on federal block grants to provide for funds for dependent children. Income and households that do not have parental care or support determine eligibility for children under age 18. The Aid to Families with Dependent Children program includes supplemental securities income, food stamps, and foster care. Now states can determine how funds are spent for programs. Applying for funds is not a positive experience for the grandparent. The process often is stigmatizing, and the grandparent for the first time may feel the need to receive welfare.

Recent changes in the welfare system mean less economic support. In addition, although the state receives a block grant, guidelines may not be followed appropriately. Although legal custody is not a requirement to receive funds, the state may mandate a legal relationship (AARP, 1995; Beltran, 2000). Minkler and Roe (1996) point out that foster care parents receive benefits not afforded to grandparents, including higher financial compensation, psychological counseling, and a clothing allowance. However, with foster care, the state or county continue to have legal custody of the children. The government makes decisions about placement and may remove the children from the foster parent. Many grandparents do not want the involvement of the government despite the financial compensation (Beltran, 2000).

Health and health care. Health and health care are also issues for the grandparent. If the younger grandparent continues to work, frequently the employee health insurance carrier will not insure the grandchild. Even if the grandparent has legal custody, the employer may or may not believe that the grandchild has any right to receive health benefits. Although views are changing, little recognition is given to nontraditional family structures. If the grandparent is 60 years or older, she is covered by Medicare. The grandchild, however, has no coverage. The grandparent must pay for health insurance or apply for Medicaid (AARP, 1993; Beltran, 2000; Chalfie, 1994; Minkler & Roe, 1996).

The health care of the grandchild requires finding a provider and relearning immunization schedules, screenings necessary for school attendance, and nutrition. The child also may have specific health-related special needs. As previously noted, the most common reason that grandparents are placed in the role of parent for the grandchild is substance abuse by the parent. Many children were born of a parent who used alcohol or cocaine, and the baby may have fetal alcohol syndrome or a cocaine addiction. The grandparent must cope with hyperactivity, respiratory problems, and emotional and behavioral problems (Barnhill, 1996; Kelley, 1993).

The health of the grandmother is also in jeopardy. Aging often is accompanied by chronic illness. Grandparents who must take on the role of raising grandchildren report a decline in health status and have exacerbations of hypertension, back pain, gastric and other gastrointestinal problems, and depression and insomnia (Miller, 1997). In addition, women also may miss appointments with health care providers because of problems with caregiving (Minkler & Roe, 1996; Miller, 1997) and have an increased use of alcohol and cigarettes after taking on the new role (Burton, 1992; Minkler, Roe, & Price, 1992).

In addition to physical problems, the grandparent must cope with psychological and emotional concerns of the grandchild and herself. The grandparent may experience resentment toward her own child for leaving the grandchild and guilt regarding her role as parent. The grandparent may resent not being able to be the traditional grandparent and the loss of plans for retirement. The grandparent also has realistic concerns about the future, including answers to the following questions. What happens to the child if something happens to me? Will I live long enough to raise the child? What suffering and ill effects will the child have because of being raised by a grandmother? Will the child's parent demand the child back? Will the child then return to an unfit home life (Chalfie, 1994)?

Social isolation. Although many grandparents report a consistent supportive network, a surprising problem experienced by grandparents raising grandchildren may be social isolation. The new role of parent may mean being able to spend less time with friends and family and may decrease outside activities such as participation in church, social organizations, and other usual activities with friends (Burton, 1992; Jendrek, 1994). Older grandparents feel isolated from their peers because they now have parenting concerns that are not shared, and older friends do not want a child around all the time (Minkler & Roe, 1996; Kelley, 1993). The older grandparent also feels too old to join younger mothers and therefore is isolated from those who could provide parenting suggestions.

Housing. Grandparents living in low-income housing may suddenly find that they may become homeless. Public housing may specify the type of household relationships that are acceptable. Usually husband and wife and children are recognized as appropriate. The grandchild is not considered acceptable unless a legal relationship exists. Also grandmothers who live in subsidized elderly housing where children are not allowed even with a legal relationship are in jeopardy. Eviction is a real possibility (AARP, 1997; Wagner, 1995).

Support. Although not widespread, programs designed for grandparents raising grandchildren seem to help decrease the stress and burden experienced. Support groups are a common type of community intervention. These groups most often are started and run by grandparents and may be sponsored by a community agency or religious organization. Although supported through an agency or organization, usually no funding is provided (Minkler & Roe, 1996).

Comprehensive programs, although few in number, provide a variety of services such as counseling, parenting classes, help for the child, and support groups. These programs are funded. If funding is generous, programs may include peer counseling and respite care. The programs differ according to the needs of the grandparents, the resources available, and the geographic location. Aid to Imprisoned Mothers works with families and tries to address the needs of the grandmothers who are now in the role of parent (Barnhill, 1996). Funding from the Administration on Aging, foundations, religious organizations, and donors enable Aid to Imprisoned Mothers to respond to a variety of needs of the grandmothers and their incarcerated daughters.

Advocacy groups and coalitions have been formed to work on the national level for reforms that address the complex needs of the grandparents as parents. Many states are initiating creative programs that include mechanisms allowing grandparents without a formal, legal relationship with the grandchildren to enroll children in schools, receive medical care, and find adequate housing (Beltran, 2000). Grandparents as parents experience physical, social, psychological, and financial problems. The nurse can help make a difference through development of programs for support, individual counseling, and health care that is sensitive to the needs of the entire family. Collaboration with the case manager helps grandparents find needed resources and ensures that they remain in the health care system. The advance practice nurse also can act as an advocate for legislation that provides grandparents with the same rights and benefits given to foster parents.

Elder Abuse

Elder abuse is not a new phenomenon. Elder abuse and neglect, a form of domestic violence, present major health care problems for women. The actual prevalence of abuse of elderly women is difficult to determine, and unfortunately, elder abuse receives little attention (Kleinschmidt, 1997). Elderly abused women have been referred to as the invisible population (Brandl & Raymond, 1996). A short review of indexes and tables of contents in a few geriatric medicine texts by noted geriatricians shows that information on elder abuse is omitted (Byyny & Speroff, 1996; Kane et al., 1999; Rowe & Kahn, 1998).

Research on abuse of older women is often in one geographic area (Brandl & Raymond, 1997; Krueger & Patterson, 1997; Rosenblatt, Cho, & Durance, 1996; Willams, 1996) and therefore cannot be generalized. More important, elder abuse is underreported. Research identifies lack of knowledge about abuse, concern about offending the patient or family, concern about repercussions aimed at the elder, lack of guidelines for assessment, lack of protocols to deal with elder abuse, and lack of knowledge about reporting requirements (Kleinschmidt, 1997; Krueger & Patterson, 1997).

Not until the 1970s did researchers attempt to define elder abuse clearly. According to Glendenning (1993), however, a lack of agreement regarding the conceptualization of abuse and neglect continues. When examining definitions since 1979, he found that topologies and conceptualizations differed between studies. As is common, the definition changes according to the research question and purpose. In addition, no agreement exists on whether elder abuse differs from other forms of domestic violence or differs from neglect and other types of abuse.

For the purpose of this chapter, the following classifications and definitions first delineated by Wolf and Pillemer (1989) are used. Theirs is one of the early attempts to differentiate between abuse and neglect. Elder abuse generally is considered the systematic mistreatment of an elder. The abuser varies according to the environment (domestic or institutional); however, the most common abuser is someone in the caregiving role.

When exploring definitions of elder abuse and neglect, the literature may use classifications other than those identified in Box 18-8.

Characteristics of the Victim

According to the *Statistical Handbook on Aging Americans* (Schick & Schick, 1994), the victims of elder abuse are predominantly female (68%). In 1991 the highest percentage of elder abused were those age 85 and older. The percentage of abused elders therefore increases as age increases. The most vulnerable are the elderly who have cognitive and communication problems (Glendenning, 1993).

Certain characteristics are common in victims (Decalmer, 1994; Kleinschmidt, 1997; Raymond, 1994). Summarizing the literature, the abused elder is most often a woman over 75 who is too poor to live independently, has physical and mental impairment, is depressed, and is socially isolated. She may take on the sick role easily,

Box 18-8 CLASSIFICATION AND DEFINITIONS OF ELDER ABUSE

Active neglect: Actual refusal or failure to carry out caregiving role, including intentional attempts to cause physical or mental distress. Example: Withholding items necessary for daily living (Hudson, 1997).

Legal mistreatment (Johnson, 1991): Material misuse of property, contracts, theft or extortion of property or contracts, denial of contracts, unnecessary guardianship, and misuse of professional role. Could be included as medical abuse and sociological mistreatment.

Material abuse: Exploitation or use of funds or resources. Includes misuse of property or money, theft, forcible admission to a nursing home, and creation of financial dependency (Krueger & Patterson, 1997; Raymond, 1994). Exploitation and financial abuse is reported to be 17% of elder abuse (Schick & Schick, 1994).

Medical abuse (Johnson, 1991): Withholding of medications or careless, improper, or unnecessary use of medications. Often encompassed in physical abuse. Also could be part of active or passive neglect.

Passive neglect: Failure or refusal to assume the caregiving role but does not include intentional attempts to inflict physical or mental distress. Example: Isolating and leaving the older person alone (Hudson, 1997; Raymond, 1994). Neglect is reported to protective service agencies as one category and accounts for 45% of elder abuse (Schick & Schick, 1994).

Physical abuse: Physical harm, injury, physical coercion, sexual molestation, physical restraint inflicted by someone else. Johnson (1991) adds to this definition medication misuse and bodily impairment such as unmet medical and physical needs. Physical abuse accounts for 19% of elder abuse and sexual abuse for 0.6% (Schick & Schick, 1994).

Psychological abuse: Mental anguish inflicted by someone else. Subclassifications by Johnson (1991) include humiliation (shame, blame, and rejection), harassment (insults, intimidation, and fear), manipulation (information withheld or untrue, emotional deprivation, and decision making prohibited). Psychological and emotional abuse represents almost 14% of reported abuse of elders (Schick & Schick, 1994).

Sociological mistreatment (Johnson, 1991): Isolation, inadequate or improper supervision, lack of privacy, poor environment, and abandonment. Wolf and Pillemer (1989) suggest sociological mistreatment may be assumed in any of the other classifications.

refusing any attempt for help. In addition, she has low self-esteem, blames herself for the abuse, and is reluctant to admit she is vulnerable or does not want to betray the family (Kleinschmidt, 1997).

Characteristics of the Abuser

Characteristically, many elderly women are abused by a loved family member (Brandl & Raymond, 1997; Lachs & Pillemer, 1995). More than 31% of abusers are adult children. Abuse by the spouse is next at 14.4%, followed by other relatives at 12.5%. Other abusers are grandchildren, service providers, friends and neighbors, and siblings (Schick & Schick, 1994). The increase in abuse with age likely results from increasing demands on the caregiver. Frequently the caregiver is the daughter or daughter-in-law. The older person lives with a family in which both parents are employed and often in households with young or teenage children. The care is often difficult and nonstop. The care places stress on the family system and on the financial, social, psychological, and physical resources of the caregiver.

Although the notion of caregiver stress is a logical conclusion as to causation of elder abuse, Brandl and Raymond (1996) and Kleinschmidt (1997) maintain that research on domestic violence in late life does not validate this hypothesis. Kleinschmidt (1997) suggests that the causative factors in abuse of older women are the emotional and financial dependency of the caregiver on the elder.

Decalmer (1994) summarized the literature and characteristics of the abuser as a relative who lives with the victim and has cared for her for at least 9 to 10 years. The relative is usually an adult child, most frequently the daughter who is having marital conflict and who uses ineffective coping mechanisms such as alcohol or drugs. In addition, the person may have given up employment to provide care and is isolated socially and depressed, angry, or hostile. The family experiences a high level of burden, including financial problems frequently requiring the victim's money or home. Communication between the victim and abuser is poor, and parent-child hostilities may have been unresolved.

Assessment

What is important is for the women's health care nurse to be aware of the types of abuse, typical victims of abuse, the characteristics of abusers, and the family situations and environments in which abuse may occur. The issues are complex, as are the strategies for assessing and managing abusive situations. Frequently the older person will not report mistreatment by family members, and families will not broach the subject readily, yet research indicates that 63% of hospitalizations are repeat admissions for severe abuse (Fulmer, McMahon, Baer-Hines, & Forget, 1992). Professionals are important in the identification of elder abuse. In the community, health care professionals report up to 35% of their elderly patients are victims of abuse (Sadler & Kurrie, 1993). The most effective factor in identification of elder abuse has been professional and public awareness (Schick & Schick, 1994).

The nurse, when interviewing the older woman, should include questions about abuse; however, the older woman may not offer information readily. Establishing an atmosphere of trust, offering to interview the woman alone, and being calm, unhurried, and nonjudgmental facilitates open conversation. In addition, using the characteristics of the victims and abusers helps identify the women at risk for abuse. Box 18-9 identifies risk factors for elder abuse and neglect by a family member or spouse.

During the interview, the clinician also may notice behaviors that might indicate a potentially abusive situation (AARP, 1996):

1. The woman is unable to provide information without presence of partner caregiver.
2. The partner demonstrates aggressive behaviors toward the woman.
3. The partner seems to control her.
4. The partner does not show affection or seems indifferent.

Signs and symptoms of abuse relate to the type of abusive situation. Many times, the older abused woman is subjected to multiple types of abuse. Physical abuse is the easiest

---

Box 18-9 RISK FACTORS FOR ELDER ABUSE AND NEGLECT BY A FAMILY MEMBER

Alcohol or drug abuse
Mental illness in the family member
History of domestic violence in the family
Control of finances by potential abuser
Cognitive problems in caregiver and/or elder
Unwanted role as caregiver
Dependency of caregiver on elder for finances and housing
Social isolation of the elder
Caregiver is a spouse or adult child
Poor housing
Lack of family or community supports

Sources: American Association of Retired Persons. (1996). Helping older women at risk of partner abuse. *Women's Initiative Fact Sheet.* Washington DC: Author. Jones, J., Holstege, C., & Holstege, H. (1997). Elder abuse and neglect: Understanding the causes and potential risk factors. *American Journal of Emergency Medicine, 15,* 579-583.

to identify. However, a complete physical examination may indicate additional types of abuse (AARP, 1996; Raymond, 1994). Box 18-10 lists some signs and symptoms for which the nurse should be alert during the physical examination. Many of the signs and symptoms may be attributed to common problems of the elderly (dizziness and falls, poor balance, and easy bruising). Therefore an awareness of the potential for abuse helps in the diagnosis of elder abuse.

Management

Once abuse is suspected, most states have mandatory reporting. In severe or dangerous situations, the older woman should be removed from the setting and, if necessary, hospitalized until the situation is made safe. The nurse needs to facilitate the provision of services. Resources to call on may be found in the geriatric interdisciplinary team, including the social worker, counselor, and case manager. Homemaking services, day programs, respite programs, and inhome support also may be available (Krueger & Patterson, 1997).

Nurses are needed to work with community agencies to assure services that have been proved effective in prevention of the first occurrence of elder abuse. The most effective measure is the provision of in-home services for the elderly. In addition, in-home respite care, community support services, counseling, and interagency coordination have been found effective preventive strategies (Krueger & Patterson, 1997; Schick & Schick, 1994).

Polypharmacy

Polypharmacy usually is defined as concurrent use of five or more different medications, often including more than one medication from the same classification.

Box 18-10 COMMON SIGNS AND SYMPTOMS OF ELDER ABUSE

Bruises and Welts
Unexplained
Several areas
Different stages of healing
Shaped like article causing the injury
Clustered

Burns
Unexplained
Rope marks
Wrists and ankles
Cigar or cigarette burns

Sexual Abuse
Problems walking or sitting
Underclothes stained, torn, or bloody
Pain and itching in genital area
Bruises and bleeding in vaginal or anal area

Neglect
Poor hygiene
Dress that is inappropriate
Lack of supervision
Unmet physical or medical needs

Psychological
Depression
Apathy
Vague physical complaints
Verbalization indicating lack of self-worth

Source: Raymond, R. (1994). Elder abuse and victimization: The hidden epidemic. *Geriatric Care and Rehabilitation, 7*, 2–8.

The problems of polypharmacy are compounded by physiological changes of aging, multiple chronic illnesses requiring complex medication regimens, the use of multiple providers that prescribe medications without thorough exploration of current medication use, and the use of more than one pharmacy. In addition, the media targets problems associated with aging to promote over-the-counter drugs. Drug misuse includes medications to counteract the side effects of other prescribed medications, inappropriate dosages, concurrent use of medications that produce drug-drug interactions or drug-patient interactions, and use of medications that are contraindicated for the elderly.

Polypharmacy, chronic disease, and the elderly go hand in hand. Polypharmacy is implicated in many issues that the older woman experiences, particularly incontinence, falls, depression, and sexuality. Currently, the elderly comprise about 12% of the population and consume 30% or more of prescription medications and over-the-counter drugs (Lassila et al., 1996; U.S. Department of Health and Human Services, 1990). As the population of older and oldest-old increases and new drugs are developed to treat chronic illness, polypharmacy will continue to grow as a problem especially for women.

Lassila and others (1996) examined prescription medications use by 1360 rural elders. The self-reported use of prescriptions showed that 71% used at least one prescribed medication and 10% reported taking five or more. Women took significantly more medications than men, including nonsteroidal antiinflammatory drugs, antidepressants, potassium supplements, and thyroid replacement medications. Findings in a large epidemiological study of medication use among persons 65 and older revealed that prescription and nonprescription medications are used more frequently among women. Prescription medications were used by 68% to 78% of women but by only 60% to 68% of the men, and nonprescription medications were used by 64% to 76% of women but only by 52% to 68% of the men (Chrischilles et al., 1992).

Problems associated with polypharmacy include alterations in fluid and electrolyte balance (Miller, 1997), hyponatremia in women using selective serotonin reuptake inhibitors (SSRIs) (Lane, 1997), hyperkalemia (Perazella & Mahnensmith, 1997), syncope (Forman & Lipsitz, 1997), falls (Koski, Luukinen, Laippala, & Livela, 1996; Monane & Avorn, 1996), delirium and other alterations in cognition (Inouye & Charpentier, 1996; Jacobson, 1997; Oxman, 1996), and increased length of hospital stays (Yuen, Zisselman, Louis, & Rovner, 1997). In addition, use of multiple medications may result in noncompliance and medication errors (Hunter, Florio, Rosmond, & Langberg, 1996).

Many of the problems are considered adverse drug reactions (ADRs) that may occur 2 to 3 times more frequently in the elderly (Jinks & Fuerst, 1995). In addition to the many reasons for medication misuse described previously, physiological changes may account for ADRs. The efficiency of the cardiovascular and nervous systems decreases, thereby changing homeostatic mechanisms; drug metabolism and excretion decreases; body tissue composition and distribution of drugs changes; and possibly drug receptor sensitivity changes (Jinks & Fuerst, 1995). Kane and others (1999) and Noyes (1997) summarized the changes in pharmacodynamics and pharmacokinetics that occur as a woman ages.

Excretion

Of the four mechanisms in drug disposition (absorption, distribution, metabolism, and excretion), excretion is the most important to consider regarding prescribing medication and potential ADRs among elderly clients. Renal function declines considerably with age as does the number of nephrons. In addition to normal physiological changes, most older persons have arteriosclerotic changes and a decrease in cardiac output. The result is a decrease of about 50% in renal perfusion and a corresponding decrease in glomerular filtration and urea clearance. The ability of the kidney to concentrate urine, conserve sodium, and clear creatinine decreases with advanced age as does tubular excretion. Any medication that relies on the kidney for excretion places the individual at risk for an ADR because of the prolongation of the plasma half-life of the drug.

Distribution

Aging is accompanied by changes in body composition, including a decrease in total body water and lean body mass and an increase in total fat. The volume of drugs primarily distributed in body water or lean body mass is decreased (e.g., digoxin), whereas highly lipid-soluble drugs (e.g., benzodiazepines) may be increased, resulting in delay of maximal effects or accumulation of the drug over time. In addition, older adults are often deficient in protein in their diets and therefore have low serum albumin. In this instance, an increase in circulating drugs binds to protein, again causing a potential ADR.

Metabolism

The liver is the main organ involved in metabolism of some drugs. With aging, liver function changes; however, the relationship between ADRs and changes in liver function is unclear. Although the relationship is equivocal, caution should be used when prescribing medications with high rates of metabolism through the hepatic system (nitrates and propranolol). As French (1996) points out, liver metabolism occurs in two phases. Phase I breaks down the drug through oxidation and the use of enzymes, and phase II renders the drug water soluble for elimination. Prolonged drug effects are found with aging and are related to the processes of phase I rather than phase II metabolism.

Homeostasis

With aging, the homeostatic mechanisms alter so that drug side effects are common. The increased incidence of side effects with age probably is caused by a combination of a decrease in synthesis of neurotransmitters, chronic illness, and altered physiological mechanisms. For instance, baroreceptor function is not efficient and the cerebral blood flow autoregulation decreases, resulting in orthostatic hypotension. This age-related change is exacerbated by drugs with sympatholytic activity and those that are volume-depleting and vasodilating.

Target Organ Sensitivity

One final complicating factor in the complexity of medications for the elderly lies in the target organ sensitivity. With aging, many physiological changes contribute to an exaggerated response to drugs (see the previous section). Decreases in neurotransmitters, diminished homeostatic responses, and declines in some of the usual inhibitory and excitatory pathways, but with preservation of others, contribute to altered pharmacodynamics and pharmacokinetics. The decrease in cholinergic pathways creates sensitivity to drugs with anticholinergic properties, creating cognitive problems such as confusion and mental fogginess. Altered target organ sensitivity occurs for heparin and warfarin in females (Jinks & Fuerst, 1995). Decreases in beta-receptor stimulation and alterations in the beta-adrenergic autonomic nervous system also occur. Beta-blockers, beta-agonists, and calcium channel blockers frequently produce less of a response in older adults compared with younger adults (French, 1996; Jinks & Fuerst, 1995; Semla, Beizer, & Higbee, 1997).

Assessment

Medications are the cause of a variety of problems in the elderly; they are the primary cause of confusion and other cognitive problems and may be the cause of depression, falls, and incontinence. For this reason, each time an elderly person is examined, current medications should be reviewed, including herbal, alternative remedies, alcohol, and over-the-counter medications. The traditional brown bag approach is a nonthreatening way to identify medication patterns. When using this approach, the older person is requested to bring *all* prescription, over-the-counter, and other medications or herbal preparations being used. At each subsequent visit, the person should be questioned about new medications, other providers, and pharmacies being used. In addition, changes in function, cognition, elimination, activity, mood, sleep, and nutrition need to be evaluated at each visit. Frequently, the elderly do not report changes they consider insignificant or a part of growing old.

Medications then need to be examined for appropriateness using the following criteria (French, 1996):

■ Length of time on the medication
■ Purpose of the medication
■ Dose appropriateness
■ Contraindications for the elderly
■ More than one medication for the same purpose or duplicate medications
■ Use of medication to counteract side effects of other medications

Although polypharmacy is a recognized problem among the elderly, one also must recognize that most medications are necessary for continued health and function. In addition, the ability to follow medication regimens is a complex task requiring cognitive and functional capacities. Research indicates that the elderly who are unable to take medications appropriately have a rapid decline in function and other indicators of health. The ability of an elder to take medications independently has been found actually to predict functional decline (Edelberg, Shallenberger, Hausdorff, & Wei, 2000). Therefore the ability of the older person to manage medications is an important part of the assessment.

Frequently the elderly do not follow the prescribed regimen, and the reasons include the high number of medications to be taken, declining cognition, poor understanding of therapeutic regimen, cost of the drugs, inability to use drug containers, decreasing or discontinuing a medication, and not taking the medication because no symptoms or problems exist. Therefore the patient needs to be questioned about the medication routine and whether the prescribed therapy is being followed.

Being able to predict or recognize a patient's ability to manage medications is an important function of the nurse. One possible approach is using an instrument designed specifically to test the ability of an older person to manage medications

(Edelberg et al., 2000). The instrument (DRUGS) involves four medication management tasks:

1. Identification of medication
2. Ability to access containers
3. Taking the proper dosage
4. Taking the medication at the correct time

Interrater and test-retest reliability of the DRUGS instrument were greater than 0.90. The self-administration of medication demonstration can be performed in the clinical setting and takes 4 to 5 minutes (see Edelberg, Shallenberger, & Wei, 1999, for more information).

If the medication regimen needs changing, the nurse must take extra time to ensure understanding and the ability of the older woman to manage the regimen independently. Reasons for changing the routine need to be discussed with the patient, family, and caregivers. Independent management capacity is facilitated if the medication routine is as simple as possible, if medication frequency is the same for a number of medications (twice daily, 3 times daily, etc.), and if the person is able to afford the medication. In addition, using daily or weekly pill containers when appropriate and making sure to include family and caregivers in the proper use of medications is also helpful in securing follow-through with the medication regimen.

Laboratory data at baseline and in the presence of changes are helpful in determining potential problems. Tests for electrolytes, serum albumin, liver function, and renal function should be included. Serum creatinine is not appropriate for the elderly because creatinine is produced by muscles. The older person may have normal serum creatinine because of the decrease in lean body mass that occurs with aging yet have severely impaired renal function. Although a 24-hour urine for creatinine is the most accurate method, obtaining a 24-hour specimen may be problematic. For that reason, using the Cockcroft-Gault formula for estimating creatinine clearance is important:

$$\text{Creatinine clearance} = \frac{(140 - \text{age}) \times (\text{mass in Kg})}{72 \times \text{serum creatinine in mg/dl}}$$

For women, the result is multiplied by 0.85.

Management

Most older persons eventually need pharmaceutical therapies (medications). However, adding new medications and discontinuing medications must be done with caution. Given the potential for problems because of prolonged half-life of a drug, an increase in medication in free circulation, changes in receptor sites, altered elimination and metabolism of drugs, a wise practitioner uses the first rule of geriatric pharmacotherapy, "start low, go slow," when prescribing. Before prescribing a new medication, one should first examine the current medications to ensure appropriateness. The beginning dose should be the lowest possible dose, even a pediatric dose for some medications.

Discontinuing medications may be possible and indeed is an important intervention. However, adverse events can be associated with stopping a medication. The most common adverse event is exacerbation of underlying disease, especially when circulatory and central nervous system drug classes are discontinued (Graves et al., 1997). As with starting medications, discontinuing them should be a gradual process with frequent monitoring.

Prescriptions

Adverse drug reactions are associated with the number of drugs taken and occur more often in women because they take more medications than men (French, 1996). Given the large amount of information provided in various drug resource manuals, discerning appropriate geriatric medications, dosages, and contraindications often is difficult. The *Geriatric Dosage Handbook* (Semla et al., 1997) and *Essentials of Clinical Geriatrics* (Kane et al., 1999) are excellent references for the advanced practice nurse. Boxes 18-11 and 18-12 list general principles in medication management of the elderly and guidelines for prescribing.

Box 18-13 lists some of these medications that are contraindicated or are to be used with caution in the elderly. For complete lists and precautions in prescribing, the nurse practitioner is referred to the *Geriatric Dosage Handbook* (Semla et al., 1997). Drugs that are contraindicated or are not the drug of choice for the elderly are so because of poor effectiveness or greater toxicity in the elderly. For further information, French (1996) or Semla and others (1997) should be consulted. In addition, two recent studies clearly identify inappropriate medications and explain reasons such as side effects and toxicity in the elderly (Aparasu & Fliginger, 1997; Beers, 1997).

Falls

Falls are a major problem for elderly women and, as with all elder syndromes, have complex causes. Many falls are related to polypharmacy and urinary incontinence. Falls cause serious injury, including hip and other fractures, and frequently result in impaired function for the long term. Falls are also the cause of mortality and morbidity and

---

Box **18-11** PRINCIPLES OF MEDICATION MANAGEMENT FOR THE ELDERLY

1. Drug pharmacology is influenced by many interrelated factors that in turn influence physiological changes of aging.
2. As with many geriatric issues, no textbook examples exist. Physiological changes that influence drug pharmacology vary greatly.
3. The clinical condition of each person and the physiological changes have an effect on drug pharmacology and must be taken into consideration. Included in assessment of the clinical status are nutritional status, hydration, renal and liver disease, and probable cardiac output.

Sources: French, D. (1996). Avoiding adverse drug reactions in the elderly patient: Issues and strategies. *Nurse Practitioner, 21,* 90–105. Stewart, J., & Cooper, J. (1994). Polypharmacy in the aged: Practical solutions. *Drugs and Aging, 4,* 449–461.

Box 18-12 GUIDELINES FOR PRESCRIBING MEDICATIONS FOR THE ELDERLY

1. Know the drugs the person is using, including over-the-counter drugs, herbs, and alcohol.
2. Evaluate cognitive status, vision, hearing, and functional status in an effort to facilitate compliance.
3. Consider the need for the drug and the risk vs. benefit.
4. Do not use one drug to treat the side effects of another drug.
5. Whenever possible, use nonpharmacological methods to manage illness.
6. Evaluate the patient and identify physiological and pathological changes that alter pharmacodynamics and pharmacokinetics.
7. Consider problems that the medication will help, those it might exacerbate or negatively affect, and those the efficacy of which it might change.
8. Clearly identify the goals of the provider, patient, family, and caregiver for using drugs.
9. Prescribe the fewest drugs possible, avoiding adverse drug reactions and making compliance easier.
10. Suspect that drugs are the cause of changes in health status.
11. Monitor changes: cognition, behavior, mood, falls, and incontinence.
12. Start with the lowest possible dose and increase slowly. Discontinue medications when possible.
13. Provide ongoing patient/family/caregiver education.
14. Use written information on the drug, the reason for using, the dose and frequency, and possible side effects to report.
15. Discuss possible interactions with other drugs, over-the-counter drugs, alcohol, caffeine, herbs and other alternative remedies, and food.
16. Discuss problems that need to be reported.
17. Encourage use of one provider and one pharmacy or collaborate with multiple providers.

Sources: French, D. (1996). Avoiding adverse drug reactions in the elderly patient: Issues and strategies. *Nurse Practitioner, 21*, 90–105. Stewart, J., & Cooper, J. (1994). Polypharmacy in the aged: Practical solutions. *Drugs and Aging, 4*, 449–461.

increase health care costs. Falls and their sequelae represent a potential area for prevention. Among the elderly, about 25% age 65 to 74 and more than 33% age 75 and older report falling in the previous year (Nevitt, 1990). Elderly may be classified as fallers or nonfallers. Multiple falls are common, and more than 66% of persons who fall will have another fall within 6 months (Hornbrook et al., 1994).

Falls tend to have more consequences for women than for men, usually because of osteoporotic changes in bone. However, compounding the problem of decreasing bone density, muscle mass and strength also decline. Leg strength in older women is 23% less than in older men (Frontera, Hughes, Lutz, & Evans, 1991). In addition, Cao, Ashton-Miller, Schultz, and Alexander (1997) found that women were less able than their male counterparts to make sudden turns successfully. Other physical factors associated with falls are strength and balance. Woolley, Czaja, and Drury (1997) found that among fallers was a significantly reduced static balance, reduced ability to walk and descend stairs, and an increase in reaction time. Wolfson, Judge, Whipple, and King (1995) found that in addition to balance and gait, falls were associated with poor knee and

Box **18-13** DRUGS CONTRAINDICATED IN OR TO BE USED WITH CAUTION FOR THE ELDERLY

Contraindicated

Benzodiazepines (long acting)
Chlordiazpoxide (Librium)
Clorazepate (Tranxene)
Diazepam (Valium)
Prazepam (Centrax)

Sedatives/Hypnotics
Flurazepam (Dalmane)
Quazepam (Doral)
Pentobarbital
Secobarbital
Meprobamate
Glutethimide (Doriden)
Ethchlorvynol (Placidyl)

Antidepressants
Amitriptyline (Elavil)
Nonsteroidal antiinflammatory drugs
Indomethacin

Analgesics
Pentazocine (Talwin)

Muscle relaxants
Orphenidrate (Norflex)
Cyclobenzaprine (Flexeril)
Carisoprodol (Soma)

Hypoglycemic agents
Chlorpropamide (Diabinese)

Use With Caution
Cardiovascular Drugs
Digoxin
Propranolol
Methyldopa
Reserpine
Volume-depleting drugs

Sources: French, D. (1996). Avoiding adverse drug reactions in the elderly patient: Issues and strategies. *Nurse Practitioner, 21,* 90–105. Kane, R., Ouslander, J., & Abrass, I. (1999). *Essentials of clinical geriatrics* (4th ed.). New York: McGraw-Hill. Semla, T., Beizer, J., & Higbee, M. (1997). *Geriatric dosage handbook* (3rd ed.). Cleveland: Lexi-Comp.

ankle strength. Finally, Richardson and Hurvitz (1995) found that the elderly with peripheral neuropathy were at a higher risk for falls than those without peripheral neuropathy. Therefore age-related and pathological changes in the musculoskeletal, neurological, and cognitive systems are implicated in assessing the risk for falls (Woollacott, 2000).

Risk Factors

Risk factors for falls usually are classified as intrinsic and extrinsic. In addition to physical changes associated with aging, intrinsic factors include vertigo, syncope, vision and hearing impairment, prior cardiovascular accident, cardiovascular disease including arrhythmias, and cognitive and neurological changes. Many intrinsic factors make adjustments to environmental risks difficult. For example, changes in vision include poor adaptation to changes in perceptual ability so that a floor may appear level when it is not, causing a trip. Another major risk involves the multiple medications individuals take for various chronic health problems. Medications can change cognition and cause orthostatic hypotension and dizziness. Multiple physiological changes also may contribute to poor nutrition and poor fluid intake, resulting in anemia and dizziness from orthostatic hypotension. Woolley and others (1997) also found that fallers significantly differed from nonfallers in the areas of static balance, walking, and stair descent. In addition, fallers had poor attention to tasks and increased reaction times.

External risk factors include environmental hazards such as inadequate lighting, loose rugs, slippery or wet floors, poor home maintenance, and objects in walkways. Hazards also may be outside the home and include uneven walkways, lack of railings on stairs, and weather hazards.

Assessment

Assessment of the older woman should always include identification or risk factors for falls. The history is crucial in the identification of causative factors and the development of possible interventions to prevent falls. Although not all older women fall, all need to be considered at risk for falls. Those women who have fallen in the past 6 weeks are at particular risk of repeat falls. The following information should be gathered on the first and subsequent visits:

1. Has the woman fallen in the past 6 weeks? (Ask for a description of the fall and circumstances and number of falls in the past year.)
2. Medication history: All medications including prescribed, over-the-counter, and those given to the client by others
3. Illnesses: Common chronic problems such as diabetes, coronary heart disease, congestive heart failure, chronic obstructive pulmonary disease
4. Exacerbations of illness
5. Ability to perform ADL, including behaviors associated with hurrying and driving
6. Nutrition and fluids
7. History of dizziness or fainting
8. History of incontinence
9. Alcohol intake

The physical examination does not differ from any complete physical. However, if the older woman has a history of falls or risk factors for falls, the nurse needs to focus on particular aspects of the examination. Box 18-14 identifies areas of focus for the physical examination of the older woman at risk for falls. In addition, diagnostic testing should include a complete blood count, urinalysis, chemical profile, thyroid function test, and electrocardiogram.

Box 18-14 PHYSICAL EXAMINATION FOR WOMEN AT RISK FOR FALLS

1. Vision and hearing screening
2. Balance and gait: Include ability to move from sitting to standing and walking, ability to make turns, and reaction time
3. Strength: Include ankle, knee, and leg
4. Sensory: Include peripheral vision
5. Cognition
6. Depression
7. Orthostatic hypotension

Management

The interdisciplinary team is invaluable in fall prevention and management programs. Depending on the cause of the falls, a case manager may be needed to coordinate the various resources. Given the extensive list of possible causes, the nurse rules out many intrinsic factors and whenever possible can identify the problem. The nurse is involved in a variety of health teaching. An exercise program as described previously in the chapter may be required to improve the woman's strength, balance, gait, and endurance.

Collaboration with a physical therapist and occupational therapist improves the outcome of any exercise program or other prescribed intervention. The physical therapist can provide a complete musculoskeletal evaluation and develop a program aimed at the functional needs of the client. The occupational therapist adds to the evaluation and then is able to teach the client safe ways to manage ADL and IADL. The entire team should make a home visit to evaluate the extrinsic factors with the client. Other possible team members may be a psychologist or other health professional appropriate for evaluation and management of mental health or cognitive problems, nutritionist for assistance with dietary needs, and a social worker for assistance with financial problems that limit home improvements or the ability to manage health promotion needs.

Sexuality

The importance of sexuality among older women often is overlooked. For women, many normal changes of aging have an affect on feelings about growing old. In American society, youth and associated beauty are revered. Aging is accompanied by outward signs such as thinner, looser, wrinkled skin; thinning, graying hair; and changes in fat distribution. Visual changes may herald a first-time need for glasses. Internally, menopause and the decrease in estrogen may create vaginal dryness and sometimes difficulty with intercourse. In addition, the decrease in estrogen and atrophic vaginitis may produce incontinence. Energy levels, strength, and endurance may decrease, particularly if planned exercise was not part of an earlier lifestyle. At every turn, women seem to be faced with their own aging. Taken in combination, a woman may feel less attractive than younger counterparts, leading to a poor self-concept and changes in feelings about intimate relationships.

Human sexuality is a basic need and does not suddenly end with menopause. Sexuality and sexual activity in older women is a function of social, psychological, moral, and physiological factors. Sexuality is multidimensional and a personal experience. Although sexuality and sexual intercourse often are used synonymously, sexual intercourse is not the sum of sexuality. Sexuality is one part of quality of life. Decline in sexual activity with aging is more the result of unavailability of a healthy partner than with physiological changes. Sexuality continues even without sexual intercourse because the need for affection, intimacy, and touch remains until death.

Physiological changes do occur. In men and women, the phases of excitation, plateau, orgasm, and resolution continue into old age. However, the following widely recognized changes in women have an effect on sexual pleasure:

Excitation: Lubrication is delayed or diminished.

               Vaginal canal has decreased elastic expansion.

Plateau: Muscle tension decreases.

               Less secretion comes from Bartholin glands.

               Less vasocongestion occurs.

Orgasm: Orgasmic contractions are fewer and less intense.

Resolution: Vasocongestion in clitoral area and orgasmic platform resolves quickly.

Although these changes occur in response to decreased estrogen and decline in sexual activity, sexual desire is not contingent on estrogen and progesterone. The adrenal gland supplies adequate amounts of androgens to sustain sexual desire, and hormone replacement therapy or vaginal estrogen cream can decrease the feeling of dryness and painful intercourse.

A major factor in sexuality in aging women is her health or her partner's health. Chronic illness may contribute to a decline in sexual desire and sexual response. Arthritis and accompanying pain, stiffness, and fatigue may decrease sexual activity. Heart disease may create a fear of MI or cardiovascular accident with sexual intercourse. Diabetes may lead to less sexual desire and lubrication in women (Katz, 1991) and impotence in men. Chronic obstructive pulmonary disease may decrease endurance and contribute to fatigue as well as inhibit expression because of coughing and dyspnea.

Women who have had a hysterectomy or mastectomy also may experience changes in sexuality Women who have had a hysterectomy may have a decrease in sexual pleasure because of the loss of movement or contraction of the cervix or uterus. However, sexuality itself is not changed with a hysterectomy. Occasionally, women have problems postoperatively that cannot be accounted for physically. A careful preoperative history and understanding of the physical aspects of a hysterectomy may help anticipate possible outcomes (Bachmann, 1990; Virtanen et al., 1993). Although no physiological changes occur with a mastectomy, women may experience a strong psychological affect. Depression, fear of rejection, and changed body image may occur and can result in loss of sexual desire.

One final area that is seldom discussed involves issues of lesbian couples, particularly older lesbian couples. Women over 60 who are lesbians tend to maintain a low profile, live alone, and are celibate but desire a relationship (Deevey, 1990). Many have been married previously and may have children, but the major part of the support system is a network of lesbian friends (Quam & Whitford, 1992). Further research on this topic is needed.

Assessment

When assessing an older woman's sexuality and sexual activity, exploring attitudes, environment, opportunity, and health of the partner as well as the physical and psychosocial concerns of the woman is important. Sexual activity in old age is a continuation of a lifelong pattern. Attitudes may be influenced by society and cohorts. Older women may not be seen as sexual beings, and health care professionals tend to omit discussions about sexual activity of the older person, particularly the woman. Environmental barriers include lack of privacy, particularly if the older woman is living with a child or in an institution. In addition, many medications alter sexual desire and sexual response.

Many health care providers hesitate to question the elderly about sexual issues. The nurse introducing the topic of sexuality by simply stating that she will be discussing sexuality and sexual functioning is often helpful. The practitioner may want to lead in with a statement about the difficulty many persons have in discussing what is considered private.

History

Because sexuality and sexual activity have lifelong patterns, starting with attitudes, beliefs, psychological issues, and family issues may be best. Questions may include those on the importance of sexual activity throughout life, current feelings about sex, and whether intimacy needs are being met. Also, the nurse should inquire as to personal, moral, and religious values that influence sexuality.

The following list of questions are part of any sexual assessment of the older woman:

■ Are you sexually active?
■ What is your sexual preference?
■ What concerns you most about your sexual life?
■ Has any change in your desire for sexual intercourse or sexual activity occurred?
■ Do you experience any discomfort with sexual activity?
■ Do you have vaginal dryness?
■ Are you able to achieve orgasm?
■ Are you and your partner healthy?
■ What type of sexual activity do you enjoy?
■ Is masturbation an option for you?
■ How satisfied are you with your current sexual activity and sexuality? (Using a scale of 1 to 10 helps.)
■ With whom do you live?
■ Does your current living environment allow an opportunity for sexual expression?

- Do you think your partner has any concerns about sexuality or problems with sexual activity?
- Are you able to discuss sexuality with your partner?

The following issues should also be addressed:

- Both the patient and her partner should be asked about medications and chronic health problems.
- The patient should be asked about her obstetrical and gynecological history.
- Information should be obtained on past or current traumatic or negative sexual experiences.

Physical Examination

The sexual response requires functioning of four systems: emotional state of excitement, nervous system pathways that control pelvic blood flow, pelvic circulation, and sex hormones. The physical examination does not differ from the normal examination. However, the practitioner needs to be alert for potential barriers to sexual expression. Box 18-15 identifies areas of the physical examination that focus on sexuality. Sexuality is an area that the older woman or couple may want to discuss. Providers do not always provide opportunities to discuss concerns. Concerns are often present and information is desired.

Incontinence

Urinary incontinence is one common problem that has a major affect on many aspects of life and may have a profound effect on sexuality. Incontinence also is known to be a causative factor in falls and can contribute to social isolation, which in turn may cause confusion and depression. Urinary incontinence in elderly women, a common and often treatable problem, may result in isolation, depression, and nursing home placement.

Box 18-15 PHYSICAL EXAMINATION WITH A FOCUS ON SEXUALITY AND THE OLDER WOMAN

General: Cognition, weight, and emotions
Skin: Impaired sensation, lesions, and turgor
HEENT: Vision and hearing
Respiratory: Cough, dyspnea, and respiratory effort with activity
Cardiovascular: Coronary heart disease, hypertension, arrhythmias, atherosclerosis, and pulses
Gastrointestinal: Abdomen—surgical scars that could cause alteration in pelvic enervation and ostomy equipment
  Bowel habits—constipation
Genitourinary: Genital lesions, inflammation, discharge, cystocele, rectocele, vaginal color, vaginal dryness, and pain
Musculoskeletal: Range of motion, pain, gait, and contractures
Laboratory: Complete blood count, chemical profile, and thyroid function

HEENT: head, eyes, ears, nose, throat.

Estimates of the scope of the problem range from 15% to 39% in community-dwelling elderly women, twice the prevalence for men (Flynn, Cell, & Luisi, 1994; U.S. Department of Health and Human Services, 1992). Incontinent episodes are not "every now and then" but usually daily or weekly.

Urinary incontinence is a universal problem among women. More than 40% of a sample of 486 community-dwelling elderly women in Spain age 65 and over reported incontinence (Iglesias et al., 2000). By age 80 the percentage increased to 48%, and among women 85 and older, 60% reported incontinence. Importantly, 50% of those who reported a problem also reported a limitation on activity because of incontinence.

Urinary incontinence has accompanying high costs in multiple ways. Medically, incontinence can result in skin irritation and infection, cystitis, falls, and fractures. Psychologically, incontinence may decrease social interaction because of embarrassment and can result in anxiety that may lead to depression, dependency, and isolation. Economically, many dollars are spent for supplies such as pads, extra laundry costs, and management of complications. Finally, incontinence places a great deal of stress on the individual, family, and friends and is often a determining factor in the decision for nursing home placement (Brandeis, Yalla, & Resnick, 1992), especially in rural areas (Coward, Horne, & Peek, 1995).

Although urinary incontinence is a major problem, particularly among elderly women, incontinence often is assessed and managed poorly. Contributing to the lack of adequate care is the reluctance of the older person to discuss the problem with the health care provider. More than 50% of those who are incontinent do not seek help, citing embarrassment or resignation (Wyman, Hawking, & Fantl, 1990). When elderly patients do report incontinence, they often are ignored and not given information about treatments or education about the problem (Goldstein, Hawthrone, & Engberg, 1992; Mitteness, 1990). McDowell, Silverman, Martin, Musa, and Keane (1994) found that physicians in the community did not always recognize mild to severe incontinence, and intervention for referral rates for incontinence were low for physicians in the community and for geriatric assessment and management teams.

Causes

The physiology of urinary control is complex and not completely understood. Control requires intact cognitive, neurological, and physical parameters as well as motivational and environmental factors.

Physiological Mechanisms for Normal Urination

The parasympathetic nervous system facilitates bladder contraction, whereas the sympathetic nervous system promotes bladder relaxation and contraction of the bladder neck and urethra. The somatic nerve influences contraction of the pelvic floor muscles. Urination is a reflex centered in the micturition center of the sacral spinal cord. Information is carried about the bladder volume to the cord. As the bladder fills, the bladder neck closes and the bladder dome relaxes allowing the bladder to expand via the sympathetic nervous system. The somatic enervation is used to maintain the tone of the pelvic floor, including the muscle around the urethra. With urination is a decrease in sympathetic and somatic tone, allowing the parasympathetic impulses to cause bladder contraction. The ultimate control of urination lies in the brainstem, cerebral cortex, and cerebellum (Kane et al., 1999; U.S. Department of Health and Human Services, 1992). Box 18-16 summarizes factors necessary for normal urination.

Aging is not a cause of incontinence. Changes occur, however, that can contribute to incontinence. Using the factors in Box 18-16 helps identify the affect of the changes. The biggest change occurs in the bladder. The ability of the bladder to expand decreases, and involuntary bladder contractions increase. In women a decrease in the ability of the bladder outlet to remain closed occurs, along with less strength and resistance of the muscles of the pelvic floor to assist the adequate closure of the bladder outlet. The urethra shortens and weakens. In addition, postvoiding residual volume increases and the ability to postpone voiding decreases.

Incontinence results from several possible factors, including (1) poor ability of the bladder to store urine, hyperactivity of the bladder, decreased resistance to pressure, or decreased ability of bladder to expand and contract appropriately; (2) decreased or increased urethral outlet resistance; and (3) a combination of (1) and (2) (Kane et al. 1999; U.S. Department of Health and Human Services, 1992).

Assessment

To assess incontinence thoroughly and manage it appropriately, the provider must have an adequate information base. Management depends on the type of incontinence and the identification of causative factors (Table 18-4).

Box 18-16 SUMMARY OF FACTORS NEEDED FOR NORMAL URINARY FUNCTION

Bladder
Appropriate neurological and physical function
Able to expand with increasing volume
Outlet must be closed
Sensation is appropriate for fullness of bladder
Lack of involuntary bladder contractions
Contractility
Unobstructed flow

Physical/Motivational
Mobility and ability for self-care in toileting
Cognitive ability for self-care in toileting
Motivation to be continent

Environment
No barriers to toileting
Caregivers available
No medications that contribute to incontinence

Source: Kane, R., Ouslander, J., & Abrass, I. (1999). *Essentials of clinical geriatrics* (4th ed.). New York: McGraw-Hill.

Table 18-4	TYPES OF INCONTINENCE	
TYPE	**PHYSIOLOGY AND CAUSE**	**SYMPTOMS**
Urge	Detrusor overactivity (involuntary detrusor contractions) Unstable bladder Detrusor hyperreflexia if associated with neurological problem Possible involuntary urethral relaxation (urethral instability) Cause: cystitis, urethritis, tumors, stones, diverticuli, cardiovascular accident, dementia, parkinsonism, suprasacral spinal injury, or disease	Sudden, strong need to void Inability to delay voiding after sensing bladder fullness Leakage of urine usually in large amounts
Stress	Displacement of urethra and bladder neck with exertion Hypermobility of urethra or bladder neck Weak pelvic floor muscles Weak bladder outlet or urethral sphincter Thinning of urethral and bladder mucosa Damage to sphincter, atrophic vaginitis, childbirth, cystocele, rectocele, or uterine prolapse	Leakage of urine, usually in small amounts when intraabdominal pressure increases Rarely occur in supine position
Overflow	Underactive or acontractile detrusor Bladder outlet obstruction Urethral obstruction Cause: drugs, fecal impaction, neurological problems, or pelvic organ prolapse	Dribbling frequently or constantly Same as urge or stress incontinence but caused by retention with overflow

From U.S. Department of Health and Human Services. (1992). *Urinary incontinence in adults: Clinical practice guidelines* (Publication No. 92-0038). Agency for Health Care Policy and Research. Washington DC: Government Printing Office.

Although urinary incontinence is common among elderly women, achieving a correct diagnosis is complex. More than one type of incontinence may be present; frequently, urge and stress are termed *combined incontinence*. The following list identifies a few common causes of urinary incontinence (U.S. Department of Health and Human Services, 1992):

■ **Delirium** is an acute confusional state that is a symptom of illness and that interferes with cognition and possibly motivation to be continent.

■ **Depression** may occur with incontinence as a symptom.

■ **Restricted mobility** may occur in an acute care facility, with side rails, inability to get to the toilet, and illness that decreases mobility. Additionally, the elderly may be slower to get to the bathroom and, if in a strange place, may be unable to find the toilet.

■ **Urinary retention** may be caused by medications, particularly adrenergic agents and anticholinergic agents. The result of retention is overflow incontinence.

■ **Urinary tract infections** cause symptoms of dysuria and urgency.

■ **Atrophic vaginitis** or **urethritis** also may cause burning, urgency, dysuria frequency, and incontinence.

■ **Fecal impaction** is a common, often overlooked cause of incontinence. In this case, feces act as an obstruction of the urethra. The patient has symptoms of overflow or urge incontinence.

Because many causes of incontinence can occur, organizing data and determining steps in diagnosing the problem is often difficult. Although the two acronyms found in Boxes 18-17 and 18-18 are from the 1980s, they remain accurate, frequently used, and helpful in differential diagnosis.

History

Many older women do not admit easily to the problem of incontinence. The provider therefore must make an effort to include questions about incontinence in the history. The history can provide clues to identify the type of incontinence and possible causes. The practitioner must keep in mind that urinary incontinence is a symptom rather than a disease and must attempt to identify the underlying cause. The *Clinical Practice Guidelines* of the U.S. Department of Health and Human Services provide the nurse with a useful reference for diagnosis and treatment of urinary incontinence. The following sections (history, physical examination, diagnostic studies, and management) represent a synopsis of the guidelines.

History of incontinence. The nurse should gather the following information:
1. Symptoms (dribbling, unable to reach toilet on time, and loss with increase abdominal pressure)
2. Duration: How long has incontinence been a problem?

Box 18-17 CAUSES OF URINARY INCONTINENCE: DRIP

D, delirium
R, restricted mobility, urinary retention
I, infection, inflammation, impaction (fecal)
P, polyuria, pharmaceutical

Source: Kane, R., Ouslander, J., Abrass, I. (1999). *Essentials of clinical geriatrics* (4th ed.). New York: McGraw-Hill.

Box 18-18 CAUSES OF URINARY INCONTINENCE: DIAPPERS

D, delirium
I, infection
A, atrophic vaginitis
P, pharmaceuticals
P, psychological
E, endocrine
R, reduced mobility
S, stool impaction

Source: Resnick, N. (1984). Urinary incontinence in the elderly. *Medical Grand Rounds, 3,* 281–294.

3. Amount of urine lost in incontinency
4. Activities, situations, events that precipitate incontinence. The nurse should ask about recent illness, new medications, urinary tract infection, trauma, surgery, or injury.
5. Frequency of problem: time of day or night and number of times per day or week
6. Causative factors
7. Mental status, including tests for cognition and depression
8. Environmental factors that might make getting to the toilet difficult
9. Physical illness
10. Bowel habits
11. Sexual function and problems
12. Fluid intake, including amount, times of the day, and type (e.g., caffeine or alcohol)

Additionally, the nurse needs to review all medications, including over-the-counter drugs. The following is a short list of medications that can contribute to incontinence:

1. Sedatives and hypnotics, including benzodiazepines and alcohol
2. Diuretics, especially loop diuretics that cause polyuria, frequency, and urgency
3. Anticholinergic drugs, including antihistamines, antidepressants, anti-parkinsonian, and antipsychotic (haloperidol) medications that cause urinary retention with overflow incontinence, sedation, and confusion.
4. Alpha-antagonists and alpha-agonists (sympathomimetics and sympatholytics) that increase and decrease sphincter tone, respectively. Alpha-antagonists for hypertension may cause stress incontinence in women.
5. Calcium channel blockers that decrease the contractibility of smooth muscle, causing retention and overflow incontinence.

Physical examination. Each patient needs a complete physical examination that focuses on potential causes of incontinence. This examination includes a thorough neurological and musculoskeletal assessment in addition to the following specific evaluation:

1. Abdominal examination: masses, fullness especially in bladder area
2. Postresidual volume and palpation of the bladder after voiding. If the bladder is palpable, overflow incontinence is a possible finding. Postresidual volume is possible to detect with abdominal palpation and percussion and bimanual examination. Catheterization allows for specific measurement, but this is not always needed.
3. Pelvic examination to assess for prolapse, vaginitis, and atrophy. The nurse should also perform provocative stress testing by having the patient cough and should note if urine leaks from the urethra. Leakage with cough indicates stress incontinence, whereas delayed leaking or continued leaking indicates detrusor overactivity (U.S. Department of Health and Human Services, 1992).
4. Rectal examination
5. Perineal sensation and autonomic reflex tone (anal sphincter tone). The nurse should check for the presence of sensation and reflex urge or stress incontinence and possibly overflow; absence indicates neurological changes. If sensation is

absent and reflex is present, neurological problems and diabetes must be considered (Byyny & Speroff, 1996).

Diagnostic studies. Although the history and physical examination are the most important aspects of evaluation of urinary incontinence, some laboratory data are also helpful:

1. A urinalysis using a dipstick may be useful to detect an underlying infection and confirm suspicion of tumor, stones, or diabetes and the need for additional studies.
2. A chemical profile is useful to identify renal function and glucose and abnormal electrolytes that might contribute to incontinence.

The nurse can use the following methods for additional assessment of urinary incontinence:

1. **Incontinence record:** The woman can assist in the basic evaluation by maintaining a voiding diary. A written account of the problem by the patient includes frequency, time, and amount of voiding. In addition, the record should include outside factors such as fluid intake, environment, and precipitating events. Examples of voiding diaries can be found in the U.S. Department of Health and Human Services *Clinical Practice Guidelines* (1992).
2. **Urodynamic studies:** Urodynamic studies usually are reserved for patients who do not respond to customary management strategies or who are in need of surgical intervention. Many urodynamic studies are available, but, when indicated, the clinician should refer the patient to a urologist knowledgeable in evaluating incontinence.

Management. Once the cause and type of incontinence is identified, the clinician is able to develop an appropriate treatment plan. Successful management is usually a combination of therapies. The first step usually involves treatment and elimination of reversible causes, which then may be followed by behavioral intervention. Behavioral techniques have been used with varying success rates. All techniques involve education, and the person must be able cognitively and motivated to follow the regimen. The techniques involve working to control detrusor and pelvic floor muscles and must be practiced. Behavioral techniques are designed for specific types of incontinence.

Bladder training is one means of managing urinary incontinence. The purpose of bladder training (or retraining) is to prolong the time between the sensation to void and voiding. The person is taught ways to postpone voiding and to urinate according to timed intervals rather than at the urge to void. In a benchmark study, Fantl and others (1991) found bladder training effective in older women with urethral sphincter weakness and detrusor instability. The women underwent a 6-week bladder training program. At the completion, incontinent episodes were decreased by 57%. After 6 months, 50% continued to report reduction in incontinence.

The basic bladder training program consists of the following steps:

1. Education regarding normal voiding and the causes of incontinence and how consciously to postpone voiding and practice distraction and relaxation techniques

2. Development of a voiding schedule in which the time interval between voiding progressively increases. The initial goal is usually 2 to 3 hours, and the ultimate goal is 4 hours between voiding.

3. Positive reinforcement

Additional techniques the woman may consider are these:

1. Habit training and prompted voiding involving *scheduled toileting* at times when voiding is most likely to happen. Education and cognitive input are not required.

2. Biofeedback

The most common behavioral intervention for stress incontinence is use of pelvic muscle exercises commonly known as Kegel exercises. The exercises are designed to increase urethral resistance and strengthen the periurethral and pelvic muscles. Muscle contraction places a force on the urethra and improves muscle support to the pelvic organs. Pelvic floor muscle exercises have been shown to cure incontinence or produce a 50% to 70% improvement (Burns, Pranikoff, Nochajski, Desotelle, & Harwook 1990; Wells, Brink, Diokno, Wolfe, & Gillis, 1991). Although generally considered the behavioral intervention of choice for stress incontinence, Kegel exercises were found useful for urge incontinence (Flynn, Cell, & Luisi, 1994) and should be taught if the woman suffers from mixed incontinence.

The basic stress incontinence prevention program consists of the following steps:

1. *Education:* Improving awareness of the pelvic muscles.

2. *Function:* First, the nurse teaches contraction or drawing in of pelvic muscles. The nurse describes contraction as trying to stop urination. The woman should be taught *not* to use abdominal, buttock, or thigh muscles at the same time. Teaching use of the exercise before and during times when incontinence may occur is often helpful.

3. *Timing:* Each contraction should be held for 10 seconds and relaxed for 10 seconds.

4. *Frequency:* The exercises should be performed 30 to 80 times per day.

5. *Duration:* The woman should practice for at least 6 weeks but may continue the exercises indefinitely.

In addition to behavioral intervention, pharmacotherapy may provide another avenue for treatment of various types of incontinence (Table 18-5).

Depression

An interrelationship exists between depression and alcoholism, polypharmacy, falls, sexuality, incontinence, and poverty. Although a common problem among elderly women, depression often goes undiagnosed or inadequately treated. Estimates of depression among the elderly vary. Possibly 10% to 20% of the elderly living in the community have a dysphoric mood, and possibly 5% have clinical depression (National Institutes of Health, 1992). Major depression, as defined by the *Diagnostic and Statistical Manual of Mental Disorders IV,* is found in from 1% to 3% of the community population over age 65 (Parmelee, Katz, & Lawton, 1992). Between the ages of 65 and 84 women are more likely than men to have severe depressive symptoms. Between the ages of 80 and 84, 17% of men and 22% of women have severe depressive symptoms.

Table 18-5   **MEDICATIONS USED TO TREAT INCONTINENCE**

TYPE OF INCONTINENCE	MEDICATION	ACTION
Combined incontinence	Estrogen, oral and/or vaginal	Restores mucosa, increases vascularity and tone, and increases bladder outlet resistance.
	Imipramine (Tofranil), 10-25 mg at bedtime up to 4 times a day	Alpha-adrenergic agonists decrease detrusor tone and increase sphincter tone.
Urge incontinence	Estrogen, oral and/or vaginal	Restores mucosa, increases vascularity and tone, and increases bladder outlet resistance.
	Oxybutynin (Ditropan), 2.5-5 mg at bedtime up to 4 times a day	Anticholinergic and smooth muscle relaxant: decreases detrusor tone.
	Propantheline (Pro-Banthine, Norpanth), 7.5-15 mg twice a day up to 4 times a day	Anticholinergic: blocks bladder contractions and decreases detrusor tone.
Stress incontinence	Estrogen, oral and/or vaginal	Restores mucosa, increases vascularity and tone, and increases bladder outlet resistance
	Phenylpropanolamine, 25 mg 4 times a day	Alpha-adrenergic agonists decrease detrusor tone.
	Best outcome is with combined alpha-adrenergic agonist (phenylpropanolamine) and estrogen.	
Overflow incontinence	Prazosin, 1-5 mg 2-4 times a day	Increases detrusor tone.
	Bethanechol (Urecholine), 5-25 mg 2-4 times a day	Decreases sphincter tone.

From U.S. Department of Health and Human Services. (1992). *Urinary incontinence in adults: Clinical practice guidelines* (Publication No. 92-0038). Agency for Health Care Policy and Research. Washington, DC: Government Printing Office.

Interestingly, by age 85 the percentages of elders with depressive symptoms equalizes (Federal Interagency Forum, 2000).

One older person per thousand is hospitalized for a major depression each year. Data taken from the Longitudinal Study of Aging by Callahan and Wolinsky (1995) showed that of the more than 7000 persons over age 70, 275 persons were hospitalized with a primary or secondary diagnosis of depression. Of these, 64% were women. In addition, women who were more likely to be hospitalized with a primary diagnosis of depression were women worried about health, women who desired more social activity, the confused or those with memory problems, those with a decrease in ADL and IADL, and African-American women (Butler, 1998).

Depression in women is not diagnosed or treated adequately for a variety of reasons. One is that the clinical presentation is often one of vague complaints and atypical symptoms. Signs and symptoms of physical illness mask depression, and an astute nurse practitioner is required to differentiate between physical illness and depression. Other reasons include the difficulty in diagnosis because of the multiple causative factors (Koenig & Blazer, 1992).

Causes

As with most problems encountered in the elderly, depression is complex and has many predisposing factors and causes. Psychosocial and economic factors unique to women and medical and physical factors contribute to placing women at risk for depression Box 18-19 gives a partial list of risk factors for the development of depression in older women.

Although women are more likely to have depression than men, the exact cause is unknown (Butler, 1998). Causes associated with depression include physiological changes of aging, medical conditions, medications, and a variety of psychosocial factors. The relationship between chronic illness and depression has been known for many years. In fact, the list of diseases associated with depression is still used today (Kane et al., 1999).

Disease states may exacerbate or cause depressive symptoms. Findings in a 1995 study validated the relationship between depression and chronic illness among African-Americans, particularly diseases of the kidney, visual problems, and cardiovascular disease (Bazargan & Hamm-Braugh, 1995). Box 18-20 gives a partial list of medical illnesses associated with depression.

Box 18-19 RISK FACTORS FOR DEPRESSION IN OLDER WOMEN

Psychosocial
Multiple losses: family or friends
Death of spouse
Isolation
Memory loss
Personality disorders

Financial
Loss of income
Decrease in income with death of spouse

Medical and Physical
Multiple diseases
Polypharmacy
Sensory deprivation
Decrease in function and independence

Sources: Byyny, R., & Speroff, L. (1996). *A clinical guide for the care of older women* (2nd ed.). Baltimore: Williams & Wilkins. Calkins, E., Ford, A., & Katz, R. (1992). *Practice of geriatrics.* Philadelphia: W. B. Saunders. Kane, R., Ouslander, J., & Abrass, I. (1999). *Essentials of clinical geriatrics* (4th ed.). New York: McGraw-Hill.

Box 18-20 MEDICAL ILLNESSES ASSOCIATED WITH DEPRESSION

Metabolic Disturbances
Dehydration
Hypoxia
Hypo- or hypernatremia
Hypo- or hypercalcemia
Any acid-base imbalance

Endocrine Disorders
Hypo- or hyperthyroidism
Diabetes mellitus
Cushing disease
Addison disease

Infectious Processes
Viral and bacterial infections
Numerous, involving any system

Cardiovascular
Congestive heart failure
Myocardial infarction

Respiratory
Chronic obstructive pulmonary disease

Musculoskeletal
Rheumatoid arthritis
Degenerative arthritis
Osteoporosis with fractures

Neurological
Cardiovascular accident
Parkinson syndrome
Early Alzheimer disease

Other
Anemia
Carcinomas
Vitamin deficiencies

Given the multiple chronic illnesses associated with aging, not surprisingly medications used to treat chronic illness may in turn contribute to depression. Medications may cause depression or a drug-drug interaction or drug-patient interaction may create depressive symptoms. Each medication must be evaluated carefully for adverse side effects individually and in combination with other medications and for side effects related to chronic illness and physiological changes with aging. The pharmacist on the interdisciplinary team is invaluable in medication assessment.

Depression is usually multifactorial. Physiological changes, disadvantaged status, financial problems, multiple stressful life events, poor self-concept, little support from friends and family, chronic illness, and medications contribute to depression among the elderly. For instance, Barzargan and Hamm-Baugh (1995) found significant relationships between depression and multiple negative life events, financial status, kidney disease, poor vision, and circulatory problems. In the end, however, depression is a biochemical imbalance.

Diagnosis

Although the *Diagnostic and Statistical Manual of Mental Disorders IV* provides criteria for diagnosing depression, the older patient may not meet standard criteria (Kane et al., 1999). Kane and others (1999) also proposed that because early socialization of the woman included keeping emotions of sadness, guilt, and anger to oneself, diagnosing depression in the elderly woman is more difficult. The most common presentation involves multiple physical symptoms and changes in cognition. Thus complaining of physical symptoms may be viewed as more acceptable to the older woman than expression of feelings. Again, a careful history and physical examination are important in the differential diagnosis. The clinical presentation of depression is atypical (Kane et al., 1999; Calkins et al., 1992). Box 18-21 identifies some common presentations.

Research also points out that the elderly women who are depressed have a negative affect compared with normal elderly women (Lawton, Parmelee, Katz, & Nesselroade, 1996). Depressed women also relate multiple negative life experiences during a life review (Fromholt, Larsen, & Larsen, 1995). They found that when the depression was resolved, the negative life events disappeared from the life review. Thus the technique of life history may be useful in identifying depression and as an outcome measure to identify the resolution of depression.

Depression Scales

A number of depression scales are available (see Box 18-4). The Geriatric Depression Scale (GDS) is useful in primary care for screening purposes although it is not particularly useful with severely demented clients. The scale helps the practitioner differentiate between a variety of symptoms. In addition, the GDS can be used many times and is useful for obtaining initial baseline data. If a change in behavior or symptoms occurs, the GDS may identify a new depression. Because a strong relationship does not exist between GDS scores and poor mental status scores, completing mental status tests with the depression scale is important (Yesavage, Brink, & Rose, 1983).

Positive findings on any screening scale warrant referral to counseling and specialists in neuropsychological and geriatric psychiatry. Because depression may present in a number of different ways, especially cognition, more definitive tests are important. Lyness, Eaton, and Schneider (1994) found a relationship between the ability to complete visuomotor scanning and depression. Visuomotor scanning was significantly less for depressed older adults than for depressed and nondepressed middle-age and old-age controls. Lichtenberg, Ross, Millis, and Manning (1995) studied the relationship between depression and cognition in 220 geriatric medical patients and found that low scores on the Dementia Rating Scale and Logical Memory were strong predictors of depression. Cognitive changes, such as the inability to perform spatial relation tasks and confusion also have multiple causes, and baseline cognitive function likely can be restored if the depression is lifted.

Box 18-21 ATYPICAL PRESENTATIONS OF DEPRESSION IN OLDER WOMEN

1. No defined period of sadness. Presentation may be apathy.
2. Confusion
3. Anxiety, somatization, and vague complaints of cognitive impairment
4. Fatigue
5. Physical symptoms: weakness, insomnia, pain (all over, back, abdominal, and chest), palpitations, dyspnea, dizziness, incontinence/frequency/urgency, headache, and weight loss

Assessment

As with any patient, for the older person who presents with an array of problems, a complete history, physical examination, and diagnostic evaluation are crucial. Given atypical presentation and the multiple factors that contribute to depressive symptoms, missing the diagnosis of depression or diagnosing and treating depression without a complete assessment is easy.

Management

Goals of management of depression are to decrease the symptoms, improve quality of life, improve health status, prevent mortality, and decrease number of relapses. The nurse needs to consider depression as a possible diagnosis for any woman. One must remember that a higher correlation exists between depression and suicide in persons over 60 than in younger adults (Osgood & Malkin, 1997). Although the advanced practice nurse is able to diagnose and treat depression in the elderly, having a psychiatrist who specializes in geriatric psychiatry (geropsychiatrist) or is familiar with the complexities of the geriatric patient evaluate and collaborate regarding appropriate treatment regimen is always wise.

Although in the past, counseling was not always considered for elderly clients, some form of counseling is important for meeting long-term goals. Supportive therapy and psychotherapy help achieve the immediate goal of symptom management and also provide a mechanism for long-term management that improves quality of life and health status and decreases relapses (French, 1996; Osgood & Malkin, 1997; Riekse & Holstege, 1996).

The following is a list of suggested supportive measures and psychotherapy:

- Education
- Support and encouragement
- Social interaction
- Physical activity
- Cognitive therapy
- Individual and group therapy

Pharmacotherapeutics

With severe symptomatology and a long duration of symptoms, medications with supportive measures and psychotherapy are necessary. Pharmacotherapy is always complex among the elderly, and medications to treat depression are no exception. Each medication has potentially harmful side effects, and each has benefits for particular symptoms. Unfortunately, medications often are used inappropriately in the outpatient setting and often in place of supportive therapy (Wells, Katon, Rogers, & Camp, 1994). In addition, the same researchers found that African-American patients were not only less likely to receive antidepressant medications but also likely to receive medication well below the therapeutic level. The following discussion of therapeutic agents is not intended to be all inclusive. Many new pharmacological agents are being introduced that may have great benefit for the older woman. In prescribing medication for depression, comparing the symptoms of the patient with the side effects of the medication is important. In addition, medications that exacerbate symptoms of age-related changes or pathological conditions should be avoided.

Selective serotonin reuptake inhibitors. SSRIs are becoming the first-line medication for depression in the elderly (Osgood & Malkin, 1997; Lustbader, Morgan, Pelayo, Vasquez, & Yuen, 1997) because they are equally as effective but do not have the adverse side effects of the tricyclic antidepressants (TCAs). In addition to fewer anticholinergic and sedative effects, the SSRIs do not interfere with cognitive function and do not contribute to orthostatic hypotension.

SSRIs usually are taken once a day, thereby increasing compliance (Terpstra & Terpstra, 1997). The practitioner must remember, however, that SSRIs have a long half-life and thus have continued effects when discontinued. The practitioner needs to consider the symptoms presented by the client with the drug profile to identify the most beneficial medication. Medications may not be effective immediately. SSRIs should be monitored every 1 to 2 weeks. If necessary, the medication can be increased gradually, a process that may take up to 8 weeks (Semla et al., 1997; Terpstra & Terpstra, 1997). The following list identifies the current recommendations for prescribing SSRIs for elderly women. However, the advanced practice nurse must remember that new SSRIs and similar medications are being developed. Recommendations will change as new, more effective drugs are introduced. The current recommendations (Terpstra & Terpstra, 1997) for prescribing SSRIs are as follows:

- ▪ *Fluoxetine:* Provides stimulating effect *but* has long half-life. Starting dosage: 10-20 mg/day
- ▪ *Paroxetine:* Provides calming, mild sedation, has beneficial effect on cognition, but causes dry mouth. Starting dosage: 10 mg/day
- ▪ *Sertraline:* Not highly recommended because it may cause more gastrointestinal problems than other SSRIs and more sexual dysfunction.

SSRIs can be taken with TCAs and other antidepressant medications. However, close monitoring of plasma concentrations of TCAs and side effects is essential for successful treatment and compliance.

Miscellaneous antidepressants. Two newer antidepressants may prove helpful for the elderly woman: bupropion (Wellbutrin) and citalopram (Celexa) (Lacy, Armstrong, Goldman, & Lance, 1999).

Bupropion can be used as adjunct for smoking cessation. The antidepressant causes seizures and insomnia; skeletal tremors are usually temporary. Doses are divided and should not be stopped abruptly. The starting dose is 50 to 100 mg/day, which can be increased only 50 mg/day and not more than once a week.

Citalopram is being evaluated as treatment for dementia, smoking cessation, alcohol abuse, obsessive-compulsive disorder, and diabetic neuropathy. Citalopram is metabolized in the liver and does not impair psychomotor performance. The starting dose is 20 mg once a day in the morning or evening; the dosage can be increased after a week if no response is observed. The woman should not receive more than 40 mg/day.

Tricyclic antidepressants. Before the introduction of SSRIs, the first-line antidepressants for older persons were the TCAs. Although still effective, the TCAs have side effects that are dangerous for the older person and should be used with caution. If a TCA is prescribed, the starting dosage is considerably less in the older adult than in young or middle-aged adults. In addition, TCAs should be used with caution in older persons with heart disease, glaucoma, urinary retention, or seizure activity (Semla et al., 1997).

Desipramine currently is recommended for the elderly. The drug has a low sedative and low anticholinergic effect and low orthostatic hypotension effect. The starting dosage is 25 to 150 mg/day.

Tricyclic antidepressants to avoid in the geriatric population include those with high to very high sedative and anticholinergic effects and those with moderate to high orthostatic hypotension effects: amitriptyline (Elavil), doxepin, and clomipramine.

Bereavement

Widowhood represents a major role transition and is more common among women than men. The loss of a husband of many years may or may not contribute to depression. Although loss of a spouse is considered a major negative life event, women tend to recover emotionally from the event within a year (Arbuckle & deVries, 1995). Physical health may decline, with most changes occurring within the first year following the loss (Bradsher, 1997).

Loneliness is a common, often serious, problem that may occur with widowhood and often is manifested as depression. Depression scores increase during the first year following the bereavement and then return to the level before widowhood (Mendes de Leon, Kasl, & Jacobs, 1994). Findings from a longitudinal study by Arbuckle and deVries (1995) indicated that the social life of widows returns to prewidowhood levels and may even increase. Also, some of the changes in social interaction come from involvement with the peer culture. Other widows provide support necessary for successful role transition. Social isolation is not always the reason for loneliness and depression in widowhood.

Women seem to be able to adapt to widowhood more easily than men. Part of adaptation is the concept of time and the fact that becoming a widow is part of the life course. Time, "on time," and "off time" were first introduced by Neugarten (1968). The life course is divided into certain events that are supposed to occur at certain times during the life cycle. When the loss of a spouse occurs on time, the impact is less than if the loss occurs off time.

Other factors that influence the ability of women to adapt to the loss of a spouse include a support network involving children, siblings, family, and friends; physical health of the spouse before death (burden of caregiving); having a confidant; possibly religious involvement; financial stability; and education. Indeed, some research, as reported by Bradsher (1997), indicates that men have more problems with health, are more socially isolated, lack a confidant, and have a smaller social network, thereby impeding role transition following the death of their spouses. Depression may be more of a long-term problem for men than for women (Umberson, Wortman, & Kessler, 1992).

Assessment and management issues are similar to depression. In addition, however, providing ongoing evaluation and treatment during the first year following the loss is especially important. Support groups, religious group connections if appropriate, counseling, and hospice bereavement groups may be sources for assisting in the adaptation to widowhood.

Alcoholism and Depression

A strong correlation exists between alcohol consumption, depression, and suicide among the elderly. Of the more than 10 million alcoholics in the United States, 50% are women (Osgood & Malkin, 1997). The AARP (Taeuber, 1996) report identifies 10% to 15% of the elderly over 65 living in the community as having a serious drinking problem. The report also states that 33% of the elders with a drinking problem began drinking after the age of 60. Alcohol abuse is associated with higher risks of mortality from accidents, breast cancer, and cirrhosis in women (Fuchs et al., 1995).

The incidence of depression among alcoholics is reported to be between 28% and 59%, and more than one third of suicides in the United States are associated with alcohol use. Although most data are from the United States, recent international studies indicate that 25% to 50% of suicides are associated with alcoholism (Osgood & Malkin, 1997). In addition to depression, risk factors for alcoholism in older women include a need for gratification, control and power, loss of a spouse, social isolation, homelessness, a family history of alcoholism, and being married to an alcoholic (Taeuber, 1996).

Alcohol is metabolized differently in women than in men. Findings indicate that although women may ingest low levels of alcohol, the blood alcohol concentration is higher than for men who ingest the same amount. A variety of physiological differences may account for this. First, men have a higher body water content, which means the alcohol is diluted to a greater extent than in women. Second, women have lower first-pass metabolism in the stomach than men, which in turn creates higher levels of alcohol in the liver (Fuchs et al., 1995; Pozzato et al., 1995).

Assessment

Because of differences in metabolism, women demonstrate impaired function and poor coordination with only small amounts of alcohol. The usual quantity considered a drink is one 12-ounce glass of beer, a 4-ounce glass of wine, or 1.5 ounces of liquor. Less than the drink quantity may impair function in elderly women (Pozzato et al., 1995). Box 18-22 outlines the history and physical examination specific for older women who may abuse alcohol (Conigliaro, 1997). During each future visit, the person should be examined for clues of alcohol abuse and questioned about habits. The nurse should always question about the use of alcohol and other drugs. The CAGE questionnaire may be used to screen for alcoholism.

Management

Counseling is often helpful in changing alcohol habits. Education about physiological changes in aging that make alcohol use more hazardous, the effects of alcohol on health,

---

Box 18-22 HISTORY AND PHYSICAL EXAMINATION SPECIFIC TO ALCOHOL ABUSE IN THE OLDER WOMAN

1. Identify risk factors
2. Family history of alcohol use
3. Observe for signs of alcohol abuse:
   Flushed face
   Trembling
   Smell of liquor, mouthwash, or mints
   Gaps in memory and confusion
   Fatigue and insomnia
   Poor hygiene
   Falls, broken bones, bruises, and burns
   Driving accidents
   Weight loss and malnutrition
   Depression and suicidal ideation
4. Chronic diseases and medication use
5. Specific questions
   a. Frequency, amount, and type of wine, beer, liquor, and other drugs
   b. General questions about alcohol (Eisendrath, 1996):
      ■ What has alcohol done to you?
      ■ Has it affected your relationships?
      ■ Does it affect the way you schedule your day? (Schedule around alcohol)
      ■ Has it affected your health?
      ■ Do you find you are preoccupied with alcohol?
   b. CAGE questionnaire (Mayfield, McLeod, & Hall, 1974):
      C. Have you ever felt the need to **cut** down on your drinking?
      A. Have people ever **annoyed** you by criticizing your drinking?
      G. Have you ever felt bad or **guilty** about drinking?
      E. Have you ever had a drink first thing in the morning to steady your nerves or get rid of a hangover (**eye-opener**)?
6. Physical
   a. Complete physical examination with particular attention to the following: throat, voice (hoarseness), and mouth (higher incidence of mouth, throat, laryngeal, and neck cancer).
   b. Abdomen and liver
   c. Breast examination
   d. Clues to alcohol abuse
7. Diagnostic evaluation
   a. Complete blood count, Chem 26 (attention to liver function, bilirubin, albumin, hemoglobin, and hematocrit)
   b. Mammogram
   c. Other tests as indicated by history and physical examination

---

and the serious side effects of alcohol use should be included in the counseling. The nurse should discuss appropriate alcohol use, such as for celebrations, and the importance of not driving for 1 to 2 hours after alcohol intake. The health care provider should also refer the heavy drinker to formal counseling or Alcoholics Anonymous.

The patient should be assessed for depression, and consideration should be given to treatment with SSRIs and counseling. Caution must be used when treating depression with medications if the person is going to continue to drink or has suicidal thoughts.

Suicide

Suicide is a potential consequence of depression that is in many cases preventable. In addition to depression, risk factors for suicide in the elderly include being male, living alone and isolated, being widowed or divorced, poor health, alcoholism, loneliness, and poor self-esteem (Osgood, 1995) The suicide rate is rising among the elderly, especially elderly men. The highest rate of completed suicide is found in males age 65 and older. The suicide rate for females rises to a peak between ages 45 and 54 and then gradually declines in old age (Osgood & Malkin, 1997).

According to the National Center for Health Statistics, persons over the age of 65 are at highest risk for suicide and commit 20% of all suicides. The American Association of Suicidology (McIntosh, 1992) reports that completed suicides for young persons are about 100:1 to 200:1, but for older persons the ratio is 4:1. Thus older persons are more successful in completing suicides, probably because of more lethal methods, poor health, less healing ability, isolation, and a high motivation to die. Elderly men are at the highest risk for completed suicides; however, women attempt suicide more often (Osgood & Malkin, 1997).

Older women, however, have behaviors that are more covert expressions of suicidal ideation. The list includes self-starvation, refusal to take medically needed medications or treatments, and withdraw from social contacts. The withdrawal from life has been called acquiescent suicide and is a widespread form of suicide among older women that frequently is overlooked (Osgood & Eisenhandler, 1994). In addition, Canetto (1995) found that women are more likely than men to be involved as victims in assisted suicide by their husbands or physicians.

Assessment

Assessment is the same as for depression and alcohol abuse because depression is the primary cause of suicide, and alcoholism and suicide are related significantly. The nurse should always ask questions specific to suicide: suicide ideation, a plan, a means. In addition, the nurse should consider questions concerning factors that may contribute to the risk of depression and suicide (Osgood & Malkin, 1997):

■ Child abuse
■ Victimization in adolescence and adulthood
■ Interpersonal difficulties
■ Financial problems
■ Alcoholism

Management

The management of suicide ideation is similar to the treatment of depression. Counseling and medication are usually successful; however, weekly monitoring may be needed to provide support and facilitate compliance with treatment plans. If alcoholism is a factor, counseling for alcohol use and depression can be given. If the person has a plan and the means, immediate referral to a psychologist, psychotherapist, or ideally a geropsychiatrist is essential.

SUMMARY

This chapter focused on the older woman and a variety of gerontological issues, including demographics, normal physiological aspects of aging, the comprehensive geriatric assessment, health promotion and disease prevention, and finally 11 areas of concern that are specific to elderly women.

The author hopes the information provided shows the complexity and the satisfaction that is possible when working with the older woman. The older woman is like an intricate jigsaw puzzle. Many pieces must find a place. When the puzzle is finished, the picture is wonderful. Often, caring for the older woman is an ongoing puzzle. Not only are the pieces difficult to fit but also the body of knowledge in the field of gerontology and particularly elderly women continues to grow.

REFERENCES

Administration on Aging. (1998). *Profile of older Americans: 1998*. Washington, D.C.: Program Resources Department, American Association of Retired Persons, & Administration on Aging, U.S Department of Health and Human Services.

American Association of Retired Persons. (1993). *Grandparents raising their grandchildren*. Grandparent Information Center. Washington DC: AARP.

American Association of Retired Persons. (1995). *Finding help untangling the web of public programs*. Grandparent Information Center. Washington DC: AARP.

American Association of Retired Persons. (1996). Helping older women at risk of partner abuse. *Women's Initiative Fact Sheet*. Washington DC: AARP.

American Association of Retired Persons Public Policy Institute. (1997, July). *Final research report on how to best reach and assist minority grandparents raising their grandchildren*. Grandparent Information Center. Washington DC:

Aparasu, R., & Fliginger, S. (1997). Inappropriate medication prescribing for the elderly by office-based physicians. *Annals of Pharmacotherapy, 31*, 823–829.

Arbuckle, N., & deVries. (1995). The long-term effects of later life spousal and parental bereavement on personal functioning. *Gerontologist, 35*, 637–647.

Bachmann, G. (1990). Psychosexual aspects of hysterectomy. *Women's Health Issues, 1*, 41–43.

Barnhill, S. (1996). Three generations at risk: Imprisoned women, their children and grandmother caregivers. *Generations, 20*, 39–48.

Bazargan, M., & Hamm-Braugh, V. (1995). The relationship between chronic illness and depression in a community of urban black elderly persons. *Journal of Gerontology, 50B*, S119–S127.

Beck, A., & Beck, R. (1972). Screening depressed patients in family practice: A rapid technique. *Postgraduate Medicine, 52*, 81–85.

Beck, A., Ward, C., Mendelson, J., Mock, J., & Ergaugh, J. (1961). An inventory for measuring depression. *Archives of General Psychiatry, 4*, 561–571.

Beers, M. (1997). Explicit criteria for determining potentially inappropriate medication use by the elderly. *Archives of Internal Medicine, 157*, 1531–1536.

Beltran, A. (2000). Grandparents and other relatives raising children: Supportive public policies. *Public Policy and Aging Report, 11*(1), 1–7.

Blass, J., Cherniak, E., & Weksler, M. (1992). Theories of aging. In E. Calkins, A. Ford, & R. Katz (Eds.), *Practice of geriatrics* (pp. 1–18). Philadelphia: W. B. Saunders.

Bradsher, J. (1997). Older women and widowhood. In J. Coyle (Ed.), *Handbook on women and aging* (pp. 418–429). Westport, CT: Greenwood Press.

Brandeis, G., Yalla, S., & Resnick, N. (1992). Urinary incontinence. In E. Calkins, A. Ford, & R. Katz (Eds.), *Practice of geriatrics* (pp. 220–228). Philadelphia: W. B. Saunders.

Brandl, B., & Raymond, J. (1996). Older abused and battered women: An invisible population. *Wisconsin Medical Journal, 95*, 298–300.

Brandl, B., & Raymond, J. (1997). Unrecognized elder abuse victims: Older abused women. *Journal of Case Management, 6*, 62–68.

Burkhauser, R. (1994). Protecting the most vulnerable: A proposal to improve social security insurance for older women. *Gerontologist, 34*, 148–149.

Burns, P., Pranikoff, K., Nochajski, T., Desotelle, P., & Harwook, M. (1990). Treatment of stress incontinence with pelvic floor exercises and biofeedback. *Journal of the American Geriatrics Society, 38*, 341–344.

Burton, L. (1992). Families and the aged: Issues of complexity and diversity. *Generations, 17*, 5–6.

Butler, R. (1998). Identifying and coping with depression. *Women and Aging Letter: National Policy and Resource Center on Women and Aging, 2*(5).

Byyny, R., & Speroff, L. (1996). *A clinical guide for the care of older women* (2nd ed.). Baltimore: Williams & Wilkins.

Calkins, E., Ford, A., & Katz, R. (1992). *Practice of geriatrics.* Philadelphia: W. B. Saunders.

Callahan, C., & Wolinsky, F. (1995). Hospitalization for major depression among older Americans. *Journals of Gerontology: Medical Sciences, 50A*, M196–M202.

Canetto, S. S. (1995). Elderly women and suicidal behavior. In S. S. Canetto & D. Lester (Eds.), *Women and suicidal behavior* (pp. 215-233). New York: Springer.

Cao, C., Ashton-Miller, J., Schultz, A., & Alexander, N. (1997). Abilities to turn suddenly while walking: The effects of age, gender, and available response time. *Journals of Gerontology: Medical Sciences, 52A*, M88–M93.

Chalfie, D. (1994). *Going it alone: A closer look at grandparents parenting grandchildren.* Washington, DC: American Association of Retired Persons Women's Initiative.

Chrischilles, E., Foley, D., Wallace, R., Lemke, J., Semla, T., Hanlon, J., et al. (1992). Use of medications by persons 65 and over: Data from the established populations for epidemiological studies of the elderly. *Journal of Gerontology: Medical Sciences, 47*, M137–M144.

Conigliaro, J. (1997). An approach to substance abuse. In L. Rucker (Ed.), *Essentials of adult ambulatory care* (pp. 73–79). Baltimore: Williams & Wilkins.

Cousins, S. (2000). "My heart couldn't take it": Older women's beliefs about exercise benefits and risks. *Journals of Gerontology: Psychological Sciences, 55B*(5), P283–P294.

Coward, R., Horne, C, & Peek, C. (1995). Predicting nursing home admissions among incontinent older adults: A comparison of residential differences across six years. *Gerontologist, 35*, 732–743.

Crystal, S., Johnson, R., Harman, J., Sambamoorthi, U., & Kumar, R. (2000). Out-of-pocket health care costs among older Americans. *Journals of Gerontology: Social Sciences, 55B*(1), S51–S62.

Dallas, M. (1997). Exercise walking for obesity management in older adult women. *Issues on Aging, 20*, 8–12.

Decalmer, P. (1994). Clinical presentation. In P. Decalmer, & F. Glendenning (Eds.), *The mistreatment of elderly people* (pp. 35–61). London: Sage Publications.

Deevey, S. (1990). Older lesbian women: An invisible minority. *Journal of Gerontological Nursing, 16*, 35–37.

Diagnostic and Statistical Manual of Mental Disorders, IV. (1994). Washington, DC: American Psychiatric Association.

Duke University Center for the Study of Aging and Human Development. (1974). *Multidimensional functional assessment: The OARS methodology.* Durham, NC: Author.

Edelberg, H., Shallenberger, E., Hausdorff, J., & Wei, J. (2000). One-year follow-up of medication management capacity in highly functioning older adults. *Journals of Gerontology: Medical Sciences, 55A*(10), M550–M553.

Edelberg, H., Shallenberger, E., & Wei, J. (1999). Medication management capacity in highly functioning community-living older adults: Detection of early deficits. *Journal of the American Geriatrics Society, 47*, 592–596.

Eisendrath, S. (1996). Psychiatric disorders. In L. Tierney, S. McPhee, & M. Padakas (Eds.), *Current medical diagnosis and treatment* (pp. 915–971). Hartford, CT: Appleton & Lange.

Fantl, J., Wyman, J., McClish, D., Harkins, S., Elswick, R., Taylor, J., et al. (1991). Efficacy of bladder training in older women with urinary incontinence. *Journal of the American Medical Association, 265*, 609–615.

Federal Interagency Forum on Aging-Related Statistics. (2000). *Older Americans 2000: Key indicators of well-being.* Hyattsville, MD: Author.

Fentem, P. (1994). Benefits of exercise in health and disease. *British Medical Journal, 308*, 1291–1295.

Ferraro, K., & Farmer, M. (1996). Double jeopardy, aging as leveler, or persistent health inequality? A longitudinal analysis of white and black Americans. *Journals of Gerontology: Social Sciences, 51B*, S319–S328.

Fillenbaum, G., (1985). Screening the elderly: A brief instrumental activities of daily living measure. *Journal of the American Geriatric Society* 33(10), 698–706.

Flynn, L., Cell, P., & Luisi, E. (1994). Effectiveness of pelvic muscle exercises in reducing urge incontinence among community residing elders. *Journal of Gerontological Nursing, 20*, 23–27.

Foley, L., & Gibson, M. (2000). *Older women's access to health care: Potential impact of Medicare reform.* Washington, D.C.: American Association of Retired Persons Public Policy Institute.

Folstein, M., Folstein, S., & McHugh, P. (1975). Mini-mental state: A practical method for grading the cognitive state of patients for the clinician. *Journal of Psychiatric Research, 12*, 189–198.

Forman, D., & Lipsitz, L. (1997). Syncope in the elderly. *Cardiology Clinics, 15*, 295–311.

Franks, P., Gold, M., & Clancy, C. (1996). Use of care and subsequent mortality: The importance of gender. *Health Services Research, 31*, 347–363.

Freedman, V. (1996). Family structure and the risk of nursing home admission. *Journals of Gerontology: Social Sciences, 51B*, 561–569.

French, D. (1996). Avoiding adverse drug reactions in the elderly patient: Issues and strategies. *Nurse Practitioner, 21*, 90–105.

Fromholt, P., Larsen, P., & Larsen, S. (1995). Effects of late-onset depression and recovery on autobiographical memory. *Journal of Gerontology: Psychological Sciences, 50B*, P74–P81.

Frontera, W., Hughes, V., Lutz, K., & Evans, W. (1991). A cross-sectional study of muscle strength and mass in 45-78 year old men and women. *Journal of Applied Physiology, 71*, 644–650.

Fuchs, C., Stampfer, M., Colditz, G., Giovannucci, E., Manson, J., Kawachi, I., et al. (1995). Alcohol consumption and mortality among women. *New England Journal of Medicine, 332*, 1245.

Fulmer, T., McMahon, D., Baer-Hines, M., & Forget, B. (1992). Abuse, neglect, abandonment, violence, and exploitation: An analysis of all elderly patients seen in one emergency department during a six-month period. *Journal of Emergency Nursing, 18*, 505–510.

Gallo, J., Reichel, W., & Andersen, L. (1995). *Handbook of geriatric assessment* (2nd ed.). Gaithersburg, MD: Aspen.

Giacomini, M. (1996). Gender and ethnic differences in hospital-based procedure utilization in California. *Archives of Internal Medicine, 156*, 217–224.

Glendenning, F. (1993). What is elder abuse and neglect? In P. Decalmer & F. Glendenning (Eds.), *The mistreatment of elderly people* (pp. 1–34). London: Sage Publications.

Goldstein, M., Hawthorne, E., & Engberg, S. (1992). Urinary incontinence: Why people do not seek help. *Journal of Gerontological Nursing, 18*, 15–19.

Graves, T., Hanlon, J., Schmader, K., Landsman, P., Samsa, G., Peiper, C., et al. (1997). Adverse events after discontinuing medications in elderly outpatients. *Archives of Internal Medicine, 157*, 2205–2210.

Hickey, T., & Stilwell, D. (1991). Health promotion for older people: All is not well. *Gerontologist, 31*(6) 822–829.

Hillner, B., Penberthy, L., & Desch, C. (1996). Variation staging and treatment of local and regional breast cancer in the elderly. *Breast Cancer Research and Treatment, 40*, 75–86.

Himes, C. (1992a). Future caregivers: Projected family structures of older persons. *Journal of Gerontology: Social Sciences, 47*, S17–S26.

Himes, C. (1992b). Social demography of contemporary families and aging. *Generations, 17*, 13–16.

Hornbrook, M., Stevens, V., Wingfield, D., Hollis, J., Greenlick, M., & Ory, M. (1994). Preventing falls among community-dwelling older persons: Results from a randomized trial. *Gerontologist, 34*, 16–23.

Hudson, M. (1997). Elder mistreatment: Its relevance to older women. *Journal of the American Medical Women's Association, 52*, 142–146.

Hunter, K., Florio, E., Rosmond, R., & Langberg, R. (1996). Pharmaceutical care for home-dwelling elderly persons: A determination of need and program description. *Gerontologist, 36*, 543–548.

Hurley, B. (1995). Age, gender, and muscular strength. *Journals of Gerontology, Series A, 50*, 41–44.

Iglesias, F., Caridad y Ocerin, J., del Molino, P., Martin, J., Gama, E., Perez, M., et al. (2000). Prevalence and psychosocial impact of urinary incontinence in older people of a Spanish rural population. *Journals of Gerontology: Medical Science, 55A*(4), M207–M214.

Inouye, S., & Charpentier, P. (1996). Precipitating factors for delirium in hospitalized elderly persons: Predictive model and interrelationship with baseline vulnerability. *Journal of the American Medical Association, 275,* 852–857.

Jacobson, S. (1997). Delirium in the elderly. *Psychiatric Clinics of North America, 20,* 91–110.

Jendrek, M. & (1994). Grandparents who parent their grandchildren: Circumstances and decisions. *Gerontologist, 34,* 206–216.

Jinks, M., & Furerst, R. (1995). Geriatric drug use and rehabilitation. In L. Young & M. Koda-Kimble (Eds), *Applied therapeutics: The clinical use of drugs* (pp. 101–113). Vancouver, WA: Applied Therapeutics.

Johnson, C. (1992). Divorced and reconstituted families: Effects on the older generation. *Generations, 17,* 17–20.

Johnson, T. F. (1991). *Elder mistreatment: Deciding who is at risk.* Westport, CT: Greenwood Press.

Kane, R., Ouslander, J., & Abrass, I. (1999). *Essentials of clinical geriatrics* (4th ed.). New York: McGraw-Hill.

Katz, L. (1991). Chronic illness and sexuality. *American Journal of Nursing, 9,* 56–59.

Katz, S., Ford, A., Moskowitz, R., Jackson, B., & Jaffee, M. (1963). Studies of illness in the aged, the index of ADL: A standardized measure of biological and psychological function. *Journal of the American Medical Association, 185,* 914–919.

Kelley, S. (1993). Caregiver stress in grandparents raising grandchildren. *Image, 25,* 331–337.

Kitzman, D., & Edwards, W. (1990). Minireview: Age-related changes in the anatomy of the normal human heart. *Journals of Gerontology: Medical Sciences, 45,* M33–M39.

Kleinschmidt, K. (1997). Elder abuse: A review. *Annals of Emergency Medicine, 30,* 463–472.

Koenig, H., & Blazer, D. (1992). Epidemiology of geriatric affective disorders. *Clinical Geriatric Medicine, 8,* 235–251.

Koski, K., Luukinen, H., Laippala, P., & Livela, S. L. (1996). Physiological factors and medications as predictors of injurious falls by elderly people: A prospective population-based study. *Age & Ageing, 25,* 29–38.

Krall, E., Dawson-Hughes, B., Hirst, K., Gallagher, J., Sherman, S., & Dalsky, G. (1997). Bone mineral density and biochemical marker of bone turnover in healthy elderly men and women. *Journals of Gerontology: Medical Sciences, 52A,* M61–M67.

Kramarow, E., Lentzner, H., Rooks, R., Weeks, J., & Saydah, S. (1999). *Health and aging chartbook: Health, United States, 1999.* Hyattsville, MD: National Center for Health Statistics.

Krueger, P., & Patterson, C. (1997). Detecting and managing elder abuse: Challenges in primary care. *Canadian Medical Association Journal, 157,* 1095–1100.

Lachs, M., & Pillemer, K. (1995). Abuse and neglect of elderly persons. *New England Journal of Medicine, 332*(7), 437–43.

Lacy, C., Armstrong, L., Goldman, M., & Lance, L. (1999). *Drug information handbook* (7th ed.). Hudson, OH: Lexi-Comp.

Lane, R. (1997). SSRIs and hyponatraemia. *British Journal of Clinical Practice, 51,* 144–146.

Lassila, H., Stoehr, G., Ganguli, M., Seaberg, E., Gilby, J., Belle, S., et al. (1996). Use of prescription medications in an elderly rural population: The MoVies project. *Annals of Pharmacotherapy, 30,* 589–595.

Lawton, M., Parmelee, P., Katz, I., & Nesselroade, J. (1996). Affective states in normal and depressed older people. *Journals of Gerontology: Psychological Sciences, 51*(6), 309–316.

Legato, M. (1997). Gender-specific physiology: How real is it? How important is it? *International Journal of Fertility 4,* 19–29.

Lexell, J. (1995). Human aging, muscle mass, and fiber type composition. *Journals of Gerontology, Series A, 50A,* 11–16.

Lichtenberg, P., Ross, T., Millis, S., & Manning, C. (1995). The relationship between depression and cognition in older adults: A cross-validation study. *Journals of Gerontology: Psychological Sciences, 50B,* P25–P32.

Lord, S., Lloyd, D., Nirui, M., Raymond, J., Williams, P., & Stewart, R. (1996). The effect of exercise on gait patterns in older women: A randomized controlled trial. *Journals of Gerontology: Medical Sciences, 51A,* M64–M70.

Lueckenotte, A. (1996). *Gerontological nursing.* St. Louis: Mosby.

Lustbader, A., Morgan, C., Pelayo, R., Vasquez, L., & Yuen, K. (1997). Psychiatry. In L. Rucker (Ed.), *Essentials of adult ambulatory care* (pp. 575–616). Baltimore: Williams & Wilkins.

Lyness, S., Eaton, E., & Schneider, L. (1994). Cognitive performance in older and middle-aged depressed outpatients and controls. *Journals of Gerontology: Psychological Sciences, 49,* P129–P136.

Mahoney, F. I., & Barthel, D. W. (1965). Functional evaluation: The Barthel Index. *Maryland State Medical Journal, 14*, 61–65.

Manton, K. (1997) Demographic trends for the aging female population. *Journal of the American Medical Women's Association, 52*, 99–105.

Markides, K. (1990). Risk factors, gender, and health. *Generations, 14*, 17–21.

Mayfield, D. G., McLeod, G., & Hall, P. (1974). The CAGE questionnaire: Validation of a new alcoholism screening instrument. *American Journal of Psychiatry, 131*, 1121–1123.

McCartney, N., Hicks, A., Martin, J., & Webber, C. (1996). A longitudinal trial of weight training in the elderly: Continued improvements in year 2. *Journals of Gerontology, 51A*, B425–B433.

McDowell, J., Silverman, M., Martin, D., Musa, D., & Keane, C. (1994). Identification and intervention for urinary incontinence by community physicians and geriatric assessment teams. *Journal of the American Geriatrics Society, 42*, 501–505.

McIntosh, J. L. (1992). *The suicide of older men and women.* Denver, CO: American Association of Suicidology.

McLaughlin, D., & Jensen, L. (2000). Work history and U. S. elders' transitions into poverty. *Gerontologist, 40*(4), 469–479.

McLaughlin, T., Soumerai, S., & Willison, D. (1996). Adherence to national guidelines for drug treatment of suspected acute myocardial infarction. *Archives of Internal Medicine, 156*, 799–805.

Mendes de Leon, C., Kasl, S., & Jacobs, S. (1994). A prospective study of widowhood and changes in symptoms of depression in a community sample of the elderly. *Psychological Medicine, 24*, 613–624.

Metter, J., Conwit, R., Tobin, J., & Fozard, J. (1997). Age-associated loss of power and strength in the upper extremities in women and men. *Journals of Gerontology, 52A*, B267–B276.

Miller, M. (1997). Fluid and electrolyte homeostasis in the elderly: Physiological changes of ageing and clinical consequences. *Clinical Endocrinology and Metabolism, 11*, 367–87.

Minkler, M., & Roe, K. (1996). Grandparents as surrogate parents. *Generations, 20*, 34–38.

Minkler, M., Roe, K., & Price, M. (1992). The physical and emotional health of grandmothers raising grandchildren in the crack cocaine epidemic. *Gerontologist, 32*(6), 752–761.

Mitteness, L. (1990). Knowledge and beliefs about urinary incontinence in adulthood and old age. *Journal of the American Geriatrics Society, 38*, 374–378.

Monane, M., & Avorn, J. (1996). Do too many cooks spoil the broth? Multiple physician involvement in medical management of elderly patients and potentially inappropriate drug combinations. *Canadian Medical Association Journal, 154*, 1177–1184.

Moon M., & Gage, B. (1997). Key Medicare provisions in the Balanced Budget Act of 1997. *Public Policy and Aging Report* (National Academy on Aging), *8*:1–5.

Mutcheler, J., & Burr, J. (1994). Racial differences in health and health care service utilization in later life: The effects of socioeconomic status. In P. Stoller & R. Gibson (Eds.), *Worlds of difference* (pp. 238–243). Thousand Oaks, CA: Pine Forge Press.

National Institutes of Health Consensus Development Panel on Depression in Late Life. (1992). Diagnosis and treatment of depression in late life. *Journal of the American Medical Association, 268*(8), 1018–1130.

Neugarten, B. (Ed.). (1968). *Middle age and aging.* Chicago: University of Chicago Press.

Nevitt, M. (1990). Falls in older persons: Risk factors and prevention. In Institute of Medicine (Ed.), *The second fifty years: Promoting health and preventing disability.* Washington, DC: National Academy Press.

Noyes, M. (1997). Pharmacotherapy for elderly women. *Journal of the American Medical Women's Association, 52*, 138–141.

Nusselder, W., & Mackenbach, J. (1997). Rectangularization of the survival curve in the Netherlands: An analysis of underlying causes of death. *Journals of Gerontology: Social Sciences, 53B*, S145–S154.

Nutrition Screening Initiative. (1991). *Report of nutrition screening 1: Toward a common view.* Washington, DC: NSI.

O'Brien, S., & Vertinsky, P. (1991). Unfit survivors: Exercise as a resource for aging women. *Gerontologist, 31*, 347–357.

Osgood, N. (1995). *Suicide in the elderly.* Rockville, MD: Aspen.

Osgood, N., & Eisenhandler, S. (1994). Gender and assisted and acquiescent suicide: A suicidologist's perspective. *Issues in Law and Medicine, 9*, 361–374.

Osgood, N., & Malkin, M. (1997). Suicidal behavior in middle-aged and older women. In J. Coyle (Ed), *Handbook of women and aging* (pp. 191–209). Westport, CT: Greenwood Press.

Oxman, T. (1996). Antidepressants and cognitive impairment in the elderly. *Journal of Clinical Psychiatry, 57*(Suppl), 34–44.

Parmelee, P., Katz, I., & Lawton, M. (1992). Depression and mortality among institutionalized aged. *Journals of Gerontology: Psychological Sciences, 47*, P3–P10.

Perazella, M., & Mahnensmith, R. (1997). Hyperkalemia in the elderly: Drugs exacerbate impaired potassium homeostasis. *Journal of General Internal Medicine, 12,* 646–646.

Pfeiffer, E. (1975). A short portable mental status questionnaire for the assessment of organic brain deficit in elderly patients. *Journal of the American Geriatrics Society, 26,* 433–441.

Phillips, S., Rook, K., Siddle, N., Bruce, S., & Woledge, R. (1993). Muscle weakness in women occurs at an earlier age than in men, but strength is preserved by hormone replacement therapy. *Clinical Science 84,* 95–98.

Pozzato, G., Moretti, M., Franzin, F., Croce, L., Lacchin, T., Bendetti, G., et al. (1995). Ethanol metabolism and aging: The role of first pass metabolism and gastric alcohol dehydrogenase activity. *Journals of Gerontology: Biological Sciences, 50A,* B135–B141.

Quam, J., & Whitford, G. (1992). Adaptation and age related expectations of older gay and lesbian adults. *Gerontologist, 32,* 367–371.

Quandt, S., McDonald, J., Arcury, T., Bell, R., & Vitoling, M. (2000). Nutritional self-management of elderly widows in rural communities. *Gerontologist, 40*(1), 86–96.

Raymond, R. (1994). Elder abuse and victimization: The hidden epidemic. *Geriatric Care and Rehabilitation, 7,* 2–8.

Richardson, J., & Hurvitz, E. (1995). Peripheral neuropathy: A true risk factor for falls. *Journals of Gerontology: Medical Sciences, 50A,* M211–M215.

Riekse, R., & Holstege, H. (1996). *Growing older in America.* New York: McGraw-Hill.

Rosenblatt, C., Cho, K., & Durance, P. (1996). Reporting mistreatment of older adults: The role of physicians. *Journal of the American Geriatrics Society, 44,* 65–70.

Rowe, J., & Kahn, R. (1997). Successful aging. *Gerontologist, 37,* 433–440.

Rowe, J., & Kahn, R. (1998). *Successful aging.* New York: Pantheon.

Sadler, P., & Kurrie, S. (1993). Australian service providers responses to elder abuse. *Journal of Elder Abuse and Neglect, 5,* 57–75.

Saltzman, A. (1992). Pulmonary disorders. In E. Calkins, A. Ford, & R. Katz (Eds.), *Practice of geriatrics* (pp. 429–435). Philadelphia: W. B. Saunders.

Schick, F., & Schick, R. (Eds.). (1994). *Statistical handbook on aging in Americans.* Phoenix, AZ: Oryx Press.

Schmidt, R. (1994). Community health: Prevention and health promotion. *Generations, 18,* 33–38.

Semla, T., Beizer, J., & Higbee, M. (1997). *Geriatric dosage handbook* (3rd ed.). Cleveland, OH: Lexi-Comp.

Sheikh, J., & Yesavage, J. (1986). Geriatric Depression Scale: Recent evidence and development of a shorter version. *Clinical Gerontology, 5,* 165–172.

Siegler, E. L., Hyer, K., Fulmer, T., & Mezey, M. (Eds.) (1998). *Geriatric interdisciplinary team training.* New York: Springer Publishing.

Snow, C., Shaw, J., Winters, K., & Witzke, K. (2000). Long-term exercise using weighted vests prevents hip bone loss in postmenopausal women. *Journals of Gerontology: Medical Sciences, 55A*(9), M489–M491.

Social Security Administration, U.S. Department of Health and Human Services (1993). *Social Security bulletin annual statistical supplement.* Washington DC: Government Printing Office.

Stoller, E., & Gibson, R. (1994). *Worlds of difference: Inequality in the aging experience.* Thousand Oaks, CA: Pine Forge Press Social Science Library.

Taeuber, C. (Ed.) (1996). *Statistical handbook on women in America* (2nd ed.). Phoenix, AZ: Oryx Press.

Terpstra, T., & Terpstra, T. (1997). Treating geriatric depression with SSRIs: What primary care practitioners need to know. *Nurse Practitioner, 22,* 118–123.

Tseng, B., Marsh, D., Hamilton, M., & Booth, F. (1995). Strength and aerobic training attenuate muscle wasting and improve resistance to the development of disability with aging. *Journals of Gerontology, Series A, 50A,* 113–119.

U.S. Bureau of the Census. (1993). *Poverty in the United States* (Current Population Reports, Series P60). Washington DC: Economics and Statistics Administration, U.S. Department of Commerce.

U.S. Bureau of the Census. (1997). *Sixty-five plus in the United States.* Washington, D.C.: Economics and Statistics Administration, U.S. Department of Commerce.

U.S. Department of Health and Human Services. (1990). *Healthy people 2000* (DHHS Publication No. 91-50212). Washington, D.C.: Government Printing Office.

U.S. Department of Health and Human Services. (1992). *Urinary incontinence in adults: Clinical practice guidelines* (Publication No. 92-0038). Washington DC: Agency for Health Care Policy and Research.

Umberson, D., Wortman, C., & Kessler, R. (1992). Widowhood and depression: Explaining long-term gender differences in vulnerability. *Journal of Health and Social Behavior, 33,* 10–24.

Virtanen, H., Makinen, J., Tenho, T., Kiilholma, P., Pitkanen, Y., & Hirvonen, T. (1993). Effects of abdominal hysterectomy on urinary and sexual symptoms. *British Journal of Urology, 72,* 868.

Wagner, D. (1995). Special report: Public policy focus on grandparents raising grandchildren. *American Association of Geriatric Education Newsletter,* pp. 5–7.

Wells, T., Brink, C., Diokno, A., Wolfe, R., & Gillis, G. (1991). Pelvic muscle exercise for stress incontinence. *Journal of the American Gerontological Society, 39,* 785–791.

Wells, K., Katon, W., Rogers, B., & Camp, P. (1994). Use of minor tranquilizers and antidepressant medications by depressed outpatients: Results from the medical outcomes study. *American Journal of Psychiatry, 151,* 694–700.

Williams, G. (1996). Elder abuse reporting and ethical dilemmas. *Iowa Medicine, 86,* 20–23.

Wolf, R., & Pillemer, K. (1989). *Helping elderly victims: The reality of elder abuse.* New York: Columbia University Press.

Wolfson, L., Judge, J., Whipple, R., & King, M. (1995). Strength is a major factor in balance, gait, and the occurrence of falls. *Journals of Gerontology, Series A, 50A,* 64–67.

Woollacott, M. (2000). Systems contributing to balance disorders in older adults. *Journals of Gerontology: Medical Sciences, 55A*(8), M424–M428.

Woolley, S., Czaja, S., & Drury. (1997). An assessment of falls in elderly men and women. *Journals of Gerontology: Medical Sciences, 52A,* M80–M87.

Wyman, J., Hawkins, S., & Fantl, J. (1990). Psychosocial input of urinary incontinence in the community-dwelling population. *Journal of the American Geriatric Society, 38,* 282–286.

Yesavage, J., Brink, T., & Rose, T. (1983). Development and validation of a geriatric depression screening scale: A preliminary report. *Journal of Psychiatric Research, 17,* 37–39.

Yuen, E., Zisselman, M., Louis, D., & Rovner, B. (1997). Sedative-hypnotic use by the elderly: Effects on hospital length of stay and costs. *Journal of Mental Health Administration, 24,* 90–97.

RESOURCES

National Institute on Aging (NIA): *www.nia.nih.gov*
The National Council on the Aging: *www.ncoa.org*
Aging & Women Getting Older: *www.4woman.gov*
American Association Retired Persons: *www.aarp.org*
American Society on Aging: *www.asaging.org*
Gerontoglogical Society of America: *www.geron.org*
American Geriatrics Society: *www.americangeriatrics.org*

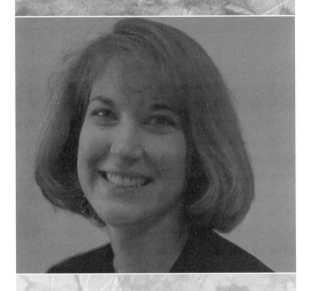

The Business of Women's Health Care

Vicki A. Lucas

Chapter 19

Caring is a powerful business advantage.

Scott Johnson

INTRODUCTION

The recognition that women's health encompasses more than reproductive health has led to changes in research and education and a reexamination of health care delivery for women (Auerbach & Figert, 1995). Women's health has been redefined as encompassing the entire life span and including health promotion, maintenance, and restoration. Besanceney (1998) identified eight aspects of women's lives that can have profound effects on their personal health: physical wellness, emotional wellness, social wellness, spiritual wellness, intellectual wellness, occupational wellness, environmental wellness, and financial wellness. The business of women's health care is complex. The administrative challenge is to know and understand women's particular needs, provide services that meet those needs, and still provide a positive financial margin (Besanceney, 1998; Expert Panel on Women's Health, 1997; Levinson, 1996).

The task of defining women's health care is complicated by the fact that the terms *sex* and *gender* often are referred to interchangeably. Sex and gender influence women's health care, but they are not interchangeable. *Sex* refers to the biologically determined differences between men and women, whereas *gender* involves culturally determined differences. Therefore women's health care should include screening, diagnosing, and managing conditions that are unique to women, are more common in women, are more serious in women, and have manifestations, risk factors, and interventions that are different for women (Jacobs Institute of Women's Health, 1993). In addition to the biological differences, women's health care must address the gender differences that affect women's health (Levinson, 1996).

Gender is a significant marker of social and economic vulnerability, which is manifest in inequalities of access to health care as well as women's and men's different positioning as users and producers of health care. Gender inequalities in health care are the consequence of the basic inequality between men and women in many societies (Castro, 1997; Doyal, 1996; Krieger, 1994; Lane, 1994; LaRosa, 1994b). Nongovernmental women's health organizations and feminist health researchers have in recent years identified major gender inequalities in access to services and in the way men and women are treated by the health care system (Hughes & Runyan, 1995; Macklin, 1996). Although women are major health care consumers and providers, they are underrepresented in decision making positions, each as presidents, CEOs, and board members (Gijsbers Van Wijk, Van Vliet, & Kolk, 1996; Standing, 1997).

Historically, women's health has been defined by men and was viewed as merely a departure from the male model of health and illness (Raftos, Mannix, & Jackson, 1997). This resulted in the medicalization of women's reproductive lives and gender bias in the management of serious, life-threatening diseases (Gijsbers Van Wijk et al., 1996). The general agreement among women's organizations is that gender-sensitive health care should be available, accessible, affordable, appropriate, and acceptable (Donahue, 1993; Expert Panel on Women's Health, 1997).

TRENDS IN WOMEN'S HEALTH CARE

Clancy and Massion (1992) describe American women's health care as a patchwork quilt with gaps. As a result of the women's movement, women's health care movement, consumer movement, and the increase in women's purchasing power, attempts have been made to reengineer women's services. Most of the reengineering attempts have failed miserably to produce anything other than a change in the decor and, in the worse cases, have resulted in the exploitation of gender-specific health care (Appleby, 1997). In fact, the facade of gender-specific health care has resulted in the false conclusion by many leaders that women's health care needs are being met in an appropriate manner. Inherent in this belief is the threat of deemphasizing women's health care and subsequently reducing the resources invested (Bernd & Reed, 1994; Kadar, 1994; Riley, 1998).

The reason women's health care has received increased emphasis in the past 20 years is simple economics. Besanceney (1998) states that women are no longer just a niche, they are the market. Women use more health services than men, make 70% to 90% of the health care decisions, and are the majority of the population (Health Care Advisory Board, 1998b).

Women are the majority consumer of health care in the United States, accounting for 66% of the 44 million annual hospital procedures, 61% of the 700 million physician visits annually, 59% of prescription drug purchases, and 75% of nursing home residents over the age of 75 (Medics Report, 1996). Women spend 66 cents of every health care dollar, and seven of the ten most frequently performed surgeries in the United States are specific to women, including four obstetrical surgeries and three surgeries on women's reproductive organs (Health Care Advisory Board, 1998b; Levine, 1994; Medics Report, 1996).

Approximately 75% of U.S. hospitals have some type of women's center (Health Care Advisory Board, 1998b). In 1991 the American Hospital Association defined a women's health center as an area set aside for coordinated education and treatment services specifically for women. According to La Fleur and Taylor (1996), hospital administrators are realizing that women's health care simply should not be a repackaging of existing services because a women's health center should deal with all aspects of women's health, not just pregnancies and childbirth. Women, not hospital administrators, should identify the services offered by hospitals. Some studies suggest the views of administrators and those of women are often different. Gravett (1989) found that administrators and women only agreed on one out of the six services/features that were the most important to be included in a women's health center. They agreed that a women's center should have a separate identity from the hospital.

Considerable controversy exists over what services should be provided, who should provide them, and where they should be provided (Freda, 1994; Friedman, Paul, & Clark, 1994). Women are faced with choices that range from feminist women's health centers with peer providers and lay midwives who provide menstrual extraction and natural childbirth to the traditional medical model where services are provided in doctor's offices or hospitals by physicians and nurses (Ernst, 1996). Many hybrid models of women's health care settings exist, such as in-hospital birthing centers, freestanding birthing centers, virtual women's health centers, in-hospital women's health centers, freestanding women's health centers, birthing/surgical centers, and women's specialty hospitals (Ernst, 1996; Health Care Advisory Board, 1998a; La Fleur & Taylor, 1996).

Table 19-1 lists examples of women's health services that may be provided and the various providers that serve women. A more recent trend is freestanding for-profit women's health centers/hospitals that are owned in part by physicians. They provide physician office space, birthing services with anesthesia and cesarean section capabilities, and surgical services with short-stay postoperative inpatient services (*Succeeding in Women's Health*, 1998). These women's centers maximize physician productivity and profitability.

The services and features that were the most important to women in Gravett's study (1989) were single-room maternity care, educational programs, separate space for counseling services, diagnostic resources made available to women as patients, and a comprehensive program of services needed throughout a woman's life. McDaniel, Graf, Brehl, and Keele (1998) found similar results in their research. They state that women's choices depend on value-added components, so issues of time, convenience, legitimacy, and availability are as important as cost. Women frequently voice a desire for a single

Table **19-1** | **EXAMPLES OF WOMEN'S HEALTH SERVICES**

CATEGORY	SERVICES	PROVIDERS
Birthing	Birthing center ■ Freestanding ■ Hospital-based Labor, delivery, and recovery rooms Labor, delivery, recovery, and postpartum rooms Home births Water births Emergency births Pain management	Nurse midwife, obstetrician, family practice physician, anesthesiologist, nurse, doula, and operating room technician
Screening	Mammogram Health risk appraisal Pap smear Ultrasound Height and weight Bone density Complete blood count Cholesterol testing Thyroid function Electrocardiogram Body fat index Genetics Physical exam Breast exam Glucose testing Alpha-fetoprotein Follicle-stimulating hormone	Radiologist, nurse practitioner, electrocardiogram technician, clinical nurse specialist, nurse midwife, nurse, medical assistant, laboratory technician, radiology technician, genetics counselor, dietitian, gynecologist, cardiologist, family practice physician, and obstetrician
Education	Childbirth education Preconception classes Women's health lectures Genetics counseling Women's health telemedicine line Women's health education events Sibling preparation classes Breast self-exam Women's health library Breast-feeding	Childbirth educator, nurse, obstetrician, nurse midwife, nurse practitioner, clinical nurse specialist, radiology technician, health educator, women's services community representative, lactation consultant, gynecologist, family practice physician, genetics counselor, doula, and dietitian
Counseling	Support groups Genetics Psychotherapy Family planning Substance abuse Domestic violence Sexual assault Image recovery	Nurse, nurse midwife, nurse practitioner, clinical nurse specialist, genetics counselor, psychologist, psychiatrist, social worker, minister/priest, family planning counselor, and therapeutic cosmetologist

Table **19-1**	EXAMPLES OF WOMEN'S HEALTH SERVICES—CONT'D	
CATEGORY	**SERVICES**	**PROVIDERS**

Wellness	Stress reduction
	Massage
	Tai chi
	Risk reduction
	Yoga
	Guided imagery
	Exercise classes
	Mind/body programs for
	  infertility and menopause
	Hypnosis
	Family planning
	Smoking cessation
	Weight reduction
		Nurse, nurse midwife, nurse practitioner,
		  clinical nurse specialist, personal trainer,
		  social worker, psychologist, family practice
		  physician, massage therapist, obstetrician,
		  gynecologist, instructor, health educator,
		  dietitian, and respiratory technician

Alternative healing,
  complementary
  medicine
	Massage
	Acupuncture
	Aroma therapy
	Biofeedback
	Reflexology
	Spinal manipulation
	Herbal and natural remedies
	Colonic therapy
	Hypnosis
	Therapeutic Touch
	Facials
		Massage therapist, acupuncturist, physical
		  therapist, chiropractor, nurse, nurse
		  midwife, nurse practitioner, clinical nurse
		  specialist, native healers, lay midwife,
		  psychologist, social worker, and
		  aesthetician

Surgical	Plastic surgery
	Abortion
	Urological surgery
	Gynecological surgery
	Liposuction
	LEEP
		Urologist, plastic surgeon, gynecologist,
		  obstetrician, dermatologist, nurse, and
		  nurse practitioner

Telemedicine	Triage Counseling Provider referral Class registration Customer service audits Hospital registration	Nurse, programmer/analyst, and communication specialist

Retail	Lactation consultation
	Breast pump rental and
	  purchase
	Nursing clothes and
	  supplies
	Baby scale
	Image recovery supplies
	Childbirth education
	Labor doula services
	Postpartum doula services
	Image recovery consultation
		Lactation consultant, childbirth educator,
		  nurse, nurse midwife, therapeutic
		  cosmetologist, volunteer, labor doula, and
		  postpartum doula

source for multiple forms of information and one-stop shopping for health care services (Appleby, 1997).

Women not only have multiple choices regarding services and settings, but they also have many choices regarding health care providers. In the past, most women received their health care services from physicians such as obstetricians, gynecologists, and family physicians. During the 1960s and 1970s, nurse midwives, lay midwives, and nurse practitioners became more prevalent in the provision of well-woman care (Sinclair, 1997). At the present time the providers in women's health care are multidisciplinary and numerous (Succeeding in Women's Health, 1998).

A debate continues in the physician community about who should provide primary health care to women: family physicians, internal medicine physicians, or obstetricians/gynecologists (Levinson, 1996). Additionally, a scholarly debate continues about which discipline owns the science of women's health: women's studies, psychology, sociology, medicine, nursing, public health, anthropology, etc. (Pinn, 1994; Schroeder, 1993; Schroeder, 1994; Sharp, 1994). The answer to scientific ownership lies in the definition of women's health. Women's health is a holistic and multidimensional phenomenon that is affected by women's progression through life. Thus multispecialty providers with multidisciplinary knowledge appear to be warranted.

Women's health care is a team sport that requires the integration of multiple sciences, settings, services, and providers (Ireland, 1996). The final question is: Who is the leader of the team? The war within medicine over the leadership role in women's health indicates a lack of understanding of the phenomenon. Simply, an examination of the philosophy of women's health clearly reveals who the leader is: the woman.

LEADERSHIP

Leadership in women's health care requires multiple skills and a knowledge base derived from multiple disciplines. Steve Covey's book *Principle-Centered Leadership* (1998) identified the following four principles of leadership: personal, interpersonal, managerial, and organizational. Personal quality is based on trustworthiness and follow-through, whereas interpersonal quality is based on trust and the building of relationships among the team members. Managerial quality is based on empowerment given by the knowledge of team relationships, and organizational quality is based on the team's ability to align its goals with organizational goals (Labovitz & Rosansky, 1997).

Margaret Wheatley (1994) developed concepts of leadership that guide organizational energy rather than attempt to control and dominate it. In organizations, real power and energy is generated through relationships (Freiberg & Freiberg, 1996). The patterns of relationships and the capacities to form them are more important than tasks, functions, roles, and positions (Greenleaf, 1997). She also believes that leaders should spend their time knowing and understanding the organization rather than in planning and attempting to control it. Collins (1999) states that although past commerce was dominated by efficient use of capital, the future is going to be dominated by knowledge industries. In the future, competitiveness is going to be a function of how well one captures the thinking potential of employees.

Wheatley and Spears (1999) also suggest that information allied to the thinking potential of individuals is going to drive change for the future. They define information as content that communicates something that requires a response. An organization can exist only in a fluid fashion if it has access to new information about external factors and internal resources. An organization must process this data constantly with high levels of self-awareness, plentiful sensing devices, and a strong capacity for self-reflection. Combing through this constantly changing information, the organization can determine what choices are available and what resources to rally in response. This is different from the more traditional organizational response to information in which priority is given to maintaining existing operating forms and information is made to fit the structure, so little change is required (Laveridge, 1996).

Persons and organizations are living systems that are intelligent, creative, adaptive, self-organizing, and meaning-seeking. Therefore leaders should focus on direction, vision, and relationships and have faith that organizations can accomplish their purposes in various ways. They should allow transient forms of the organization to emerge and disappear in response to information (Wheatley & Myron, 1996). Leadership in women's health care requires passionately living a philosophy of women's health that creates a women-centered culture for the provision of women's services (Schaps, Linn, Wibonles, & Wilbanks, 1993; Stichler, 1999).

A women-centered culture creates an environment that is experientially different from traditional health care for the providers and the patients. The culture balances fiscal responsibility with relationship building and caring (Peppers & Rogers, 1997). Quality of life issues for the patients and providers are equally as important as quality of care issues; the two are inseparable, and the culture works to find a balance between them. Accountability is integrated into one's sense of self, and successful outcomes are a matter of self-respect and personal pride (Phillips, Himwich, & Fitzgerald, 1999).

Women's health care leadership requires alignment strategies and incentive management. Employees and providers need to be aligned with the overall goals of the organization. This requires excellent communication skills, reinforcement, and rewards. Goals and expectations must be communicated clearly and must be measurable through performance standards based on the critical success factors of the organization (Labovitz & Rosansky, 1997). Critical success factors for women's health care organizations are customer satisfaction, employee partnership, provider partnership, community partnership, financial performance, and clinical quality. The true success of leadership is realized when the employees and providers have internalized the philosophy of women's health care and have integrated it with the goals of the organization. Such integration results in ownership and personal accountability for the success of the organization (Peppers & Rogers, 1997).

Strong nursing leadership in women's health care is absolutely critical during this period of rapid change in health care (Laveridge, 1996). Nurses have the ability to integrate clinical knowledge with business knowledge and effectively translate it to the various stakeholders (Kuzajian, 1998). The nursing body of knowledge is derived from multiple disciplines and integrates the art and science of nursing. Leadership in women's health care requires the same integration skills. Nurses are qualified uniquely as leaders in the field and must step forward as the ultimate women's health care advocates (Lucas, 2000).

HEALTH CARE FINANCE: INSTITUTIONAL PERSPECTIVE

Money is a pivotal factor in the business of women's health. The old adage "No margin, no mission" is still relevant today. If women's services do not produce a positive financial margin (profit), funds will not be available to pay for programs to meet the mission to improve the health status of women (Phillips, Himwich, & Fitzgerald, 1999).

Health care finance has evolved from self-payment, family care, and charity care to military benefits in the 1940s, employee benefits in the 1950s, and a perceived right to universal health care with the enactment of Medicare and Medicaid in the 1960s. The 1960s and 1970s are known as the golden age of health care because health care spending and growth were unprecedented. In the 1980s, legislators and leaders realized that an ever-increasing portion of the U.S. Gross National Product was being spent on health care with only minimal regulations and accountability for outcomes. The U.S. government is the largest purchaser of health care in the United States. Therefore budget cutbacks and the concerns over the Gross National Product led to federal legislation that dramatically changed the way health care is financed in the United States (Lucas, 2000).

The 1980s and 1990s produced many forms of regulation to reduce health care consumption and ultimately costs. Initially hospital length of stay was targeted, with case management departments and outcome coordinators. This evolved into precertification and primary care physicians known as the gatekeepers to control access to acute inpatient care. An emphasis was placed on nonurgent care, ambulatory care, home care, and outpatient care. In other words, mechanisms were used to reduce the consumption of urgent care and inpatient care. These mechanisms had financial incentives and disincentives through premiums, copayments, and deductibles (Lucas, 2000).

Payers evolved from an indemnity model into a managed care model. The phrase "the bed is dead" was proclaimed by health care futurists, and the industry responded by closing inpatient units, closing hospitals, investing in home care and rehabilitation units, downsizing their inpatient workforce, changing the focus of health care education to a wellness public health model, and forming integrated health care delivery systems. Many hospitals developed their own insurance products and provider networks hypothetically to capture more of the health care dollar through elimination of the middle man. The goals of integrated health care systems were to control more of the health care dollar and have greater leverage over the payers (Keshner, 1996).

The end of the 1990s into the 2000s have seen a public backlash against managed care and the failure to control health care costs, resulting in a loosening of managed care regulations and in the growth of inpatient and acute care services. Many hospitals have capacity issues and severe staffing shortages. "The bed is back" appears to be a new resurgence of an old trend. Table 19-2 summarizes the paradigm shifts in health care.

The basic assumptions of a free enterprise system are violated when the model is applied to health care. In a free enterprise model, a person (consumer) identifies a need and then seeks to meet that need by identifying producers of the product or service needed (vendor). The consumer compares vendors based on their specifications, selects a vendor, negotiates the price, and pays for the product or service before receipt. The consumer has significant control over the process and freedom of choice. The vendor has control over price, product, and distribution.

In a health care enterprise model, a consumer identifies a need and then seeks a provider. The consumer's choice of a provider usually is restricted based on the payer. Unlike a free enterprise model in which the consumer is the payer, in the health care enterprise the payer is often a third party. The consumer receives services from the provider, which may include prescriptive instructions to obtain more products and services. Once again the consumer's choices are restricted because of the payer and reliance on the expertise of the provider. Consumer control and freedom are significantly different in a health care enterprise model. Additionally, payment is different. In a free enterprise model, payment is rendered by the consumer before receipt of goods or services. Therefore the vendor has minimal risk regarding payment. In a health care enterprise model, payment is not received until after the goods and services are received and are paid for by a third party, not the consumer. Therefore the vendor is at significant risk for nonpayment or late payment. Thus health care enterprise violates the consumer need/direct payment assumption and the consumer need/vendor choice assumption. The bottom line is that consumers have less freedom and control and the vendors have more risk in a health care enterprise model.

Table 19-2 PARADIGM SHIFTS IN HEALTH CARE

1960s	2000
Health care as a privilege	Health care as a right
Expansion of health care dollars	Shrinking of health care dollars
Minimal health care technology	Explosion in health care technology
Stable demand for services	Huge increase in demand and complexity
Stable costs of supplies, medicines, equipment, and personnel	Explosive growth in supplies, medicines, equipment, and personnel
Surplus of nurses	Shortage of nurses
Shortage of doctors	Surplus of doctors
Minimal regulations	Highly regulated
Simple finance system	Complex finance system
Collection rate of fees charged 95% or more	Collections 50% or less
Indemnity insurance	Preferred provider organizations and health maintenance organizations
Generalists	Specialists

Health care finance dramatically affects women's health care as a business (Phillips, Himwich, & Fitzgerald, 1999). The payers, not the consumers, determine what they will pay for and how much they will pay. Although philosophically most of us believe that prevention, wellness, and complementary medicine are priorities in women's health care, the payers and consumers do not value these services as evidenced by their unwillingness to pay for them. A belief is not a value without action. The action that is missing is the willingness to purchase these services. Hospitals also are unwilling to pay for such services unless they can obtain revenue from them. Hospitals are in the business to provide acute care services; therefore they would be foolish from a business perspective to provide services that reduce the need for acute care services. That is how they make their money.

Most of the revenue in health care is operating revenue or revenue from operations. This is money received from services rendered. Nonoperating revenue is money earned from sources other than the primary business, such as interest income. Direct revenue is analogous to operating revenue from direct services. Indirect revenue is operating revenue but from indirect services such as the radiology department and the laboratory. Downstream revenue is money made later from services provided earlier. An example of downstream revenue may be gynecological surgery several years after the provision of obstetrical services to the same patient. Lifetime value is the potential revenue stream generated from a woman throughout her life span. Table 19-3 summarizes the types of revenue, and Table 19-4 lists the sources of revenue for health care providers. Table 19-5 summarizes popular women's health products and analyzes revenue potential for each of them from a hospital perspective. Lifetime value revenue streams and downstream revenue are both vitally important for documenting the value of women's services to an organization. The average obstetricion/gynecologist refers 200 patients per year to the following specialists: gastroenterologists, cardiologists, surgeons, urologists, oncologists, and psychiatrists. These specialists use diagnostic, laboratory, inpatient, ambulatory, and outpatient services of hospitals and other health care organizations. This business actually originated in women's services and should be included in a complete financial analysis of women's services.

Obstetrics is a very low-profit margin service because of the high fixed costs of delivery care. Gynecology has a reasonable profit margin. However, the real financial payoff for women's services is in the lifetime value and downstream revenue of the service. In other words, hospitals need obstetrics to bring women into their front doors, but they must harvest the long-term revenue streams to justify obstetrics as an investment. Figure 19-1 (p. 775) gives a revenue stream model for women's services.

Downstream revenue is also revenue from sources provided to the woman's family that result from her referring them for services (Figure 19-2, p. 776). For example, a woman who receives obstetrical care at a hospital often uses their pediatric services for her baby.

A financial statement documents revenue and expenses. A balance sheet illustrates the difference between the revenue and the expenses. The financial goal is to document a positive number on the bottom line of a balance sheet, which represents a profit margin.

Table 19-3 **TYPES OF REVENUE**

TYPE	EXAMPLE	GOOD SOURCES	POOR SOURCES
Operating revenue	Part A Part B copayments	Surgery Inpatient services Indemnity insurance Per diem rates Cancer Emergency room Pharmacy Neonatal Intensive Care Unit Cardiovascular Orthopedics Infertility Antenatal Testing Unit (ATU) Increased risk disorders	Outpatient services Physician practices Ambulatory services Capitation Obstetrics Home care Rehabilitation Mammography Bone density Wellness services Preventive services Decreased risk disorders
Nonoperating revenue	Donations Grants Partnerships Investment income Rebates In-kind donations	Foundations Vendors Community Research (indirect) Special projects Volunteers Capital campaign	Routine operations
Downstream revenue	Gynecological surgeries Pediatrics Cancer Cardiovascular Orthopedics Specialty services Specialty practices Perinatology Neonatal Intensive Care Unit	Obstetrics/gynecology practices Family practice Ambulatory services Prevention services Wellness services Medicine practices Community education	Subspecialty practices Hospital-based practices Specialty services Emergency room
Lifetime value	Geriatrics Long-term care Cardiovascular Repeat business Orthopedics Cancer Senior services Medicine Intermediate care	Employers Volunteer services Primary care providers Community boards Membership programs Advisory boards Operating room	Specialty services Emergency room Hospital-based practices Community education

Table 19-4 **SOURCES OF REVENUE**

PURCHASERS	PRODUCTS	PLACE
Payers	Services	Hospitals
Patients	Retail goods	Home health company
Providers	Supplies	Durable medical equipment company
Vendors*	Pharmacy	Long-term care centers
Employers	Equipment	Community
Volunteers*	Insurance	Ambulatory services
Businesses*	Laboratory	Senior living centers
Foundations	Radiology	Women's centers
Government	Food	Surgery centers
Community†	Space office/meetings	Office building
	Parking	Employers
	Education	Malls
	Tax-free bonds	Businesses
	Public relations	U.S. and state capitals
	Marketing	Churches
	Advertising	Community center
	Consultation	
	Advocacy	
	Providers	

*In-kind contributions result in expense avoidance and increased net revenue.
†Community financial benefit for not-for-profit status needs to be documented. Tax exemption results in expense avoidance and increases net revenue.

Expense categories are similar to types of revenue. Direct expenses are the costs incurred to provide the direct service. In health care the highest direct expense is patient care staff. Indirect expenses also known as overhead are the indirect costs incurred to be in business. Examples of indirect expenses are electricity and financial services. Variable expenses are those that vary by volume. The higher the volume, the greater the expense, such as for food and staff. Fixed expenses are those that do not vary based on volume. For example, the rent for the office is the same whether the provider has 100 patients per day or none at all. A capital expense is usually equipment that has a value greater than $500 and has a life expectancy of greater than 7 years. Capital expenses are depreciated and expensed over 7 to 10 years. The reason for this method is to have financial statements that more accurately represent the financial health of the organization. A large expense incurred all at once can deflate the profit margin of an organization artificially.

In summary, health care finance is pivotal to the business of women's health. Therefore any business model in women's health must be based on the realities of health care finance and the health care industry today (Lucas, 2000; Phillips, Himwich, & Fitzgerald, 1999). The realities of health care are: payers affect choice, providers

Table 19-5	NEW SERVICE OPPORTUNITIES IN WOMEN'S HEALTH CARE ANALYSIS OF REVENUE POTENTIAL (HOSPITAL PERSPECTIVE)	
OPPORTUNITY	**REVENUE POTENTIAL**	**FACTORS**
Midlife Women's Center (Services: Education, screening, and prevention)	Low-direct Low-indirect	Violates primacy of provider-patient relationship Reimbursement issues Absence of procedure/surgical revenue Out of pocket expenses for patients Need mechanism to build loyalty Need mechanism to track downstream revenue Geographic movement with retirement
Complementary Women's Health Center (Services: Massage, herbal, acupuncture, yoga, and tai chi)	Low-direct Low-indirect Moderate downstream	Reimbursement issues Out of pocket expense Absence of procedure/surgical revenue Goal is avoidance of traditional health measures Potential retail revenue with vitamins, herbs, etc. Loyalty-building strategies Tracking downstream and indirect revenue Cost avoidance with employee health, managed care, etc.
Specialty Women's Hospital (Services: Obstetrics, gynecology, cosmetic surgery, and urology)	High-direct Low-indirect Low-downstream	Joint venture model with providers Skimming and cherry picking Limited offerings Not full service: emergency room, etc. Limited indirect and downstream revenue unless part of a partnership with traditional system Volume and efficiency are critical Limited loyalty building except repeat women's services
Women's Heart Programs/ Centers (Services: Education, screening, diagnostics, surgery, rehabilitation, and support groups)	High-direct Moderate-indirect Moderate-downstream	High procedure/surgical revenue Loyalty-building strategies necessary for indirect and downstream revenue Tie in with women's service program to cross-sell and build loyalty Holistic approach to women's heart program—feminine edge Prevention and screening used as a funnel for procedures and surgeries
Breast Centers (Services: Mammography, diagnostics, education, prevention, and support groups)	Low-direct Moderate-indirect High-downstream	Must capture breast cancer cases for downstream revenue Must capture diagnostics Loyalty-building strategies Part of women's services program: cross-sell cancer services

Continued

Table 19-5	NEW SERVICE OPPORTUNITIES IN WOMEN'S HEALTH CARE ANALYSIS OF REVENUE POTENTIAL (HOSPITAL PERSPECTIVE)—CONT'D	
OPPORTUNITY	REVENUE POTENTIAL	FACTORS
		Avoid cancer identity Women's cancer center vs. breast center Steerage issues Managed care turf issues: preferred care provider vs. radiologist vs. surgeon vs. oncologist Volume and efficiency are critical Multispecialty support team approach usually not a cost-effective option for providers
Retail Centers (Services: Lactation, obstetrics, breast care, image recovery, cosmetic care, complementary care, and support groups)	Moderate-direct Low-direct Low-downstream	Indirect and downstream potential depend on placement and partnerships (remote vs. on-site) Loyalty-building strategies

affect choice, consumers have less freedom of choice than it appears, consumer choices are affected more by providers than any other factor, hospitals are in the business of providing acute care services, and neither consumers nor payers will pay for wellness services. Therefore I believe that changes in the business of women's health care will be incremental, not revolutionary. Although the changes over the last 20 years may appear revolutionary, I believe that they are merely cosmetic. "Necessity is the mother of invention," and right now consumers do not perceive a need for change great enough to value them and act.

BUSINESS TRENDS IN WOMEN'S HEALTH CARE

The business of women's health care has become increasingly more complex with the managed care movement. Managed care has emphasized cost reduction and quality improvement. Cost reduction strategies have resulted in some significant changes in women's health care (Weisman, 1996).

The most noteworthy change in women's health care is the shortened length of hospital stays for obstetrical patients. In 1996, normal vaginal delivery patients were being discharged in 24 hours and cesarean section patients were being discharged in 48 to 72 hours. This practice resulted in major public outcry, a managed care backlash, and the passage of federal legislation with mandatory maternity lengths of stay (Newborns' and Mothers' Health Protection Act, 1997). The interim federal rules were effective January 1, 1999 (Department of Health and Human Services, Department of the Treasury, and Department of Labor, 1999), although before this, 40 states already had passed legislation that mandated maternity lengths of stay (American Hospital Association, 1999). Managed care organizations were mandated

Revenue Stream Model for Women's Services

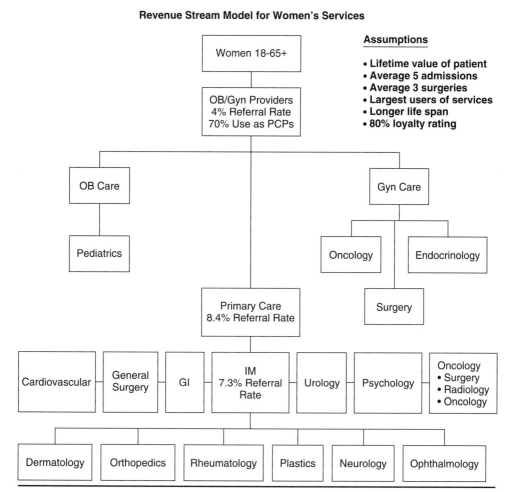

Figure 19-1 Revenue stream model for women's services. *IM,* internal medicine. (Courtesy V. Lucas, 2003.)

to pay for 48 hours of care for vaginal delivery patients and 96 hours of care for cesarean section patients. This legislation effectively doubled the maternity lengths of stay.

The ripple effects from both ends of the spectrum on maternity length of stay have been dramatic. The decreased length of stay before the legislated mandate and the movement toward patient-centered care influenced many administrators to convert inpatient maternity units to single-room maternity delivery systems. The setting for this system is usually labor, delivery, recovery, and postpartum all in one rooms. Such rooms are expensive to build at the front end but theoretically have cost savings on the back end through more efficient cross-trained staffing, fewer room transfers (which results in decreased room turnover), and fewer total rooms needed. Unfortunately, most single-room maternity units were planned using the 24- to 72-hour length of stay model. The

Downstream Revenue Model for Women's Services

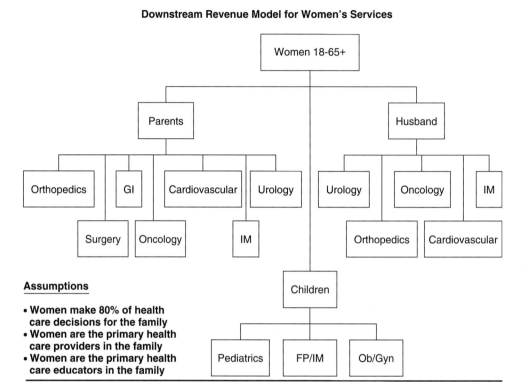

Figure 19-2 Downstream revenue model for women's services. *IM*, internal medicine. *FP*, family practice. (Courtesy V. Lucas, 2003.)

new mandatory lengths of stay have resulted in bed shortages in many of these units, negatively affecting patient and provider satisfaction.

Patient and provider dissatisfaction is multifaceted with the single-room maternity model. Continually declining reimbursement for maternity services has resulted in productivity standards and strict staffing guidelines. Although staffing levels continue to decrease, patient acuity levels have increased. Cross-trained staff models struggle to have the correct mix of staff expertise to manage the patients safely. Additionally, critics of cross training argue that each area in maternity nursing (labor and delivery, postpartum, and nursery) has a unique knowledge base with specialized care competencies and that cross training merely results in a dilution of the staff expertise. Single-room maternity models overlook the psychological transition to motherhood that women experience during the labor, birthing, and postpartum (reintegration) process. Women in labor are focused on the work of safe passage for themselves and their newborns. In the immediate recovery period, inspection and reassurance are followed by relief and elation. After the woman is reassured that all is well, she focuses on her most basic needs. During this period the mother needs intense physical and emotional nurturing: food, sleep, praise, touch. After the mother is revitalized, she is ready to integrate her birthing experience through socially interacting with others and learning about her newborn. Critics of the single-room maternity units believe that these emotional stages cannot possibly occur in such a distracting environment. They also believe that physically moving the mother to a postpartum room is a rite of passage and actually helps facilitate the reintegration process. Single-room maternity delivery systems and changes in maternity lengths of stay are examples of changes in the care delivery system that were not based on adequate empirical evidence. The arguments for these changes appeared to be so logical, almost common sense, that the changes were integrated into practice without adequate scientific scrutiny (Shuster, 1996).

Cost reduction also has resulted in fewer gynecological surgeries, more outpatient surgeries, fewer patient choices, more complex approval processes, and higher copayments and deductibles. For many women, higher copayments and deductibles are real barriers to health care. Collins and Simon (1996) discuss the potential for women to delay preventative well-women care and to seek care only when the disease state is more advanced.

Most of the health maintenance organizations (HMOs) do pay for well-woman preventative care. Theoretically, the HMOs have more incentives to keep women healthy through their capitation financing structure. The HMO receives a specified dollar amount per member per month regardless of the member's use of services. Thus if the member stays healthy or if a diagnosis is made early and the treatment is limited, the HMO should make a profit. Preferred provider organizations, however, provide women with more choices than HMOs do and are more flexible regarding the referral process through the primary care provider, but they often include well-women care in the deductible, which means that most women pay for this care out of their own pocketbooks. Preferred provider organizations generally pay providers on a discounted fee-for-service basis, not on a capitation model. Fee-for-service means that providers submit a bill (charges) for the services provided, and the insurance company pays all or part of the bill (Keshner, 1996).

Kadar (1994) argues that women receive more than their fair share of health care because statistics demonstrate that women do consume more health services than men. He argues that the debate over women's access to care is unfounded based on the difference in use patterns between the sexes. This argument is flawed because it does not address the issues of appropriateness or acceptability of care.

The total quality improvement movement in health care has resulted in increased accountability for women's health outcomes. Cesarean section rates are the most visible outcome data tracked by managed care payers. Physicians have been held accountable for their cesarean section rates, yet nurses have not had to face that level of professional scrutiny. Close scrutiny has resulted in significant improvements of cesarean section rates. In 1990 the national average was 30%, and, in 1998, it dropped to 22%. The Centers for Disease Control and Prevention goal for the year 2000 is a cesarean section rate of 15% (McGlynn, 1997).

The motivation behind decreasing cesarean section rates was clearly financial. Managed care payers were paying significantly more to providers and hospitals for cesarean section patients (McGlynn, 1997). Many women remain uneducated about the risks of cesarean sections and may believe that cesarean sections are safer for mothers and babies. Consumers may pressure providers into repeat cesarean sections. Also the fear of lawsuits may influence the provider's decision.

Outcome measurement is often the tool used to quantify clinical quality or to measure the results of a total quality improvement or process improvement intervention. Simply put, outcome measurement is the product of evaluation research (Greenberger, 1998). The goal of evaluation research should be to measure the baseline and subsequently measure the change or lack of change resulting from an intervention in the real world practice situation. Some frequently used outcome measures in women's health care are Papanicolaou (Pap) smear rate, mammography rate, cesarean section rate, customer satisfaction rating, consumer awareness rating, readmissions rate, market share, birth volume, gynecological surgery volume, cost per case, mammogram volume, induction rate, epidural rate, breast-feeding rate, and vaginal birth after cesarean attempted and success rate (Anonymous, 1997; Houston & Fleschler, 1997). These outcomes do not address the full range of women's health perspective and are limited to the traditional reproductive health and cost indexes (Shuster, 1996).

Pittman and Hartigan (1996), LaRosa (1994a), and Sharp (1994) state that gender indicators need to be incorporated into quality assessment research and management, although others argue that biological and social determinants of health from a gender perspective need to be measured (Abou Zahr, Vlassoff, & Kumar, 1996; Schroeder, 1993). Many women's health care leaders are questioning the questions. Are the correct questions that measure quality in women's health care being asked (Cassel, 1997)? The questions to ask may be, for example, what the stage of cancer is at diagnosis and the 5-year breast cancer survival rates of members of HMOs rather than merely asking what the mammography rates are. Certainly studying cesarean section rates is inappropriate without also monitoring maternal and infant morbidity and mortality rates. Do the outcome measures answer the questions of appropriate, acceptable, affordable, accessible, and available women's health care?

Health care organizations are experiencing widespread variation in practice behaviors and subsequent outcomes of care. Managed care settings are struggling with the same spiraling costs as are the fee-for-service settings. Clinicians are asking for assistance to give consistent, evidence-based care to their patients. Finally, payers (insurance companies) are demanding data about clinical outcomes as well as cost. Shamansky (1996) believes that population-based managed care is a strategy that can be used to improve clinical and financial outcomes. Population-based managed care is a systematic, planned approach to caring for patients who have common, predictable health care needs. The intent is to achieve the best health and satisfaction outcomes while using health care resources cost effectively. Women's health is a population-based clinical specialty. Cost-effective health care identifies waste and the root causes of defects and inefficiency to eliminate variability, repetition, and unnecessary work. In other words, population-based health care seeks to control the sources of variability, which are patient, provider, payer, and setting. Reduction of variability through quality control and the standardization of care should result in consistently better clinical and cost outcomes.

Women in various age groups or women with certain risk factors or conditions such as pregnancy could be managed as a population. However, Shamansky (1996) cautions that nurses have to be careful, lest the person gets lost in the population. Populations consist of individuals and individual providers of care for individuals. The goal is to have predictable, quality clinical outcomes and profitable financial outcomes while maintaining a woman-centered culture of care.

HEALTH CARE FINANCE: MANAGED CARE

Health care finance has been changing rapidly over the past 20 years. Before that, health care never encountered the typical business pressures of a capitalistic, competitive enterprise. In the past, most women had indemnity health insurance through their husbands' work-related health plans and women's services were reimbursed at 100% of charges on a fee-for-service basis. In other words, the physician determined what needed to be done, performed the service, billed for the service, and was paid 100% of the bill. The same was true for hospitals. Provider charges were called Part B gross revenue and hospital charges were called Part A gross revenue. No gatekeepers existed and basically no internal control or accountability was exercised. The cost of health care and subsequently the cost of health insurance continued to rise at a shocking rate.

When women started entering the job market in large numbers over the past three decades, health care coverage became a highly sought-after workforce benefit. As divorce rates rose over the same time period, many women found themselves without health care coverage for themselves and their children. Despite the fact that more women are in the labor force now than ever before in the history of the United States, women and their children disproportionately lack access to health care coverage. The major reasons for this access problem are that more women than men are in low wage, part-time jobs that do not offer health care benefits, or the health care coverage is not affordable. In response to this growing number of uninsured women and children, the U.S. Congress has passed numerous forms of legislation that expand Medicaid for woman and children and most recently established the Children's Health Insurance Program in 1998.

The first attempt to control the rising cost of health care was the establishment of a gatekeeping function by the payers. The gatekeeping function started with reviews of use in which the payers set limits on what constituted a reasonable length of stay in the hospital. If the patient exceeded the limits set by the payer, the hospital did not get paid for the additional days. Precertification is the process for hospitalization, procedures, and anything other than the routine prespecified care outlined in the benefit package. In addition to these controls, managed care organizations started to limit their provider and facility panels by negotiating discounted rates, per diem rates, and global case rates (Lucas, 2000).

Discounted rates are a percentage discount from charges. For example, a hospital may have a negotiated rate of 80% of reasonable and customary charges. Therefore the payer would pay 80% of the Part A gross revenue (charges) and would save 20% off of the bill. The 20% discount is called a deduction from gross revenue. Fee-for-service and discount from charges agreements are forms of retrospective reimbursement. The bill (charges) is submitted after the care is provided, and the provider is expecting full payment based on the contractual arrangement. The amount of charges submitted in this type of reimbursement model can vary considerably. Per diem rates are a negotiated fee per day for hospital care regardless of the charges. Global case rates are a fee based on a diagnosis, not based on the charges, such as one payment for all of the hospital care for a normal vaginal delivery. Most women's services are reimbursed using global case rates. For example, a hospital may be reimbursed anywhere from $1500 to $3000 for a normal vaginal delivery. Every woman's service bill has two parts. Part A is for the hospital, and Part B is for the provider. Providers may be reimbursed anywhere from $1000 to $2500 for a normal vaginal delivery. This provider case rate includes all of the antepartum, intrapartum, and postpartum care. Case rates or rates based on diagnosis-related groups are a form of prospective payment. Before the provision of care, rates already have been negotiated and contractually set.

More recently, payers have negotiated package prices or have bundled charges into one bill. For example, a package price for obstetrics may include the obstetric provider, hospital for mother, anesthesia services, hospital for baby, and pediatric provider. This is often more convenient for the payer and limits the paperwork and overhead for all parties involved.

In addition to packaged payments, HMOs use a capitation payment strategy. Basically, the primary care provider receives a certain amount of money per member per month, and, if a woman is pregnant, she is referred to an obstetric provider (specialist). These providers are paid one of two ways: they may receive a small amount of capitation dollars per member per month as a specialist to be available to provide women's health care for all of the members, or they may receive a negotiated case rate for their services. The average capitation payment to preferred care providers is $15 to $17 per member per month, and the average payment to specialists is $2 to $3 per member per month. The advantage of capitation for the providers is that income is steady every month, which helps to stabilize the cash flow. The risk for the providers is if use exceeds the predicted levels, which results in decreased profitability. Hospitals usually receive a negotiated case rate for services to capitated patients unless they have a full-risk contract. A full-risk contract means that the hospital shares in the monthly capitation dollars and provides hospital services for all of the members. The contract is a prepaid health plan in which hospitals and providers are paid for their services in advance. Again, if use exceeds predicted levels, profitability suffers.

In a more recent trend, hospitals are developing their own insurance products and are becoming the payer and the provider. Hospitals believe that by becoming payers, they can have more control over outcomes, can have more control over the process, can cut out the middleman, and can keep more money to pay providers and improve care. Thus far, the transition for most hospitals has been difficult, and many have abandoned their insurance products because of significant financial losses. Many hospitals did not select this strategy because they were fearful they would be boycotted by the traditional payers if they were perceived as direct competitors.

For-profit and not-for-profit hospitals provide women's health care. Not-for-profit hospitals are owned by the community and are tax-exempt. They are required by law to provide care to everyone, regardless of a person's ability to pay. They also are required to reinvest their profits into uncompensated care, community services, and capital improvements in the hospital. Capital improvements are the purchase of a significant piece of equipment or improvement in the facility that costs more than $500 and has a life expectancy of greater than 7 years (Payne, 1995). For-profit hospitals are owned by stockholders, and they turn their profit into dividends for their stockholders. They are not tax-exempt and do not have an uncompensated care requirement.

During the 1990s, the trend was toward large for-profit health care corporations in response to the decreasing reimbursement rates, shrinking profits, intense competition, and the need to become more cost-efficient. Many for-profit hospitals also merged into large health care systems. The major advantage that for-profit systems had during this period of mergers and buyouts was their abundant access to capital (money) by selling stock. The not-for-profit systems had to rely on issuing tax-free bonds to raise capital, which is more highly regulated and is a much slower process (Mieling & Keshner, 1996). The for-profit segment buying spree has slowed down, but the not-for-profit segment is still merging, buying, and trying to find ways to reduce costs through economies of scale and to leverage the market with size, geographic coverage, and comprehensive services.

Leverage means the ability to influence the payers to negotiate better rates or to steer more business to fewer providers, thus increasing profitability and market share (Keshner, 1996). What does this have to do with women's services? First of all, stand-alone women's specialty hospitals are at risk of extinction if they are not part of a larger system. Payers do not want to carve out women's services to one provider if they have other options. They want one provider who can provide comprehensive services, including women's services, with good geographic coverage. If providers do not have women's services, they have a problem competing for managed care contracts unless they have a regional or national market with superb subspecialty services and little competition.

Women will have fewer choices as the managed care market evolves and consolidates. In fact, long-standing patient-provider relationships may be at risk because of managed care contracting. Lastly, that providers of women's services be held accountable for clinical quality, customer service outcomes, and cost-effectiveness is critical. This information should be in the public domain so that the leader of the team, the woman, can make informed choices for herself and her family.

INTEGRATION OF WOMEN'S SERVICES

The integration of women's services is essential for the success of health care organizations. Women's health service lines and product lines and women's centers have several current mechanisms to integrate services. Integration strategies in women's services can improve greatly the critical success factors of financial performance, clinical quality, customer satisfaction, employee partnership, provider partnership, and community partnership. Financial performance and profitability must be improved in women's services to survive in such a competitive market (Conner, Hanold, Lee, Robb, & Lucas, 2000).

Over the past 10 years, reimbursements for women's services have continued to decline, while expenses to provide services have continued to rise. Reimbursement minus expenses equals profit or loss. Women's services have a small profit margin and in many hospitals are considered a loss leader. A loss leader is a necessary service of doing business but one that consistently loses the most money. Hospitals offset their losses through the more profitable services such as cardiovascular and cancer services (Graf, 1999). As the profit margins continue to decline for all services, hospitals may be forced to discontinue women's services or actually face bankruptcy and closure. Justification strategies for the investment in women's services are managed care contracting requirements, downstream revenue from referral business directly or indirectly from women's services, and the lifelong value of women customers as the family decision makers for health care services. Women's health care administrators must use expert business skills to balance the demands of technological advances and economic concerns with the provision of humane, empathetic, and ethical health care services for women (Lucas, 2000).

An integration strategy that can improve profitability greatly is standardized productivity targets across the system. Salaries account for 60% of most expense budgets; therefore controlling salary costs through maximizing productivity and flexing staff hours down based on volumes will add millions of dollars to the bottom line.

Table 19-6 and Box 19-1 give examples of productivity targets that are valid and reliable for a patient-focused care delivery system. Validity tests how accurate the measurement is, and reliability tests how stable the measurement is over time. Table 19-7 lists productivity targets for advanced practice nurses and physicians.

The Joint Commission on Accreditation of Healthcare Organizations (1998) publishes staffing standards in the provision of care section. The Perinatal Guidelines (1997), jointly developed by the American College of Obstetricians and Gynecologists, the American Academy of Pediatrics, and the Association of Women's Health, Obstetric and Neonatal Nurses' Standards of Care (1997), address the issue of staffing guidelines. Standardized productivity targets not only help control labor costs, but they set the expectations for uniform productivity that should be translated into parity in compensation.

Compensation should be based on productivity. For example, a new obstetrician/gynecologist out of residency should have an annual base salary of

Table 19-6   PRODUCTIVITY TARGETS FOR PATIENT CARE UNITS

UNIT	TARGET*
Labor and delivery	16-18 hours of care per delivery 5.3 hours per encounter†
Postpartum	8-9 hours of care per patient day
Routine nursery	6 hours of care per patient day
Neonatal intensive care unit level II	12 hours of care per patient day
Neonatal intensive care unit level III	16 hours of care per patient day
Gynecology surgery	8 hours of care per patient day
Antepartum inpatient	10 hours of care per patient day

*Patient-focused care model. Targets include total worked hours of all direct and indirect staff, including orientation and education hours.
†Refer to Box 19-1 for labor and delivery encounters.

Table 19-7   WOMEN'S HEALTH PROVIDER PRODUCTIVITY TARGETS

PROVIDER	TARGET
Obstetrician	120-140 deliveries/year
Nurse midwife	80-100 deliveries/year
Gynecologist	60-80 major gynecological surgeries/year
Gynecologist	80-100 minor gynecological surgeries/year
Physician	30-40 office visits/8-hour day
Certified nurse midwife or nurse practitioner	20-30 office visits/8-hour day
Obstetrician/gynecologist	$500,000 gross revenue/year

$110,000 to $130,000, an obstetrician/gynecologist with 3 to 5 years of experience should have a base salary of $130,000 to $160,000, and one with 5 to 10 years of experience should have a base salary of $150,000 to $180,000. The average certified nurse midwife has a salary of $70,000 to $90,000, and the average women's health care nurse practitioner has a salary of $55,000 to $70,000. The productivity targets for each provider translate into revenue that further substantiates the parity in compensation. For example, medical doctors receive significant revenue from surgery and complex procedures that certified nurse midwives and nurse practitioners do not have the credentials to perform. In addition to the base salary, productivity-based bonuses should be structured to reward those providers who exceed their productivity targets and contribute additional revenue. Gain sharing of the additional revenue should occur (HFMA, 1999). For example, a common physician productivity bonus

BOX 19-1 BIWEEKLY MANAGEMENT REPORT DATA

Dept. Name: *Labor & Delivery* Dept. No. _____ Payroll Week Ending _____

MVI Title	MVI Volume	Serves Audit Date %
Encounters		
Vaginal Delivery	_____	
Cesarean Section	_____	
Nonstress Test	_____	
Oxytocin Challenge Test	_____	
Prostaglandin Gel	_____	
Observation Patient	_____	
Special Drips	_____	
Epidural Insertion	_____	
Recovery/Vaginal	_____	
Recovery/Cesarean Section	_____	
Surgical Procedure	_____	
Pitocin Induction/Augment	_____	
Concentrated Care	_____	
Newborn Care (1/4 encounter)	_____	
Total Encounters	_____	

Contract Hours Worked:_____

Prepared by: _____   Approved by: _____

Procedure:
Purpose: Input to Management Reporting System (MRS)
Frequency: Biweekly due the day following the end of the payroll period
Responsibility: Manager and Approval
Flow: To MRS Data Input Center

---

formula is 25% of any net revenue (gross revenue minus deductions) above the amount that covers salary, benefits, and practice expenses. This is an incentive for physicians to control their expenses and increase their productivity.

Financial performance also can be improved through revenue enhancement. Three basic ways to enhance revenue are to reduce costs, increase prices, and increase volume (BDC Advisors, 1999). Using productivity targets to control salary expenses is an example of a strategy to reduce costs. As discussed previously, health care has four categories of expenses: fixed, variable, direct, and indirect. Fixed expenses are those that are the same regardless of volume, such as a salaried manager. Variable expenses are those that vary with volume, such as an hourly staff nurse. Managers who are salaried receive their full pay regardless of volume; whereas hourly staff nurses could be flexed down: either cancelled or sent home if the volume is low. Direct expenses are those items involved in direct services, such as clinical staff and supplies. Indirect expenses are expenses incurred to support direct operations, such as information systems, marketing, and finance. Indirect expenses also are known as overhead. Clinical managers have control over direct, variable expenses and can reduce them to improve financial performance. Other examples of cost reduction strategies are standardization of supplies and equipment; limited formulary; standardized clinical protocols; just-in-time inventory; reducing the richness of the staff mix; call back bonuses instead of call pay; bonus incentives instead of cost-of-living raises; reduced overtime, turnover, and sick time; reduced agency staff use; and renegotiating service contracts. Clinical managers do not have direct control over indirect, fixed expenses unless they choose to eliminate salaried managerial positions within their departments.

In an era in which reduced reimbursement is the standard, raising prices to payers is worthless in terms of revenue enhancement. Also, because most of the reimbursement in women's services is based on a case rate methodology, raising prices or charging for additional services is also not effective for revenue enhancement. Increasing volume enhances revenue if costs are well controlled and the additional volume results in an economy of scale. At a certain volume the cost per case drops as the maximum productivity is realized. This is the definition of economy of scale. An example of this concept is a labor and delivery core staff that handles 1000 births but really can manage 1200 births at maximum productivity. Therefore the unit produces additional revenue without adding additional staffing costs.

Provider partnership is another critical success factor that will benefit from integration strategies. In addition to compensation, major issues for providers are on-call time, call coverage, practice expansion, succession planning, vacation time, support staff, managed care credentialing, overhead, paperwork, billing, different providers' level of compatibility with practice philosophy, proximity of practice location, and efficiency with time management. Obstetricians/gynecologists must maximize the efficiency of their time in the office, operating room, and labor and delivery to maximize their profits. Providers also have been affected negatively by declining reimbursements and increasing overhead expenses. Liability insurance continues to be a significant expense for providers, especially if they are practicing obstetrics. The average obstetrician/gynecologist pays $30,000 annually for liability coverage. Two types of liability insurance policies are claims made and occurrence policies. The advantage of an occurrence policy is that the provider is covered on all prior exposure even after a change of employment without having to purchase a "liability tail." A liability tail is a costly liability policy that covers all prior exposures and can cost as much as $100,000.

Women of the twenty-first century want women providers (Clinton, 1999). In response to that demand, more women providers have been prepared. Presently, 60% to 80% of all obstetrics/gynecology residents are women, and nearly 100% of all certified nurse midwives and women's health nurse practitioners are women (Barran, Lazaroff, & Osborne, 1995; Brooks & Phillips, 1996; Welch, 1996). Women providers are more likely to make quality of life issues a high priority when making career choices such as on-call time, philosophy of practice issues, and call coverage. Women providers select their practice settings based on a balance of compensation and quality of life issues rather than on compensation alone. An ideal practice situation for most female obstetricians/gynecologists is an all-women practice group of five providers that allows them to limit their on-call time to every fifth night and every fifth weekend.

Integration strategies in provider development are critical to the prudent management of this expensive and essential resource. Physicians are the most expensive providers in the delivery of health care. Some strategies for the integration of physician practices are as follows:

- Form large single-specialty groups
- Form multispecialty groups
- Provide start-up or expansion support
- Form independent practice associations
- Provide management services organizations (MSOs)
- Form call coverage groups
- Form limited liability companies
- Form physician-hospital organizations (PHOs)
- Provide shared office space
- Form advisory committees
- Provide systemwide medical staff credentialing
- Provide office efficiency and management consultation
- Provide information systems support
- Provide education to office staff
- Provide low-cost benefits to office staff
- Subsidize office space
- Provide marketing support
- Provide low-cost liability coverage
- Provide medical school loan forgiveness contracts
- Provide extra income for in-house or emergency room call coverage
- Provide shared investment opportunities
- Provide education support
- Provide emotional support (the most important element)

In a not-for-profit system, monetary support of any kind to a provider must be substantiated by a documented community need or a contractual agreement for services.

A major form of support for providers is to form a network of interdisciplinary providers of women's health services. Women are multidimensional and complex and so are their health care needs. No one discipline or provider can meet the complex needs of women completely. Therefore providers of women's services need a network of interdisciplinary women's health specialists for referrals and a mechanism to integrate services for women. One example of an integration mechanism for services is a women's health telephone line staffed by nurses who serve as personal services coordinators to educate, triage, refer, and integrate services for each woman. Managed care has affected the providers of women's services greatly, and they are uncertain about their financial futures. They are essential members of the team and are critical to the success of any organization providing women's services (Graf, 1999).

The integration of women's services can affect customer satisfaction positively. Integration strategies can control effectively the critical processes that affect customer satisfaction. Hundreds of processes occur when a women accesses the health care system. Women desire one-stop shopping for services with convenient accessibility. A freestanding women's center integrates all services into one space; however, this one location may not be convenient for all women in the area. Therefore a virtual women's center that integrates processes in a variety of locations may still serve the one-stop shopping desire through an integration strategy of a personal services coordinator on a women's services telephone line.

Women's services are driven by customer satisfaction because the number one method of new customer acquisition is through personal referral (Ireland, 1999). A satisfied customer tells five others, and a dissatisfied customer tells 25 others. The goal in women's services customer satisfaction should be to score at or above the 75th percentile nationally in an independent, national customer satisfaction survey. Customer satisfaction is critical to leading in customer loyalty. One should remember the major profits in women's health are from downstream revenue, not the initial service that is often maternity care.

The cornerstone of customer satisfaction is employee satisfaction and partnership. Employees must feel valued and rewarded consistently. Employees cannot internalize the customer service philosophy if their own needs are not met. The leaders must be servants to the employees so that the employees then can serve the customers (Customer Service Group, 1995). In a women-centered business culture, employee needs are equally as important as customer needs. Integration strategies such as an incentive management program for employees across the continuum of women's health care can enhance employee satisfaction and employee partnership. Examples of an incentive management program can be quarterly bonuses based on performance standards or as simple as management tool kits with thank-you notes and little gifts.

Community partnership can be enhanced through the integration strategy of having a community service requirement for the employee incentive management program. This strategy integrates the employees into the community to improve the health of the community. Other examples of community partnership strategies are women's services community representatives employed by the hospital, a community advisory board, seminars, screenings, health fairs, telephone line education, charitable donations, board memberships, newsletters, media partnerships, Web site education mentoring programs, parish nursing programs, school partnerships, and grocery store partnerships.

Integration can be made operational through a formal structure such as service line/product line management or an informal structure such as systemwide or hospitalwide committees. Integration can occur through a physical location such as a separate women's center or through a virtual women's center. Service line/product line management usually implies an executive-level position with the responsibility to manage the entire product life cycle: research and development, new product development, product testing, marketing, production, distribution, product portfolio analysis, and financial analysis. The major principle, regardless of the structure, is to focus on women consumers as the centerpiece (Levinson, 1996). Four major themes associated with all women-centered care delivery systems are symmetry in provider-patient relationships, access to information, shared decision making, and social change (Andrist, 1997). These themes require developing programs that meet the gap in care, coordinating care, providing essential women's health services, and ensuring a smooth continuum of care between inpatient, outpatient, home, and community programs (Besanceney, 1998). Integrating women's services also means providing multidisciplinary providers with the opportunity to build the integrative science of women's health through collaborative research and scholarly endeavors (Walker & Tinkle, 1996). An ideal practice site is one where a team of multidisciplinary providers work synergistically to produce the optimum outcomes for each woman while working in totality to improve the health of all women through the integration of practice, education, and research.

LEGAL AND ETHICAL ISSUES

The well-managed corporation is the most significant commercial invention of the twentieth century, more significant than electrical lighting, the Model T, jet aircraft, the computer, or the Internet, according to Collins of *USA Today* (September 23, 1999). He states that without well-managed corporations, we could not have had these innovations in the first place. The point is that well-managed corporate entities, be they for-profit or not-for-profit, have become the dominant productive vehicle in society. Collins believes that as government continues to lose moral authority and practical effectiveness, the corporate state will increase its value-shaping role. With the corporate model as the dominant vehicle of human productivity, corporations may need to shift from being socially responsible (adhering to society's values and rules) to socially progressive (consciously shaping societal values). The business of women's health care is based on a corporate model; therefore, as women's health care leaders, nurses have the responsibility to become socially progressive in consciously shaping societal values about women and women's health care.

Ethics is the discipline dealing with what is good and bad and with moral duty and obligation. Women's health care providers and leaders confront ethical issues every day. Three major principles form the basis of ethical decision making in which a belief may ultimately result in a value (an action based on a belief). The three principles are autonomy, beneficence, and nonmaleficence.

Autonomy is the state of being self-governing with moral independence. Beneficence is to do good. Maleficence is the act of committing harm, and nonmaleficence is to do no harm. In the United States, the overriding principle is autonomy, which comes from the Bill of Rights. However, individual autonomy will not be the prevailing principle if society will be harmed. This is called the justice principle, which weighs the various principles against each other (McFadden, 1996).

Many ethical aspects derive from the application of reproductive control in women's health (Schenker & Eisenberg, 1997). For example, induced abortion raises ethical issues related to the rights of the woman versus the rights of the fetus. For those who consider life to begin at conception, abortion always equals murder and therefore is forbidden. Those who believe in the absolute autonomy of the woman over her body take the other extreme. When ethical issues move into the legislative and legal systems to resolve the controversy, profound outcomes may occur on both sides of the debate. The legislative and legal systems were not established to deal with such ethical dilemmas. A commonly held belief is that morality cannot be legislated. Yet when medical technology, as in the case of artificial reproductive technology, advances beyond the development of society's moral belief system, health policies and legal precedents attempt to resolve the controversy. Ideally, if autonomy is the prevailing principle, then the controversy should be resolved individually in one's own conscience, and the issue should only enter the legislative or legal system if society will be profoundly affected.

Informed consent for medical procedures, the provision of care, and participating in research are examples in which legal statutes have been developed to protect the prevailing principle of autonomy. The protection of research subjects through informed consent occurred in 1966 in the United States (McCarthy, 1994). Genuine informed consent involves discussion of all relevant medical issues with the patient so that she understands the ramifications of the diagnosis, treatment, risks, and benefits of undergoing or of refusing treatment, and this enables the patient to make a reasoned autonomous decision (Cummings, 1994).

In the past, women have been denied their right of autonomous decision making regarding their participation in medical research. They have been excluded almost entirely from medical research over the past 100 years (Merkatz, 1998.) Because of this exclusion, the body of knowledge on long-term women's health is woefully inadequate. The original Nurses' Health Study, which began in the 1970s, has become established as the single most important source of information on lifestyle factors and women's health (*Nurses' Health Study Newsletter*, 1999; Speizer & Willett, 1999). This is the only database more than 20 years old that deals with women's health longitudinally.

RESEARCH ISSUES

In response to the critical need for long-term clinical research on women's health, women's health care leaders, legislators, and consumers adopted a strong advocacy position that resulted in new health policy and the funding of the Office of Research on Women's Health within the National Institutes of Health in 1990 and the funding of the Women's Health Initiative in 1991 (Healy, 1999; Schroeder, 1993; Schroeder, 1994). The Office for Women's Services at the Substance Abuse and Mental Health Services Administration was established in 1992, and the Office of Women's Health at the Centers for Disease Control and Prevention was established in 1994. The Women's Health Initiative is a longitudinal clinical research study on women's health that will span 14 years and has a budget of $625 million. The Office of Research on Women's Health now has a $4 billion budget to fund research and to perform its oversight function to ensure women are included appropriately in all research funded by the National Institutes of Health. The three major mandates of the Office of Research on Women's Health are these:

1. To strengthen, develop, and increase research into diseases, disorders, and conditions that are unique to, more prevalent among, or more serious in women or for which risk factors are different for women than for men
2. To ensure that women are represented appropriately in biomedical and biobehavioral research studies, especially clinical trials, that are supported by the National Institutes of Health
3. To direct initiatives to increase the number of women in biomedical careers (Pinn, 1994)

The last decade has been marked by a rapid growth in the women's health movement. Many advances have been made in medical technology, health policy, and women's health research. Yet few changes actually have occurred in the women's health delivery system. Despite the corporate structure of women's health, the care delivery system is still predominantly a patriarchal medical model in which women are dissected into their body parts. Unfortunately, not much has changed except the wallpaper and the facade of holistic preventative women's health care. The challenge for women's health care leaders is to be socially progressive and consciously to reshape societal values related to women's health care. According to Wuest (1993), for health policy to be responsive to women's needs, it must be based on research that considers the social complexity of ordinary women's lives.

SUMMARY

Women's health is complex, multidimensional, and relational and is affected by changes across the life span (Besanceney, 1998). The business of women's health care is a conundrum because it requires the blending of a holistic women's health philosophy and a women-centered culture with the critical business success factors of health care organizations. Women need strong leaders in women's health care who possess a passion for the field. Women's health advocates are persons who can obtain the resources necessary to improve the health of women. Women's health care administrators manage billions of dollars annually and have the potential to elevate the health status of women everywhere if they stay focused on their business, the business of women's health.

REFERENCES

Abou Zahr, L., Vlassoff, J., & Kumar, V. (1996). Maternal mortality. *World Health Statistical Quarterly, 48,* 77–87.

American College of Obstetricians and Gynecologists & American Academy of Pediatrics (1997). *Guidelines for perinatal care* (4th ed.). Elk Grove Village, IL and Washington, DC: Authors.

American Hospital Association. (1999). *Draft Advisory on Newborns' and Mothers' Health Protection Act Regulations.* Chicago, IL: Author.

Andrist, L. (1997). A feminist model for women's health care. *Nursing Inquiry, 4,* 268–274.

Anonymous. (1997). Identifying goals and measures for women's health strategies. *Quality Letter for Healthcare Leaders, 9,* 16–18.

Appleby, C. (1997). Marketing to women: Clinics with a feminine touch. *Hospitals and Health Networks, 71,* 100.

Association of Women's Health, Obstetric and Neonatal Nurses. (1997). *Standards of care.* Washington, DC: Author.

Auerbach, J. D., & Figert, A. E. (1995). Women's health research: Public policy and sociology. *Journal of Health and Social Behavior*, pp. 115–131.

Barran, M. L., Lazaroff, P., & Osborne, C. (1995). The role of the nurse practitioner in ambulatory women's health. *Journal of Perinatal and Neonatal Nursing, 9*, 1–9.

BDC Advisors. (1999, April 16). Enhancing profitability through payor, product, and pricing strategies. *Point of View*, pp. 1–5.

Bernd, D. L., & Reed, N. M. (1994). Re-engineering women's services. *Healthcare Forum Journal, 37*, 63–67.

Besanceney, S. (1998, July/August). Developing a high-performance women's health program. *Ireland Report on Succeeding in Women's Health*, pp. 1–22.

Brooks, F., & Phillips, D. (1996). Do women want women health workers? Women's views of the primary care services. *Journal of Advanced Nursing, 23*, 1207–1211.

Cassel, C. K. (1997). Policy implications of the Human Genome Project for women. *Women's Health Issues, 7*, 225–229.

Castro, I. (1997, Spring). Worth more than we earn. *Gender and Equity* (Supplement to *National Forum*), 17–22.

Clancy, C. M., & Massion, C. T. (1992). American women's health care: A patchwork quilt with gaps. *Journal of the American Medical Association, 268*, 191–192.

Clinton, H. R. (1999, Spring/Summer). The next frontier. *Newsweek*, pp. 94–95.

Collins, J. (1999, September 23). Corporations will shape our future values. *USA Today*, p. 19A.

Collins, K. S., & Simon, L. J. (1996). Women's health and managed care: Promises and challenges. *Women's Health Issues, 6*, 39–44.

Connor, B., Hanold, K., Lee, G., Robb, A., & Lucas, V. (2000). *Desperately seeking synergy.* Washington, DC: Jacobs Institute on Women's Health.

Covey, S. (1998). *Principle-centered leadership.* New York: Summit Books.

Cummings, N. B. (1994). Ethical issues and the breast cancer patient. *Archives of Pathology and Laboratory Medicine, 118*, 1077–1080.

Customer Service Group. (1995, February). Managers' role in team building: Share the power. *Customer Service Newsletter, 23*, 1–3.

Department of Health and Human Services, Department of the Treasury, and Department of Labor. (1999). Interim rules implementing the 1996 Newborns' and Mothers' Health Protection Act. *Federal Register, 20*, 575–576.

Donahue, A. H. (1993). Women's health: A national plan for action. *Journal of Dental Education, 57*, 738–741.

Doyal, L. (1996). The politics of women's health: Setting a global agenda. *International Journal of Health Services, 26*, 47–65.

Editorial Staff. (1997, Spring). Gender and equity. *National Forum*, pp. 1–48.

Edmunds, M. (1995). Policy research: Balancing vigor with relevance. *Women's Health, 1*, 97–119.

Ernst, E. K. M. (1996). Midwifery birth centers and health care reform. *Journal of Obstetric, Gynecologic, and Neonatal Nursing, 25*, 433–439.

Expert Panel on Women's Health. (1997). Women's health and women's health care: Recommendations of the 1996 AAN Expert Panel on Women's Health. *Nursing Outlook, 45*, 7–15.

Freda, M. C. (1994). Childbearing, reproductive control, aging women and health care: The projected ethical debates. *Journal of Obstetric, Gynecologic, and Neonatal Nursing, 23*, 144–152.

Freiberg, K., & Freiberg, J. (1996). *Nuts!* Austin, Texas: Bard Press.

Friedman, E., Paul, H., Clark, M., et al. (1994, January/February). Health Herstory. *Healthcare Forum Journal*, pp. 1–74.

Gijsbers Van Wijk, C. M., Van Vliet, K. P., & Kolk, A. M. (1996). Gender perspectives and quality of care: Towards appropriate and adequate health care for women. *Social Science and Medicine, 43*, 707–720.

Graf, M. A. (1999, May/June). New trends in women's services. *Ireland Report, 1*, 17–22.

Gravett, W. (1989, July 5) Women's centers: 10 common misconceptions. *Hospitals*, pp. 2–4.

Greenberger, P. (1998). What works for women: Outcomes research. *Journal of Women's Health, 7*, 4–11.

Greenleaf, R. K. (1997). *Servant leadership.* New York: Paulist Press.

Health Care Advisory Board. (1998a, Summer). Alternative obstetrics programs. *Issue Tracking Services*, pp. 1–50.

Health Care Advisory Board. (1998b, March). Women's centers. *Fact Brief*, pp. 1–13.

Healthcare Financial Management Association. (1999, January). Rethinking specialist integration strategies. *BDC Advisor.*

Healy, B. (1999, Spring/Summer). A medical revolution. *Newsweek*, pp. 64–65.

Houston, S., & Fleschler, R. (1997). Outcomes management in women's health. *Journal of Obstetric, Gynecologic, and Neonatal Nursing, 26*, 342–350.

Hughes, D. C., & Runyan, S. J. (1995). Prenatal care and public policy: Lessons for promoting women's health. *Journal of American Medical Women's Association, 50*, 56–159, 163.

Ireland, R. C. (1996, May/June). Using the umbrella concept to create women's health services. *Ireland Report, 1*, 18–22.

Ireland, R. C. (1999, March/April). Creating a culture of customer service: Satisfied customers build volume and revenue. *Ireland Report, 1*, 18–22.

Jacobs Institute of Women's Health. (1993, Summer). Conference on women's health centers: review, assessment, and goals. *Women's Health Issues*, 49–54.

Kadar, A. C. (1994). Medicine short changes women? Not at all. *Medical Economics, 71*, 35–36.

Keshner, J. O. (1996). Keys to success in managed care. *Healthcare Financial Management, 50*, 46–60.

Krieger, N. (1994). Man-made medicine and women's health: The biopolitics of sex/gender and race/ethnicity. *International Journal of Health Services, 24*, 265–283.

Kuzajian, A. (1998). Understanding women's health through data development and data linkage: Implications for research and policy, *CMAJ, 159*, 342–345.

Labovitz, G., & Rosansky, V. (1997). *The power of alignment.* New York: John Wiley and Sons.

LaFleur, E., & Taylor, S. (1996). Women's health centers and specialized services. *Journal of Health Care Marketing, 16*, 16–23.

Lane, S. D. (1994). From population control to reproductive health: An emerging policy agenda. *Social Science and Medicine, 39*, 1303–1314.

LaRosa, J. H. (1994a). Office of Research on Women's Health, National Institutes of Health, and the women's health agenda. *Annals of the New York Academy of Science, 736*, 96–204.

LaRosa, J. H. (1994b). Women's health: Science and politics. *Annals of Epidemiology, 4*, 84–88.

Laveridge, C. E. (1996). *Nursing management in the new paradigm.* Gaithersburg, MD: Aspen Publishers.

Levine, C. (1994). Ethics, epidemiology, and women's health. *Annals of Epidemiology, 4*, 159–165.

Levinson, S. (1996). Multidisciplinary women's health centers: A viable option? *International Journal of Fertility, 41*, 132–135.

Lucas, V. A. (2000). *Health care finance for nurses.* White Plains, NY: MGI Management Institute & Association of Women's Health, Obstetric and Neonatal Nurses.

Macklin, R. (1996). Ethics and reproductive health: A principled approach. *World Health Statistics Quarterly, 49*, 148–153.

McCarthy, C. R. (1994). Historical background of clinical trials involving women and minorities. *Academic Medicine, 69*, 695–698.

McDaniel, K., Graf, M. A., Brehl, M. S., & Keele, R. (1998, July/August). Thank you, Dr. Lamaze. *Ireland Report*, pp. 3–16.

McFadden, E. A. (1996). Moral development and reproductive health decisions. *Journal of Obstetric, Gynecologic, and Neonatal Nursing, 25*, 507–512.

McGlynn, E. A. (1997). *Quality of care for women: A review of selected clinical conditions and quality indicators.* Santa Monica, CA: RAND.

Medics Report. (1996, Second Quarter). Women's health, obstetrics, and perinatology. *Healthcare Industry Research*, pp. 1–39.

Merkatz, R. B. (1998). Inclusion of women in clinical trials. *Journal of Obstetric, Gynecologic, and Neonatal Nursing, 27*, 78–84.

Mieling, T. M., & Keshner, J. O. (1996). Accessing capital for integrated delivery systems. *Healthcare Financial Management, 50*, 32–45.

Newborns' and Mothers' Health Protection Act. (1997). Washington, DC: U.S. Federal Registry.

Nurses' Health Study Newsletter. (1999). *Nurses' Health Study II celebrates tenth anniversary.* Boston, MA: Channins Laboratory.

Payne, C. T. (1995). *Strategic capital planning for health care organizations.* Burr Ridge, VT: Irwin Professional Publishing.

Peppers, D., & Rogers, M. (1997). *Enterprise one to one.* New York: Doubleday.

Phillips, C. R., Himwich, D. B., & Fitzgerald, C. (1999, April/May). The business of women's health. *AWHONN Lifelines*, pp. 22–30.

Pinn, V. W. (1994). The role of NIH's Office of Research on Women's Health. *Academic Medicine, 69,* 698–702.

Pittman, P., & Hartigan, P. (1996). Gender inequity: An issue for quality assessment, researching, and managers. *Health Care for Women International, 17,* 469–486.

Raftos, M., Mannix, J., & Jackson, D. (1997). More than motherhood? A feminist exploration of women's health in papers indexed by CINAHL 1993-1995. *Journal of Advanced Nursing, 26,* 1142–1149.

Riley, K. (1998, March 2). Companies exploit opportunities in women's health care as interest in "gender-specific" medicine increases. *Clinica,* p. 14.

Schaps, M. J., Linn, E.S., Wibonles, E. D., Wilbanks, E. K. (1993). Women-centered care: Implementing a philosophy. *Women's Health Issues, 3,* 52–54.

Schenker, J. G., & Eisenberg, V. H. (1997). Ethical issues relating to reproduction control and women's health. *International Journal of Gynecology and Obstetrics, 58,* 167–176.

Schroeder, P. (1993). Legislation to further women's health research. *Women's Health Issues, 3,* 93–94.

Schroeder, P. (1994). Women's health care turns a corner in Congress. *American Nurse, 26,* 15.

Shamansky, S. L. (1996). Population-based managed care to improve outcomes. *Nursing Economics, 14,* 245–249.

Sharp, N. (1994). Women's Health Equity Act of 1990. *Nursing Management, 21,* 21–22.

Shuster, E. (1996). For her own good: Protecting (and neglecting) women in research. *Cambridge Quarterly of Healthcare Ethics, 5,* 346–361.

Sinclair, B. P. (1997). Advanced practice nurses in integrated healthcare systems. *Journal of Obstetric, Gynecologic, and Neonatal Nursing, 26,* 217–223.

Speizer, F., & Willett, W. (June, 1999). Nurses' health study update. *Nurses Health Study Newsletter, 6,* 1–14.

Standing, H. (1997). Gender and equity in health sector reform programs: A review. *Health Policy and Planning, 12,* 12–18.

Stichler, J. (1999, April). The principles of leadership. *Stichler Ink, 2,* 1–2.

Succeeding in Women's Health. (1998, July/August), *Ireland Report,* pp. 1–24.

Walker, C. O., & Tinkle, M. B. (1996, June). Toward an integrated science of women's health. *Journal of Obstetric, Gynecologic, and Neonatal Nursing, 6,* 379–382.

Weisman, C. S. (1996). Proceedings of women's health and managed care: Balancing cost, access, and quality. *Women's Health Issues, 6,* 1–28.

Welch, H. (1996). Nurse midwives as primary care providers for women. *Clinical Nurse Specialist, 10,* 121–124.

Wheatley, M. J. (1994). *Leadership and the new science: Learning about organization from an orderly universe.* San Francisco: Berrett-Koehler.

Wheatley, M. J., & Myron, K. R. (1996). *A simpler way.* San Francisco: Berrett-Koehler.

Wheatley, M. J., & Spears, L. (1999). Work as a calling. In L. C. Spears (Ed.), *Insights on leadership: Service, stewardship, spirit, and servant leadership.* San Francisco: Berrett-Koehler.

Woods, N. F. (1994). The United States women's health research agenda analysis and critique. *Western Journal of Nursing Research, 16,* 467–479.

Wuest, J. (1993). Institutionalizing women's oppression: The inherent risk of health policy that fosters community participation. *Health Care for Women International, 14,* 407–417.

RESOURCES

National Women's Health Resource Center, Inc.
120 Albany Street, Suite 820
New Brunswick, NJ 08901
(877) 986-9472
www.healthywomen.org

Snowmass Institute
The Ireland Report and
Succeeding in Women's Health
8694 East Mineral Circle
Englewood, CO 80112-2746
(303) 771-4044
www.snowmassinstitute.com

National Association for Women's Health
300 W. Adams Street, Suite 328
Chicago, IL 60606-5101
(312) 786-1468
www.nawh.org

Association of Women's Health, Obstetrics and Neonatal Nurses Consulting Group
2000 L Street, NW, Suite 740
Washington, DC 20036
(202) 261-2400
www.awhonn.org

American Hospital Association
Section for Maternal and Child Health
One North Franklin
Chicago, IL 60606-3421
(312) 422-3000
www.aha.org

Society for Women's Health Research
1828 L Street, NW, Suite 628
Washington, DC 20036
(202) 223-8224
www.womancando.org

National Women's Health Information Center
8550 Arlington Blvd., Suite 300
Fairfax, VA 22031
(800) 994-9662
www.4woman.org

National Women's Health Network
514 10th Street, NW
Washington, DC 20004
(202) 347-1140
www.womenshealthnetwork.org

Agency for Health Care Policy and Research
(800) 358-9295
www.ahcpr.gov/consumer/utensil.htm

Office of Women's Health
U. S. Department of Health and Human Services
200 Independence Avenue, SW
Room 728 F
Washington, DC 20201
(202) 690-7650
www.womenshealth.cos.com

The Jacobs Institute of Women's Health
Women's Health Issues
State Profiles on Women's Health (1998)
409 12th Street, SW
Washington, DC 20024-2188
(202) 863-1990
www.jiwh.org

American College of Nurse Practitioners
Nurse Practitioner World News
The American Journal for Nurse Practitioners
Nurse Practitioners Communications LLC
109 South Main Street
Cranbury, NJ 08512
(609) 371-5085 (phone)
(609) 371-5086 (fax)

National Women's Law Center
Making the Grade on Women's Health (2000)
11 Dupont Circle, NW
Suite 800
Washington, DC 20036
(202) 588-5180 (Phone)
(202) 588-5185 (Fax)
www.nwlc.org

FOCUS on Health and Leadership for Women
Center for Clinical Epidemiology and Biostatistics
University of Pennsylvania School of Medicine
423 Guardian Drive
Blockley Hall, Room 932
Philadelphia, PA 19104-8897
(215) 573-8897 (phone)
(215) 573-2265 (fax)

Children's, Women's, Infant's Specialty Hospital (WISH): *www.cwish.org*
Voluntary Hospitals of America (VHA): *www.vha.com/public/*
AWHONN Consulting Group: *www.awhonn.org*
American College of Nurse Midwives: *www.midwife.org*
American Academy of Nurse Practitioners: *www.aanp.org*
American Nurses Association Primary Care Council: *www.nursing world.org*
Health Care Advisory Board: *www.advisoryboardcompany.com*
Nurse Practitioners in Reproductive Health: *www.npwh.org*

Index